MW00857009

ADHD IN ADOLESCENTS

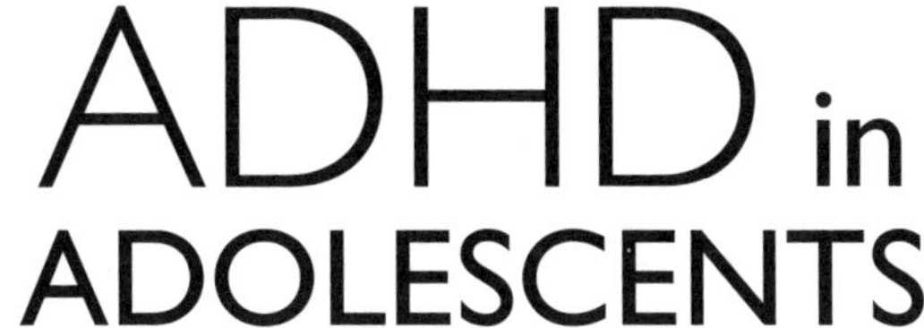

ADHD in ADOLESCENTS

Development, Assessment, and Treatment

Edited by
Stephen P. Becker

Foreword by Russell A. Barkley

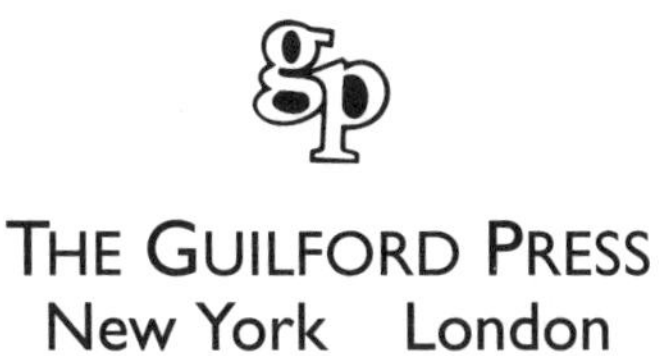

THE GUILFORD PRESS
New York London

A Division of Guilford Publications, Inc.
370 Seventh Avenue, Suite 1200, New York, NY 10001
www.guilford.com

Printed in the United States of America

This book is printed on acid-free paper.

Last digit is print number: 9 8 7 6 5 4 3 2 1

The authors have checked with sources believed to be reliable in their efforts to provide information that is complete and generally in accord with the standards of practice that are accepted at the time of publication. However, in view of the possibility of human error or changes in behavioral, mental health, or medical sciences, neither the author, nor the editor and publisher, nor any other party who has been involved in the preparation or publication of this work warrants that the information contained herein is in every respect accurate or complete, and they are not responsible for any errors or omissions or the results obtained from the use of such information. Readers are encouraged to confirm the information contained in this book with other sources.

Library of Congress Cataloging-in-Publication Data

Names: Becker, Stephen P., editor.
Title: ADHD in adolescents : development, assessment, and treatment / edited by Stephen P. Becker.
Description: New York : The Guilford Press, 2020. | Includes bibliographical references and index.
Identifiers: LCCN 2019041782 | ISBN 9781462541836 (hardcover)
Subjects: LCSH: Attention-deficit disorder in adolescence. | Attention-deficit disorder in adolescence—Diagnosis. | Attention-deficit disorder in adolescence—Treatment.
Classification: LCC RJ506.H9 A33674 2019 | DDC 618.92/8589—dc23
LC record available at *https://lccn.loc.gov/2019041782*

To Joy, for everything

About the Editor

Stephen P. Becker, PhD, is Associate Professor of Pediatrics in the Division of Behavioral Medicine and Clinical Psychology at Cincinnati Children's Hospital Medical Center and the Department of Pediatrics at the University of Cincinnati College of Medicine. His research examines attention-deficit/hyperactivity disorder (ADHD), sluggish cognitive tempo, and sleep in children and adolescents. Dr. Becker's focus is on better understanding the developmental pathways of ADHD, co-occurring psychopathologies, and functional impairments. He has published over 125 articles on these and related topics. Dr. Becker serves on the editorial boards of the *Journal of Abnormal Child Psychology*, *Journal of Attention Disorders*, *Journal of Youth and Adolescence*, and *Adolescent Research Review*, and on the advisory board of *The ADHD Report*.

Contributors

Arthur D. Anastopoulos, PhD, Department of Psychology, University of North Carolina Greensboro, Greensboro, North Carolina

Stephen P. Becker, PhD, Division of Behavioral Medicine and Clinical Psychology, Cincinnati Children's Hospital Medical Center, and Department of Pediatrics, University of Cincinnati College of Medicine, Cincinnati, Ohio

William B. Brinkman, MD, Division of General and Community Pediatrics, Cincinnati Children's Hospital Medical Center, Cincinnati, Ohio

Nóra Bunford, PhD, Department of Ethology, Eötvös Loránd University (ELTE), Institute of Biology, Budapest, Hungary

Jennifer A. Burbridge, PhD, Department of Psychiatry, Harvard Medical School, Boston, Massachusetts

Naomi Ornstein Davis, PhD, Department of Psychiatry and Behavioral Sciences, Duke University Medical Center, Durham, North Carolina

Joshua Doidge, PhD candidate, Department of Psychology, York University, Toronto, Ontario, Canada

George J. DuPaul, PhD, College of Education, Lehigh University, Bethlehem, Pennsylvania

Jeffery N. Epstein, PhD, Division of Behavioral Medicine and Clinical Psychology, Cincinnati Children's Hospital Medical Center, Cincinnati, Ohio

Steven W. Evans, PhD, Department of Psychology, Ohio University, Athens, Ohio

Nicholas D. Fogleman, PhD, The Carolina Institute for Developmental Disabilities, University of North Carolina at Chapel Hill, Carrboro, North Carolina

Tanya E. Froehlich, MD, Division of Developmental and Behavioral Pediatrics, Cincinnati Children's Hospital Medical Center, Cincinnati, Ohio

Annie A. Garner, PhD, Department of Psychology, Saint Louis University, St. Louis, Missouri

Cathrin D. Green, PhD candidate, Department of Psychology, Virginia Commonwealth University, Richmond, Virginia

Stephen P. Hinshaw, PhD, Department of Psychology, University of California, Berkeley, Berkeley, California

Traci M. Kennedy, PhD, Department of Psychiatry, University of Pittsburgh, Pittsburgh, Pennsylvania

Kristen Kipperman, MA, Department of Education and Human Sciences, Lehigh University, Bethlehem, Pennsylvania

Joshua M. Langberg, PhD, Department of Psychology, Virginia Commonwealth University, Richmond, Virginia

Henrik Larsson, PhD, Department of Medical Epidemiology and Biostatistics, Karolinska Institute, Stockholm, Sweden

Kirsten M. P. McKone, BA, Department of Psychiatry, University of Pittsburgh, Pittsburgh, Pennsylvania

Julia D. McQuade, PhD, Department of Psychology, Amherst College, Amherst, Massachusetts

John T. Mitchell, PhD, Department of Psychiatry and Behavioral Sciences, Duke University Medical Center, Durham, North Carolina

Brooke S. G. Molina, PhD, University of Pittsburgh School of Medicine, Pittsburgh, Pennsylvania

Melissa Mulraney, PhD, Community Health Services Research, Murdoch Children's Research Institute, Parkville, Victoria, Australia

Emma E. Rogers, BA, Department of Psychology, Ohio University, Athens Ohio

Wafa Saoud, PhD candidate, Department of Psychology, York University, Toronto, Ontario, Canada

Emma Sciberras, PhD, School of Psychology, Deakin University, Burwood, Victoria, Australia

Margaret H. Sibley, PhD, Department of Psychiatry and Behavioral Sciences, University of Washington, and Seattle Children's Research Institute, Seattle, Washington

Zoe R. Smith, PhD candidate, Department of Psychology, Virginia Commonwealth University, Richmond, Virginia

Susan E. Sprich, PhD, Department of Psychiatry, Massachusetts General Hospital, Boston, Massachusetts

Maggie E. Toplak, PhD, Department of Psychology, York University, Toronto, Ontario, Canada

Saskia Van der Oord, PhD, Department of Psychology, Katholieke Universiteit Leuven, Leuven, Belgium

Judith Wiener, PhD, Ontario Institute for Studies in Education/ University of Toronto, Toronto, Ontario, Canada

Erik G. Willcutt, PhD, Department of Psychology and Neuroscience, University of Colorado Boulder, Boulder, Colorado

Foreword

Despite a tremendous body of research on attention-deficit/hyperactivity disorder (ADHD), there remains a limited number of studies that focus on ADHD in adolescents. Thousands of studies exist on children with ADHD and hundreds more on adults. Having conducted clinical research on adolescents myself, both cross-sectionally and in my longitudinal research, I think the reason for the more limited research perhaps lies in the greater difficulty we experience in recruiting such samples for study or even clinical services. While parents may agree to participate, getting the cooperation of their teens with ADHD is no easy matter.

A number of reasons stand in the way of conducting research with adolescents and ADHD. First, teens tend to markedly underreport their degree of ADHD symptoms and associated impairments. They apparently view themselves as functioning far better than they do in reality, disclaiming that they do indeed have a neurodevelopmental disorder. Second, many adolescents believe their problems stem from parental control over their lives or from teachers' expectations regarding academic performance and comportment at school. Third, many teens are highly sensitive to peer perceptions, which makes them avoid any association with psychiatric or psychological research or clinical providers in these fields. The fear or reality of stigma remains a problem for this age group, even if it seems that adults with ADHD are increasingly willing to disclose their disorder, among them celebrities such as Adam Levine, Justin Timberlake, Ty Pennington, Simone Biles, Bubba Watson, and Michael Phelps. Fourth, many adolescents have reported their personal challenges in owning their disorder as a teenager. Finally, given that teens are in a developmentally appropriate process of individuating from parental influence, in order to maintain their own sense of autonomy, they understandably seek to have more decision-making power and therefore resist the efforts of parents to enroll them in clinical research or services. Regardless, experienced researchers and clinicians are likely to confide that gaining the cooperation of this age group can be quite challenging and thus slow the acquisition of clinical and research-based knowledge about them.

It is therefore cause for great celebration to see an entire volume devoted to ADHD in adolescents. Research results have indicated that adolescence is an incredibly important developmental stage for those with ADHD. Recent follow-up studies have shown that most of the risks and outcomes of adults with ADHD by midlife or later can be traced back not to their childhood years so much as to their adolescent stage of development. In addition, during adolescence, teens are exposed for the first time to adult-like activities, which can put them into high-risk situations. This major change provides the first glimpse as to how teens will manage their behavior in these new domains, which include driving, sexual activity, independence outside the home, managing money, part- or full-time employment, access to substances, peer groups, and the other new challenges to be found in middle school and high school. In this volume, chapters that cite the growing body of research indicate that these areas pose challenges for adolescents in handling the responsibility for the consequences of their choices. As we know from adult studies, people with ADHD often take far greater risks without fear of the consequences of their actions. Perhaps this is why some longitudinal research suggests that while the symptoms of ADHD may decline in frequency or severity across development and into adolescence, the degree of impairment associated with ADHD may increase in pervasiveness and severity. The importance of this developmental stage of ADHD demands a textbook focused on how the effects of ADHD can be mitigated to help teens with ADHD, and provide support to their families.

This text offers a welcome rebuttal to the idea that was pervasive at the time I entered the field of ADHD (then termed *hyperactive child syndrome* or *minimal brain dysfunction*) in the 1970s. During that period, ADHD was seen as a condition limited to children, an inaccurate assumption embraced by professionals and their national organizations, and concretized in the second edition of the *Diagnostic and Statistical Manual of Mental Disorders* (DSM-II). No one thought that ADHD existed in adolescents or adults. As a result, academic institutions were not expected or required to serve students with ADHD, which guaranteed that many children and teens with ADHD would fail or quit school. When Mariellen Fischer and I initiated our own Milwaukee longitudinal study of children with ADHD, we were not surprised to find that approximately one-third of subjects never completed high school, nearly half were engaged in sufficient antisocial activities to be considered conduct disordered, and only approximately one-fourth of them continued to receive any treatments for ADHD by medical or mental health services as they moved into late adolescence and early adulthood. Dispelling the views of the time, we documented the persistence of nearly 80% of full disorder over the first 10 years of follow-up into mid-adolescence. Our reports of such findings and those of other longitudinal researchers provided a stunning rebuke to the unfortunate assumptions of researchers and practitioners. This shift over the last 45 years of research has ushered in a new period that documents the validity and seriousness of ADHD in both this adolescent and later adult stages of life.

Kudos to Stephen Becker and his colleagues for providing readers with a volume of tremendous significance focused on adolescents with ADHD. The authors represent a "who's who" list of experts on topics that are the focus of each of their chapters. Their standing in the field ensures that their work represents state-of-the-art summations of what is currently known in their specialized areas. Akin to my own handbook on the diagnosis and treatment of ADHD in children and adults, this book covers a panoply of areas related to ADHD. Chapters focus on not only what is known about symptoms, course, etiologies, comorbidities, peer relationships, families, and education, among other topics, but also cover clinical areas that will help readers evaluate, assess, and manage treatment of youth with ADHD. All this guarantees that this book will be the desk reference on the topic of adolescents with ADHD for clinicians, researchers, and graduate students for years to come.

RUSSELL A. BARKLEY, PHD
Clinical Professor of Psychiatry,
Virginia Center for Children
and Virginia Commonwealth
University School of Medicine

Preface

I never thought I would study attention-deficit/hyperactivity disorder (ADHD), let alone edit a book about it. I started my doctoral work examining possible mechanisms by which trauma and posttraumatic stress lead to adolescent delinquency. Even after my advisor, Patricia Kerig, moved to a different university, I steadfastly collected my thesis data every Saturday morning at a local juvenile detention center. In 2009, as data collection was wrapping up and I was on the lookout for local research opportunities, students in my program received an e-mail from Dr. Joshua Langberg at the nearby Center for ADHD at Cincinnati Children's Hospital. With little knowledge of ADHD and no idea where it would lead, I jumped at the chance to volunteer on a federally funded study of school-based interventions for teens with ADHD. I was hooked, and 10 years later, here we are.

We all have stories like this. They illuminate the paths we each take, some straight and some winding. Detours and roadblocks, as well as scenic byways, are possible at any point in development, but perhaps no more so than in adolescence. This is certainly true for teens with ADHD, who must navigate the perils and promises of adolescence alongside deficits in self-regulation and a history often marked by difficulties in multiple areas of functioning. Navigating this period of development is challenging for parents, teachers, and clinicians alike, and, of course, for adolescents themselves. Yet I am once again reminded of the teens I interviewed as part of my research in the juvenile detention center—teens with unfavorable and at times horrific pasts—who were determined to change the paths of their own trajectories but clearly needed strong supports and interventions along the way. These adolescents are the inspiration for this volume.

Two decades ago, Arthur Robin wrote an influential book on ADHD in adolescence, a book that played an important role in my own thinking and certainly contributed to the field's increased attention to ADHD during this developmental period. Building from this work, this book includes 18 chapters that provide an up-to-date, authoritative overview of the rapidly accumulating research and intervention work specific to adolescents with ADHD. The contributors to this volume are all experts in the topics at hand. Each was tasked with taking on an area of major importance to adolescents with ADHD and ensuring that developmental factors were considered prominently throughout. The opening chapter, by Stephen P. Hinshaw and me, provides an overview of the interplay of ADHD and adolescence, and the core tenets of developmental psychopathology that set the stage for the following chapters. In the remaining chapters, Part I focuses on the trajectories and impairments of ADHD in the context of adolescence, and Part II focuses on assessing and treating adolescents with ADHD. I am deeply appreciative of the care the contributors took in writing their chapters, doing so by finding time in their already busy schedules.

In college I was a vocal performance music major and did not take a single psychology class. I spent my days memorizing German lieder and practicing Mozart recitatives, not running subjects, entering data, or conducting analyses. A terminal master's degree in counseling psychology ignited my passion for research, but I desperately needed patient and thoughtful guidance. I was exceedingly fortunate to have a trio of excellent mentors early in my training and professional development—my own mentorship triple threat, so to speak. Patricia Kerig introduced me to developmental psychopathology, Josh Langberg introduced me to ADHD, and Aaron Luebbe helped me learn to integrate the two. I am also indebted to other wonderful colleagues who have each pushed my work into new and exciting territories and made the work infinitely more fun in the process. I want to especially thank my colleagues in the Cincinnati Children's Center for ADHD, particularly Jeff Epstein, Richard Loren, Leanne Tamm, and Aaron Vaughn, who each played important roles in my training. At The Guilford Press, Kitty Moore has been an indefatigable sounding board, and Carolyn Graham has provided invaluable support for this book from conception to fruition.

Most of all, I thank my family members for their unrelenting support. My wife, Joy, has provided encouragement and a listening ear, so much so that I am confident she now knows the difference between moderation and mediation. More importantly, she has been my champion throughout the completion of this book, even when I wondered if our young children would be adolescents themselves before it was completed. Our children, Charlotte, Andrew, and Milo, have given me a lively and fresh perspective on child development, and I count it my greatest privilege to watch their own paths unfold.

Contents

CHAPTER 1

Toward a Developmental Psychopathology Approach for Understanding, Assessing, and Treating ADHD in Adolescents

Stephen P. Hinshaw
Stephen P. Becker

The two major topics addressed in this book—attention-deficit/hyperactivity disorder (ADHD) and adolescence—are steeped in lore and myth. Adolescence, for example, has been posited as a period of inevitable *sturm und drang* (storm and stress). ADHD has often been described as a social construction related to poor parenting and schooling. Far too many parents, teachers, clinicians, and member of the general public can become swayed by the inaccuracies.

In fact, although often challenging, adolescence is not inevitably tumultuous, and the psychobiological reality of ADHD is undoubted. Moreover, it is now clear that neither adolescence nor ADHD is a static category, but instead are highly dynamic processes shaped by the confluence of biology and transacting contextual forces. Official scientific and/or clinical recognition for both topics has emerged only within the past century-plus (e.g., Hall, 1904; Still, 1902). Finally, in recent years both adolescence and ADHD have been subjects of intense interest from the perspectives of science, clinical intervention, and policy, interest that has finally begun to place knowledge of each domain on a firm scientific foundation.

This volume marks the huge need for integration of findings related to ADHD—its manifestations, causal factors, development, and response to intervention—during the crucial developmental period of adolescence. Until quite recently, the intersection of these domains was extremely small. Indeed, psychiatry and clinical psychology assumed that the symptoms of ADHD (or what was formerly termed *minimal brain dysfunction, hyperkinesis,* or *hyperactivity*) largely vanished following puberty. Accumulating evidence, however, reveals that despite age-normative declines in overtly hyperactive behavior patterns, impairing levels of impulsivity and inattention persist in an overwhelming majority of children with diagnosable ADHD through the teenage years, and often beyond (Sibley, Mitchell, & Becker, 2016). In fact, the spiraling transactional patterns linked to ADHD during childhood often magnify with the onset of adolescence, resulting in an escalation and intensification of academic and social impairments, a broadening and deepening of comorbid psychopathology, and the presentation of major challenges for those interested in mounting and sustaining effective treatment strategies.

In this opening chapter, we provide a necessarily brief overview of basic points about both ADHD and adolescence before discussing the confluence of these crucial topics within the framework of developmental psychopathology. Such a framework is essential, we believe, given that reciprocal, interactive, and transactional forces typify the unfolding of ADHD-related problems—and, we hope, protective factors—during adolescence. We conclude with an overview of the volume's remaining contents.

At the outset, we are of the strong opinion that it is high time for increased consideration of ADHD and adolescence in tandem. Imagine entering the life-altering hormonal surge of puberty and the vast expansion of social expectations marking the adolescent years with a history of poor self-regulation and deficient impulse control, struggles in school, difficulties with peers, and strained family relationships. The challenges would be considerable indeed, requiring the best of scientific and clinical knowledge.

Attention-Deficit/Hyperactivity Disorder

Scientific findings about ADHD, along with controversies surrounding the entire topic, have grown exponentially in recent years (e.g., Barkley, 2015). Historically, following the advent of compulsory education during the 19th century, children's problems in attention span and behavioral deportment became salient to the medical community. Within the past 50 years, increasing academic pressures of postindustrial life and ready access to stimulant medications have prompted an explosion of concern and controversy over ADHD in national and international dialogue (Hinshaw & Scheffler, 2014). Overall, it is hard to conceive a clinical topic garnering the amounts of interest, debate, and (too often) misinformation that ADHD has generated.

Readers should note that ADHD is a global phenomenon. Issues of dysregulated attention and impulsive behavior occur at surprisingly similar rates in youth around the world (see Polanczyk, de Lima, Horta, Biederman, & Rohde, 2007; Polanczyk, Willcutt, Salum, Kieling, & Rohde, 2014). It can no longer be contended that this diagnostic condition is a sole product of U.S. values and cultural mores, a point that rings true for adolescent manifestations as well. The underlying behavioral features cluster into the domains of (1) inattention–disorganization and (2) hyperactivity–impulsivity (American Psychiatric Association, 2013). Developmentally extreme manifestations of these symptoms—when accompanied by clear functional impairments and not better accounted for by a different psychiatric condition—qualify the individual in question for a diagnosis. Yet without careful assessment procedures, ADHD can be both underdiagnosed and overdiagnosed (Hinshaw & Scheffler, 2014). Evidence-based evaluation strategies are therefore a priority, and the special considerations of adolescence with respect to assessment and diagnosis are featured in this book.

Beyond the core symptom domains, underlying processes related to self-regulation, executive function, intrinsic motivation and reward sensitivity, and emotion regulation are salient in differing subgroups of individuals with ADHD (see Brown, 2013; Sonuga-Barke, Bitsakou, & Thompson, 2010). With regard to neural underpinnings, multiple brain regions and circuits are involved (Castellanos & Proal, 2012), and maturational deficits in prefrontal gray matter are highly implicated in relevant symptom patterns (Shaw et al., 2007). Heritability is strong for the relevant behavioral and attention-related symptoms. Even more, a host of additional early-onset, biologically related triggers are also salient, exemplifying the developmental psychopathology principle of equifinality, whereby several different etiological pathways may yield similar symptom profiles (Cicchetti & Rogosch, 1996; for findings related to ADHD, see Nigg, 2017). Crucially, transactions between biological vulnerabilities and contextual influences such as parenting practices, school settings, and wider sociocultural factors influence both rates of diagnosis and outcomes of individuals with underling vulnerabilities, either favorably or unfavorably (e.g., Beauchaine & McNulty, 2013; Fulton, Scheffler, & Hinshaw, 2015). In short, ADHD is simultaneously a biological, social, and cultural construct.

This lightning-round overview does not begin to do justice to the multiple perspectives and levels of analysis related to full understanding ADHD (see Hinshaw, 2018). In fact, ADHD comprises far more than a homogenous diagnostic category of children, adolescents, or adults. Every aspect of ADHD is multifactorial, developmentally complex, and transactional in nature, and at no time in life is this truism more accurate than the adolescent years.

ADOLESCENCE

Many cultures have recognized a period of development from the time of physical and sexual maturation to the full adoption of adult roles and financial independence. Yet it took the publication of G. Stanley Hall's two-volume book, *Adolescence,* at the beginning of the 20th century, to mark the official pronouncement of this developmental epoch (Hall, 1904). Prescient in key respects yet almost comically inaccurate in others, these volumes opened up the age period in question—roughly spanning puberty to the early 20s—for scientific study, as well as educational and psychological scrutiny (see Arnett, 2006, for a cogent overview of the strengths and weaknesses of Hall's conceptions). For a lucid and readable overview of a host of issues related to adolescence, see Steinberg (2014).

The time span of adolescence is a moving target. Given that (1) puberty occurs much earlier, on average, than it did 150 years ago; (2) full independence in industrialized nations does not automatically take place at age 18; and (3) brain development (particularly in the frontal lobes) does not become adult-like until the mid-20s or beyond, adolescence has an ever-increasing scope. In fact, the life period now termed *emerging adulthood,* stretching from the late teen years to the mid-20s (Arnett, 2000), may actually constitute an extended period of adolescence. Like ADHD, adolescence is a construct embedded in the worlds of both biology (e.g., puberty) and social-contextual forces (e.g., delayed entry into full independence).

A key paradox is that adolescence is a time period of unprecedented cognitive and physical prowess *and,* simultaneously, of greatly enhanced vulnerability for physical injury, risk-taking behaviors, sleep problems, and the onset or intensification of many forms of mental disorder. The World Health Organization (2016) has recently become quite invested in promoting adolescent physical and mental health, given the population surge of adolescents worldwide, particularly in developing nations.

In science and policy, the adolescent years mark a second "inflection point" in individual physical, cognitive, and social development, following the huge expansion of abilities during the first few years of life. Ellis et al. (2012) frame this shift in evolutionary terms: Following puberty, individuals become intensely oriented toward attaining social status and developing reproductive strategies, guided by natural selection to propagate the species. Casey, Jones, and Hare (2008) describe the cascade of brain-related changes in development during adolescence, discussing the mismatch of "bottom-up" motivations from limbic regions with slower-developing "top-down" cognitive control (see also Steinberg et al., 2008). More broadly, Forbes and Dahl (2010) argue that pubertal maturation spurs a reorientation of the individual's social and motivational tendencies, enhancing the drive for sensation seeking and pressing youth toward both peers and potential romantic partners. Newfound cognitive skills (e.g., the attainment of formal operations), changing attitudes toward authority and conformity, surges in risky decision making and risky behavior, individuation from one's family of origin, and major shifts in identity development are hallmarks of this period of life (see also Crone & Dahl, 2012).

Indeed, the influence of peers grows precipitously during adolescence. The classic experimental work of Gardner and Steinberg (2005) revealed that in the period of middle to late adolescence, the presence of agemates strongly magnifies risky behavior and risky decision making, a finding not present in adults. Given the peer-related difficulties surrounding youth with ADHD, this is a particularly fertile area for research—and clinical intervention.

The Confluence of ADHD and Adolescence

Synthesizing findings from these two domains, this volume features consideration of multiple aspects of ADHD during the adolescent years: clinical features, developmental trajectories, delineation of underlying mechanisms, evidence-based assessment practices, and effective and emerging intervention strategies. A focus on adolescent manifestations of ADHD is crucial given that ADHD beyond the childhood years has not received anywhere near the scientific and clinical scrutiny it so urgently requires.

In fact, the cumulative problems generated by ADHD-linked symptoms and problems often gain momentum following the major shifts in psychobiology and social expectations related to puberty. Consider, for example, the potential for escalating patterns of academic dysfunction—and resulting school disengagement—when academic material becomes more difficult and abstract, and when multiple teachers fill one's school day. Consider as well the pernicious social exclusion that can occur as peer groups coalesce and intimate relationships form during the teen years, along with growing opportunity for antisocial behavior and substance use during the transitional years of adolescence—particularly when children enter adolescence with preexisting vulnerabilities linked to impulse control. Risk for mood-related disorders and self-injury is also highly salient as emotion dysregulation becomes increasingly problematic during the teenage and early-adult years, particularly for youth with poor attentional filters and poor inhibitory control (e.g., Hinshaw et al., 2012; Owens et al., 2017). Moreover, these problems may all be compounded by increasingly shortened sleep duration across the adolescent years, in part due to early school start times in most high schools (American Academy of Pediatrics, 2014; Becker, Langberg, & Byars, 2015). In short, the passage through puberty, with its accompanying pressures for independence and self-sufficiency in the context of widening social networks—and in a world increasingly preoccupied with social media and academic pressure—makes adolescence a critical time period. It also prioritizes compiling and synthesizing the many scientific and clinical advances related to adolescents who have underlying problems in self-regulation.

The biological maturation linked to puberty pushes young teens to explore, seek thrills, and express themselves sexually at earlier ages than during most epochs of recent history. At the same time, the press for ever-greater educational and vocational training in much of the developed world—in an era of declining incomes for the majority of families and the unprecedented reality of lower income levels for young adults compared to their parents—means that adolescence appears to be extending longer than ever before. In the current era of rapid advances in our device-driven information landscape, with social media predominating many interpersonal exchanges, it is undoubtedly the case that intensive concentration needed for academic and social success may be both enhanced and hindered by the digital world in ways that still defy full comprehension. It is also likely that individuals with attention-related and impulsive styles may be quite vulnerable to the seduction of the digital world. The digital world may intersect in dangerous ways with the start of driving for many teens age 16 and upward, which is itself a key developmental challenge that becomes particularly salient when deficits in self-control and lapses in attention are part of the clinical picture (Barkley, Murphy, & Fisher, 2008; Narad et al., 2013).

Beyond ADHD per se, adolescent mental health has become a major topic. Data from the World Health Organization (2014) reveal that the leading cause of death, globally, for girls ages 15–19 years is now suicide. The age of onset of serious mood disorders appears to be dropping, signaling the importance of contextual "push" in unearthing vulnerability (Hinshaw, 2009). In both the developing and developed worlds, serious mental disorder in youth portends major life consequences and even tragedy (Sawyer et al., 2002). Even more, recent findings reveal links between a range of mental disorders and a long list of chronic physical illnesses (Scott et al., 2016). Emerging evidence suggests this linkage applies to ADHD as well, including predictions of lowered life expectancy (Barkley et al., 2008; Barkley & Fisher, 2019). Once again, adolescence marks a phase of life characterized by extreme promise and extreme risk.

Developmental Psychopathology Framework

To provide a conceptual framework for the entire volume, we now convey several core principles of developmental psychopathology (DP), the optimal lens through which ADHD and associated impairments during adolescence should be viewed. Indeed, we believe it takes a theorctical model that encompasses reciprocal, dynamic, transactional models of influence to yield full understanding of an age period marked by intensive transactional processes that transpire on a daily basis.

For the past four decades, the perspectives of DP have provided an integrative framework for understanding typical and atypical development.

A small sampling of historical works includes Achenbach (1974), Cicchetti (1984, 1990), Rutter and Sroufe (2000), and Sroufe and Rutter (1984); for current volumes of state-of-the art conceptualizations, see Cicchetti (2016) and Lewis and Rudolph (2014). In a nutshell, DP models blend developmental psychology and the clinical disciplines in a unique synthesis, whereby atypical behavior emanates from early vulnerability (either biological or psychosocial), which is compounded by spiraling transactions with widening environmental influences to result in deviations from typical developmental paths. In other cases, protective factors and processes may deflect the at-risk individual toward a healthier set of outcomes. Inherent in the study of these processes is the need to consider *multiple levels of analysis,* spanning molecular, brain-based, intraindividual, familial, school-related, neighborhood, and wider societal–cultural influences. Our concise review of core axioms and principles shows clearly that static models, rigid categorical conceptions of diagnosis, and unidimensional perspectives are simply not up to the task of explaining mental disorders, including ADHD, in a convincing or clinically satisfactory manner.

DP perspectives are no longer considered radical, as they have become the mainstream models for understanding pathways to healthy versus less healthy developmental outcomes. In fact, the DP focus on the interplay between biology and context and on multilevel influences has come to dominate current models of psychopathology (e.g., Beauchaine & Hinshaw, 2016). Key guiding principles include cross-disciplinary perspectives, multilevel processes, and systems-level, often nonlinear change processes that ultimately lead to developmental aberrations (Hinshaw, 2017).

At the outset, it is essential to realize that multiple pathways to pathology exist. Indeed, a key problem with static nosologies is their implicit assumption that everyone receiving a similar psychiatric diagnosis has parallel, if not identical, risk factors for and underlying processes related to psychopathology. In fact, however, disparate routes may lead to behaviorally similar conditions or outcomes, exemplifying the construct of *equifinality* (Cicchetti & Rogosch, 1996). For example, ADHD may result from strong genetic liability, from prenatal alcohol exposure or low birthweight, from difficult temperament interacting with environmental risk, or even—rarely—from horrific deprivation in early caregiving. Similarly, *multifinality* pertains when a given vulnerability, risk factor, or initial state fans out into disparate outcomes across different individuals (Cicchetti & Rogosch, 1996). Thus, neither difficult temperament nor child abuse or neglect inevitably leads to maladaptation, depending on a host of intervening factors. In terms of the current subject matter, heritable vulnerability for ADHD does not inevitably portend clinical levels of symptoms. Moreover, ADHD is itself heterogeneous in its presentation, whereby any given vulnerability may lead to widely varying clinical presentations.

The following list of principles represents one means of synthesizing DP formulations, adapted and shortened from the discussion in Hinshaw

(2017). Other conceptualizations posit additional axioms and formulations; in the interest of brevity, we provide the following summation.

Normal and Atypical Development: Mutually Informative

DP models emphasize that clinical phenomena represent aberrations in continua of normal developmental pathways and processes—in other words, they constitute *adaptational failures* (Sroufe, 1997). Accordingly, without understanding typical development, the study of pathology will remain incomplete and decontextualized. For example, comprehending ADHD requires knowledge of the normative development of attention, impulse control, and self-regulation (e.g., Barkley, 2015; Hinshaw & Scheffler, 2014; Nigg, 2017; Owens & Hinshaw, 2016; Sonuga-Barke et al., 2010). One cannot study (or adequately treat) mental disorder without real understanding of normative developmental processes. At the same time, DP envisions a two-way street, as investigations of pathological conditions can and should, in parallel, provide a unique perspective on normative development. Atypical developmental processes may therefore provide an essential window on general models of human development.

This core tenet—of the mutual interplay between normality and pathology—is espoused widely. Indeed, examples are prevalent in neurology, where the study of disrupted neural systems enhances understanding of healthy brain functioning, and vice versa (Gazzaniga, Ivry, & Magnun, 2014). In neurology, however, single lesions or single genes can often be isolated, whereas mental disorder is inherently multifactorial (see Kendler, 2005). Still, accumulating evidence suggests that at the levels of genes, harshly aberrant environments, reward mechanisms, empathy "modules," and many more examples, examination of pathological development may yield key clues to normative pathways.

Developmental Continuities and Discontinuities

Here, a key conception is that, across development, traits and behavior may unfold in lawful ways, but the surface behavioral manifestations may well change with maturity and opportunity; that is, continuity of behavior may be *heterotypic*. In the realm of antisocial behavior, for example, extremes of difficult temperament (e.g., intense and frequent tantrums) may give way to verbal aggression in preschool, physical assaults in elementary school, sexual aggression and robbery during adolescence, and partner violence by adulthood. The "surface" behaviors change as an underlying antisocial trait changes form with time. In other words, brain maturation, growing cognitive skills, and widening social and cultural opportunities converge to propel the emergence of heterotypically continuous behavior patterns over time, in keeping with the dynamic tenets of DP models.

With ADHD, for example, defiance and overt hyperactivity early in development typically yield academic problems and peer rejection during grade school, with multiple forms of impulsivity and disorganization becoming salient by the teen years. Even more, other disorders (e.g., substance abuse, antisocial personality) may become apparent. By adulthood, pathways may branch even further. Of extreme importance, girls with ADHD (particularly those with early-emerging impulsivity) are at high risk for displaying clinically significant levels of self-harm by adolescence (see Hinshaw et al., 2012; for additional information on predictor and mediator variables, see Guendelman, Owens, Galan, Gard, & Hinshaw, 2016; Meza, Owens, & Hinshaw, 2016; Swanson, Owens, & Hinshaw, 2014). Indeed, Guendelman et al. (2016) showed that childhood ADHD in the presence of maltreatment yields extraordinarily high rates of suicide attempts by late adolescence in girls. Thus, (1) heterotypic continuity may encompass behavior patterns that are dissimilar to their *phenotypic* precursors but lawfully emerge from core *developmental* precursors; (2) the adolescent years are likely to witness important examples of the emergence of heterotypically continuous problems in youth with ADHD; (3) the individual's biological sex may serve as a moderator of differing patterns of heterotypic continuity; and (4) biological vulnerability (e.g., impulsivity) is likely to interact with psychosocial risk (e.g., maltreatment) to yield particularly salient impairment and pathology.

Risk and Protective Factors

A key focus of DP—with the term *psychopathology* embedded in its title—is discovery of the nature and roots of behavioral and emotional problems. But many argue that it is equally (if not more) important to uncover those protective influences that may transform risk into *resilience,* defined as unexpectedly good outcomes, or competence, in the face of adversity or risk (see Luthar, 2006; Masten & Cicchetti, 2016). Indeed, the concept of multifinality, noted previously, directly implies that depending on a host of biological, environmental, and contextual factors, variegated outcomes may well emanate from the same risk factor across individuals, with the distinct possibility of resilience and positive adaptation in some cases.

DP is therefore involved centrally in the search for what have been called *protective factors:* variables and processes that mitigate vulnerability/risk and promote more successful outcomes than would be expected in their presence. Controversy surrounds the construct of resilience, the nature of protective factors, and the definitions of competent functioning (see Burt, Coatsworth, & Masten, 2016). Perhaps there is no need to invoke a set of special processes that are involved in resilience, as a certain percentage of any high-risk sample is likely to show better-than-expected outcomes. Also, protective factors are too often viewed as the opposite poles of risk variables or vulnerabilities (e.g., higher rather than lower IQ; easier rather than more difficult temperament; warm and structured rather than cold and lax parenting). Yet it is essential to examine processes involved in promoting competence and strength rather than disability and despair; such processes may be harnessed for prevention efforts and may provide key conceptual leads toward the understanding of both pathology and competence.

Reciprocal, Transactional, and Ontogenic Process Models

Linear models of causation, whereby static psychological or psychobiological risk factors respond in invariant ways to the influence of additional variables, cannot fully explain psychopathology and its development (see Richters, 1997, for elaboration). Pathways to adolescent and adult functioning are marked by reciprocal patterns or chains, in which children influence parents, teachers, and peers, who in turn shape the further development of the child (for a classic formulation, see Bell, 1968). Such mutually interactive processes evolve over time into *transactional models*. It is little wonder that static categories of mental disorder are hard-pressed to do justice to such dynamic, interactive processes. Sensitive data-analytic strategies and innovative research designs are crucial essential for fostering greater understanding of these phenomena.

Incorporation of these processes can elucidate patterns of equifinality and multifinality, as described earlier. Moreover, recognition of the problems with current categorical nosologies prompted the genesis of the National Institute of Mental Health (NIMH) Research Domain Criteria (RDoC; Insel et al., 2010), a dimensional means of accounting for psychopathology that embraces a multiple-levels-of-analysis approach and emphasizes neural circuitry in interaction with contextual influences. Clearly, the field is seeking the kinds of models and paradigms that can optimally incorporate the complexity and multifaceted nature of mental disorder.

In parallel, *ontogenic* process models of psychopathology have witnessed a resurgence (see Beauchaine & Hinshaw, 2016; Beauchaine & McNulty, 2013). Here, heritable vulnerabilities transact with environmental forces (e.g., coercive family interactions; violent neighborhoods) to yield psychopathology. In such models, what appear to be the emergence of discrete, "comorbid" disorders across development may in fact represent heterotypic continuity. Indeed, apparent *comorbidity* (the joint presence of two or more independent conditions) may in many cases be artifactual, representing instead the unfolding of transactional, DP-related processes. Once again, static and/or linear models of influence must yield to reciprocal, dynamic chains of influence.

Psychobiological Vulnerability and Context

The genomic era fully emerged in 2001, when the strands of DNA comprising the human genome were finally decoded. At the same time, progressions in brain imaging research have made the developing brain far more accessible to scientific view than ever before. These advances flew in the face of the predominant models of the 20th century, which emphasized parenting and other aspects of socialization as the core drivers of development. Rather than pitting biology against context, DP prioritizes interactive and transactional models of the ways in which early biological risk is potentiated (or redirected) by complex, multilevel contextual influences (e.g., see Hyde, 2015).

For example, gene–environment correlation recognizes the inextricable confounding of genes and contexts in shaping development within biological families. Genetically informative research investigations are therefore crucial to understanding risk and protection. Regarding ADHD, Harold et al. (2013) leveraged two adoption designs to disentangle heritable from contextual influences. In brief, even in adoptive families, which remove the influence of gene–environment correlation, children's disruptive behaviors evoked harsh maternal responses, which in turn predicted subsequent ADHD behavior patterns. Thus, although the heritable nature of ADHD is clear, psychosocial processes within families are still highly influential in terms of development and clinical manifestation.

The area of gene × environment interplay provides an additional, if sometimes contentious, example. The underlying idea is that genotypes moderate the effects of environmental context on the development of psychopathology, such that contextual risk is most pronounced for only certain configurations of genetic–biological vulnerability (for elaboration, see Dodge & Rutter, 2011). Might it be the case that risk for ADHD-related impairment is most pronounced for only certain genotypes in the context of certain environments? Core critiques of this concept have been argued. For instance, Dick et al. (2015) outline essential recipes for avoiding the major issue of false-positive findings in research on gene × environment interactions; Keller (2014) adds the cautionary note that many gene–environment researchers will overestimate such interactive power unless they take into account the potentially confounding effects of passive gene–environment correlation. Crucially, it may also be the case that some "vulnerability" genes are actually "susceptibility" genes, which means that they are particularly responsive to either extremely good or poor environments in yielding optimal versus pathological outcomes (see Belsky & Pluess, 2009; Ellis, Boyce, Belsky, Bakermans-Kranenburg, & van IJzendoorn, 2011). The potential for resilience is fascinating to consider within this framework.

Summary

These principles converge on the major theme that the development of psychopathological functioning, including ADHD, is multidetermined, complex, interactive, transactional, and in many instances nonlinear. When the life period of adolescence becomes part of the mix, with its inherent complexities and dynamics, the need for DP models becomes even more apparent. In fact, we consider the DP perspective an essential framework for readers who are intrigued by the diverse clinical presentations of various pathological conditions, like ADHD, across childhood and adolescence; for those who are fascinated with how much remains to be learned about risk and maintaining factors; and for those looking for ways to assess and treat adolescent forms of ADHD with maximum impact. With this consideration in mind, we now turn to providing an overview of the following chapters that examine the confluence of ADHD and adolescence within a DP framework.

Overview of the Book's Contents

The contributors to this book were encouraged to carefully consider the previously discussed review on the DP of ADHD in adolescence as they prepared their chapters. The result is a compendium of chapters on ADHD that each take seriously the developmental context of adolescence. This book is divided into two sections. Part I focuses on ADHD in the context of adolescence and adolescent development, and Part II focuses on assessing and treating ADHD in adolescence. Immediately following this chapter, Henrik Larsson (Chapter 2) provides an overview of the developmental course of ADHD across adolescence and into early adulthood. He covers important questions regarding the trajectory of ADHD across adolescence, including both diagnostic persistence and symptom dimensions, and also reviews the recent controversial literature on the possibility of an adult-onset ADHD that is distinct from childhood-onset ADHD. In Chapter 3, Erik G. Willcutt summarizes behavioral genetic studies of ADHD with a particular focus on adolescence, including new analyses from two twin samples conducted for this chapter. He also reviews literature on molecular genetic and environmental risk factors, observing the need for etiologically informative longitudinal designs that may help identify factors associated with the persistence or decline of ADHD symptoms across adolescence. Next, Joshua Doidge, Wafa Saoud, and Maggie E. Toplak (Chapter 4) provide a review of the executive function and decision-making research in ADHD. Particular attention is given to temporal discounting, risky decision making, and ADHD presentations/co-occurring psychopathologies. In Chapter 5, Nóra Bunford covers the area of emotion regulation and its importance to conceptualizations of ADHD. In doing so, she reviews key definitional and measurement issues, considers overlapping biological and psychosocial vulnerabilities, and emphasizes the important role of emotion regulation for functioning in adolescents with ADHD.

The remaining chapters in Part I shift to the social experiences, co-occurring difficulties, and adolescent-salient domains of functioning. In Chapter 6, Judith Wiener considers the family context of adolescents with ADHD. She builds on the larger literature on families of children with ADHD before reviewing the extant literature on adolescents specifically, including bidirectional associations, parenting cognitions, parental ADHD, and parent involvement in interventions for adolescents with ADHD. Chapter 7, by Julia D. McQuade, shifts to the peer relationships that take on increased priority and consume more time during adolescence. In reviewing the literature on peer relationships in adolescents with ADHD, attention is given to the larger peer group, dyadic friendships, and romantic relationships, in addition to both in-person and online relationships. She also summarizes the very limited intervention research focused on the peer relationships of adolescents with ADHD, an area ripe for much-needed attention. Steven W. Evans, Saskia Van der Oord, and Emma E. Rogers (Chapter 8) then turn our attention to the school setting in which adolescents spend much of their day and frequently struggle. The authors consider pathways to academic difficulties in adolescents with ADHD and review the rapidly growing body of intervention research specifically targeting academic impairments in adolescents with ADHD. In Chapter 9, Stephen P. Becker and Nicholas D. Fogleman review psychopathologies that frequently co-occur with ADHD (comorbidity). Prevalence rates of co-occurring internalizing and externalizing psychopathologies in adolescence are reviewed, in addition to risk factors and developmental pathways. Attention is given to domains of psychopathology that need additional scrutiny in adolescence, including autism spectrum disorder (ASD), sluggish cognitive tempo (SCT), eating pathology, and self-harm and suicide. Research examining co-occurring psychopathologies as outcomes, predictors, or moderators of intervention for adolescents with ADHD are also reviewed. Sleep difficulties are also common in youth with ADHD, and sleep is the focus of Chapter 10 by Melissa Mulraney, Emma Sciberras, and Stephen P. Becker. Although the sleep problems of children with ADHD have been documented for some time, only recently has there been significant interest in the sleep of adolescents with ADHD. Mulraney and colleagues review recent research in this area and possible biological and psychosocial contributors to poor and insufficient sleep in adolescents with ADHD, in addition to likely transactional processes and assessment–intervention considerations. Next, Traci M. Kennedy, Kirsten M. P. McKone, and Brooke S. G. Molina (Chapter 11) review the extensive literature on substance use in adolescents with ADHD. The authors give important attention to assessment and measurement issues before reviewing evidence for problematic substance use in adolescents with ADHD. Developmental pathways, moderators and protective effects, and treatment implications are carefully considered. The final chapter (Chapter 12) in Part I focuses on a key domain that first emerges in adolescence: driving. Annie A. Garner first provides an important backdrop on driving risk and driving problems in adolescence broadly, before reviewing the literature examining driving behaviors and outcomes in adolescents with ADHD specifically. Risk and protective factors are thoroughly reviewed, and possible interventions to improve the driving of adolescents with ADHD are discussed.

In Part II, we turn our attention more directly to the assessment and treatment of adolescents with ADHD. George J. DuPaul, Arthur D. Anastopoulos, and Kristen Kipperman (Chapter 13) start this section off with a comprehensive review of the process, methods, and measures used to assess and diagnose ADHD in adolescence. Their chapter also includes several case examples that highlight key issues in the assessment of ADHD in adolescents and young adults. In Chapter 14, Margaret H. Sibley addresses the key issue of motivation when treating adolescents with ADHD. She reviews the complex causal pathways implicated in the complex pathways of ADHD that often give rise to organization, time management, and planning problems as well as volitional, self-efficacy, and/or motivation difficulties. Various treatment approaches to target these multifaceted difficulties are discussed, including the Supporting Teens' Autonomy Daily (STAND) intervention, which is a parent–adolescent therapy targeting executive function and motivation deficits. Intervention approaches targeting homework problems are the focus of Chapter 15 by Joshua M. Langberg, Zoe R. Smith, and Cathrin D. Green. Using the homework completion cycle as their guide, the authors consider homework problems across development, the assessment of homework problems, and core treatment strategies for improving homework problems in adolescents with ADHD. Research on treating these problems in adolescents with ADHD is reviewed, including interventions implemented in afterschool, in-school, and clinic settings: the Challenging Horizons Program (CHP) and the Homework, Organization, and Planning Skills (HOPS) and STAND interventions. Next, Susan E. Sprich and Jennifer A. Burbridge (Chapter 16) briefly review psychosocial treatments for adult ADHD and the theoretical and developmental rationale to extend cognitive-behavioral approaches down to adolescence. They describe modifying their adult cognitive-behavioral therapy (CBT) treatment protocol for use with adolescents with ADHD, which consists primarily of individual sessions augmented by two parent–adolescent sessions and optional parent-only sessions. Two case examples offer insights for implementing a CBT approach when working with adolescents with ADHD. In Chapter 17, Naomi Ornstein Davis and John T. Mitchell provide an overview of mindfulness-based interventions and their extension to adolescents before providing a rationale for applying these interventions to individuals with ADHD. They then review the small but growing body of research evaluating mindfulness-based interventions for adolescents with ADHD and provide important considerations for this nascent area. In the final chapter (Chapter 18), William B. Brinkman, Tanya E. Froehlich, and Jeffery N. Epstein shift our focus to the important area of medication treatment in adolescents with ADHD. The authors review the evidence for medication treatment in this population, including effects on ADHD symptoms and functional impairments, as well as side effects and possible adverse consequences such as misuse and diversion. Issues related to medication adherence are detailed, and recommendations are provided for clinicians working with adolescents with ADHD, with two case examples illustrating how clinicians can help support medication continuity while also fostering autonomy.

Together, the chapters in this book integrate a large volume of research to help us better understand, assess, and treat adolescents with ADHD. Yet each chapter also points to the need for far more research devoted to ADHD during this crucial developmental period. A DP approach is especially well-suited to examining the inherent complexities of ADHD in adolescence, and it is our hope that others will join us in this endeavor of major empirical and clinical importance.

References

Achenbach, T. M. (1974). *Developmental psychopathology*. New York: Ronald Press.

American Academy of Pediatrics. (2014). School start times for adolescents. *Pediatrics, 134*, 642–649.

American Psychiatric Association. (2013). *Diagnostic and statistical manual of mental disorders* (5th ed.). Arlington, VA: Author.

Arnett, J. J. (2000). Emerging adulthood: A theory of development from the late teens through the twenties. *American Psychologist, 55*, 469–480.

Arnett, J. J. (2006). G. Stanley Hall's *Adolescence: Brilliance and nonsense. History of Psychology, 9*, 186–197.

Barkley, R. A. (Ed.). (2015). *Attention deficit hyperactivity disorder: A handbook for diagnosis and treatment* (4th ed.). New York: Guilford Press.

Barkley, R. A., & Fischer, M. (2019). Hyperactive child syndrome and estimated life expectancy at young adult follow-up: The role of ADHD persistence and other potential predictors. *Journal of Attention Disorders, 23*(9), 907–923.

Barkley, R. A., Murphy, K., & Fisher, M. (2008). *ADHD in adults: What the science says*. New York: Guilford Press.

Beauchaine, T. P., & Hinshaw, S. P. (Eds.). (2016). *The Oxford handbook of externalizing spectrum disorders*. New York: Oxford University Press.

Beauchaine, T. P., & McNulty, T. (2013). Comorbidities and continuities as ontogenic processes: Toward a developmental spectrum model of externalizing psychopathology. *Development and Psychopathology, 25*, 1505–1528.

Becker, S. P., Langberg, J. M., & Byars, K. C. (2015). Advancing a biopsychosocial and contextual model of sleep in adolescence: A review and introduction to the special issue. *Journal of Youth and Adolescence, 44*, 239–270.

Bell, R. Q. (1968). A reinterpretation of the direction of effects in studies of socialization. *Psychological Review, 75*, 81–95.

Belsky, J., & Pluess, M. (2009). Beyond diathesis stress: Differential susceptibility to environmental influences. *Psychological Bulletin, 135*(6), 885–908.

Brown, T. E. (2013). *A new understanding of ADHD in children and adults: Executive function impairments*. New York: Routledge.

Burt, K. B., Coatsworth, J. D., & Masten, A. S. (2016). Competence and psychopathology in development. In D. Cicchetti (Ed.), *Developmental psychopathology: Vol. 4. Risk, resilience, and intervention* (3rd ed., pp. 435–484). New York: Wiley.

Casey, B. J., Jones, R. M., & Hare, T. A. (2008). The adolescent brain. *Annals of the New York Academy of Sciences, 1124,* 111–126.

Castellanos, F. X., & Proal, E. (2012). Large-scale brain systems in ADHD: Beyond the prefrontal–striatal model. *Trends in Cognitive Science, 16,* 17–26.

Cicchetti, D. (1984). The emergence of developmental psychopathology. *Child Development, 55,* 1–7.

Cicchetti, D. (1990). An historical perspective on the discipline of developmental psychopathology. In J. Rolf, A. Masten, D. Cicchetti, K. Neuchterlein, & S. Weintraub (Eds.), *Risk and protective factors in the development of psychopathology* (pp. 2–28). New York: Cambridge University Press.

Cicchetti, D. (Ed.). (2016). *Developmental psychopathology* (Vols. 1–4). Hoboken, NJ: Wiley.

Cicchetti, D., & Rogosch, F. (1996). Equifinality and multifinality in developmental psychopathology. *Development and Psychopathology, 8,* 597–600.

Crone, E. A., & Dahl, R. E. (2012). Understanding adolescence as a period of social–affective engagement and goal flexibility. *Nature Reviews Neuroscience, 13,* 636–650.

Dick, D. M., Agrawal, A., Keller, M. C., Adkins, A., Aliev, F., Monroe, S., . . . Sher, K. J. (2015). Candidate gene–environment interaction research: Reflections and recommendations. *Perspectives on Psychological Science, 10,* 37–59.

Dodge, K. A., & Rutter, M. (Eds.). (2011). *Gene–environment interactions in developmental psychopathology.* New York: Guilford Press.

Ellis, B. J., Boyce, W. T., Belsky, J., Bakermans-Kranenburg, M. J., & van IJzendoorn, M. (2011). Differential susceptibility to the environment: An evolutionary neurodevelopmental theory. *Development and Psychopathology, 23*(1), 7–28.

Ellis, B. J., del Guidice, M., Dishion, T. J., Figueredo, A. J., Gray, P., Griskevicius, P., . . . Wilson, D. S. (2012). The evolutionary basis of risky adolescent behavior: Implications for science, policy, and practice. *Developmental Psychology, 48,* 598–623.

Forbes, E. E., & Dahl, R. E. (2010). Pubertal development and behavior: Hormonal activation of social and motivational tendencies. *Brain and Cognition, 72,* 66–72.

Fulton, B. D., Scheffler, R. M., & Hinshaw, S. P. (2015). State variation in increased ADHD prevalence: Links to NCLB school accountability and state medication laws. *Psychiatric Services, 66,* 1074–1082.

Gardner, M., & Steinberg, L. (2005). Peer influence on risk taking, risk preference, and risky decision making in adolescence and adulthood: An experimental study. *Developmental Psychology, 41,* 625–635.

Gazzaniga, M. S., Ivry, R. B., & Mangun, G. R. (2014). *Cognitive neuroscience: The biology of the mind* (4th ed.). New York: Norton.

Guendelman, M., Owens, E. B., Galan, C., Gard, A., & Hinshaw, S. P. (2016). Early adult correlates of maltreatment in girls with ADHD: Increased risk for internalizing problems and suicidality. *Development and Psychopathology, 28,* 1–14.

Hall, G. S. (1904). *Adolescence: Its psychology and its relations to physiology, anthropology, sociology, sex, crime, religion, and education* (Vols. 1 & 2). New York: Appleton.

Harold, G. T., Leve, L. D., Barrett, D., Elam, K., Neiderhiser, J. M., Natsuaki, N. M., . . . Thapar, A. (2013). Biological and rearing mother influences on child ADHD symptoms: Revisiting the developmental interface between nature and nurture. *Journal of Child Psychology and Psychiatry, 54*(10), 1038–1046.

Hinshaw, S. P. (2017). Developmental psychopathology as a scientific discipline: A

21st-century perspective. In T. P. Beauchaine & S. P. Hinshaw (Eds.), *Child and adolescent psychopathology* (3rd ed., pp. 3–32). Hoboken, NJ: Wiley.

Hinshaw, S. P. (2018). Attention deficit-hyperactivity disorder (ADHD): Controversy, developmental mechanisms, and multiple levels of analysis. *Annual Review of Clinical Psychology, 14,* 291–316.

Hinshaw, S. P., with Kranz, R. (2009). *The triple bind: Saving our teenage girls from today's pressures.* New York: Ballantine.

Hinshaw, S. P., Owens, E. B., Zalecki, C., Huggins, S. P., Montenegro-Nevado, A., Schrodek, E., & Swanson, E. N. (2012). Prospective follow-up of girls with attention-deficit hyperactivity disorder into young adulthood: Continuing impairment includes elevated risk for suicide attempts and self-injury. *Journal of Consulting and Clinical Psychology, 80,* 1041–1051.

Hinshaw, S. P., & Scheffler, R. M. (2014). *The ADHD explosion: Myths, medication, money, and today's push for performance.* New York: Oxford University Press.

Hyde, L. W. (2015). Developmental psychopathology in an era of molecular genetics and neuroimaging: A developmental neurogenetics approach. *Development and Psychopathology, 27,* 587–613.

Insel, T., Cuthbert, B., Garvey, M., Heinssen, R., Pine, D. S., Quinn, K., . . . Wang, P. (2010). Research domain criteria (RDoC): Toward a new classification framework for research on mental disorders. *American Journal of Psychiatry, 167,* 748–751.

Keller, M. C. (2014). Gene × environment interaction studies have not properly controlled for potential confounders: The problem and the (simple) solution. *Biological Psychiatry, 75*(1), 18–24.

Kendler, K. S. (2005). "A gene for . . . ": The nature of gene action in psychiatric disorders. *American Journal of Psychiatry, 162,* 1243–1252.

Lewis, M., & Rudolph, K. D. (Eds.). (2014). *Handbook of developmental psychopathology* (3rd ed.). New York: Springer.

Luthar, S. S. (2006). Resilience in development: A synthesis of research across five decades. In D. Cicchetti & D. J. Cohen (Eds.), *Developmental psychopathology: Vol 3. Risk, disorder, and adaptation* (2nd ed., pp. 739–795). Hoboken, NJ: Wiley.

Masten, A. S., & Cicchetti, D. (2016). Resilience in development: Progress and transformation. In D. Cicchetti (Ed.), *Developmental psychopathology: Vol 4. Risk, resilience, and intervention* (3rd ed., pp. 271–333). Hoboken, NJ: Wiley.

Meza, J., Owens, E. B., & Hinshaw, S. P. (2016). Response inhibition, peer preference and victimization, and self-harm: Longitudinal associations in young adult women with and without ADHD. *Journal of Abnormal Child Psychology, 44,* 323–334.

Narad, M., Garner, A. A., Brassell, A. A., Saxby, D., Antonini, T. N., O'Brien, K. M., . . . Epstein, J. N. (2013). Impact of distraction on the driving performance of adolescents with and without attention-deficit/hyperactivity disorder. *JAMA Pediatrics, 167,* 933–938.

Nigg, J. T. (2017). Attention-deficit/hyperactivity disorder. In T. P. Beauchaine & S. P. Hinshaw (Eds.), *Child and adolescent psychopathology* (3rd ed., pp. 407–448). Hoboken, NJ: Wiley.

Owens, E. B., & Hinshaw, S. P. (2016). Pathways from neurocognitive vulnerability to co-occurring internalizing and externalizing problems among women with and without ADHD followed prospectively for 16 years. *Development and Psychopathology, 28,* 1013–1031.

Owens, E. B., Zalecki, C., Gillette, P., & Hinshaw, S. P. (2017). Girls with childhood ADHD as adults: Cross-domain outcomes by diagnostic status. *Journal of Consulting and Clinical Psychology, 85,* 723–736.

Polanczyk, G., de Lima, M. S., Horta, B. L., Biederman, J., & Rohde, L. A. (2007). The worldwide prevalence of ADHD: A systematic review and metaregression analysis. *American Journal of Psychiatry, 164,* 942–948.

Polanczyk, G. V., Willcutt, E. G., Salum, G. A., Kieling, C., & Rohde, L. A. (2014). ADHD prevalence estimates across three decades: An updated systematic review and meta-regression analysis. *International Journal of Epidemiology, 43,* 434–442.

Richters, J. E. (1997). The Hubble Hypothesis and the developmentalist's dilemma. *Development and Psychopathology, 9,* 193–229.

Rutter, M., & Sroufe, L. A. (2000). Developmental psychopathology: Concepts and challenges. *Development and Psychopathology, 12,* 265–296.

Sawyer, M. G., Whaites, L., Rey, J. M., Hazell, P. L., Graetz, B. W., & Baghurst, P. (2002). Health-related quality of life of children and adolescents with mental disorders. *Journal of the American Academy of Child and Adolescent Psychiatry, 41*(5), 540–537.

Scott, K. M., Lim, C., Al-Hamzawi, A., Alonso, J., Bruffaerts, R., Caldas-de-Almeida, J. M., . . . Kessler, R. C. (2016). Association of mental disorders with subsequent chronic physical conditions: World mental health surveys from 17 countries. *JAMA Psychiatry, 73*(2), 150–158.

Shaw, P., Eckstrand, K., Sharp, W., Blumenthal, J., Lerch, J. P., Greenstein, D., & Rapoport, J. L. (2007). Attention deficit/hyperactivity disorder is characterized by a delay in cortical maturation. *Proceedings of the National Academy of Sciences of the USA, 104,* 19649–19654.

Sibley, M. H., Mitchell, J. T., & Becker, S. P. (2016). Method of adult diagnosis influences estimated persistence of childhood ADHD: A systematic review of longitudinal studies. *Lancet Psychiatry, 3,* 1157–1165.

Sonuga-Barke, E., Bitsakou, P., & Thompson, M. (2010). Beyond the dual pathway model: Evidence for the dissociation of timing, inhibitory, and delay-related impairments in attention-deficit/hyperactivity disorder. *Journal of the American Academy of Child and Adolescent Psychiatry, 49,* 345–355.

Sroufe, L. A. (1997). Psychopathology as an outcome of development. *Development and Psychopathology, 9,* 261–268.

Sroufe, L. A., & Rutter, M. (1984). The domain of developmental psychopathology. *Child Development, 55,* 17–29.

Steinberg, L. (2014). *Age of opportunity: Lessons from the new science of adolescence.* New York: Mariner Books.

Steinberg, L., Albert, D., Cauffman, E., Banich, M., Graham, S., & Woolard, J. (2008). Age differences in sensation seeking and impulsivity as indexed by behavior and self-report: Evidence for a dual systems model. *Developmental Psychology, 44,* 1764–1778.

Still, G. F. (1902). Some abnormal psychical conditions in children: The Goulstonian lectures. *Lancet, 1,* 1008–1012.

Swanson, E. N., Owens, E. B., & Hinshaw, S. P. (2014). Pathways to self-harmful behaviors in young women with and without ADHD: A longitudinal investigation of mediating factors. *Journal of Child Psychology and Psychiatry, 44,* 505–515.

World Health Organization. (2014). *Health for the world's adolescents: A second chance in the second decade.* Geneva, Switzerland: Author.

World Health Organization. (2016). Global Accelerated Action for the Health of Adolescents (AA-HA!). Retrieved February 20, 2017, from *www.who.int/maternal_child_adolescent/topics/adolescence/framework-accelerated-action/en.*

PART I

ADHD IN THE CONTEXT OF ADOLESCENCE

CHAPTER 2

Developmental Course of ADHD across Adolescence and into Young Adulthood

Henrik Larsson

Attention-deficit/hyperactivity disorder (ADHD) was long considered a childhood disorder, but increasingly it is being recognized as a lifespan condition (Asherson, Buitelaar, Faraone, & Rohde, 2016). Clinically based longitudinal studies that have followed up on preadolescents with ADHD into adolescence and adulthood have been instrumental in documenting impairment in psychiatric, educational, occupational, and health-related outcomes. As discussed in many chapters in this book, studies indicate that ADHD is associated with outcomes such as poor academic performance (e.g., lower grade point average and increased rates of grade retention; Galera, Melchior, Chastang, Bouvard, & Fombonne, 2009), and lower rates of high school graduation and postsecondary education (Galera et al., 2009; Klein et al., 2012; Mannuzza, Klein, Bessler, Malloy, & LaPadula, 1993). ADHD is also associated with occupational outcomes such as unemployment (Biederman et al., 2006; Klein et al., 2012), having trouble keeping a job (Barkley, Fischer, Smallish, & Fletcher, 2006; Biederman et al., 2006), financial problems (Barkley et al., 2006; Klein et al., 2012), and work incapacity in terms of absence due to sickness (Kleinman, Durkin, Melkonian, & Markosyan, 2009; Secnik, Swensen, & Lage, 2005). Longitudinal studies have also shown that individuals with ADHD are at increased risk for poor social outcomes such as high rates of separation and divorce

(Biederman et al., 2006; Klein et al., 2012), residential moves (Barkley et al., 2006), and early parenthood (Barkley et al., 2006).

There is recent interest in better understanding the developmental trajectories of ADHD from childhood to adulthood. An improved understanding of the developmental course of ADHD has clear implications for both research and clinical practice. First, accurate knowledge about the developmental trajectories of ADHD and the expected prevalence estimates across developmental stages is essential for both effective screening and diagnosis, and prediction. Second, an increased understanding of the developmental course of ADHD is needed to create developmentally sensitive diagnostic tools (e.g., *Diagnostic and Statistical Manual of Mental Disorders* [DSM] and *International Classification of Diseases* [ICD]). Finally, a better understanding of ADHD across the lifespan may help avoid a misinformed and at times polarized debate in which ADHD on the one hand is conceptualized as a condition that children will eventually outgrow, and on the other as a chronic neurodevelopmental disorder that does not change with development.

This chapter explores four questions that are relevant to the developmental course of ADHD:

1. Is childhood ADHD a persistent disorder?
2. Do ADHD symptom presentations change across time?
3. Is adult ADHD a childhood-onset neurodevelopmental disorder?
4. What factors predicts persistent and remitting ADHD?

Is Childhood ADHD a Persistent Disorder?

Longitudinal studies of children diagnosed with ADHD and followed into adolescence consistently show high persistence rates. For example, a study based on 296 individuals (85.5% male), ages 11–17 years, who were diagnosed with DSM-IV ADHD at the mean age of 6.7 years, reported a persistence rate of 63% at the follow-up in adolescence (Gau et al., 2010). A similar persistence rate of 69% was found in a sample of girls with ADHD, ages 6–12 years, who were followed for 5 years into adolescence (Hinshaw, Owens, Sami, & Fargeon, 2006). An ADHD persistence rate of 76% was reported in a U.K. study of children and adolescents (mean age 11.8 years, 87% males) diagnosed with DSM-IV ADHD combined type (Cheung et al., 2015). Another study of 126 boys with ADHD, ages 6–17 years old, revealed that 85% of the children with ADHD continued to have the disorder, and 15% remitted at the 4-year follow-up assessment. Of those who remitted, half did so in childhood and the other half did so in adolescence (Biederman et al., 1996). In contrast to other studies, the 8-year follow-up (mean age 16.8 years) from the Multimodal Treatment of ADHD (MTA) study found a persistence rate of 30%, which the authors suggested may be due to the lack of age-appropriate symptom cutoffs (Molina et al., 2009).

In part because symptoms of ADHD, particularly hyperactivity–impulsivity, decrease with age, lower persistence rates are usually observed when participants are followed up in adulthood. Another notable finding is that longitudinal studies of children diagnosed with ADHD and followed into adulthood present a wide range of ADHD persistence rates. For example, in two separate follow-up studies of boys with a clinical diagnosis of ADHD, Mannuzza, Klein, Bessler, Malloy, and LaPadula (1998) estimated the persistence rate of ADHD as 4% by a mean age of 24 years, whereas Weiss, Hechtman, Milroy, and Perlman (1985) reported a 66% persistence rate of ADHD by a mean age of 25 years. There is an ongoing debate about reasons for this discrepancy across studies.

Several factors may explain the discrepancy in ADHD persistence rates across studies. The ADHD persistence rate is typically higher in clinical samples than in population-based samples, because clinical samples include more severe cases that present with more comorbidity and symptom impairment. In contrast, individuals with more severe problems are often lost at follow-up in population-based setting (i.e., selective attrition). For example, Barkley, Fischer, Smallish, and Fletcher (2002) examined the persistence of ADHD into young adulthood using a clinically based follow-up study of 147 ADHD cases and 71 community controls. Using a developmentally referenced criterion for ADHD (scoring +2 *SD* above the population mean), the observed persistence rate of ADHD was estimated to be 66%. In contrast, in a population-based study of all children born in Pelotas, Brazil, in 1993, who were assessed using the Hyperactivity scale of the Strengths and Difficulties Questionnaire at age 11, and again using structured interviews at age 18 or 19, the persistence rate of ADHD was estimated as 17% (Caye, Rocha, et al., 2016).

Another important complicating factor is that there is no developmentally sensitive "gold standard" objective test for ADHD. There are, therefore, considerable differences across studies in the definitions and assessments of ADHD at follow-up. Using a meta-analysis of published follow-up studies of ADHD, Faraone, Biederman, and Mick (2006) examined how differences in the definition and assessments of ADHD persistence may matter. To be included in the analysis, the studies had to clarify whether the diagnosis of ADHD at follow-up was based on full criteria or modified criteria that required some ADHD symptoms or evidence of residual and impairing signs of the disorder. This information was used to assess separately the persistence of ADHD for full diagnoses versus subthreshold diagnoses. When persistence was defined as meeting criteria for a full ADHD diagnosis, the rate of persistence was low (15%) at age 25 years. In contrast, when persistence was defined in line with DSM-IV criteria of ADHD in partial remission, the rate of persistence was much higher (65%). Results from a prospective, 10-year follow-up study of 110 boys with ADHD and 105 non-ADHD controls supported a similar conclusion (Biederman, Petty, Evans, Small, & Faraone, 2010). This study showed that although 65% of boys with ADHD no longer met full DSM-IV criteria for ADHD at the 10-year follow-up (boys were ages 6–17 years at ascertainment), 78% of subjects met at least one of the definitions of persistence: 35% continued to meet full DSM-IV criteria for ADHD, 22% met subthreshold criteria, 15% were functionally impaired, and 6% were treated for ADHD even though they no longer met criteria for ADHD and were functioning well.

More recently, Sibley, Swanson, et al. (2017) explored how sources (parent vs. self-report), methods (rating scale vs. interview) and symptom thresholds (DSM- vs. norm-based) used for the assessment of ADHD may result in substantial variability across studies in estimates of ADHD persistence rates. Using parent-reports and self-reports of symptoms and impairment on rating scales and structured interviews from the MTA study, the investigators found that when using combined parent reports and self-reports, the balance between diagnostic sensitivity and specificity was optimized by a rating scale method and a norm-based symptom threshold (i.e., four symptoms of either inattention or hyperactivity–impulsivity). Sibley, Swanson, et al. (2017) also reported that the persistence of ADHD in young adulthood was approximately 60%, with 41% of the adults diagnosed with ADHD in childhood meeting both the optimized persistence criteria and presence of impairment. Recent result from a systematic review have further clarified how variability in diagnostic methods influences adult ADHD persistence estimates (Sibley, Mitchell, & Becker, 2016). To reduce the number of factors that could cause variability in persistence and thereby better isolate the effect of diagnostic methods, this systematic review only included studies that used DSM-based assessments of ADHD (i.e., childhood diagnosis of ADHD or a research diagnostic protocol that matched DSM standards) combined with baseline case ascertainment from childhood (i.e., mean childhood age younger than 12.0 years, with no participants older than 18.0 years) and follow-up case ascertainment from adulthood (i.e., mean adult age of 18.0 years or older, with no participants younger than 17.0 years). This inclusion criteria resulted in 12 included samples. Despite strict inclusion criteria estimates of ADHD, persistence ranged from 4 to 77%. Methods of diagnosing ADHD in adulthood varied substantially among these studies with respect to source of information, diagnostic instruments (e.g., rating scales, interviews), diagnostic symptom threshold, and whether impairment was required for diagnosis. Analyses of heterogeneity of the included studies revealed that reliance on self-reports only and a strict threshold of six DSM symptoms generated very low persistence estimates, which indicate that recommended methods for determining adult persistence of ADHD include collecting self- and informant ratings, requiring the presence of impairment, and using an age-appropriate symptom threshold.

The available longitudinal studies of children diagnosed with ADHD and followed into adulthood via adolescence have clearly demonstrated that ADHD is serious condition associated with impairment across the lifespan. Precise and robust estimates clarifying how stable ADHD is from childhood to adulthood have been more difficult to obtain, in part because such estimates depend on how *persistence* is defined. Yet regardless of definition, all longitudinal studies suggest that ADHD is persistent to some extent, but that it lessens with age.

Do ADHD Symptom Presentations Change Across Time?

Several cross-sectional studies exploring prevalence differences in the three ADHD subtypes (i.e., primarily hyperactive–impulsive type, primarily inattentive type, and combined type) across time suggest age-related changes in ADHD symptoms (Graetz, Sawyer, Hazell, Arney, & Baghurst, 2001). These studies have generally reported that in very young children, the primarily hyperactive–impulsive type is more frequently observed than the primarily inattentive type, whereas the opposite pattern has been found in adolescents.

Several longitudinal studies suggest that symptoms of inattention tend to persist from childhood into adolescence to a greater extent than do symptoms of hyperactivity–impulsivity. For example, Hart, Lahey, Loeber, Applegate, and Frick (1995) used a sample of youth ($N = 106$) that fulfilled DSM-III-R diagnostic criteria for ADHD. These participants were assessed regarding their ADHD symptoms multiple times across development, with multiple informants (i.e., parents, teachers). The longitudinal analyses revealed that hyperactive–impulsive symptoms significantly declined with increasing age, whereas inattentive symptoms did not. Several longitudinal studies have replicated the finding that symptoms of inattentiveness are more persistent throughout development than symptoms of hyperactivity–impulsivity (Biederman, Mick, & Faraone, 2000; Hinshaw et al., 2006; Larsson, Lichtenstein, & Larsson, 2006; Leopold et al., 2016; Nagin & Tremblay, 1999; van Lier, van der Ende, Koot, & Verhulst, 2007).

Nagin and Tremblay (1999) applied trajectory modeling approaches on teacher-rated hyperactivity symptoms in children ages 6–15 and found that the majority of youth followed either a low or moderate declining trajectory, whereas a small percentage of children (6% of the sample) followed a chronic high-hyperactivity trajectory. The observed decline in hyperactivity–impulsivity symptoms across time might reflect a true developmental change in the underlying hyperactivity–impulsivity trait. An alternative explanation for the observed decline is the use of developmentally insensitive diagnostic criteria including age-inappropriate symptoms.

Only a few longitudinal studies have explored how the three ADHD subtypes/presentations develop over time. Using 1,450 Swedish twin pairs, Larsson, Dilshad, Lichtenstein, and Barker (2011) investigated the developmental trajectories of inattentive and hyperactive–impulsive symptoms across childhood and adolescence. Data were available for three time points, when the children were ages 8–9, 13–14, and 16–17 years. For the inattentive symptoms, a trajectory of low scores was found at all time points, as well as a second trajectory characterized by *increasing* inattentive symptoms across time. The hyperactive–impulsive symptoms showed a different pattern: a stable low trajectory but also a trajectory of high hyperactive–impulsive symptoms that *decreased* over time. The combinations of these trajectories lend developmental insight into how children shift from (1) a combined to predominantly inattentive subtype/presentation, and (2) a predominantly hyperactive–impulsive to a combined subtype/presentation. Lahey, Pelham, Loney, Lee, and Willcutt (2005) found similar results in a longitudinal study based on a volunteer sample of 118 children ages 4–6 years who met DSM-IV criteria for ADHD. In the longitudinal follow-up assessments of DSM-IV ADHD subtypes, the authors found that 37% of the children with the combined subtype of ADHD and 50% of those with the predominantly inattentive subtype met criteria for a different subtype at least twice in the next six assessments. Children with the predominantly hyperactive–impulsive subtype of ADHD were even more likely to shift to a different subtype over time. Similar results were observed in a study by Todd et al. (2008), who reported that the 5-year ADHD subtype stability was poor to modest and ranged from 11 to 24% for the three DSM-IV ADHD subtypes. Taken together, this line of research suggests that the ADHD subtypes cannot be viewed as discrete and stable categories. Rather, individual variation in the development course of ADHD must be considered. This is now also clearly emphasized in DSM-5, in which the concept of trait-like "subtypes" now is conceptualized as states known as "presentations."

Is Adult ADHD a Childhood-Onset Neurodevelopmental Disorder?

As noted earlier, for a long time, ADHD was primarily conceptualized as a childhood-onset disorder. This is now reflected in DSM-5, which includes the diagnostic criteria for ADHD in the neurodevelopmental disorders section. Since the publication of DSM-5, three population-based longitudinal studies in diverse cultures have challenged the notion that ADHD has its onset only in childhood, suggesting the existence of a large proportion of individuals who report onset of ADHD symptoms and impairments after childhood (Caye, Swanson, et al., 2016).

In a study based on the Dunedin sample, follow-back analyses of adult cases revealed that these individuals had few ADHD symptoms during childhood, and only mild elevations during adolescence (Moffitt et al., 2015). In a study based on the Pelotas sample, about 12% of individuals meeting ADHD criteria as adults met criteria as children (Caye, Rocha, et al., 2016). Finally, in a sample of over 2,000 U.K. twins rated in childhood for parent-reported, and again during adulthood using a self-reported symptom checklist, the majority of individuals meeting ADHD symptom criteria as adults did not do so as children (Agnew-Blais et al., 2016). Based on these results, it was suggested, with different degrees of certainty, that ADHD onset may occur in adulthood and that the adult-onset form of the disorder is distinct from the childhood-onset form. Although interesting hypotheses, these suggestions may seem premature, as all three studies had clear limitations (Faraone & Biederman, 2016).

First, one of the studies assessed ADHD using DSM-III criteria during childhood, and adult ADHD using DSM-IV criteria, which means that it is unclear whether secular changes in the ADHD diagnosis contributed to the results (Moffitt et al., 2015). Second, two of the studies switched from parent reports of ADHD symptoms during childhood to self-reports during adulthood (Agnew-Blais et al., 2016; Caye, Rocha, et al., 2016). Parent reports and self-reports of ADHD correlate only modestly (Merwood et al., 2013), leading to the question of whether the switch in rater led to the lack of overlap between childhood and adulthood ADHD. In addition, one of the previous studies found a low heritability estimate for self-reported ADHD symptoms in adults (Agnew-Blais et al., 2016). A more thorough assessment of ADHD symptom in adulthood using a combination of parent ratings and self-ratings has recently been found to be a useful approach for resolving such puzzling twin study results (Brikell, Kuja-Halkola, & Larsson, 2015). As reviewed in Chapter 3, twin studies in childhood have for a long time consistently reported high heritability estimates of 60–90%, while a couple of more recent studies of adult samples have showed moderate heritability of 30–40% when estimated from self-ratings. The substantial difference in heritability could suggest differences in the etiological underpinnings of ADHD between children and adults. However, more recent studies of adult twins that combined self- and parent reports to assess ADHD or used clinical diagnoses as a measure of ADHD reported substantial heritability estimates of 70–80%, in line with the findings for children. These results suggest that the reported low heritability of ADHD in adults is unlikely to reflect a distinct etiology for ADHD in childhood. Instead, the attenuated heritability is better explained by rater effects related to a switch from using one rater (parent–teacher) in childhood and adolescence to relying on self-ratings (each twin rating him- or herself) of ADHD symptoms in adults.

Over and above the previously mentioned limitations of the three earlier studies, there are also alternative explanations to the observed adult-onset ADHD cases. Faraone and Biederman (2016) suggest that many cases of adult-onset ADHD may be due to the existence of subthreshold childhood ADHD. In order to explore alternative explanations to adult-onset ADHD, Sibley, Rohde, et al. (2017) examined psychiatric assessments administered longitudinally to the local normative comparison group of the MTA study. The findings from this study indicated that adult-onset ADHD is rare, and that most people exceeding the symptom threshold for diagnosis in adulthood, but not childhood, on closer examination, are false positives; that is, only 1 out of 24 adult-onset ADHD cases could not be explained by the presence of other psychiatric disorders (Sibley, Rohde, et al., 2017). The most common explanation was symptoms or impairment occurring exclusively in the context of heavy substance use. Most late-onset cases displayed onset in adolescence and an adolescence-limited presentation. There was no evidence for adult-onset ADHD independent of a complex psychiatric history. This alternative explanation was not fully explored in the previous three studies, as a participant was defined as having adult-onset ADHD only if full diagnostic criteria for ADHD had not been fulfilled at prior assessments, despite the fact that many of the adult-onset cases had evidenced other psychiatric problems in childhood.

In summary, the available longitudinal studies suggest that a distinct adult-onset form of ADHD most likely is rare and is most often strongly associated with some type of childhood-onset form, but additional research is warranted to shed more light on this issue. Clinically, the available research highlights the importance of performing detailed assessments of individuals displaying symptoms of ADHD who first come to clinical attention as adults, which should take account of the patient's history.

What Predicts Persistent and Remitting ADHD?

It remains largely unknown why symptoms persist in some individuals and remit in others. Quantitative genetic studies suggest that persistence and remittance in ADHD may be underpinned by partially different genetic factors. Family studies have found evidence for higher familial risk in relatives of persistent ADHD cases. More specifically, studies have reported a 57% prevalence of ADHD in children of parents with ADHD (Biederman et al., 1995), a higher risk in siblings of adults cases with ADHD compared to family members of those with childhood cases (Manshadi, Lippmann, O'Daniel, & Blackman, 1983), and higher prevalence among relatives of children with ADHD that persisted into adolescence, compared to relatives of children with remitting ADHD (Biederman et al., 1996). This suggest that persistent ADHD may be associated with a higher genetic load compared to the remitting type of ADHD. Chang, Lichtenstein, Asherson, and Larsson (2013) used twin modeling in a sample of 1,480 twin pairs who were prospectively followed up from childhood to young adulthood. Symptoms were obtained using parent ratings and self-ratings of the Attention Problems scale from the Child Behavior Checklist (CBCL) and the Youth Self-Report (YSR) at ages 8–9, 13–14, 16–17, and 19–20 years. The finding that childhood genetic factors explained a moderate amount (24%) of the variation in early adulthood provides strong support for genetic stability. However, in line with a "developmentally dynamic" hypothesis, new sources of genetic effects on ADHD symptoms emerged over development (i.e., genetic innovation), and the genetic factors that act in childhood declined in influence with age (i.e., genetic attenuation). The finding of stable and dynamic genetic influences over the course of the development suggest that molecular genetic studies of ADHD symptoms in adults will identify genes that are shared with childhood ADHD and represent not only developmentally stable genetic influences but also those that are newly arising, perhaps involving processes that lead to persistence or remission of the disorder as children with ADHD grow older. The findings regarding the stable and dynamic nature of the genetic risks may also link to the neurodevelopmental model of Halperin, Trampush, Miller, Marks, and Newcorn (2008), which postulates that ADHD is associated with early-appearing and enduring subcortical dysfunctions, while persistence over the course of development is associated with prefrontally mediated executive control functions. These two factors may mediate the observed genetic stability and innovation, with innovative genetic influences being related to cortical maturation and the degree of cognitive control.

Evidence of both stable and dynamic genetic influences over the course of development has also been observed in longitudinal twin studies of younger children (Kuntsi, Rijsdijk, Ronald, Asherson, & Plomin, 2005; Larsson et al., 2006; Rietveld, Hudziak, Bartels, van Beijsterveldt, & Boomsma, 2004). Another twin study further suggests that genetic factors that underpin ADHD symptoms in childhood are largely independent of those contributing to individual differences in developmental trajectories of ADHD symptoms (Pingault et al., 2015).

In addition to family and twin studies, a recent longitudinal molecular genetic study also indicates that genetic factors are important for the persistence of ADHD. Riglin et al. (2016) used data from the Avon Longitudinal Study of Parents and Children to examine the associations between genetic risk variants and trajectories of ADHD symptoms from childhood to adolescence. They found that persistence of ADHD symptoms across childhood and adolescence in the general population was associated with higher polygenic risk scores for ADHD.

Another line of research suggests that neurodevelopment maturation may be associated with differential developmental trajectories in ADHD

(Shaw et al., 2013). Longitudinal neuroimaging data have shown that children with ADHD attain peak cortical thickness and surface area 2–3 years later than do controls, which suggests that ADHD may be related to delayed, but otherwise normal, brain development (Shaw et al., 2007). Similar results have been found in normally developing children, in whom higher levels of hyperactivity–impulsivity have been associated with slower rates of cortical maturation (Shaw et al., 2011). Interestingly, data also suggest that the remittance of ADHD symptoms is associated with development catch-up and convergence toward normative neurodevelopment, whereas persistence is associated with atypical trajectories of fixed–accelerated cortical thinning and reduced volumes of the subcortical, inferior–posterior cerebellar lobes (Shaw et al., 2013).

A previous study of 140 ADHD probands and 120 controls found that family history of ADHD, psychosocial adversity, and psychiatric comorbidity may be useful predictors of which children with ADHD are at risk for ADHD persistence into adolescence (Biederman et al., 1996). Other researchers found that the course of ADHD across childhood and adolescence did not differ between males and females (Monuteaux, Mick, Faraone, & Biederman, 2010).

One longitudinal case–control study assessed participants when they were ages 7–11 years old, and again at ages 16–22, to explore the role of personality characteristics in persistence of ADHD into adolescence. This study indicated that childhood ADHD was associated with lower scores on the Conscientiousness subscale of the NEO Personality Inventory in adolescents/young adults irrespective of the degree of ADHD persistence. In contrast, ratings of Neuroticism and Agreeableness appeared to be more closely linked to adolescent status, in which those with persisting ADHD symptoms only exhibited increased Neuroticism and decreased Agreeableness (Miller, Miller, Newcorn, & Halperin, 2008).

Caye, Spadini, et al. (2016) conducted a systematic review of childhood predictors of ADHD persistence into adulthood. The study identified data from 16 studies and performed meta-analyses of all predictors that were evaluated by at least three studies, which resulted in the following potential predictors: female gender, ADHD treatment, severe ADHD, comorbid oppositional defiant disorder, comorbid conduct disorder, comorbid major depressive disorder, single-parent family, socioeconomic status, and IQ. Among those predictors, severity of ADHD, treatment for ADHD, comorbid conduct disorder, and comorbid major depressive disorder emerged as predictors for ADHD persistence. This systematic review illustrates that the question of predictors for ADHD persistence is overlooked in ADHD research literature, as very few studies were identified, and these studies evaluated a mixed set of factors that in many cases do not enable enough comparisons or meaningful conclusions. Thus, several potentially important predictors for persistence remain to be investigated.

Two previous studies suggest that not only ADHD symptom severity and childhood comorbidity but also parental mental health predicts persistence of ADHD symptoms into adulthood (Biederman, Petty, Clarke, Lomedico, & Faraone, 2011; Roy et al., 2017). Some convergence for markers of ADHD persistence and remission is potentially also starting to emerge across cognitive and neuroimaging domains. For example, ADHD remitters show reduced reaction time variability compared to persisters (Cheung et al., 2016; Michelini et al., 2016). In addition, it has been found that impairments in executive function do not distinguish individuals with remitting versus persistent ADHD (Cheung et al., 2016; Michelini et al., 2016).

Further large-scale studies are needed to explore the potential role of such predictors. Family–environmental risks, prenatal exposures, and genetic risk variants are other potential predictors that need to be explored in future studies.

Conclusions

Based on the available longitudinal studies, there can be no doubt that ADHD is characterized by a strong, stable component that causes ADHD to be a chronic condition for many, but not all, individuals with ADHD. More work is definitely needed to better characterize the nature of the stable component and how it interacts with other factors to cause variability in ADHD persistence across individuals. The available longitudinal studies have illustrated that thorough assessments of ADHD, including objective cognitive and neurophysiological data and multiple raters across the different developmental stages will be crucial for the field to move forward.

References

Agnew-Blais, J. C., Polanczyk, G. V., Danese, A., Wertz, J., Moffitt, T. E., & Arseneault, L. (2016). Evaluation of the persistence, remission, and emergence of attention-deficit/hyperactivity disorder in young adulthood. *JAMA Psychiatry, 73*(7), 713–720.

Asherson, P., Buitelaar, J., Faraone, S. V., & Rohde, L. A. (2016). Adult attention-deficit hyperactivity disorder: Key conceptual issues. *Lancet Psychiatry, 3*(6), 568–578.

Barkley, R. A., Fischer, M., Smallish, L., & Fletcher, K. (2002). The persistence of attention-deficit/hyperactivity disorder into young adulthood as a function of reporting source and definition of disorder. *Journal of Abnormal Psychology, 111*(2), 279–289.

Barkley, R. A., Fischer, M., Smallish, L., & Fletcher, K. (2006). Young adult outcome of hyperactive children: Adaptive functioning in major life activities. *Journal of the American Academy of Child and Adolescent Psychiatry, 45*(2), 192–202.

Biederman, J., Faraone, S., Mick, E., Spencer, T., Wilens, T., Kiely, K., . . . Warburton, R. (1995). High risk for attention deficit hyperactivity disorder among children of parents with childhood onset of the disorder: A pilot study. *American Journal of Psychiatry, 152*(3), 431–435.

Biederman, J., Faraone, S., Milberger, S., Curtis, S., Chen, L., Marrs, A., . . . Spencer, T. (1996). Predictors of persistence and remission of ADHD into adolescence: Results from a four-year prospective follow-up study. *Journal of the American Academy of Child and Adolescent Psychiatry, 35*(3), 343–351.

Biederman, J., Faraone, S. V., Spencer, T. J., Mick, E., Monuteaux, M. C., & Aleardi, M. (2006). Functional impairments in adults with self-reports of diagnosed ADHD: A controlled study of 1001 adults in the community. *Journal of Clinical Psychiatry, 67*(4), 524–540.

Biederman, J., Mick, E., & Faraone, S. V. (2000). Age-dependent decline of symptoms of attention deficit hyperactivity disorder: Impact of remission definition and symptom type. *American Journal of Psychiatry, 157*(5), 816–818.

Biederman, J., Petty, C. R., Clarke, A., Lomedico, A., & Faraone, S. V. (2011). Predictors of persistent ADHD: An 11-year follow-up study. *Journal of Psychiatric Research, 45*(2), 150–155.

Biederman, J., Petty, C. R., Evans, M., Small, J., & Faraone, S. V. (2010). How persistent is ADHD?: A controlled 10-year follow-up study of boys with ADHD. *Psychiatry Research, 177*(3), 299–304.

Brikell, I., Kuja-Halkola, R., & Larsson, H. (2015). Heritability of attention-deficit hyperactivity disorder in adults. *American Journal of Medical Genetics B: Neuropsychiatric Genetics, 168*(6), 406–413.

Caye, A., Rocha, T. B., Anselmi, L., Murray, J., Menezes, A. M., Barros, F. C., . . . Rohde, L. A. (2016). Attention-deficit/hyperactivity disorder trajectories from childhood to young adulthood: Evidence from a birth cohort supporting a late-onset syndrome. *JAMA Psychiatry, 73*(7), 705–712.

Caye, A., Spadini, A. V., Karam, R. G., Grevet, E. H., Rovaris, D. L., Bau, C. H., . . . Kieling, C. (2016). Predictors of persistence of ADHD into adulthood: A systematic review of the literature and meta-analysis. *European Child and Adolescent Psychiatry, 25*(11), 1151–1159.

Caye, A., Swanson, J., Thapar, A., Sibley, M., Arseneault, L., Hechtman, L., . . . Rohde, L. A. (2016). Life span studies of ADHD: Conceptual challenges and predictors of persistence and outcome. *Current Psychiatry Reports, 18*(12), 111.

Chang, Z., Lichtenstein, P., Asherson, P. J., & Larsson, H. (2013). Developmental twin study of attention problems: High heritabilities throughout development. *JAMA Psychiatry, 70*(3), 311–318.

Cheung, C. H., Rijdijk, F., McLoughlin, G., Brandeis, D., Banaschewski, T., Asherson, P., & Kuntsi, J. (2016). Cognitive and neurophysiological markers of ADHD persistence and remission. *British Journal of Psychiatry, 208*(6), 548–555.

Cheung, C. H., Rijdijk, F., McLoughlin, G., Faraone, S. V., Asherson, P., & Kuntsi, J. (2015). Childhood predictors of adolescent and young adult outcome in ADHD. *Journal of Psychiatric Research, 62*, 92–100.

Faraone, S. V., & Biederman, J. (2016). Can attention-deficit/hyperactivity disorder onset occur in adulthood? *JAMA Psychiatry, 73*(7), 655–656.

Faraone, S. V., Biederman, J., & Mick, E. (2006). The age-dependent decline of attention deficit hyperactivity disorder: A meta-analysis of follow-up studies. *Psychological Medicine, 36*(2), 159–165.

Galera, C., Melchior, M., Chastang, J. F., Bouvard, M. P., & Fombonne, E. (2009). Childhood and adolescent hyperactivity–inattention symptoms and academic achievement 8 years later: The GAZEL Youth study. *Psychological Medicine, 39*(11), 1895–1906.

Gau, S. S., Ni, H. C., Shang, C. Y., Soong, W. T., Wu, Y. Y., Lin, L. Y., & Chiu, Y. N.

(2010). Psychiatric comorbidity among children and adolescents with and without persistent attention-deficit hyperactivity disorder. *Australian and New Zealand Journal of Psychiatry, 44*(2), 135–143.

Graetz, B. W., Sawyer, M. G., Hazell, P. L., Arney, F., & Baghurst, P. (2001). Validity of DSM-IV ADHD subtypes in a nationally representative sample of Australian children and adolescents. *Journal of the American Academy of Child and Adolescent Psychiatry, 40*(12), 1410–1417.

Halperin, J. M., Trampush, J. W., Miller, C. J., Marks, D. J., & Newcorn, J. H. (2008). Neuropsychological outcome in adolescents/young adults with childhood ADHD: Profiles of persisters, remitters and controls. *Journal of Child Psychology and Psychiatry, 49*(9), 958–966.

Hart, E., Lahey, B., Loeber, R., Applegate, B., & Frick, P. (1995). Developmental change in attention-deficit hyperactivity disorder in boys: A four-year longitudinal study. *Journal of Abnormal Child Psychology, 23*(6), 729–749.

Hinshaw, S. P., Owens, E. B., Sami, N., & Fargeon, S. (2006). Prospective follow-up of girls with attention-deficit/hyperactivity disorder into adolescence: Evidence for continuing cross-domain impairment. *Journal of Consulting and Clinical Psychology, 74*(3), 489–499.

Klein, R. G., Mannuzza, S., Olazagasti, M. A., Roizen, E., Hutchison, J. A., Lashua, E. C., & Castellanos, F. X. (2012). Clinical and functional outcome of childhood attention-deficit/hyperactivity disorder 33 years later. *Archives of General Psychiatry, 69*(12), 1295–1303.

Kleinman, N. L., Durkin, M., Melkonian, A., & Markosyan, K. (2009). Incremental employee health benefit costs, absence days, and turnover among employees with ADHD and among employees with children with ADHD. *Journal of Occupational and Environmental Medicine, 51*(11), 1247–1255.

Kuntsi, J., Rijsdijk, F., Ronald, A., Asherson, P., & Plomin, R. (2005). Genetic influences on the stability of attention-deficit/hyperactivity disorder symptoms from early to middle childhood. *Biological Psychiatry, 57,* 647–654.

Lahey, B. B., Pelham, W. E., Loney, J., Lee, S. S., & Willcutt, E. (2005). Instability of the DSM-IV Subtypes of ADHD from preschool through elementary school. *Archives of General Psychiatry, 62*(8), 896–902.

Larsson, H., Dilshad, R., Lichtenstein, P., & Barker, E. D. (2011). Developmental trajectories of DSM-IV symptoms of attention-deficit/hyperactivity disorder: Genetic effects, family risk and associated psychopathology. *Journal of Child Psychology and Psychiatry, 52*(9), 954–963.

Larsson, H., Lichtenstein, P., & Larsson, J. O. (2006). Genetic contributions to the development of ADHD subtypes from childhood to adolescence. *Journal of the American Academy of Child and Adolescent Psychiatry, 45*(8), 973–981.

Leopold, D. R., Christopher, M. E., Burns, G. L., Becker, S. P., Olson, R. K., & Willcutt, E. G. (2016). Attention-deficit/hyperactivity disorder and sluggish cognitive tempo throughout childhood: Temporal invariance and stability from preschool through ninth grade. *Journal of Child Psychology and Psychiatry, 57*(9), 1066–1074.

Mannuzza, S., Klein, R. G., Bessler, A., Malloy, P., & LaPadula, M. (1993). Adult outcome of hyperactive boys: Educational achievement, occupational rank, and psychiatric status. *Archives of General Psychiatry, 50*(7), 565–576.

Mannuzza, S., Klein, R., Bessler, A., Malloy, P., & LaPadula, M. (1998). Adult psychiatric status of hyperactive boys grown up. *American Journal of Psychiatry, 155*(4), 493–498.

Manshadi, M., Lippmann, S., O'Daniel, R. G., & Blackman, A. (1983). Alcohol abuse and attention deficit disorder. *Journal of Clinical Psychiatry, 44*(10), 379–380.

Merwood, A., Greven, C. U., Price, T. S., Rijsdijk, F., Kuntsi, J., McLoughlin, G., . . . Asherson, P. J. (2013). Different heritabilities but shared etiological influences for parent, teacher and self-ratings of ADHD symptoms: An adolescent twin study. *Psychological Medicine, 43*(9), 1973–1984.

Michelini, G., Kitsune, G. L., Cheung, C. H., Brandeis, D., Banaschewski, T., Asherson, P., . . . Kuntsi, J. (2016). Attention-deficit/hyperactivity disorder remission is linked to better neurophysiological error detection and attention–vigilance processes. *Biological Psychiatry, 80*(12), 923–932.

Miller, C. J., Miller, S. R., Newcorn, J. H., & Halperin, J. M. (2008). Personality characteristics associated with persistent ADHD in late adolescence. *Journal of Abnormal Child Psychology, 36*(2), 165–173.

Moffitt, T. E., Houts, R., Asherson, P., Belsky, D. W., Corcoran, D. L., Hammerle, M., . . . Caspi, A. (2015). Is adult ADHD a childhood-onset neurodevelopmental disorder?: Evidence from a four-decade longitudinal cohort study. *American Journal of Psychiatry, 172*(10), 967–977.

Molina, B. S. G., Hinshaw, S. P., Swanson, J. M., Arnold, L. E., Vitiello, B., Jensen, P. S., . . . MTA Cooperative Group. (2009). The MTA at 8 years: Prospective follow-up of children treated for combined-type ADHD in a multisite study. *Journal of the American Academy of Child and Adolescent Psychiatry, 48,* 484–500.

Monuteaux, M. C., Mick, E., Faraone, S. V., & Biederman, J. (2010). The influence of sex on the course and psychiatric correlates of ADHD from childhood to adolescence: A longitudinal study. *Journal of Child Psychology and Psychiatry, 51*(3), 233–241.

Nagin, D., & Tremblay, R. E. (1999). Trajectories of boys' physical aggression, opposition, and hyperactivity on the path to physically violent and nonviolent juvenile delinquency. *Child Development, 70*(5), 1181–1196.

Pingault, J., Viding, E., Galéra, C., Greven, C. U., Zheng, Y., Plomin, R., & Rijsdijk, F. (2015). Genetic and environmental influences on the developmental course of attention-deficit/hyperactivity disorder symptoms from childhood to adolescence. *JAMA Psychiatry, 72*(7), 651–658.

Rietveld, M. J., Hudziak, J. J., Bartels, M., van Beijsterveldt, C. E., & Boomsma, D. I. (2004). Heritability of attention problems in children: Longitudinal results from a study of twins, age 3 to 12. *Journal of Child Psychology and Psychiatry, 45*(3), 577–588.

Riglin, L., Collishaw, S., Thapar, A. K., Dalsgaard, S., Langley, K., Smith, G. D., . . . Thapar, A. (2016). Association of genetic risk variants with attention-deficit/hyperactivity disorder trajectories in the general population. *JAMA Psychiatry, 73*(12), 1285–1292.

Roy, A., Hechtman, L., Arnold, L. E., Swanson, J. M., Molina, B. S. G., Sibley, M. H., . . . MTA Cooperative Group. (2017). Childhood predictors of adult functional outcomes in the Multimodal Treatment Study of Attention-Deficit/Hyperactivity Disorder (MTA). *Journal of the American Academy of Child and Adolescent Psychiatry, 56*(8), 687–695.

Secnik, K., Swensen, A., & Lage, M. J. (2005). Comorbidities and costs of adult patients diagnosed with attention-deficit hyperactivity disorder. *Pharmacoeconomics, 23*(1), 93–102.

Shaw, P., Eckstrand, K., Sharp, W., Blumenthal, J., Lerch, J. P., Greenstein, D., . . . Rapoport, J. L. (2007). Attention-deficit/hyperactivity disorder is characterized by a delay in cortical maturation. *Proceedings of the National Academy of Sciences of the USA, 104*(49), 19649–19654.

Shaw, P., Gilliam, M., Liverpool, M., Weddle, C., Malek, M., Sharp, W., . . . Giedd, J. (2011). Cortical development in typically developing children with symptoms of hyperactivity and impulsivity: Support for a dimensional view of attention deficit hyperactivity disorder. *American Journal of Psychiatry, 168*(2), 143–151.

Shaw, P., Malek, M., Watson, B., Greenstein, D., de Rossi, P., & Sharp, W. (2013). Trajectories of cerebral cortical development in childhood and adolescence and adult attention-deficit/hyperactivity disorder. *Biological Psychiatry, 74*(8), 599–606.

Sibley, M. H., Mitchell, J. T., & Becker, S. P. (2016). Method of adult diagnosis influences estimated persistence of childhood ADHD: A systematic review of longitudinal studies. *Lancet Psychiatry, 3*(12), 1157–1165.

Sibley, M. H., Rohde, L. A., Swanson, J. M., Hechtman, L. T., Molina, B. S. G., Mitchell, J. T., . . . MTA Cooperative Group. (2017). Late-onset ADHD reconsidered with comprehensive repeated assessments between ages 10 and 25. *American Journal of Psychiatry, 175*, 140–149.

Sibley, M. H., Swanson, J. M., Arnold, L. E., Hechtman, L. T., Owens, E. B., Stehli, A., . . . MTA Cooperative Group. (2017). Defining ADHD symptom persistence in adulthood: Optimizing sensitivity and specificity. *Journal of Child Psychology and Psychiatry, 58*(6), 655–662.

Todd, R. D., Huang, H., Todorov, A. A., Neuman, R. J., Reiersen, A. M., Henderson, C. A., & Reich, W. C. (2008). Predictors of stability of attention-deficit/hyperactivity disorder subtypes from childhood to young adulthood. *Journal of the American Academy of Child and Adolescent Psychiatry, 47*(1), 76–85.

van Lier, P. A., van der Ende, J., Koot, H. M., & Verhulst, F. C. (2007). Which better predicts conduct problems?: The relationship of trajectories of conduct problems with ODD and ADHD symptoms from childhood into adolescence. *Journal of Child Psychology and Psychiatry, 48*(6), 601–608.

Weiss, G., Hechtman, L., Milroy, T., & Perlman, T. (1985). Psychiatric status of hyperactives as adults: A controlled prospective 15-year follow-up of 63 hyperactive children. *Journal of the American Academy of Child and Adolescent Psychiatry, 24*(2), 211–220.

CHAPTER 3

The Etiology of ADHD in Adolescents

Behavioral and Molecular Genetic Approaches

Erik G. Willcutt

Although over 99% of the deoxyribonucleic acid (DNA) sequence that comprises the human genetic code is identical in all people, the genetic sequence varies at millions of locations across the remainder of the human genome. Many of these sequence differences, or *polymorphisms,* cause individual differences in protein production, which may then lead to individual differences in neural development or brain functioning if the polymorphism is in a gene that is expressed in the central nervous system.

The past two decades have produced an exponential increase in research examining the genetic and environmental factors that contribute to the development of attention-deficit/hyperactivity disorder (ADHD). This rapid accumulation of new knowledge illustrates the potential impact of behavioral and molecular genetic methods. However, results of these studies have also underscored the complexity of the etiological pathways to ADHD and related disorders and demonstrate clearly how much is yet to be learned.

Behavioral genetic studies have demonstrated conclusively that genetic influences play a role in the etiology of ADHD, as is true for virtually all psychological traits and disorders (e.g., Knopik, Niederhiser, DeFries, & Plomin, 2017). Similarly, environmental factors also play an important role in the etiology of ADHD. Therefore, the question is no longer whether ADHD is due to nature or nurture. Instead, the focus of behavioral and molecular genetic studies has shifted to the estimation of the relative impact of genetic and environmental influences, and the identification of the specific genetic and environmental risk factors that increase susceptibility to ADHD.

Given this focus in the field, I have four primary objectives in this chapter. In the first section, I summarize family, adoption, and twin studies of ADHD, with a specific focus on studies of adolescents. In the second section and throughout the chapter, I describe new analyses, completed for this chapter, that extend these methods to address more complex questions regarding the etiology of ADHD in adolescents, including the developmental course of ADHD, the validity of ADHD subtypes across development, and the causes of the frequent co-occurrence of ADHD and other disorders in adolescence. In the third section, I summarize the results of molecular genetic studies of ADHD, including analyses that have tested for interactions between genetic and environmental risk factors. I then discuss in the fourth and final section the clinical implications of these results and describe several areas in which additional research is needed to develop a comprehensive understanding of the etiology of ADHD in adolescence and across the lifespan.

Samples Allowing for New Analyses in Adolescence

In addition to summarizing the existing literature, this chapter includes new analyses of samples from two of our ongoing studies to illustrate several key methodological approaches. To set the stage for these analyses, these two samples are first described briefly in this section.

Colorado Learning Disabilities Research Center

In collaboration with administrators in 22 Colorado school districts, parent and teacher ratings were obtained for all consenting twin pairs in each district to screen for ADHD or learning difficulties (e.g., Willcutt et al., 2013, 2014). If either member of a twin pair met DSM-IV criteria for ADHD, the pair was then invited to participate in the full study by completing an extensive test battery that includes diagnostic measures of ADHD and other psychopathology, standardized measures of general cognitive ability and academic achievement, and extensive measures of neuropsychological functioning. Our overall sample included over 400 pairs of twins with ADHD, but the new analyses conducted for this chapter focus on 175 pairs of adolescent twins (ages 13–18 years) in which at least one twin meets criteria for ADHD, along with a comparison sample of 225 pairs of adolescent twins without ADHD.

International Longitudinal Twin Study of Early Reading and Attention

This is a longitudinal twin study of the development of reading and attention (e.g., Leopold et al., 2016; Willcutt, Betjemann, Wadsworth, et al., 2007). As part of the overall battery of measures, parents completed ratings of DSM-IV ADHD symptoms regarding their twins during the summer prior to the start of kindergarten, then again during the summer after the twins completed kindergarten, first grade, second grade, fourth grade, and ninth grade. The Colorado component of the study was used for the longitudinal behavioral genetic analyses reported in this chapter (total N = 459 twin pairs), with the primary assessment during adolescence occurring at the end of ninth grade, when participants were 14–15 years of age.

Behavioral Genetic Studies of ADHD

Individuals cannot be randomly assigned to different environmental or genetic backgrounds. Therefore, family, adoption, and twin studies take advantage of naturally occurring events to estimate the relative influence of genetic and environmental factors on a trait or disorder (for a detailed overview of these methods, see Knopik et al., 2017). The influence of genes is quantified by estimating *heritability* (h^2), the proportion of the total phenotypic variance in a trait that is attributable to genetic influences. The proportion of variance due to environmental factors can be subdivided into *shared environmental influences* (c^2) and *nonshared environmental influences* (e^2). Shared environmental influences are those that increase the similarity of individuals within a family in comparison to unrelated individuals in the population. These effects may potentially include environmental influences within the home, such as parenting, family nutrition, or any other shared experiences such as mutual friends or shared teachers. In contrast, nonshared environmental influences are those that lead to differences among individuals in a family (the estimate of e^2 also includes measurement error). For example, nonshared environmental risk factors might include a head injury or other accident, a traumatic event, or exposure to physical or sexual abuse (if other family members were not similarly exposed). This section summarizes the results of studies that have applied these methods to test the etiology of ADHD.

Family Studies

In a family study, individuals with and without a specific disorder are identified, then the rate of the disorder in their biological family members is compared. If ADHD occurs more frequently in the relatives of individuals with ADHD than in relatives of individuals without ADHD, this suggests that familial factors increase risk for ADHD.

Previous studies demonstrate clearly that ADHD is familial (e.g., Faraone, Biederman, & Friedman, 2000; Friedman, Chhabildas, Budhiraja, Willcutt, & Pennington, 2003). Approximately 30–35% of the full siblings of ADHD probands also meet criteria for ADHD, indicating that the relative risk for ADHD is six to eight times higher among first-degree relatives of individuals with ADHD than the base rate of ADHD in the population (Willcutt, 2012).

New analyses were completed in the Colorado Learning Disabilities Research Center (CLDRC) to test whether the familiality of ADHD differs in childhood versus adolescence. Probands selected for ADHD were subdivided into a sample of children (8–12 years old) and adolescents (13–18 years old), and the rate of ADHD in their biological family members was compared. The prevalence of ADHD was very similar in the family members of probands with ADHD during childhood (31% of siblings and 21% of parents) and adolescence (33% of siblings and 20% of parents), suggesting that the familiality of ADHD may be similar across development.

Overall, these results indicate that familial factors clearly contribute to the development of ADHD in both childhood and adolescence. However, because biological relatives living in the same home share both their home environment and some of their genes, family studies cannot be used to test whether these familial influences are genetic or environmental. Therefore, other methods, such as twin studies, are needed to disentangle the relative contributions of genetic and family environmental influences on ADHD.

Twin Studies

Identical twins are also called *monozygotic* (MZ) twins because they come from a single egg, and therefore have the same DNA sequence across the genome. In contrast, fraternal (*dizygotic,* or DZ) twins share half of their genetic sequence in regions of the genome that vary across people, the same as a pair of biological siblings. By comparing the similarity of pairs of MZ and DZ twins, twin studies provide direct estimates of the extent to which a disorder is due to genetic or environmental influences.

Concordance Rates

The most straightforward analysis of twin data assesses how frequently both twins in a pair meet criteria for ADHD, indicating that the pair is "concordant" for the disorder. If genetic influences play an important role in the development of ADHD, MZ twin pairs should be concordant for ADHD significantly more often than DZ pairs. Nearly all twin studies of ADHD that reported concordance rates reported higher concordance in

MZ pairs (58–82%) than in DZ pairs (25–38%) in combined samples of children and adolescents (e.g., Levy, Hay, McStephen, Wood, & Waldman, 1997; Willcutt, Pennington, & DeFries, 2000; see systematic review by Willcutt, Pennington, et al., 2010).

Similarly, new analyses of adolescent twin pairs from the CLDRC and International Longitudinal Twin Study of Early Reading and Attention (ILTS) conducted for this chapter indicated that the rate of concordance for ADHD was significantly higher in pairs of identical twins (67–71%) than in pairs of same-sex fraternal twins (28–32%). However, the concordance rate in identical twins was approximately 10% lower in adolescents than in younger children (78–82%). While it is important to interpret this fairly subtle difference with caution, it may potentially reflect the developmental decline in symptoms (particularly symptoms of hyperactivity–impulsivity) that occurs for some individuals in adolescence (see Chapter 2 and review by Willcutt et al., 2012), leading a subset of co-twins to fall below the symptom cutoff for ADHD. Alternatively, environmental risk factors could potentially become more important as adolescents are exposed to a wider range of environments and potential environmental risk factors.

Etiology of Individual Differences in ADHD Symptoms

While the simplicity of a comparison of concordance rates is appealing, compelling evidence suggests that ADHD and most other complex disorders are defined by a diagnostic threshold imposed upon a quantitative measure that is continuously distributed in the population (Larsson, Anckarsater, Rastam, Chang, & Lichtenstein, 2012; Willcutt et al., 2012; Willcutt, Pennington, et al., 2010). The transformation of a continuous measure such as ADHD symptoms into a categorical variable (i.e., presence or absence of ADHD) throws away important information about both individual differences below the threshold for ADHD and differences in severity among individuals who meet criteria for the disorder. As an alternative, variance components analysis of unselected samples and multiple regression analysis of selected samples have been developed to provide greater statistical power and versatility by using information about the entire continuum of ADHD behaviors.

Several large population-based twin studies have assessed the etiology of individual differences in ADHD symptoms (e.g., Chang, Lichtenstein, Asherson, & Larsson, 2013; Greven, Asherson, Rijsdijk, & Plomin, 2011; Sherman, McGue, & Iacono, 1997; see reviews in Willcutt, 2014; Willcutt, Pennington, et al., 2010). Despite important differences in study designs, sampling procedures, and measures of ADHD, the results of these studies are strikingly consistent. All studies found that individual differences in ADHD symptoms are largely attributable to genetic influences, with an average heritability of approximately .70 across all studies. The phenotypic variance in ADHD symptoms that is not accounted for by genetic influences is primarily attributable to nonshared environmental influences, whereas shared environmental influences are not significant in most studies.

In terms of adolescence in particular, the analyses conducted for this chapter replicate the findings of studies that examined the etiology of individual differences in ADHD symptoms in large samples of adolescents in Sweden (e.g., Larsson, Lichtenstein, & Larsson, 2006) and the United Kingdom (e.g., Greven et al., 2011). Analyses of both the CLDRC and the ILTS revealed moderate to high heritability for individual differences in inattention, hyperactivity–impulsivity, and overall ADHD symptoms during adolescence (h^2 = .65–.74). Thus, even though ADHD symptoms may decline as a whole across adolescence, particularly hyperactive–impulsive symptoms, these new analyses indicate that dimensional ADHD symptoms continue to demonstrate a large degree of heritability.

Etiology of Clinically Significant Elevations of ADHD Symptoms

Although studies of individual differences in ADHD symptoms in unselected samples are an important starting point, the diagnosis of ADHD is defined by symptom levels that extend above a diagnostic threshold at the extreme tail of the distribution. Therefore, DeFries and Fulker (1985, 1988) developed a multiple regression method to test the etiology of the extreme scores that define clinical disorders. This model is based on the differential regression of MZ and DZ co-twin scores toward the population mean when probands are selected for ADHD. Although scores of both MZ and DZ co-twins are expected to regress toward the population mean, scores of DZ co-twins should regress further than scores of MZ co-twins, to the extent that the proband deficit is influenced by genes. The magnitude of this differential regression by zygosity provides an estimate of the heritability of the extreme ADHD scores of the proband group (h^2_g).

To illustrate this approach and test the etiology of ADHD in adolescents for this chapter, a multiple regression model was fitted to DSM-IV ADHD symptom counts in twin pairs between 13 and 18 years of age in the CLDRC. For each of the three separate multiple regression analyses, all twins who exceeded the diagnostic threshold on the relevant measure of ADHD (i.e., inattention symptoms, hyperactivity–impulsivity symptoms, or the overall ADHD symptom composite) were selected as probands. As shown in Table 3.1, the selected MZ and DZ probands exhibited a similar number of symptoms for all three measures of ADHD, providing important confirmation that the severity of the proband deficit was similar across zygosity. On each measure of ADHD, the mean number of symptoms exhibited by MZ co-twins was higher than the mean score of the DZ co-twins, indicating that MZ co-twins regressed less toward the population mean, providing compelling support for the hypothesis that extreme ADHD scores are due to genetic influences. Indeed, when the multiple regression model was fitted, the resulting estimates of group heritability were highly significant for all three measures of ADHD (h^2_g = .76–.90). Furthermore, the heritability estimates for extreme scores are similar to the estimates obtained for individual differences in ADHD symptoms, consistent with the hypothesis that the same genetic influences may contribute to both extreme ADHD scores and individual differences in ADHD symptoms across the entire population. Once again, these new findings indicate that even if ADHD symptoms as a whole decrease across adolescence (see next section and Chapter 2), the most extreme scores continue to be driven largely by genetic factors.

Extensions of Behavioral Genetic Analyses

In addition to yielding important information about the etiology of ADHD during adolescence, extensions of these methods provide useful approaches to answer key questions about the etiology and diagnostic nosology of ADHD and related disorders. This section briefly summarizes the use of behavioral genetic methods to test the developmental etiology of ADHD, the validity of diagnostic subtypes, and the etiology of the frequent comorbidity between ADHD and other disorders during adolescence.

The Developmental Etiology of ADHD

Longitudinal studies of twins provide an important extension of cross-sectional behavioral genetic analyses by testing the etiology of stability and

TABLE 3.1. Multiple Regression Analyses to Test the Heritability of Clinically Significant Elevations on DSM-IV ADHD Symptom Dimensions

	MZ pairs		DZ pairs			
Symptom dimension	Proband *M* (*SD*)	Co-twin *M* (*SD*)	Proband *M* (*SD*)	Co-twin *M* (*SD*)	h^2_g (*SE*)	*t*
Inattention	7.8 (1.2)	5.5 (3.3)	7.7 (1.1)	3.0 (3.6)	.78 (.17)	4.6*
Hyperactivity–Impulsivity	7.3 (1.3)	4.9 (2.9)	7.3 (1.4)	2.4 (3.0)	.75 (.22)	3.4*
Total ADHD	12.5 (3.5)	10.1 (5.7)	12.0 (3.6)	4.9 (4.9)	.74 (.12)	6.2*

Note. Number of selected twin pairs = 76 MZ, 78 DZ for inattention; 45 MZ, 40 DZ for hyperactivity–impulsivity; 112 MZ, 110 DZ for total ADHD.

*$p < .001$.

change in symptoms of ADHD between childhood and adolescence. For this chapter, new analyses were conducted in the CLDRC and ILTS samples to examine the developmental course of inattention and hyperactivity–impulsivity across development.

Longitudinal phenotypic analyses in both samples indicated that symptoms of inattention are generally stable between preschool and ninth grade, whereas mean levels of hyperactivity–impulsivity decline starting in late childhood. This pattern replicates the results of our meta-analysis of longitudinal studies of DSM-IV ADHD (Willcutt et al., 2012). Furthermore, longitudinal behavioral genetic analyses in both of our samples and other large twin studies (e.g., Greven et al., 2011) indicated that nearly all of the stability in ADHD symptoms between childhood and adolescence is due to genetic influences. While no twin studies have followed individuals with ADHD into adulthood, these results provide important support for the developmental continuity of ADHD, and suggest that the same genetic influences contribute to ADHD symptoms across development.

Understanding Diagnostic Heterogeneity: Etiology of ADHD Subtypes

Etiologically informative methods also provide a powerful tool to understand the heterogeneity that characterizes ADHD. For example, the criteria for ADHD in DSM-IV and DSM-5 describe three discrete subtypes (DSM-IV; American Psychiatric Association, 2000) or symptom presentations (DSM-5; American Psychiatric Association, 2013). The predominantly inattentive type or presentation (ADHD-I) is characterized by elevations of inattention symptoms but not hyperactivity–impulsivity symptoms, whereas individuals with the predominantly hyperactive–impulsive type or presentation (ADHD-H) exhibit elevations of hyperactivity–impulsivity symptoms but not inattention, and the combined type or presentation (ADHD-C) is defined by elevations on both symptom dimensions.

To examine the validity of these diagnostic subgroups, we completed new analyses that examined MZ and DZ concordance rates for the DSM-IV ADHD subtypes in adolescent twin pairs from the CLDRC (see Figure 3.1). Two specific findings would support the validity of the three-subtype model. First, the high heritability of the overall ADHD diagnosis suggests that each subtype should also be strongly influenced by genes. If one of the subtypes is primarily due to environmental influences, it may call into question the validity of the subtype, or at least suggest that it may be better conceptualized as a different disorder. Second, if the distinction between the subtypes is valid, the subtypes should "breed true," such that co-twins tend to meet criteria for the same subtype as the selected proband and not one of the other subtypes.

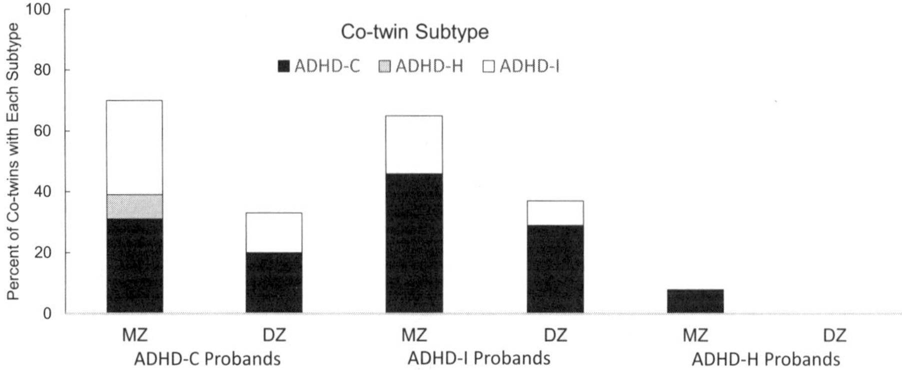

FIGURE 3.1. Rates of DSM-IV ADHD subtypes in the MZ and DZ co-twins of probands selected for ADHD-C, ADHD-I, and ADHD-H.

Whether probands were selected for the combined type or inattentive type, the overall rate of ADHD was significantly higher in MZ co-twins than in DZ co-twins (70 vs. 33% for ADHD-C and 65% vs. 37% for ADHD-I). ADHD-I also breeds true in adolescent twin pairs to some extent (46% of MZ co-twins versus 19% of DZ co-twins of probands with ADHD-I also met criteria for ADHD-I). However, co-twins of probands with ADHD-I were also significantly more likely to meet criteria for ADHD-C than expected based on the population base rate, and co-twins of probands with ADHD-C were equally likely to meet criteria for ADHD-C or ADHD-I. These results suggest that ADHD-C and ADHD-I are influenced by both unique and shared genetic influences in adolescence, a finding that is consistent with results across several other levels of analysis in our meta-analytic review of the correlates of ADHD-I and ADHD-C across the lifespan (Willcutt et al., 2012).

Results for the hyperactive–impulsive type were quite different. The ADHD-H subtype was rare among adolescents (12% of all probands with ADHD), a finding that is consistent with the decline in hyperactivity–impulsivity symptoms that is consistently observed between childhood and adolescence (e.g., Willcutt et al., 2012). Furthermore, analyses of concordance rates indicated that the rate of any ADHD subtype was extremely low in the co-twins of adolescent probands selected for ADHD-H (MZ = 8%, DZ = 0%), and none of the pairs was concordant for the hyperactive–impulsive type (Figure 3.1). These results suggest that the hyperactive–impulsive type is neither familial nor heritable, a finding that is also consistent with the overall conclusions of our meta-analysis (Willcutt et al., 2012). Therefore, while the results from our sample should be interpreted with caution due to the relatively small sample of adolescents with ADHD-H, these findings add to a growing literature that challenges the validity of ADHD-H after preschool.

Etiology of Comorbidity

As summarized by Becker and Fogleman (Chapter 9, this volume), comorbidity is the rule rather than the exception for adolescents with ADHD. Population-based studies indicate that in comparison to individuals without ADHD, individuals with ADHD exhibit significantly higher rates of learning disabilities; externalizing disorders, such as oppositional defiant disorder (ODD) and conduct disorder (CD); and internalizing disorders, such as depression and anxiety disorders. Several recent studies suggest that ADHD symptoms are also correlated with symptoms of autism spectrum disorder and psychosis (studies of comorbidity with DSM-IV ADHD are reviewed by Becker and Fogleman in Chapter 9 and in the meta-analysis by Willcutt et al., 2012). Furthermore, the presence of one or more comorbid disorders is often associated with greater impairment in a range of important academic, behavioral, social, and neuropsychological domains (e.g., Connor, Steeber, & McBurnett, 2010; Waschbusch, 2002; Willcutt, Betjemann, Pennington, et al., 2007).

Multivariate behavioral genetic analyses can extend phenotypic studies of comorbidity by assessing the extent to which genetic and environmental influences contribute to the co-occurrence of ADHD and other disorders. Results from our samples and others indicate that shared genetic influences account for nearly all of the phenotypic covariance between ADHD and learning disabilities, particularly for symptoms of inattention (e.g., Willcutt, Betjemann, et al., 2010). Shared genetic influences also accounted for a significant portion of the phenotypic covariance between ADHD symptoms and elevations of internalizing disorders, externalizing disorders, and autism spectrum disorder in studies that included both children and adolescents (e.g., Neale et al., 2010; Thapar, Harrington, & McGuffin, 2001; Willcutt, 2014).

New analyses conducted for this chapter not only confirm these overall findings but also underscore important differences in the pattern of results for the DSM-IV ADHD symptom dimensions. Specifically, our results in both children and adolescents consistently indicate that genetic influences on inattention symptoms are more strongly associated with academic difficulties and symptoms of depression than hyperactivity–impulsivity symptoms, and genetic correlations during adolescence are especially high between inattention and higher-order academic skills, such as reading comprehension and math word problems. In contrast, genetic influences that lead to high levels of hyperactivity–impulsivity are strongly associated with comorbid aggressive and delinquent behaviors across development, but these effects are weaker in adolescence than during childhood.

Testing the Etiology of the Relation between ADHD and a New Symptom Dimension

In addition to testing the etiology of comorbidity between ADHD and other DSM disorders, behavioral genetic methods provide a powerful approach to evaluate the validity of newly discovered clinical constructs and test their association with ADHD. As described in more detail by Becker and Fogleman (Chapter 9, this volume) and elsewhere (Becker, Marshall, & McBurnett, 2014; Willcutt et al., 2012), initial factor analyses of ADHD symptoms identified dimensions of inattention and hyperactivity–impulsivity, along with a third factor characterized by cognitive sluggishness, drowsiness, and lethargic and apathetic behavior that was labeled sluggish cognitive tempo (SCT). Although SCT has never been included in the criteria for a formal disorder, our recent meta-analysis provides strong support for the internal validity, longitudinal stability, and external validity of SCT, along with the discriminant validity of SCT and DSM-IV ADHD inattention (Becker et al., 2016).

In contrast to the growing literature that supports the internal and external validity of SCT, only one previous study has examined the etiology of SCT or its covariation with ADHD (Moruzzi, Rijsdijk, & Battaglia, 2014). Questions regarding etiology are especially important to examine in adolescence, because SCT symptoms increase in adolescence (Leopold et al., 2016), longitudinally predict adolescent outcomes (Becker, Burns, Leopold, Olson, & Willcutt, 2018), and are associated with key developmental outcomes that increase dramatically during adolescence, such as suicide risk (Becker, Holdaway, & Luebbe, 2018). Therefore, as a first step to understand the developmental etiology of SCT and its covariance with ADHD, new twin analyses were completed for this chapter in both children and adolescents drawn from the CLDRC and ILTS samples.

The single published twin study of SCT focused on three SCT items drawn from the Achenbach Child Behavior Checklist (Moruzzi et al., 2014). Individual differences in SCT on this measure were significantly heritable, but the estimated heritability of SCT in the best-fitting model (h^2 = .28) was lower than the heritability of ADHD symptoms in the same sample (h^2 = .45–.57) or in the broader literature of twin studies of ADHD, and the estimate of nonshared environmental influences was substantially higher (e^2 = .72). In contrast, new twin analyses in both of our samples indicated that individual differences in SCT symptoms are moderately heritable in both children (h^2 = .55–.66) and adolescents (h^2 = .56–.62), although slightly less heritable than symptoms of ADHD. The remaining variance was also explained by nonshared environmental influences or measurement error in our samples, but these estimates were smaller in magnitude (e^2 = .35–.45) than the estimates reported by Moruzzi and colleagues (2014).

The most likely explanation for differences between the estimates obtained across studies may be the reliability of the measures of SCT. The composite score based on the three Child Behavior Checklist items is correlated with other measures of SCT, but it tends to be somewhat less reliable than more extensive measures of SCT that include a larger number of items (Becker et al., 2016), including the five- to seven-item scales that were available in our twin samples.

Results from our twin samples also provide additional evidence that SCT symptoms are highly correlated with DSM-IV inattention in both childhood and adolescence (r = .58–.68), and multivariate analyses indicate that inattention and SCT are due in part to shared genetic influences, along with significant independent genetic and environmental influences that are uniquely associated with each dimension. In contrast, the smaller correlation with DSM-IV hyperactivity–impulsivity (r = .31–.40) was no longer significant in phenotypic or behavioral genetic models after inattention was controlled. Taken together, these findings support a model in which SCT and ADHD are etiologically related but separable constructs in both children and adolescents, and illustrate the potential utility of behavioral genetic methods to inform diagnostic models of ADHD and related disorders.

Summary of Behavioral Genetic Studies

Behavior genetic studies indicate that ADHD is significantly familial, and that this familiality is primarily due to genetic influences that also lead to the frequent comorbidity between ADHD and a range of other disorders. Nonshared environmental factors specific to the individual account for nearly all of the remaining risk for ADHD, and estimates of shared environmental influences are not significant in most twin studies. Based on these results, subsequent studies have attempted to identify the specific environmental or genetic factors that increase the likelihood that a child will develop ADHD.

Studies of Specific Measured Genetic and Environmental Risk Factors

Molecular Genetic Studies

The high heritability of ADHD and other developmental disorders led to initial optimism that identification of specific genes would explain a large proportion of the risk for each disorder. However, results of molecular genetic studies have turned out to be much more complicated than anticipated. This section first summarizes results of studies that used one of two main approaches to attempt to identify genes that increase susceptibility to ADHD, then reviews studies that tested for significant associations between ADHD and specific environmental risk factors.

Candidate Gene Studies

The candidate gene approach investigates the role of a specific gene identified because it is part of a biological system that is associated with a disorder. For example, because psychostimulant medication increases dopamine availability by blocking reuptake at the synapse, many early molecular genetic studies of ADHD examined polymorphisms in genes that influence the dopamine pathway (for an early meta-analytic review, see Faraone et al., 2005). Although results of candidate gene studies were inconsistent and frequently contradictory, a meta-analytic review reported small but significant effects for polymorphisms in three genes in the dopamine system, two genes that play a role in serotonin transmission, and a gene coding for a synaptic vesicle regulating protein (Gizer, Ficks, & Waldman, 2009). However, small effect sizes indicated that each of these risk factors accounts for a very small proportion of the total genetic risk for ADHD, and few studies have focused specifically on adolescents.

Genomewide Analyses

Because most of the genetic variance in ADHD symptoms was not explained by the polymorphisms included in initial candidate gene studies, the next generation of molecular genetic studies took advantage of advances in DNA technology that made it possible to screen the entire human genome for chromosomal regions that may contain genes that increase risk for ADHD. This systematic approach tests for associations between ADHD and millions of DNA markers spaced relatively evenly across the genome. Because each marker is tested individually, the large number of statistical tests required for this approach is a key limitation, and very large samples are required to obtain adequate statistical power to detect effects after controlling for multiple testing. To date no published genomewide association studies have identified any loci that were significant after researchers controlled for the number of statistical tests across the genome (e.g., Hinney et al., 2011; Middeldorp et al., 2016; Neale et al., 2010), although small effects approached significance for several genes involved in neuronal development (Middeldorp et al., 2016).

Conclusions from Molecular Genetic Studies

In contrast to initial models suggesting that single genetic risk factors would account for most or all of the genetic risk for ADHD, results of molecular genetic studies clearly suggest that the genetic etiology of ADHD is much more complex. Both candidate gene and genomewide association studies indicate that genetic risk for ADHD reflects the combined effects of a large number (potentially hundreds) of genetic risk factors, each of which leads to a small increase in risk in isolation.

Environmental Influences and Gene × Environment Interactions

Studies of environmental variables suggests that ADHD may have small associations with environmental risk factors that include prenatal or perinatal complications, specific prenatal exposure to nicotine or other substances, and potentially exposure to lead or other environmental toxins (e.g., Froehlich et al., 2009; Milberger, Biederman, Faraone, Guite, & Tsuang, 1997; Nigg, Nikolas, Mark Knottnerus, Cavanagh, & Friderici, 2010; reviewed by Froehlich et al., 2012). However, much like the results of molecular genetic studies, effects are small and inconsistent across studies, and interpretation is complicated by several key methodological issues. Important potential confounds include psychometric weaknesses in measures of environmental risk, potential biases due to retrospective reports in samples identified through clinics, and the fact that many putative environmental risk factors are partially heritable (including parenting behavior, social support, and exposure to prenatal stressful life events and parental substance use during pregnancy; e.g., Kendler & Baker, 2007). Future research is needed that uses etiologically informative designs that prospectively assess population-based samples and control for the potential heritability of environmental risk factors.

Gene × Environment Interactions

In addition to studies of environmental influences alone, recent studies have begun to incorporate genetic polymorphisms and environmental measures in the same analyses to test for gene × environment (G × E) interactions, which occur if the expression of a gene varies as a function of the specific environment. For example, diathesis–stress interactions occur when the co-occurrence of a genetic vulnerability (the diathesis) and an environmental risk factor results in more severe symptomatology than would be expected based on their additive combination.

Several studies of ADHD have reported significant diathesis–stress interactions between dopamine system genes or other candidate genes and prenatal exposure to nicotine or alcohol (reviewed by Nigg, Nikolas, & Burt, 2010). These significant G × E interactions are intriguing and warrant additional research. However, many initially positive G × E interactions have replicated inconsistently in studies of ADHD and other psychopathology, leading several authors to urge caution in the interpretation of G × E results (e.g., Duncan & Keller, 2011).

Epigenetics

An additional way that environmental influences can impact the effect of genes is epigenetic effects. Broadly, *epigenetics* refers to changes in the activity and expression of a particular gene due to an environmental event that changes gene activation without changing the underlying DNA sequence (for a more detailed overview of epigenetics, see Kiser, Rivero, & Lesch, 2015). These effects can occur due to environmental exposures in the womb or later in life.

Only a handful of studies has investigated epigenetic effects in ADHD to date, but this initial work has yielded some intriguing results. For example, a recent prospective study suggested that differences in methylation, a measure of gene activation, in several regions of the genome at birth were associated with different early trajectories of attention development at age 7 (Walton et al., 2017). Much more work remains to be done to replicate these results and fully understand the nature of these and other epigenetic effects, including their extension to adolescence and adolescent-salient outcomes, but these initial results suggest that epigenetic approaches may be a fruitful direction for future research.

Conclusions

Results of studies that incorporate environmental measures must be interpreted in the context of a range of important design considerations, and additional research is needed on adolescent samples with ADHD. Nonetheless, initial results suggest that specific prenatal environmental factors may increase susceptibility to ADHD, possibly in combination with specific genetic risk factors. If the effect of genetic risk factors is indeed moderated by environmental influences, then this may help to explain the small effect sizes and inconsistent replication of results for specific genetic polymorphisms despite the high heritability of ADHD.

CONCLUSIONS AND FUTURE DIRECTIONS

Family and twin studies clearly show that ADHD is familial and heritable in adolescence, and shared genetic influences account for much of the co-occurrence of ADHD and other disorders. Despite the high heritability of ADHD and other disorders, each individual genetic polymorphism appears to explain a very small proportion of the total population variance in ADHD symptoms. This pattern of results suggests that dozens or even hundreds of genes act in combination with a range of environmental risk factors to lead to the development of ADHD. This final section of this chapter examines the broader implications of this pattern of results and reviews several potential next steps for behavioral and molecular genetic studies in light of these results.

Future Directions for Behavioral Genetic Studies of ADHD in Adolescence

Developmental Trajectories of ADHD

Longitudinal twin data provide important support for the developmental continuity of ADHD symptoms from early childhood through at least early adolescence. Longitudinal studies that extend this research into early adulthood and beyond will provide an important extension of these results to facilitate the development of a comprehensive model of the developmental etiology of ADHD across the lifespan. Etiologically informative longitudinal designs may also help to identify the factors associated with the persistence or decline of ADHD symptoms in different individuals during adolescence and early adulthood. Finally, longitudinal studies of unselected samples that systematically include measures of ADHD symptoms will be uniquely positioned to assess the frequency, etiology, and correlates of any cases of ADHD that emerge later in development.

Etiology of Comorbidity during Adolescence

The data summarized earlier in this chapter illustrate the value of behavioral and molecular genetic methods to understand the etiology of comorbidity. In the future, it may be fruitful to use these approaches to test whether the etiological influences on the most frequent comorbidities with ADHD during childhood (e.g., anxiety and mood disorders, learning disorders, ODD and CD) are similar to those that lead to comorbidity later in adolescence or adulthood. Furthermore, etiologically informative studies of adolescents and young adults will provide an important opportunity to test the etiology of comorbidity between ADHD and disorders that often emerge later in development, such as schizophrenia spectrum disorders, eating disorders, and panic disorder.

ADHD and Functional Impairment

Cross-sectional studies clearly show that ADHD is associated with significant functional impairment in a range of domains, but far fewer studies have examined the developmental relations between ADHD symptoms and functional impairment during adolescence. Future etiologically informative studies that systematically assess these measures will provide important new information regarding the etiological influences that contribute to developmental associations between ADHD and functional impairment, including aspects of functioning that may first become relevant during adolescence, such as driving ability and management of money.

Clinical Implications and Future Collaborative Research

There is currently no valid genetic test for ADHD and, in my view, it is unlikely that a definitive diagnostic test will be developed in the near future. Because ADHD and other developmental disorders have polygenic, multifactorial etiologies in which each risk factor confers only a small increase in susceptibility, it is unlikely that any specific risk factor will have sufficient predictive power to be useful as a diagnostic measure. Having said this, it may eventually be possible to develop probabilistic risk profiles that combine information from all genetic risk factors to provide a measure of overall genetic risk. These risk profiles could be used to identify individuals who are at higher risk for ADHD, facilitating primary prevention or early intervention to reduce the probability that the child will eventually develop ADHD.

Furthermore, even if behavioral and molecular genetic studies do not identify a definitive genetic test for ADHD or other disorders, these methods are still likely to have important clinical benefits in the future. Studies that integrate these approaches in neuropsychological or neuroimaging studies are likely to improve models of the pathophysiology of ADHD, and may eventually inform the development of tertiary pharmacological or psychosocial treatments that directly target the physiological and psychological mechanisms that are compromised.

In closing, it is worth noting that procedures for DNA collection and genetic analysis continue to become more automated and efficient. It is rapidly becoming possible for researchers with relatively modest budgets and minimal specific training in behavioral or molecular genetics to collaborate with experts in DNA analysis to incorporate genetically informative methods as one part of their study. In the future, the capacity to easily apply these methods more broadly is likely to facilitate an extraordinary kind of collaborative synergy between behavioral and molecular genetic researchers and investigators focusing on other aspects of ADHD in adolescence, strengthening research across all levels of analysis.

References

American Psychiatric Association. (2000). *Diagnostic and statistical manual of mental disorders* (4th ed., text rev.). Washington, DC: Author.

American Psychiatric Association. (2013). *Diagnostic and statistical manual of mental disorders* (5th ed.). Arlington, VA: Author.

Becker, S. P., Burns, G. L., Leopold, D. R., Olson, R. K., & Willcutt, E. G. (2018). Differential impact of trait sluggish cognitive tempo and ADHD inattention in early childhood on adolescent functioning. *Journal of Child Psychology and Psychiatry, 59,* 1094–1104.

Becker, S. P., Holdaway, A. S., & Luebbe, A. M. (2018). Suicidal behaviors in college students: Frequency, sex differences, and mental health correlates including sluggish cognitive tempo. *Journal of Adolescent Health, 63,* 181–188.

Becker, S. P., Leopold, D. R., Burns, G. L., Jarrett, M. A., Langberg, J. M., Marshall, S. A., . . . Willcutt, E. G. (2016). The internal, external, and diagnostic validity of sluggish cognitive tempo: A meta-analysis and critical review. *Journal of the American Academy of Child and Adolescent Psychiatry, 55,* 163–178.

Becker, S. P., Marshall, S. A., & McBurnett, K. (2014). Sluggish cognitive tempo in abnormal child psychology: An historical overview and introduction to the Special Section. *Journal of Abnormal Child Psychology, 42,* 1–6.

Chang, Z., Lichtenstein, P., Asherson, P. J., & Larsson, H. (2013). Developmental twin study of attention problems: High heritabilities throughout development. *JAMA Psychiatry, 70,* 311–318.

Connor, D. F., Steeber, J., & McBurnett, K. (2010). A review of attention-deficit/hyperactivity disorder complicated by symptoms of oppositional defiant disorder or conduct disorder. *Journal of Developmental and Behavioral Pediatrics, 31,* 427–440.

DeFries, J. C., & Fulker, D. W. (1985). Multiple regression analysis of twin data. *Behavior Genetics, 15,* 467–473.

DeFries, J. C., & Fulker, D. W. (1988). Multiple regression analysis of twin data: Etiology of deviant scores versus individual differences. *Acta Geneticae Medicae et Gemellologiae, 37,* 205–216.

Duncan, L. E., & Keller, M. C. (2011). A critical review of the first 10 years of candidate gene-by-environment interaction research in psychiatry. *American Journal of Psychiatry, 168*(10), 1041–1049.

Faraone, S. V., Biederman, J., & Friedman, D. (2000). Validity of DSM-IV subtypes of attention-deficit/hyperactivity disorder: A family study perspective. *Journal of the American Academy of Child and Adolescent Psychiatry, 39,* 300–307.

Faraone, S. V., Perlis, R. H., Doyle, A. E., Smoller, J. W., Goralnick, J. J., Holmgren, M. A., & Sklar, P. (2005). Molecular genetics of attention-deficit/hyperactivity disorder. *Biological Psychiatry, 57,* 1313–1323.

Friedman, M. C., Chhabildas, N., Budhiraja, N., Willcutt, E. G., & Pennington, B. F. (2003). Etiology of the comorbidity between RD and ADHD: Exploration of the non-random mating hypothesis. *American Journal of Medical Genetics B: Neuropsychiatric Genetics, 120,* 109–115.

Froehlich, T. E., Anixt, J. S., Loe, I. M., Chirdkiatgumchai, V., Kuan, L., & Gilman, R. C. (2012). Update on environmental risk factors for attention-deficit/hyperactivity disorder. *Current Psychiatry Reports, 13,* 333–344.

Froehlich, T. E., Lanphear, B. P., Auinger, P., Hornung, R., Epstein, J. N., Braun, J., & Kahn, R. S. (2009). Association of tobacco and lead exposures with attention-deficit/hyperactivity disorder. *Pediatrics, 124,* e1054–e1063.

Gizer, I. R., Ficks, C., & Waldman, I. D. (2009). Candidate gene studies of ADHD: A meta-analytic review. *Human Genetics, 126,* 51–90.

Greven, C. U., Asherson, P., Rijsdijk, F. V., & Plomin, R. (2011). A longitudinal twin study on the association between inattentive and hyperactive–impulsive ADHD symptoms. *Journal of Abnormal Child Psychology, 39,* 623–632.

Hinney, A., Scherag, A., Jarick, I., Albayrak, O., Putter, C., Pechlivanis, S., . . . Psychiatric GWAS Consortium: ADHD Subgroup. (2011). Genome-wide association study in German patients with attention deficit/hyperactivity disorder. *American Journal of Medical Genetics B: Neuropsychiatric Genetics, 156,* 888–897.

Kendler, K. S., & Baker, J. H. (2007). Genetic influences on measures of the environment: A systematic review. *Psychological Medicine, 37,* 615–626.

Kiser, D. P., Rivero, O., & Lesch, K. P. (2015). Annual research review: The (epi)genetics of neurodevelopmental disorders in the era of whole-genome sequencing—unveiling the dark matter. *Journal of Child Psychology and Psychiatry, 56,* 278–295.

Knopik, V. S., Niederhiser, J. M., DeFries, J. C., & Plomin, R. (2017). *Behavioral genetics.* New York: Worth.

Larsson, H., Anckarsater, H., Rastam, M., Chang, Z., & Lichtenstein, P. (2012). Childhood attention-deficit hyperactivity disorder as an extreme of a continuous trait: A quantitative genetic study of 8,500 twin pairs. *Journal of Child Psychology and Psychiatry, 53,* 73–80.

Larsson, H., Lichtenstein, P., & Larsson, J. O. (2006). Genetic contributions to the development of ADHD subtypes from childhood to adolescence. *Journal of the American Academy of Child and Adolescent Psychiatry, 45,* 973–981.

Leopold, D. R., Christopher, M. E., Burns, G. L., Becker, S. P., Olson, R. K., & Willcutt, E. G. (2016). Attention-deficit/hyperactivity disorder and sluggish cognitive tempo throughout childhood: Temporal invariance and stability from preschool through ninth grade. *Journal of Child Psychology and Psychiatry, 57,* 1066–1074.

Levy, F., Hay, D. A., McStephen, M., Wood, C., & Waldman, I. (1997). Attention-deficit hyperactivity disorder: A category or a continuum?: Genetic analysis of a large-scale twin study. *Journal of the American Academy of Child and Adolescent Psychiatry, 36,* 737–744.

Middeldorp, C. M., Hammerschlag, A. R., Ouwens, K. G., Groen-Blokhuis, M. M., Pourcain, B. S., Greven, C. U., . . . Boomsma, D. I. (2016). A genome-wide association meta-analysis of attention-deficit/hyperactivity disorder symptoms in population-based pediatric cohorts. *Journal of the American Academy of Child and Adolescent Psychiatry, 55,* 896–905.

Milberger, S., Biederman, J., Faraone, S. V., Guite, J., & Tsuang, M. T. (1997). Pregnancy, delivery and infancy complications and attention deficit hyperactivity disorder: Issues of gene–environment interaction. *Biological Psychiatry, 41,* 65–75.

Moruzzi, S., Rijsdijk, F., & Battaglia, M. (2014). A twin study of the relationships among inattention, hyperactivity/impulsivity and sluggish cognitive tempo problems. *Journal of Abnormal Child Psychology, 42,* 63–75.

Neale, B. M., Medland, S. E., Ripke, S., Asherson, P., Franke, B., Lesch, K. P., . . . Psychiatric GWAS Consortium: ADHD Subgroup. (2010). Meta-analysis of genome-wide association studies of attention-deficit/hyperactivity disorder. *Journal of the American Academy of Child and Adolescent Psychiatry, 49,* 884–897.

Nigg, J. T., Nikolas, M., & Burt, S. A. (2010). Measured gene-by-environment interaction in relation to attention-deficit/hyperactivity disorder. *Journal of the American Academy of Child and Adolescent Psychiatry, 49,* 863–873.

Nigg, J. T., Nikolas, M., Mark Knottnerus, G., Cavanagh, K., & Friderici, K. (2010). Confirmation and extension of association of blood lead with attention-deficit/hyperactivity disorder (ADHD) and ADHD symptom domains at population-typical exposure levels. *Journal of Child Psychology and Psychiatry, 51,* 58–65.

Sherman, D. K., McGue, M. K., & Iacono, W. G. (1997). Twin concordance for attention deficit hyperactivity disorder: A comparison of teachers' and mothers' reports. *American Journal of Psychiatry, 154,* 532–535.

Thapar, A., Harrington, R., & McGuffin, P. (2001). Examining the comorbidity of ADHD-related behaviours and conduct problems using a twin study design. *British Journal of Psychiatry, 179,* 224–229.

Walton, E., Pingault, J. B., Cecil, C. A., Gaunt, T. R., Relton, C. L., Mill, J., & Barker,

E. D. (2017). Epigenetic profiling of ADHD symptoms trajectories: A prospective, methylome-wide study. *Molecular Psychiatry, 22,* 250–256.

Waschbusch, D. A. (2002). A meta-analytic examination of comorbid hyperactive–impulsive–attention problems and conduct problems. *Psychological Bulletin, 128,* 118–150.

Willcutt, E. G. (2012). The prevalence of DSM-IV attention-deficit/hyperactivity disorder: A meta-analytic review. *Neurotherapeutics, 9,* 490–499.

Willcutt, E. G. (2014). Using behavior genetic methods to understand the etiology of comorbidity. In S. Rhee & A. Ronald (Eds.), *Behavior genetics of psychopathology* (pp. 231–252). New York: Springer.

Willcutt, E. G., Betjemann, R. S., McGrath, L. M., Chhabildas, N. A., Olson, R. K., DeFries, J. C., & Pennington, B. F. (2010). Etiology and neuropsychology of comorbidity between RD and ADHD: The case for multiple-deficit models. *Cortex, 46,* 1345–1361.

Willcutt, E. G., Betjemann, R. S., Pennington, B. F., Olson, R. K., DeFries, J. C., & Wadsworth, S. J. (2007). Longitudinal study of reading disability and attention-deficit/hyperactivity disorder: Implications for education. *Mind, Brain, and Education, 4,* 181–192.

Willcutt, E. G., Betjemann, R. S., Wadsworth, S. J., Samuelsson, S., Corley, R., DeFries, J. C., . . . Olson, R. K. (2007). Preschool twin study of the relation between attention-deficit/hyperactivity disorder and prereading skills. *Reading and Writing, 20,* 103–125.

Willcutt, E. G., Chhabildas, N., Kinnear, M., Defries, J. C., Olson, R. K., Leopold, D. R., . . . Pennington, B. F. (2014). The internal and external validity of sluggish cognitive tempo and its relation with DSM-IV ADHD. *Journal of Abnormal Child Psychology, 42,* 21–35.

Willcutt, E. G., Nigg, J. T., Pennington, B. F., Solanto, M. V., Rohde, L. A., Tannock, R., . . . Lahey, B. B. (2012). Validity of DSM-IV attention-deficit/hyperactivity disorder dimensions and subtypes. *Journal of Abnormal Psychology, 121,* 991–1010.

Willcutt, E. G., Pennington, B. F., & DeFries, J. C. (2000). Etiology of inattention and hyperactivity/impulsivity in a community sample of twins with learning difficulties. *Journal of Abnormal Child Psychology, 28,* 149–159.

Willcutt, E. G., Pennington, B. F., Duncan, L., Smith, S. D., Keenan, J. M., Wadsworth, S. J., & DeFries, J. C. (2010). Understanding the complex etiology of developmental disorders: Behavioral and molecular genetic approaches. *Journal of Developmental and Behavioral Pediatrics, 31,* 533–544.

Willcutt, E. G., Petrill, S. A., Wu, S., Boada, R., DeFries, J. C., Olson, R. K., & Pennington, B. F. (2013). Implications of comorbidity between reading and math disability: Neuropsychological and functional impairment. *Journal of Learning Disabilities, 46,* 500–516.

CHAPTER 4

Executive Functions and Decision Making in Adolescents with ADHD

Joshua Doidge
Wafa Saoud
Maggie E. Toplak

An emerging distinction between cognitive abilities (e.g., executive functions and intelligence) and judgment and decision-making skills in the cognitive science literature (Stanovich, 1999, 2009a) is becoming increasingly recognized in the developmental literature (Albert & Steinberg, 2011; Stanovich, West, & Toplak, 2012). Judgment and decision-making skills, in particular, have been used to explain several phenomena during adolescence, such as engagement in risky behaviors (Reyna & Farley, 2006). The study of cognitive abilities, especially executive functions, has been well-studied in the field of attention-deficit/hyperactivity disorder (ADHD), but there has been relatively less emphasis on the study of decision making in ADHD. Temporal discounting and risky decision-making have been the most well-studied constructs in ADHD, perhaps because impulsivity and engagement in risky behaviors have been well documented in individuals with ADHD (American Psychiatric Association, 2013; Barkley, 2006). In this chapter, we provide a review of the executive function and decision-making research in ADHD, with an emphasis on the period of adolescence. We discuss how studies of typical development can be used to advance our understanding of the development of these competencies in adolescents with ADHD.

DISTINGUISHING EXECUTIVE FUNCTIONS FROM JUDGMENT AND DECISION MAKING

The idea of "smart people doing foolish things" has progressed from a folk psychological concept to an area of study grounded in empirical research (Sternberg, 2002; Stanovich, 2009a). For example, we are surprised when intelligent adolescents make poor choices by subjecting themselves to risk factors such as substance abuse, sexually transmitted diseases, and unsafe driving (Reyna & Farley, 2006). This paradox in competencies has also been expressed in the popular press literature on ADHD (e.g., Brown, 2005; Kelly & Ramundo, 2006). Another example comes from empirical findings related to performance versus ratings of executive function (Toplak, West, & Stanovich, 2013; Lambek et al., 2010); that is, we are surprised to find youth who are not impaired on performance-based measures of executive function but report high impairment on activities that require executive function skills in everyday activities. These discrepancies are difficult for us to explain in our current neuropsychological models of ADHD. Self-regulation and executive function models of ADHD provide an exhaustive description of the difficulties experienced by individuals with ADHD (Barkley, 2006). These difficulties include behavioral inhibition, self-awareness, self-questioning, problem solving, moral reasoning, and self-regulation of arousal in the service of goal-directed action. However, our models of executive function do not seem to provide the proper operational definitions needed to assess these behaviors (Barkley, 2006). It seems that what is happening in the executive function and ADHD literature is parallel to what has happened in the field of intelligence, regarding the "broad" and "narrow" sense of the term intelligence:

> What is happening here is that we are bumping up against an old controversy in the study of cognitive ability—the distinction between broad and narrow theories of intelligence. Broad theories include aspects of functioning that are captured by the vernacular term intelligence (adaptation to the environment, showing wisdom and creativity, etc.) whether or not these aspects are actually measured by existing tests of intelligence. Narrow theories, in contrast, confine the concept of intelligence to the set of mental abilities actually tested on extant IQ tests. Narrow theories adopt the operationalization of the term that is used in psychometric studies of intelligence, neurophysiological studies using brain imaging, and studies of brain disorder. This definition involves a statistical abstraction from performance on established tests and cognitive ability indicators. (Stanovich, 2009a, p. 12)

This distinction between the broad and narrow sense helps us to explain the seeming discrepancy in competencies, such as smart people doing foolish things. A similar phenomenon has occurred in the study of executive functions. We often use the term *executive functions* in the broad sense (e.g., failures due to impulsivity in decision making, poor self-discipline, and inability to pursue goals) rather than referring to what is actually measured on these tests (e.g., trying to name colors on the Stroop test, while ignoring the inclination to read the words). Our models of ADHD have the challenge of trying to explain our complex behavioral clinical observations of individuals with ADHD (broad characteristics), but we often fall short in explaining these behaviors when relying exclusively on actual neuropsychological performance-based measures (narrow sense). The construct of executive functions has been criticized by ADHD researchers for being overly broad and weakly defined (Halperin, 2016; Pennington & Ozonoff, 1996; Sergeant, Geurts, Huijbregts, Scheres, & Oosterlaan, 2003) and lack of a satisfying operational definition (Barkley, 2006). This distinction between the broad and narrow sense can be used to develop models that can explain discrepancies in different competencies, including the potential that both cognitive failures and competencies can co-occur in individuals with ADHD (Sagvolden, Johansen, Aase, & Russell, 2005).

Moving forward, what is needed are conceptual distinctions that allow us to generate testable hypotheses about why certain competencies tend to co-occur or not. Recent models in cognitive science have differentiated between decision making and other cognitive abilities, such as intelligence and performance-based measures of executive function (Stanovich, 2009a; Toplak, Sorge, Benoit, West, & Stanovich, 2010). Neuropsychological assessments measure cognitive abilities, including intelligence and executive function performance. These cognitive ability measures capture computational resources that are assessed under highly structured conditions in which the examiner sets the parameters for optimal performance (Stanovich, 2009b). Alternatively, judgment and decision-making skills are conceptually unique from cognitive abilities. Cognitive science theories of decision making use experimental methods to illustrate thinking errors in which people fail to successfully track the world (e.g., knowledge calibration) or fail to achieve their goals (e.g., maximize expected utility). Rational temporal discounting and risky decision making are two tasks in which successful performance requires overriding the tendency to select the immediate or a risky choice that may lead to a lower return or expected value (Stanovich, 1999, 2009a). Performance on several decision-making tasks has been correlated with cognitive abilities (Stanovich & West, 2008; Stanovich, 1999, 2009a; Toplak, West, & Stanovich, 2011), as the processing requirements of inhibition (or interference control) and working memory are required to permit consideration and generation of alternative hypotheses in decision-making tasks. However, correlations tend to be modest with individual tasks, suggesting that there is room for dissociation between cognitive abilities and decision-making performance. The useful implication for models of ADHD is the potential to explain both relative competencies and relative deficits in the same individual; that is, deficits in executive functions do not necessarily lead to cognitive failures on decision-making measures. We focus on the conceptual distinction between executive functions and decision making, and the implications for understanding these competencies in adolescents with ADHD.

Executive Functions and Intellectual Abilities in Adolescents with ADHD

Performance-based measures of executive function are usually grouped in three core domains: inhibitory control, working memory, and flexibility (Diamond, 2013; Miyake et al., 2000; Miyake & Friedman, 2012). *Inhibitory control* is the process of stopping a response, as well as the ability to cancel an ongoing action or thoughts, or selectively attend to information while inhibiting interfering information (Logan, Cowan, & Davis, 1984; Schachar & Logan, 1990; Diamond, 2013). Examples of performance-based measures of executive function include the stop-signal task and the Stroop test to measure response inhibition (Logan et al., 1984; Schachar & Logan, 1990; Soreni, Crosbie, Ickowicz, & Schachar, 2009) and interference control (MacLeod, 1991; Stroop, 1935). *Working memory,* the ability to manipulate and temporarily store information in day-to-day life (Kane et al., 2007), can be measured using spatial or auditory stimuli. *Mental flexibility,* or set-shifting tasks, involves the ability to change between tasks or mental sets (Miyake et al., 2000). The Trail Making Test (Part B) is a set-shifting task, in which the participants are required to connect a series of circles based on matching both letters and numbers as quickly as possible (Reitan, 1971). Other executive functioning abilities include *planning,* which is the ability formulate a plan, evaluate and sequence thoughts, as well as *vigilance,* or the ability to sustain attention over a long period of time, such as performance on the continuous-performance test (CPT; Diamond, 2013; Barkley, Edwards, Laneri, Fletcher, & Metevia, 2001).

Performance-based measures of executive function are administered under highly standardized and structured testing conditions. These measures are different than ratings of executive function, which involve an informant reporting on how well an individual carries out everyday tasks involving executive functions (Toplak et al., 2013). On performance-based measures, accuracy and response time are the typical dependent measures. In this chapter, we focus on performance-based measures of executive function.

Executive Functioning in Adolescents with ADHD

Several studies have now documented significant differences between individuals with ADHD and controls on performance-based measures of executive function, including a meta-analysis by Willcutt, Doyle, Nigg, Faraone, and Pennington (2005) that included thousands of children and adolescents with ADHD, and typically developing individuals, and examined performance on an extensive set of executive function measures (inhibition, vigilance, inhibition, set-shifting, working memory, planning). They obtained significant group differences on 109 out of 168 comparisons, which is 65% of the studies. The largest effects were found on the stop-signal task and on the CPT. Differences were also found on planning tasks, visual–spatial working memory tasks, the Stroop task, and the Wisconsin Card Sorting Test (WCST), but relatively weaker effects than on the other measures. They concluded that approximately up to half of individuals with ADHD in these studies display impairments on any one (or more) performance-based measure of executive function (Loo et al., 2007; Biederman et al., 2004). Overall, no single performance-based measure of executive functioning has been consistently identified as impaired across samples with those with ADHD (Nigg et al., 2005; Willcutt et al., 2005), suggesting that no single deficit or common set of deficits characterize individuals with ADHD (Halperin & Schulz, 2006; Willcutt et al., 2005) and that there are individual differences in the correlated deficits among individuals with ADHD (e.g., Sonuga-Barke, Bitsakou, & Thompson, 2010). Determining the diagnosticity of performance on these measures is further complicated by the fact that impairments in executive functioning skills also occur in community-based samples (Lambek et al., 2011).

Relative to research with children with ADHD, there is limited information on how executive functioning abilities change in the adolescent years (Blakemore & Choudhury, 2006; Seidman, 2006). Developmental level and/or age were not examined as moderators in the meta-analysis by Willcutt et al. (2005). Of the studies in this meta-analysis, typically developing adolescents tended to outperform adolescents with ADHD on measures of executive function, including inhibitory control (and response inhibition), working memory and set shifting, but this has not been consistent across all measures and samples. Even among adolescents, there is a lack of homogeneity in individuals with ADHD in executive function deficits. Among these studies, relatively little attention has been given to developmental considerations.

There is evidence to suggest that executive functions develop in samples of typically developing children (Davidson, Amso, Anderson, & Diamond, 2006; Lamm, Zelazo, & Lewis, 2006; Salthouse & Davis, 2006). ADHD-related difficulties in childhood, as reported by teacher reports in typically developing samples, have also been shown to predict executive function performance longitudinally in adolescents (Friedman et al., 2007). Halperin and Schulz (2006) proposed a developmental model in order to explain neurocognitive development in ADHD. They hypothesized that childhood ADHD is due to early developmental noncortical neural dysfunction and that this dysfunction remains relatively stable over the lifespan. They further hypothesized that development of the prefrontal cortex and related neural systems can compensate for these subcortical deficits. This model suggests that the development of these prefrontal processes leads to a reduction in ADHD symptoms in adolescents and young adults. To test this model, this group examined the neurocognitive profile of children with ADHD, who were followed longitudinally approximately 10 years later when they were entering early adulthood (Halperin, Trampush, Miller, Marks, & Newcorn, 2008). At the longitudinal follow-up, those children who continued to meet criteria for ADHD were called "persisters," and those who no longer met criteria for ADHD were called "remitters." Nearly half of the sample were remitters (40%), which means that they met criteria in childhood but no longer met criteria in young adulthood. The results indicated that remitters scored better on several indices of the CPT and working memory measures compared to the persisters. In another recent longitudinal study, Murray, Robinson, and Tripp (2017) reported parallel findings, with children in a partial remission group outperforming those in a persistent ADHD group on measures of attentional control, information processing, cognitive flexibility. and goal setting. However, a systematic review of 18 studies revealed that ADHD persisters and remitters remained equally impaired in neurocognitive functioning, and that neurocognitive functioning appeared to be unrelated to the developmental course of ADHD (van Lieshout, Luman, Buitelaar, Rommelse, & Oosterlaan, 2013). However, it is difficult to draw conclusions about the associations among ADHD, neurocognitive functioning, and ADHD symptom persistence based on these extant studies. One of the complicating factors is that standardized measures that provide age-corrected scores can be problematic for examining trends in developmental samples (Rizeq, Flora, & Toplak, 2017), which were not systematically examined in these studies but may importantly alter the data patterns and conclusions.

Determining the effect size of performance on measures of executive functions in ADHD is also impacted by the practice of statistically controlling for differences in intellectual abilities when examining executive function deficits in ADHD samples (Willcutt et al., 2005). It has been well documented that those with ADHD tend to have lower Full-Scale IQs (Frazier, Demaree, & Youngstrom, 2004), and it has also been demonstrated that statistically controlling for intellectual abilities can greatly reduce the group differences found on performance-based measures such as working memory (Jonsdottir, Bouma, Sergeant, & Scherder, 2006, Martel, Nikolas, & Nigg, 2007; Willcutt et al., 2005; Barkley et al., 2001). Researchers have discouraged the practice of covarying for IQ scores in studies of neurodevelopmental disorders such as ADHD (Dennis et al., 2009), as statistical control of intellectual ability scores may remove some of the variation in the experimental measures under study that is due to the difficulties observed in ADHD samples.

Overall, a working hypothesis in the ADHD literature suggests that children who display more improvement in their performance on measures of executive function over the course of development into adolescence will display fewer ADHD symptoms. As in samples of typically developing youth (Salthouse, Atkinson, & Berish, 2003; Davidson et al., 2006; Zelazo & Carlson, 2012), individuals with ADHD may also display improvements and growth in executive function skills. The fact that some youth have remitted symptoms and others continue to have an ADHD diagnosis suggests that there are individual differences in the trajectories of these youth.

Decision Making in Adolescents with ADHD

Clinical characterizations of ADHD include poor decision making, such as failing to achieve goals and to recognize how one's own difficulties impact others (Barkley, 2006). There has been less work examining decision making in ADHD relative to performance-based measures of executive function and intelligence (Castellanos, Sonuga-Barke, Milham, & Tannock, 2006), but neuroeconomic models rooted in decision-making perspectives are beginning to gain attention in ADHD (Sonuga-Barke & Fairchild, 2012). Temporal discounting (also related are delay of gratification and delay aversion tasks) and risky decision making are the most commonly studied areas of decision making in ADHD. *Temporal discounting* involves choosing between various guaranteed rewards and risky decision-making tasks that involve choices between uncertain probable rewards. Similar to the literature on executive function performance, relatively less work has been done with adolescents with ADHD than with children.

Temporal Discounting, Delay of Gratification, and Delay Aversion

There is a long history documenting the impulsive tendencies of individuals with ADHD (American Psychiatric Association, 2013). One way to quantify these impulsive tendencies has been through the observation that children with ADHD tend to prefer a small, immediate reward over a larger, delayed reward, which has been most extensively addressed by the delay aversion hypothesis in the ADHD literature (Sonuga-Barke, Taylor, Sembi, & Smith, 1992) which focuses on a motivational style that is associated with alterations in reward mechanisms (Sonuga-Barke, 2002). Delay aversion deficits in ADHD have been linked to neural circuits that link ventral striatum (nucleus accumbens) to frontal regions (including the anterior cingulate and orbitofrontal cortex; Sonuga-Barke, Sergeant, Nigg, & Willcutt, 2008). For this chapter, we highlight the behavioral choice of whether to maximize expected value on temporal discounting tasks as an indicator of decision making.

Temporal discounting involves asking participants to make a series of choices between smaller, immediate rewards or substantially larger, delayed rewards. To "temporally discount" is to give less value to larger, delayed rewards in the future when offered the choice between a smaller, immediate reward or a substantially larger, delayed reward (Shamosh & Gray, 2008). For example, if offered the choice between $10 today or $15 in a month, many people would choose the option of $10 today. People tend to "discount" the larger $15 in a month, because temporally it is too far off, even though it might be in their long-term interests to choose the delayed option. Several variants of this paradigm have been used, including delay aversion and delay of gratification paradigms. In delay of gratification, participants choose a larger, delayed reward and must wait out the complete delay time of the trial to get the reward before they can continue to the next trial. This method is very similar to the choice-delay task, which is used to assess delay aversion (e.g., Solanto et al., 2001). The difference between "only choosing" (temporal discounting) and "choosing and waiting" (delay of gratification and delay aversion) makes these tasks experimentally and conceptually somewhat different (Toplak, Hosseini, & Basile, 2016; Stanovich, 2011).

Across all of the paradigms that have been used to measure the preference for the smaller, immediate reward over the larger, delayed reward, the selection of the larger, delayed reward is typically scored as more optimal (Ainslie, 2001; Basile & Toplak, 2015; Kirby, 1997). These paradigms have been conceptualized as a component of instrumental rationality, pertaining to an individual's goal fulfillment (Stanovich, 2011). From an expected utility perspective, maximizing reward would be in line with instrumental rationality. In our own work, we have found that preference for the larger, delayed reward is significantly associated with cognitive abilities, including intellectual abilities and performance-based measures of executive function (Basile & Toplak, 2015; Toplak et al., 2016).

Individuals with ADHD have also been found to make more choices for immediate over delayed rewards on temporal discounting, delay aversion, and delay of gratification tasks (Patros et al., 2016; Jackson & MacKillop, 2016; Doidge, Flora, & Toplak, 2018). In a recent meta-analytic review, Jackson and MacKillop (2016) reported that developmental level (whether the participants were over or under 18 years of age) was not found to be a significant moderator. Patros et al. (2016) compared ADHD samples' preferences to a typically developing control group in both school-age children (8.00 to 12.99 years) and adolescents (13.00 to 17.99 years) on both temporal discounting and delay of gratification tasks. They found that the effect size for adolescents was nearly equivalent to that of the children with ADHD, but the number of studies with adolescents was five compared to 19 studies for school-age children. In studies that have included adolescents with ADHD, the findings quite consistently show that adolescents with ADHD tend to prefer immediate rewards significantly more than do typically developing adolescents. Another recent meta-analysis revealed a lack of temporal discounting differences between adults with ADHD (Mowinckel, Pedersen, Eilertsen, & Biele, 2015). These studies, however, may not be inconsistent, taking into account developmental factors.

Several studies have examined temporal discounting paradigms in typically developing samples. Steinberg and colleagues (2009) examined temporal discounting in a sample of 935 participants between ages 10 and 30. Their delay discounting task used a constant delayed reward of $1,000, with six delay periods (1 day, 1 week, 1 month, 3 months, 6 months, and 1 year). They reported age-related differences in temporal discounting choices. Participants age 13 years and younger were more likely to choose a smaller, immediate reward than a larger, delayed reward than were participants age 16 years and older. Other researchers have also reported more steep discounting in children than in adolescents (Green, Fry, & Myerson, 1994; Prencipe et al., 2011), showing that older children and youth tend to wait for the larger, delayed reward more often than do younger children.

The association between temporal discounting and delay of gratification paradigms with measures of cognitive ability has been examined in typically developing and ADHD samples. In typically developing samples, choices on temporal discounting and delay of gratification tasks have been correlated with having better executive functioning performance (working memory, set shifting, and inhibition) and higher intellectual abilities (Basile & Toplak, 2015; Shamosh et al., 2008). Steinberg et al. (2009) also examined the association between delay discounting and executive functions (Tower of London test and Stroop task) in a typically developing sample, and found a marginal relationship, perhaps attributable to controlling for intelligence scores in this analysis. Toplak et al. (2016) examined developmental differences in temporal discounting and associations with cognitive abilities in a sample of typically developing youth ages 8–14 years. Older youth were significantly more likely to choose the larger, delayed reward compared to younger youth. The preference for the larger, delayed reward was significantly associated with cognitive abilities, including intellectual abilities and executive functions (interference control, working memory, and set shifting), and all scores on these measures were not age-corrected. The sizes of the correlation were in the .18 ($p < .01$) to .30 ($p < .001$) range using the indifference point dependent measure, which were statistically significant but also relatively modest correlations. These modest correlations suggest that there is room for dissociations on these measures.

The association between temporal discounting-type paradigms and measures of cognitive ability in ADHD samples has been mixed. For example, Vloet et al. (2010) found that choosing the immediate reward was negatively correlated with intelligence scores in a sample of children with ADHD and typically developing children. Alternatively, Bitsakou, Psychogiou, Thompson, and Sonuga-Barke (2009) found that statistically controlling for intelligence scores eliminated the significant group difference between the ADHD and typically developing samples of children on a choice-delay task, but such an effect was not reported in other studies (Marco et al., 2009; Paloyelis, Asherson, Mehta, Faraone, & Kuntsi, 2010; Sonuga-Barke et al., 2010; Barkley et al., 2001). The findings with measures of executive functioning are also mixed. Sonuga-Barke et al. (2010) found a significant correlation between performance on a delay aversion task and the Stroop task, but no significant association with the stop-signal or working memory tasks.

The distinction between the stop-signal task (executive function performance) and the choice-delay task (measure of delay aversion) as separable indicators related to impulsivity has been described in models of ADHD (Solanto et al., 2001; Sonuga-Barke, 2002; Sonuga-Barke et al., 2008). The stop-signal task was conceptualized as an indicator of the ability to inhibit a prepared motor response, whereas the choice-delay task was instead "the result of a rational choice to avoid delay, which the individual finds aversive" (Solanto et al., 2001, p. 217). While these tasks were originally presented as potentially competing explanations of impulsive behaviors in ADHD, the results of this study demonstrated that accurate classification of children with and without ADHD improved from 70% with the individual tasks to 85% when using both tasks. These results acknowledge the separability of these constructs and their unique contribution in discriminating children with and without ADHD.

In summary, temporal discounting, delay of gratification, and delay aversion paradigms have been well-studied in ADHD samples. A consistent pattern of findings has shown that children and adolescents with ADHD tend to choose a smaller, immediate reward over a larger, delayed reward compared to typically developing controls. There seems to be a changing developmental trajectory, which suggests that the preference for a delayed reward may emerge in adulthood. This developmental path has been demonstrated in typically developing samples, and some evidence suggests that this may also be the case in ADHD samples (especially adults). Temporal discounting paradigms have also been shown to be positively associated with cognitive abilities in typically developing samples, but this pattern is less clear in ADHD samples. Developmental considerations may help to explain individual differences in temporal discounting choices in both typically developing and ADHD samples.

Risky Decision Making

Individuals with ADHD have been documented to engage in more risk taking than do individuals without ADHD, including elevated rates of substance use, risky sexual behaviors, criminal activities, gambling problems, and risky driving (Jerome, Segal, & Habinski, 2006; Pratt, Cullen, Blevins,

Daigle, & Unnever, 2002; Lee, Humphreys, Flory, Liu, & Glass, 2011; Flory, Molina, Pelham, Gnagy, & Smith, 2006; Faregh & Derevensky, 2011). Given these risk-taking behaviors in ADHD samples, risky decision-making tasks provide a useful operationalization to characterize these tendencies.

Risky decision making is typically assessed using laboratory gambling tasks (see Dekkers, Popma, van Rentergem, Bexkens, & Huizenga, 2016; Groen, Gaastra, Lewis-Evans, & Tucha, 2013). In laboratory gambling tasks, participants are typically offered the choice between options that differ in magnitude and probability of gains and losses. Generally, making choices that result in a high probability of large loss is indicative of risky decision making. In the Iowa Gambling Task (IGT), which is among the most commonly used laboratory gambling tasks, participants are asked to collect as much money as possible by choosing cards from one of four decks (A, B, C, or D). The amount of money won or lost varies between decks. For example, Decks A and B represent disadvantageous choices that result in overall loss, while Decks C and D represent advantageous choices that result in overall gain. The Hungry Donkey Task (HDT) is the child/youth version of the IGT. In another risky decision-making task, the Balloon Analogue Risk Task (BART), participants are told that they will have the opportunity to win money by inflating balloons on a computer screen without popping them. Participants may choose to stop pumping and collect the money earned from the trial at any time. Since each pump increases the risk of the balloon popping, resulting in loss of money, greater numbers of balloon pumps indicate greater levels of risk taking.

Groen et al. (2013) conducted a literature review of 14 studies and reported that children and adolescents with ADHD made riskier choices on risky decision-making tasks than controls, but that no differences were obtained in adults. Dekkers et al. (2016) conducted a meta-regression analysis of 37 studies and reported that individuals with ADHD displayed riskier decision making than controls. They also reported that developmental level (less than 12 years of age, 12–18 years of age, or over 18 years of age) did not have a significant impact on this relationship, suggesting that individuals with ADHD tend to make riskier choices on laboratory tasks regardless of age.

Relatively few studies have examined risky decision making in adolescents with ADHD. Of the few studies that have been conducted in adolescent populations, the available research suggests that adolescents with ADHD tend to make riskier choices on decision-making tasks than adolescents without ADHD. Among approximately 40 studies conducted on risky decision making in ADHD samples, five studies have examined adolescent populations using the IGT or the BART. In most of these studies, adolescents with ADHD were consistently reported to make riskier choices on the laboratory gambling tasks than adolescents without ADHD (Ernst et al.,

2003; Hobson, Scott, & Rubia, 2011; Skogli, Egeland, Andersen, Hovik, & Øie, 2014; Toplak, Jain, & Tannock, 2005), with the exception of one study (Weafer, Milich, & Fillmore, 2011).

Skogli et al. (2014) compared a group of children with ADHD and typically developing controls on performance-based measures of executive function (working memory, inhibition, and cognitive flexibility) and a risky decision-making task (HDT) at two time points, when the participants were 11 and 13 years of age. The authors reported that both groups displayed gains in executive function performance over time, but that the ADHD group continued to perform relatively more poorly than the typically developing control group. Neither group displayed improved performance on the HDT over time, and no group differences were observed on this task. The different developmental patterns with the executive function and risky decision-making tasks support the separation between these domains.

The development of risky decision making in typically developing samples provides an important reference point for efforts to understand this in special populations such as individuals with ADHD. Steinberg (2010) examined IGT performance on a modified version of the original IGT in a typically developing sample ranging from ages 10–30 years. Selections from advantageous and disadvantageous decks were examined separately. A curvilinear relationship with age was reported for selections from the advantageous decks, with an increase between early and midadolescence, then a decline between midadolescence and adulthood. Alternatively, a linear relationship between age and selections from the disadvantageous decks was obtained, indicating a decrease in these selections over time. In a more recent study, pubertal maturation was found to predict selections from advantageous decks (reward approach) on the IGT, whereas age was found to predict selections from disadvantageous decks (cost avoidance) on the IGT in a large cross-sectional sample of adolescents ages 9–17 years (Icenogle et al., 2017). Another paradigm, the Cups Task, has been used to examine risky decision making in typically developing samples. Sensitivity to expected value is varied with risky choices (Weller, Levin, & Denburg, 2011). In this study of participants ranging in age from 5 to 85 years, risky choices were found to decrease in the gain domain, whereas risky choices stayed constant in the loss domain. In addition to these developmental considerations, there is evidence to suggest that reinforcement contingencies may operate differently in individuals with ADHD than in controls (Luman, Oosterlaan, & Sergeant, 2005). It was reported in a follow-up study that boys with ADHD were unaffected by frequency and magnitude of reward relative to typically developing controls on a stimulus–response learning task (Luman, Van Meel, Oosterlaan, Sergeant, & Geurts, 2009). The interface between the development of risky decision making with the possibility of altered reward mechanisms is an area for further research in ADHD.

Some researchers have examined associations between cognitive abilities and risky decision making on laboratory gambling tasks in ADHD. Impaired performance on the risky decision-making tasks was found to be unrelated to cognitive abilities, such as intelligence and executive functions, in samples of ADHD and controls (Toplak et al., 2005; Ernst et al., 2003). These findings are consistent with a review of studies that have examined associations between IGT performance and cognitive abilities across typically developing and special populations, as only a small proportion of these studies reported a significant association (Toplak et al., 2010).

In summary, children and adolescents with ADHD tend to make riskier choices than typically developing youth on risky decision-making tasks. Older youth tend to make fewer risky choices than younger youth, but the developmental trajectory in youth with ADHD is unclear. Like temporal discounting, risky decision making has small to modest correlations with cognitive abilities, indicating that dissociations between these measures may not be uncommon.

Impact of ADHD Presentations/Dimensions and Comorbid Disorders

ADHD-I, ADHD-H, and ADHD-C presentations used to clinically characterize ADHD have been less central in the most recent DSM criteria (DSM-5; American Psychiatric Association, 2013), as literature reviews of ADHD presentations (subtypes) have revealed weak evidence for the distinction between the ADHD-I and ADHD-C presentations, as well as instability of subtype designation in longitudinal studies (Willcutt et al., 2012). In terms of executive function performance, there has been evidence to suggest that the inattentive symptoms, not hyperactive–impulsive symptoms, predicted performance on processing speed, vigilance, and inhibition, but that these differences were not apparent when inattentive and combined subtypes were compared in the analysis (Chhabildas, Pennington, & Willcutt, 2001). Some research in risky decision making has suggested that hyperactive–impulsive symptoms were more related to risky choices on the IGT in adolescents with ADHD, rather than inattentive symptoms (Toplak et al., 2005). The relative contributions of inattention and hyperactive–impulsive symptoms from a dimensional perspective remain an important research question for future investigations, and will likely yield more conclusive patterns than subtype comparisons.

The impact of comorbid disorders may also be importantly related to executive function and decision-making performance. The impact of comorbid disorders is complicated by empirical findings that indicate executive function performance and decision-making differences in several disorders (Pennington & Ozonoff, 1996). Efforts have been made to delineate executive function performance profiles between ADHD and other conditions by directly comparing performance between these groups, including comorbid groups. For example, Purvis and Tannock (1997) reported that children with ADHD displayed difficulties with the organization and monitoring of their storytelling, whereas children with reading disabilities displayed difficulties on receptive and expressive semantic language abilities on language processing tests. Nigg and Huang-Pollock (2003) reported that individuals with CD and ADHD both exhibit inhibition deficits, but that verbal abilities separate CD from ADHD. It is difficult to draw conclusions on the specificity of executive function performance and other comorbid conditions.

In the study of decision-making constructs, the presence of CD and ODD has been examined as relevant comorbidities. On temporal discounting tasks, studies indicate that ADHD and comorbid ODD and CD do not significantly affect results compared to ADHD samples without ODD and CD (Jackson & MacKillop, 2016; Antonini, Becker, Tamm, & Epstein, 2015). Fewer empirical findings are available on ADHD and comorbidity in adolescents in terms of delay of gratification tasks. With regards to risky decision-making tasks, externalizing symptoms may increase risky choices in individuals with ADHD, such as ODD (Luman, Sergeant, Knol, & Oosterlaan, 2010). Dekkers et al. (2016) demonstrated that disruptive behavior disorders (DBD) had a significant moderating influence on risky decision making, as individuals with ADHD and comorbid DBD tended to take more risks than individuals with ADHD alone. Hobson et al. (2011) demonstrated that although adolescents with ADHD and comorbid ODD–CD made riskier choices than adolescents without ADHD, ODD–CD symptoms were independently related to risky decision making, while ADHD symptoms were not.

Summary

Based on the cognitive science literature, we make a conceptual distinction between cognitive abilities (including executive functions and intellectual abilities) and decision making. This conceptual separation allows us to begin understanding why discrepancies between performances may occur on these tasks, such as in ADHD samples. In addition to this conceptual distinction, developmental patterns in both typically and atypically developing samples also provide a basis for understanding why performance on some of these tasks are more related than performance on others.

Adolescents with ADHD tend to perform less well on performance-based measures of executive function than do typically developing youth (Willcutt et al., 2005). Similarly, studies on risky decision making and temporal discounting suggest that individuals with ADHD tend to perform less well (and tend to prioritize immediate rewards rather than wait for a better, delayed choice) compared to typically developing individuals. However, across these constructs, there is considerable variability in performance, indicating that not all individuals with ADHD display executive function deficits and necessarily show lower performance on these decision-making tasks. Developmental changes in cognitive abilities that have been documented in adolescents with ADHD and typically developing youth may also be associated with remission of symptoms in youth with ADHD. The developmental shift from childhood to adolescence, and the shift from adolescence to adulthood, is becoming an increasingly important period for study with respect to decision-making constructs such as temporal discounting and risky decision making. There is evidence to suggest that particular changes in adolescence, such as the onset of puberty, may impact the selection of advantageous versus disadvantageous choices on risky decision-making tasks. These changes in development, coupled with changes in cognitive abilities, offer a lens through which to understand individual differences in ADHD and why some youth may be more impaired or display competence on different indicators of cognitive abilities and decision making.

References

Ainslie, G. (2001). *Breakdown of will.* Cambridge, UK: Cambridge University Press.

Albert, D., & Steinberg, L. (2011). Judgment and decision-making in adolescence. *Journal of Research on Adolescence, 21*(1), 211–224.

American Psychiatric Association. (2013). *Diagnostic and statistical manual of mental disorders* (5th ed.). Arlington, VA: Author.

Antonini, T. N., Becker, S. P., Tamm, L., & Epstein, J. N. (2015). Hot and cool executive functions in children with attention-deficit/hyperactivity disorder and comorbid oppositional defiant disorder. *Journal of the International Neuropsychological Society, 21*(8), 584–595.

Barkley, R. A. (2006). *Attention-deficit hyperactivity disorder: A handbook for diagnosis and treatment* (3rd ed.). New York: Guilford Press.

Barkley, R. A., Edwards, G., Laneri, M., Fletcher, K., & Metevia, L. (2001). Executive functioning, temporal discounting, and sense of time in adolescents with attention deficit hyperactivity disorder (ADHD) and oppositional defiant disorder (ODD). *Journal of Abnormal Child Psychology, 29*(6), 541–556.

Basile, A. G., & Toplak, M. E. (2015). Four converging measures of temporal discounting and their relationships with intelligence, executive functions, thinking dispositions, and behavioral outcomes. *Frontiers in Psychology, 6*(728), 1–13.

Biederman, J., Monuteaux, M. C., Doyle, A. E., Seidman, L. J., Wilens, T. E., Ferrero, F., . . . Faraone, S. V. (2004). Impact of executive function deficits and attention-deficit/hyperactivity disorder (ADHD) on academic outcomes in children. *Journal of Consulting and Clinical Psychology, 72*(5), 757–766.

Bitsakou, P., Psychogiou, L., Thompson, M., & Sonuga-Barke, E. J. (2009). Delay aversion in attention deficit/hyperactivity disorder: An empirical investigation of the broader phenotype. *Neuropsychologia, 47*(2), 446–456.

Blakemore, S. J., & Choudhury, S. (2006). Development of the adolescent brain:

Implications for executive function and social cognition. *Journal of Child Psychology and Psychiatry, 47*(3–4), 296–312.
Brown, T. E. (2005). *Attention deficit disorder: The unfocused mind in children and adolescents*. New Haven, CT: Yale University Press.
Castellanos, F. X., Sonuga-Barke, E. J., Milham, M. P., & Tannock, R. (2006). Characterizing cognition in ADHD: Beyond executive dysfunction. *Trends in Cognitive Sciences, 10*(3), 117–123.
Chhabildas, N., Pennington, B. F., & Willcutt, E. G. (2001). A comparison of the neuropsychological profiles of the DSM-IV subtypes of ADHD. *Journal of Abnormal Child Psychology, 29*(6), 529–540.
Davidson, M. C., Amso, D., Anderson, L. C., & Diamond, A. (2006). Development of cognitive control and executive functions from 4 to 13 years: Evidence from manipulations of memory, inhibition, and task switching. *Neuropsychologia, 44*(11), 2037–2078.
Dekkers, T. J., Popma, A., van Rentergem, J. A. A., Bexkens, A., & Huizenga, H. M. (2016). Risky decision-making in attention-deficit/hyperactivity disorder: A meta-regression analysis. *Clinical Psychology Review, 45*, 1–16.
Dennis, M., Francis, D. J., Cirino, P. T., Schachar, R., Barnes, M. A., & Fletcher, J. M. (2009). Why IQ is not a covariate in cognitive studies of neurodevelopmental disorders. *Journal of the International Neuropsychological Society, 15*(3), 331–343.
Diamond, A. (2013). Executive functions. *Annual Review of Psychology, 64*, 135–168.
Doidge, J. L., Flora, D. B., & Toplak, M. E. (2018). A meta-analytic review of sex differences on delay of gratification and temporal discounting tasks in ADHD and typically developing samples. *Journal of Attention Disorders*. [Epub ahead of print]
Ernst, M., Grant, S. J., London, E. D., Contoreggi, C. S., Kimes, A. S., & Spurgeon, L. (2003). Decision-making in adolescents with behavior disorders and adults with substance abuse. *American Journal of Psychiatry, 160*(1), 33–40.
Faregh, N., & Derevensky, J. (2011). Gambling behavior among adolescents with attention deficit/hyperactivity disorder. *Journal of Gambling Studies, 27*(2), 243–256.
Flory, K., Molina, B. S., Pelham, W. E., Jr., Gnagy, E., & Smith, B. (2006). Childhood ADHD predicts risky sexual behavior in young adulthood. *Journal of Clinical Child and Adolescent Psychology, 35*(4), 571–577.
Frazier, T. W., Demaree, H. A., & Youngstrom, E. A. (2004). Meta-analysis of intellectual and neuropsychological test performance in attention-deficit/hyperactivity disorder. *Neuropsychology, 18*(3), 543–555.
Friedman, N. P., Haberstick, B. C., Willcutt, E. G., Miyake, A., Young, S. E., Corley, R. P., & Hewitt, J. K. (2007). Greater attention problems during childhood predict poorer executive functioning in late adolescence. *Psychological Science, 18*(10), 893–900.
Green, L., Fry, A. F., & Myerson, J. (1994). Discounting of delayed rewards: A life-span comparison. *Psychological Science, 5*(1), 33–36.
Groen, Y., Gaastra, G. F., Lewis-Evans, B., & Tucha, O. (2013). Risky behavior in gambling tasks in individuals with ADHD–a systematic literature review. *PLOS ONE, 8*(9), e74909.
Halperin, J. M. (2016). Editorial: Executive functioning—A key construct for understanding developmental psychopathology or a "catch-all" term in need for some rethinking? *Journal of Child Psychology and Psychiatry, 57*(4), 443–445.
Halperin, J. M., & Schulz, K. P. (2006). Revisiting the role of the prefrontal cortex in the pathophysiology of attention-deficit/hyperactivity disorder. *Psychological Bulletin, 132*(4), 560–581.
Halperin, J. M., Trampush, J. W., Miller, C. J., Marks, D. J., & Newcorn, J. H. (2008). Neuropsychological outcome in adolescents/young adults with childhood ADHD:

Profiles of persisters, remitters and controls. *Journal of Child Psychology and Psychiatry, 49*(9), 958–966.

Hobson, C. W., Scott, S., & Rubia, K. (2011). Investigation of cool and hot executive function in ODD/CD independently of ADHD. *Journal of Child Psychology and Psychiatry, 52*(10), 1035–1043.

Icenogle, G., Steinberg, L., Olino, T. M., Shulman, E. P., Chein, J., Alampay, L. P., . . . Chang, L. (2017). Puberty predicts approach but not avoidance on the Iowa Gambling Task in a multinational sample. *Child Development, 88*(5), 1598–1614.

Jackson, J. N., & MacKillop, J. (2016). Attention-deficit/hyperactivity disorder and monetary delay discounting: A meta-analysis of case-control studies. *Biological Psychiatry: Cognitive Neuroscience and Neuroimaging, 1*(4), 316–325.

Jerome, L., Segal, A., & Habinski, L. (2006). What we know about ADHD and driving risk: A literature review, meta-analysis and critique. *Journal of the Canadian Academy of Child and Adolescent Psychiatry, 15*(3), 105–125.

Jonsdottir, S., Bouma, A., Sergeant, J. A., & Scherder, E. J. (2006). Relationships between neuropsychological measures of executive function and behavioral measures of ADHD symptoms and comorbid behavior. *Archives of Clinical Neuropsychology, 21*(5), 383–394.

Kane, M. J., Brown, L. H., McVay, J. C., Silvia, P. J., Myin-Germeys, I., & Kwapil, T. R. (2007). For whom the mind wanders, and when: An experience-sampling study of working memory and executive control in daily life. *Psychological Science, 18*(7), 614–621.

Kelly, K., & Ramundo, P. (2006). *You mean I'm not lazy, stupid or crazy?!: The classic self-help book for adults with attention deficit disorder.* New York: Scribner.

Kirby, K. (1997). Bidding on the future: Evidence against normative discounting of delayed rewards. *Journal of Experimental Psychology: General, 126*(1), 54–70.

Lambek, R., Tannock, R., Dalsgaard, S., Trillingsgaard, A., Damm, D., & Thomsen, P. H. (2010). Validating neuropsychological subtypes of ADHD: How do children with and without an executive function deficit differ? *Journal of Child Psychology and Psychiatry, 51*(8), 895–904.

Lambek, R., Tannock, R., Dalsgaard, S., Trillingsgaard, A., Damm, D., & Thomsen, P. H. (2011). Executive dysfunction in school-age children with ADHD. *Journal of Attention Disorders, 15*(8), 646–655.

Lamm, C., Zelazo, P. D., & Lewis, M. D. (2006). Neural correlates of cognitive control in childhood and adolescence: Disentangling the contributions of age and executive function. *Neuropsychologia, 44*(11), 2139–2148.

Lee, S. S., Humphreys, K. L., Flory, K., Liu, R., & Glass, K. (2011). Prospective association of childhood attention-deficit/hyperactivity disorder (ADHD) and substance use and abuse/dependence: A meta-analytic review. *Clinical Psychology Review, 31*(3), 328–341.

Logan, G. D., Cowan, W. B., & Davis, K. A. (1984). On the ability to inhibit simple and choice reaction time responses: A model and a method. *Journal of Experimental Psychology: Human Perception and Performance, 10*(2), 276–291.

Loo, S. K., Humphrey, L. A., Tapio, T., Moilanen, I. K., McGough, J. J., McCracken, J. T., . . . Smalley, S. L. (2007). Executive functioning among Finnish adolescents with attention-deficit/hyperactivity disorder. *Journal of the American Academy of Child and Adolescent Psychiatry, 46*(12), 1594–1604.

Luman, M., Oosterlaan, J., & Sergeant, J. A. (2005). The impact of reinforcement contingencies on AD/HD: A review and theoretical appraisal. *Clinical Psychology Review, 25*(2), 183–213.

Luman, M., Sergeant, J. A., Knol, D. L., & Oosterlaan, J. (2010). Impaired decision-making in oppositional defiant disorder related to altered psychophysiological responses to reinforcement. *Biological Psychiatry, 68*(4), 337–344.

Luman, M., Van Meel, C. S., Oosterlaan, J., Sergeant, J. A., & Geurts, H. M. (2009). Does reward frequency or magnitude drive reinforcement-learning in attention-deficit/hyperactivity disorder? *Psychiatry Research, 168*(3), 222–229.

MacLeod, C. M. (1991). Half a century of research on the Stroop effect: An integrative review. *Psychological Bulletin, 109*(2), 163–203.

Marco, R., Miranda, A., Schlotz, W., Melia, A., Mulligan, A., Müller, U., . . . Medad, S. (2009). Delay and reward choice in ADHD: An experimental test of the role of delay aversion. *Neuropsychology, 23*(3), 367–380.

Martel, M., Nikolas, M., & Nigg, J. T. (2007). Executive function in adolescents with ADHD. *Journal of the American Academy of Child and Adolescent Psychiatry, 46*(11), 1437–1444.

Miyake, A., & Friedman, N. P. (2012). The nature and organization of individual differences in executive functions four general conclusions. *Current Directions in Psychological Science, 21*(1), 8–14.

Miyake, A., Friedman, N. P., Emerson, M. J., Witzki, A. H., Howerter, A., & Wager, T. D. (2000). The unity and diversity of executive functions and their contributions to complex "frontal lobe" tasks: A latent variable analysis. *Cognitive Psychology, 41*(1), 49–100.

Mowinckel, A. M., Pedersen, M. L., Eilertsen, E., & Biele, G. (2015). A meta-analysis of decision-making and attention in adults with ADHD. *Journal of Attention Disorders, 19*(5), 355–367.

Murray, A. L., Robinson, T., & Tripp, G. (2017). Neurocognitive and symptom trajectories of ADHD from childhood to early adolescence. *Journal of Developmental and Behavioral Pediatrics, 38*(7), 465–475.

Nigg, J. T., & Huang-Pollock, C. L. (2003). An early-onset model of the role of executive functions and intelligence in conduct disorder/delinquency. In B. B. Lahey, T. E. Moffitt, & A. Caspi (Eds.), *Cause of conduct disorder and juvenile delinquency* (pp. 227–253). New York: Guilford Press.

Nigg, J. T., Stavro, G., Ettenhofer, M., Hambrick, D. Z., Miller, T., & Henderson, J. M. (2005). Executive functions and ADHD in adults: Evidence for selective effects on ADHD symptom domains. *Journal of Abnormal Psychology, 114*(4), 706–717.

Paloyelis, Y., Asherson, P., Mehta, M. A., Faraone, S. V., & Kuntsi, J. (2010). DAT1 and COMT effects on delay discounting and trait impulsivity in male adolescents with attention deficit/hyperactivity disorder and healthy controls. *Neuropsychopharmacology, 35*(12), 2414–2426.

Patros, C. H., Alderson, R. M., Kasper, L. J., Tarle, S. J., Lea, S. E., & Hudec, K. L. (2016). Choice-impulsivity in children and adolescents with attention-deficit/hyperactivity disorder (ADHD): A meta-analytic review. *Clinical Psychology Review, 43,* 162–174.

Pennington, B. F., & Ozonoff, S. (1996). Executive functions and developmental psychopathology. *Journal of Child Psychology and Psychiatry, 37*(1), 51–87.

Pratt, T. C., Cullen, F. T., Blevins, K. R., Daigle, L., & Unnever, J. D. (2002). The relationship of attention deficit hyperactivity disorder to crime and delinquency: A meta-analysis. *International Journal of Police Science and Management, 4*(4), 344–360.

Prencipe, A., Kesek, A., Cohen, J., Lamm, C., Lewis, M. D., & Zelazo, P. D. (2011). Development of hot and cool executive function during the transition to adolescence. *Journal of Experimental Child Psychology, 108*(3), 621–637.

Purvis, K. L., & Tannock, R. J. (1997). Language abilities in children with attention deficit hyperactivity disorder, reading disabilities, and normal controls. *Journal of Abnormal Child Psychology, 25*(2), 133–144.

Reitan, R. M. (1971). Trail making test results for normal and brain-damaged children. *Perceptual and Motor Skills, 33*(2), 575–581.

Reyna, V. F., & Farley, F. (2006). Risk and rationality in adolescent decision-making: Implications for theory, practice, and public policy. *Psychological Science, 7*(1), 1–44.

Rizeq, J., Flora, D. B., & Toplak, M. E. (2017). Changing relations among cognitive abilities across development: Implications for measurement and research. *Clinical Neuropsychologist, 31*(8), 1353–1374.

Sagvolden, T., Johansen, E. B., Aase, H., & Russell, V. A. (2005). A dynamic developmental theory of attention-deficit/hyperactivity disorder (ADHD) predominantly hyperactive/impulsive and combined subtypes. *Behavioral and Brain Sciences, 28*(3), 430–440.

Salthouse, T. A., Atkinson, T. M., & Berish, D. E. (2003). Executive functioning as a potential mediator of age-related cognitive decline in normal adults. *Journal of Experimental Psychology: General, 132*(4), 566–594.

Salthouse, T. A., & Davis, H. P. (2006). Organization of cognitive abilities and neuropsychological variables across the lifespan. *Developmental Review, 26*(1), 31–54.

Schachar, R., & Logan, G. D. (1990). Impulsivity and inhibitory control in normal development and childhood psychopathology. *Developmental Psychology, 26*(5), 710–720.

Seidman, L. J. (2006). Neuropsychological functioning in people with ADHD across the lifespan. *Clinical Psychology Review, 26*(4), 466–485.

Sergeant, J. A., Geurts, H., Huijbregts, S., Scheres, A., & Oosterlaan, J. (2003). The top and the bottom of ADHD: A neuropsychological perspective. *Neuroscience and Biobehavioral Reviews, 27*(7), 583–592.

Shamosh, N. A., DeYoung, C. G., Green, A. E., Reis, D. L., Johnson, M. R., Conway, A. R., . . . Gray, J. R. (2008). Individual differences in delay discounting: Relation to intelligence, working memory, and anterior prefrontal cortex. *Psychological Science, 19*(9), 904–911.

Shamosh, N. A., & Gray, J. R. (2008). Delay discounting and intelligence: A meta-analysis. *Intelligence, 36*(4), 289–305.

Skogli, E. W., Egeland, J., Andersen, P. N., Hovik, K. T., & Øie, M. (2014). Few differences in hot and cold executive functions in children and adolescents with combined and inattentive subtypes of ADHD. *Child Neuropsychology, 20*(2), 162–181.

Solanto, M. V., Abikoff, H., Sonuga-Barke, E., Schachar, R., Logan, G. D., Wigal, T., . . . Turkel, E. (2001). The ecological validity of delay aversion and response inhibition as measures of impulsivity in AD/HD: A supplement to the NIMH multimodal treatment study of AD/HD. *Journal of Abnormal Child Psychology, 29*(3), 215–228.

Sonuga-Barke, E. (2002). Psychological heterogeneity in AD/HD—A dual pathway model of behavior and cognition. *Behavioural Brain Research, 130*(1–2), 29–36.

Sonuga-Barke, E., Bitsakou, P., & Thompson, M. (2010). Beyond the dual pathway model: Evidence for the dissociation of timing, inhibitory, and delay-related impairments in attention-deficit/hyperactivity disorder. *Journal of the American Academy of Child and Adolescent Psychiatry, 49*(4), 345–355.

Sonuga-Barke, E. J. S., & Fairchild, G. (2012). Neuroeconomics of attention-deficit/hyperactivity disorder: Differential influences of medial, dorsal, and ventral prefrontal brain networks on suboptimal decision-making? *Biological Psychiatry, 72*(2), 126–133.

Sonuga-Barke, E. J. S., Sergeant, J. A., Nigg, J., & Willcutt, E. (2008). Executive dysfunction and delay aversion in attention deficit hyperactivity disorder: Nosologic and diagnostic implications. *Child and Adolescent Psychiatric Clinics of North America, 17*(2), 367–384.

Sonuga-Barke, E. J. S., Taylor, E., Sembi, S., & Smith, J. (1992). Hyperactivity and delay aversion—I. The effect of delay on choice. *Journal of Child Psychology and Psychiatry, 33*(2), 387–398.

Soreni, N., Crosbie, J., Ickowicz, A., & Schachar, R. (2009). Stop signal and Conners' continuous performance tasks: Test–retest reliability of two inhibition measures in ADHD children. *Journal of Attention Disorders, 13*(2), 137–143.

Stanovich, K. E. (1999). *Who is rational?: Studies of individual differences in reasoning.* Mahwah, NJ: Erlbaum.

Stanovich, K. E. (2009a). *What intelligence tests miss: The psychology of rational thought.* New Haven, CT: Yale University Press.

Stanovich, K. E. (2009b). Distinguishing the reflective, algorithmic, and autonomous minds: Is it time for a tri-process theory? In J. Evans & K. Frankish (Eds.), *In two minds: Dual processes and beyond* (pp. 55–88). Oxford, UK: Oxford University Press.

Stanovich, K. E. (2011). *Rationality and the reflective mind.* Oxford, UK: Oxford University Press.

Stanovich, K. E., & West, R. F. (2008). On the relative independence of thinking biases and cognitive ability. *Journal of Personality and Social Psychology, 94*(4), 672–695.

Stanovich, K. E., West, R. F., & Toplak, M. E. (2012). Judgment and decision-making in adolescence: Separating intelligence from rationality. In V. Reyna, S. Chapman, M. Dougherty, & J. Confrey (Eds.), *The adolescent brain: Learning, reasoning, and decision-making* (pp. 337–378). Washington, DC: American Psychological Association.

Steinberg, L. (2010). A dual systems model of adolescent risk-taking. *Developmental Psychobiology, 52*(3), 216–224.

Steinberg, L., Graham, S., O'Brien, L., Woolard, J., Cauffman, E., & Banich, M. (2009). Age differences in future orientation and delay discounting. *Child Development, 80*(1), 28–44.

Sternberg, R. J. (2002). *Why smart people can be so stupid.* New Haven, CT: Yale University Press.

Stroop, J. R. (1935). Studies of interference in serial verbal reactions. *Journal of Experimental Psychology, 18*(6), 643–662.

Toplak, M. E., Hosseini, A., & Basile, A. G. (2016). Temporal discounting and associations with cognitive abilities and ADHD-related difficulties in a developmental sample. In M. E. Toplak & J. Weller (Eds.), *Individual differences in judgment and decision making: A developmental perspective* (pp. 85–106). London: Psychology Press.

Toplak, M. E., Jain, U., & Tannock, R. (2005). Executive and motivational processes in adolescents with attention deficit-hyperactivity disorder (ADHD). *Behavioral and Brain Functions, 1*(1), 8.

Toplak, M. E., Sorge, G. B., Benoit, A., West, R. F., & Stanovich, K. E. (2010). Decision-making and cognitive abilities: A review of associations between Iowa Gambling Task performance, executive functions, and intelligence. *Clinical Psychology Review, 30*(5), 562–581.

Toplak, M. E., West, R. F., & Stanovich, K. E. (2011). The Cognitive Reflection Test as a predictor of performance on heuristics and biases tasks. *Memory and Cognition, 39*(7), 1275–1289.

Toplak, M. E., West, R. F., & Stanovich, K. E. (2013). Practitioner Review: Do performance-based measures and ratings of executive function assess the same construct? *Journal of Child Psychology and Psychiatry, 54*(2), 131–143.

van Lieshout, M., Luman, M., Buitelaar, J., Rommelse, N. N. J., & Oosterlaan, J. (2013). Does neurocognitive functioning predict future or persistence of ADHD?: A systematic review. *Clinical Psychology Review, 33*(4), 539–560.

Vloet, T. D., Marx, I., Kahraman-Lanzerath, B., Zepf, F. D., Herpertz-Dahlmann, B., & Konrad, K. (2010). Neurocognitive performance in children with ADHD and OCD. *Journal of Abnormal Child Psychology, 38*(7), 961–969.

Weafer, J., Milich, R., & Fillmore, M. T. (2011). Behavioral components of impulsivity predict alcohol consumption in adults with ADHD and healthy controls. *Drug and Alcohol Dependence, 113*(2), 139–146.

Weller, J. A., Levin, I. P., & Denburg, N. L. (2011). Trajectory of risky decision-making for potential gains and losses from ages 5 to 85. *Journal of Behavioral Decision Making, 24*(4), 331–344.

Willcutt, E. G., Doyle, A. E., Nigg, J. T., Faraone, S. V., & Pennington, B. F. (2005). Validity of the executive function theory of attention-deficit/hyperactivity disorder: A meta-analytic review. *Biological Psychiatry, 57*(11), 1336–1346.

Willcutt, E. G., Nigg, J. T., Pennington, B. F., Solanto, M. V., Rohde, L. A., Tannock, R., . . . Lahey, B. B. (2012). Validity of DSM-IV attention deficit/hyperactivity disorder symptom dimensions and subtypes. *Journal of Abnormal Psychology, 121*(4), 991–1010.

Zelazo, P. D., & Carlson, S. M. (2012). Hot and cool executive function in childhood and adolescence: Development and plasticity. *Child Development Perspectives, 6*(4), 354–360.

CHAPTER 5

Emotion Regulation in Adolescents with ADHD

Nóra Bunford

Emotion regulation, broadly conceptualized, is the process by which an emotional state is modified either in that is it attenuated/decreased or that it is increased/strengthened (Cole, Marin, & Dennis, 2004). Emotion *dys*regulation (ED) occurs when any of the processes involved in the emotion regulatory process—physiological, experiential, or behavioral—are excessive or insufficient given short- or long-term adaptation[1] goals. ED is transdiagnostic, in that it is associated with externalizing (e.g., oppositional defiant disorder [ODD]), internalizing (e.g., anxiety, depression), and neurodevelopmental disorders (Bunford, Evans, & Wymbs, 2015; Mazefsky et al., 2013). Attention-deficit/hyperactivity disorder (ADHD) is one neurodevelopmental disorder with which ED is associated (Bunford et al., 2017; Bunford, Evans, & Langberg, 2014; Bunford, Evans, Becker, & Langberg, 2015; Graziano & Garcia, 2016; Okado & Mueller, 2016; Sjöwall, Backman, & Thorell, 2015), and the association between ADHD and ED in adolescence—from the perspectives of conceptualization, relation to functional impairments and negative outcomes, measurement, and intervention—is the focus of this chapter.

[1] *Adaptation,* as I intend to use it here, is a phenotypic trait or process of an organism that allows it to successfully meet environmental challenges and survive in its ecological niche.

EMOTION REGULATION AND ED IN ASSOCIATION WITH ADHD

As ED is transdiagnostic, some manifestations of it are shared across disorders and others are unique to specific disorders (Bunford, Evans, & Wymbs, 2015). In the case of ADHD, although differences across definitions exist, in accordance with a recent conceptualization building on Barkley's (2010) pioneering theory and successive empirical research,

> emotion regulation is an individual's ability to modulate (1) the speed with which and degree to which the physiological, experiential, and behavioral expression of an emotion escalates, (2) the intensity of the physiological, experiential, and behavioral expression of an emotion, and (3) the speed with which and degree to which physiological, experiential, and behavioral expression of an emotion deescalates in a manner congruent with an optimal level of functioning. (Bunford, Evans, & Wymbs, 2015, p. 188)

In turn, ED is any dysfunction in emotion regulation that is associated with functional impairment. As such,

> emotion dysregulation is an individual's inability to exercise any or all aspects of the emotion regulation modulatory processes, to such a degree that the inability results in the individual failing to successfully adapt to and meet environmental challenges and goals and thus functioning meaningfully below his or her baseline. (p. 188)

The specific manifestation or pattern of ED varies inter- and intraindividually across development or different situations. In addition, any given individual's emotional baseline may change over time (Fruzzetti, Shenk, & Hoffman, 2005). (For additional discussion and examples, see Bunford, Evans, & Wymbs, 2015.)

EMOTION REGULATION ACROSS DEVELOPMENT

Acquiring age-appropriate emotion regulatory skills is an important task across development. Although from infancy through middle toddlerhood, a meaningful portion of emotion regulation is external to the child (i.e., a mother or other caregiver soothes the infant or toddler) (Bowlby, 1969, 1973), during the preschool years, an increase in adult–child coregulation (Cole, Michel, & Teti, 1994), accompanied by a differentiation and diversification of emotion expression and regulation skills (Kopp, 1989), is observable. By middle childhood, owing in part to changes in cognitive, perceptual, and verbal skills, emotion regulation primarily takes the form of child self-regulation (Coyne & Downey, 1991). Middle childhood ends around puberty, which marks the beginning of adolescence. By the time they reach adolescence, typically developing teens are equipped with multiple ways to express and regulate their emotions and are able to receive and integrate feedback on their emotion expression and regulation into their behavioral repertoires (Bunford & Evans, 2017). Although deficits in emotion regulation can have a significant impact on children's ability to function in school and socially, adolescence is a period that is unique *insofar as* the reasons underlying how and why ED can be impairing as well as some of the consequences or correlates of ED.

Adolescence, ED, and ADHD: Overlapping Biological and Psychosocial Vulnerabilities

Regarding how and why ED can be impairing in adolescence, first, teens experience more psychological turmoil than do children and adults, and this often manifests in intense and labile emotions (Silk, Steinberg, & Morris, 2003). Second, these (turmoil and emotions) occur in a context wherein asynchronicity between brain development and self-regulatory (behavioral, cognitive, and emotional) skills development is combined with decreased input from the adults (e.g., parents, teachers) who had previously provided regulatory guidance and structure, and with increased environmental demands for self-regulation (Steinberg, 2005). This asynchronicity, decreased input, and increased demands correspond in turn to suboptimal actions and decisions that result in a host of negative outcomes, such as increased incidence of unintentional injuries and pregnancy, violence, and of alcohol and other drug misuse and sexually transmitted diseases (Casey, Jones, & Hare, 2008).

Some of the brain regions that undergo the most prolonged and striking changes during adolescence—summarized next—are the ones associated with emotion processing, including emotion recognition and regulation. Specifically, there appears to be differential development of bottom-up limbic systems, implicated in emotional and incentive processing, to top-down control systems during the teenage years (Arain et al., 2013).

Regarding relevant biological changes in adolescence, first, there is a second surge of synaptogenesis (dendritic pruning and myelinogenesis) during the teenage years, making adolescence one of the most dynamic periods of human development and growth, second only to infancy in terms of the rate of developmental changes in the brain (Arain et al., 2013). Second, neurocircuitry remains structurally and functionally unstable, in part due to vulnerability to considerable increases in sex hormones (i.e., estrogen, progesterone, and testosterone). Indeed, a significant portion of brain development and growth in adolescence is the construction and strengthening of regional neurocircuitry and pathways, manifesting, in particular, as active maturation of the basal ganglia, cerebellum, occipital lobe, parietal lobe, temporal lobe, and—as perhaps most characteristically and frequently cited—frontal lobe (Arain et al., 2013). Third, neurotransmission (e.g., gamma-aminobutyric acid [GABA]), particularly in the prefrontal cortex, remains under construction, and there is a decrease in dopamine (resulting in difficulty with emotion regulation and mood swings) and serotonin (resulting in decreased impulse control) levels (Arain et al., 2013).

The processes and systems in which these changes occur are not only relevant to adolescence, but, as noted earlier, are also implicated in ED (Arain et al., 2013) and, what is more, in some of the psychiatric disorders with which ED is associated, such as ADHD. For example, several candidate genes for ADHD are involved in synaptogenesis and neuronal alignment and adhesion. Indeed, it has been suggested that altered synaptic extinction and reinforcement is related to characterization of an endophenotype of ADHD that can be dimensionally related to differences in inattention, hyperactivity, and impulsivity levels (Vadalá, Giugni, Pichiecchio, Balottin, & Bastianello, 2011).

Furthermore, neuroscience studies show abnormalities in a number of brain areas implicated in the frontostriatal circuit in ADHD, with structural and functional abnormalities in the basal ganglia—in particular the caudate (Semrud-Clikeman et al., 2000) and globus pallidus (Castellanos et al., 2001; Castellanos, Giedd, Hamburger, Marsh, & Rapoport, 1996). Importantly, the basal ganglia are also implicated in (motor and) emotion regulation (Johnson, Hurley, Benkelfat, Herpertz, & Taber, 2003). The frontolimbic system is also implicated in ADHD, although it is currently unclear whether the primary deficit in that system is bottom-up (e.g., associated primarily with the amygdala), reflects poor emotion processing (Herrmann et al., 2009; Williams et al., 2008), and thus constitutes a "lower" level dysfunction; or is top-down (e.g., associated with lateral and medial prefrontal cortex and anterior cingulate cortex, as suggested perhaps by the findings mentioned earlier) and constitutes a higher-order processing or regulatory problem (Bush, Valera, & Seidman, 2005; Krauel et al., 2007). The frontolimbic system is also implicated in the generation and regulation of emotions (Banks, Eddy, Angstadt, Nathan, & Phan, 2007). As final examples, associations have been observed between ADHD and reduced GABA concentration in primary motor and somatosensory cortices (Edden, Crocetti, Zhu, Gilbert, & Mostofsky, 2012), abnormal dopaminergic functioning in multiple brain regions (Forssberg, Fernell, Waters, Waters, & Tedroff, 2006) and lower dopamine (D_2 and D_3) receptor availability in the left caudate (Volkow et al., 2007). In addition, variations at the serotonin transporter gene have been shown to influence susceptibility to ADHD (Kent et al., 2002). As with the frontostriatal and frontolimbic systems, these neurostransmitters are also implicated in emotion regulation and ED (GABA: Thayer & Lane, 2000; dopamine: Laviolette, 2007; serotonin transporter gene: Canli & Lesch, 2007).

In combination with key biological changes during adolescence, the overlap between ED and ADHD in etiological considerations (e.g., with regard to brain regions and processes implicated) and in the consequences or associated features thereof during this developmental phase, such as immature and impulsive behavior, alcohol and drug misuse, and risky behavior (e.g., risky driving and sex) is striking and underscore the clinical and scientific significance of the co-occurrence of the two phenomena in teens.

ED, ADHD, and Relevant Outcomes

Despite key links between ED and ADHD, there is relatively little research on the association between ED and ADHD in adolescents, or on the relation of that association to functional impairment or negative outcomes. Findings that could be relevant or informative for the next generation of studies in this area can be categorized into three main groups: data linking the same phenomenon (e.g., aggression, family conflict, or romantic difficulties) to both ED and ADHD but not to ED in an ADHD sample specifically; data linking the same phenomenon to ED in a nonadolescent ADHD sample; and data indicating that ED is associated with functional impairment or a negative outcome, above and beyond symptoms of the disorder, in an adolescent ADHD sample. Prior to summarizing the pertinent findings in the indicated order, a discussion of the clinical or phenotypic manifestation of ED in youth with ADHD may be helpful in placing the considered functional impairments and negative outcomes into context.

Some youth with ADHD have been described in the literature as being prone to excessive displays of both negative and positive emotions. These descriptions include characterizations of these youth as being emotionally immature, overly exuberant, rambunctious, and as having low tolerance for anger and frustration (Barkley, 2010; Barkley, Anastopoulos, Guevremont, & Fletcher, 1992; Henker & Whalen, 1989; Hoy, Weiss, Minde, & Cohen, 1978; Landau & Moore, 1991). In our clinical experience, this overexcitability in response to negative and/or positive emotions is often paired with emotional intensity that is atypical for the youth's age- and/or gender group or inappropriate for the provocation or the situation. Furthermore, when experiencing such intense emotion, it takes some youth with ADHD longer to alter the course or intensity of the emotion and its expression than socially and situationally appropriate. These elements of ED result in some youth with ADHD exhibiting behavioral displays of emotions that are disruptive, offensive, developmentally inappropriate (most often immature), or incongruent with environmental and situational demands. As such, it is not surprising that ED, in association with ADHD, confers risk for a host of functional impairments and negative outcomes. Although some of these have already received empirical attention and are detailed next, it stands to reason that there are additional impairments and outcomes worthy of research and clinical focus (e.g., academic and occupational functioning).

First, both ADHD and ED are associated with aggression (physical and verbal); family conflict and problems (e.g., more stressful and conflicted family environments, poorer parenting practices); romantic difficulties (e.g., decreased romantic relationship satisfaction, intimate partner violence); and risky behaviors, including risky sexual (e.g., greater number of lifetime sexual partners, frequency of sex with strangers and failure to use condoms, or having sex with someone under the influence of alcohol/drugs; Bunford, Evans, & Wymbs, 2015) and driving behavior (ADHD: Fischer, Barkley, Smallish, & Fletcher, 2007; ED: Ŝeibokaité, Endriulaitiené, Sullman, Markŝaityté, & Žardeckaité–Matulaitiené, 2017; Trógolo, Melchior, & Medrano, 2014). Yet the the impact of ED, above and beyond ADHD, on these outcomes (i.e., aggression, family conflict and problems, romantic difficulties, and risky behaviors) has not been examined, including in adolescents. This is a noteworthy limitation of the literature, as some of these outcomes are especially relevant in adolescence. For instance, it is during the teenage years that youth debut the dating world and begin experiencing romantic relationships (see McQuade, Chapter 7, this volume), and begin learning to drive (see Garner, Chapter 12, this volume). Equally importantly, the noted biological changes during adolescence and the asynchronicity thereof with affective and cognitive development negatively impact decision making and thus often contribute to risky behaviors. Specifically, the changing neurocircuitry and neural plasticity increase adolescents' vulnerability to making improper decisions (e.g., via increasing difficulty to engage in critical and rational thinking prior to making complex decisions; Arain et al., 2013).

Second, in addition to ample research indicating that both ADHD and ED are associated with alcohol and other substance abuse and misuse, the data suggest that among adults and young adults at-risk for/with ADHD, emotional lability (i.e., involving overly frequent and excessive behavioral displays of emotions and mood), a characteristic related to ED, is associated with alcohol misuse and cigarette smoking (Bunford, Wymbs, Dawson, & Shorey, 2017; Mitchell et al., 2012). Regarding alcohol misuse, childhood emotional neglect has been shown to increase risk for alcohol problems in young adults at-risk for ADHD who exhibit high/very high emotional lability, but not for those who exhibit very low–moderate levels. Furthermore, in the same sample, childhood emotional abuse decreased risk for alcohol problems among men very low–low on emotional lability but not among men who who are moderate–very high on emotional lability, or among women (Bunford, Wymbs, et al., 2017). In another sample, a positive association was observed between ADHD symptoms and an attempt to increase (i.e., up-regulate) positive emotions via cigarette smoking (Mitchell et al., 2012). Although these data certainly indicate progress in this area of research, the impact of ED on alcohol misuse or cigarette smoking has not been examined in adolescents with ADHD, and there is no research on the degree to which ED, in association with ADHD, increases risk for drug use, despite the documented greater prevalence of drug and polysubstance use in youth with ADHD, relative to youth without ADHD (Molina & Pelham, 2003; see Kennedy, McKone, & Molina, Chapter 11, this volume).

Third, ED, in association with ADHD, is related to social impairment such as that in peer relationships and prosocial behaviors. In two observational studies involving experimental paradigms aimed to elicit disappointment and frustration, observable ED conferred risk for parent and teacher ratings of social status in children with ADHD (Maedgen & Carlson, 2000; Melnick & Hinshaw, 2000). Across two other studies, three aspects of ED, namely, low threshold for emotional excitability/impatience, behavioral dyscontrol in the face of strong emotions, and inflexibility/slow return to baseline, predicted parent- and self-rated social skills and parent-rated social problems, above and beyond comorbid ODD (Bunford, Evans, Becker, et al., 2015; Bunford et al., 2018). Potential next steps in this line of research include, of course, replication and also assessment of the observed relationships using other measures of the same type (e.g., other rating scales) or of different types (e.g., brain circuit or physiological indicators of emotion regulation). Similarly, the concept of social functioning is complex, and one of the most pervasive and primary domains of impairment in individuals with ADHD, and investigations of the relationship of ED to indices of social functioning should be expanded to include measures reflecting the broad social functioning construct, such as taking part in home life; interacting with family members and peers; making friends; developing and exercising physical, cognitive and social skills; attending school; abiding by rules at home and at school; and pursuing spare-time interests (John, 2001). As examples, measured indices might include ones of social competence and motivation, focusing beyond social skills and problems on beliefs and goals that lead to adaptive and maladaptive functioning.

Relatedly, a domain of functioning that, albeit highly relevant, has received little to no attention in the literature to date on ED in association with ADHD in adolescents, is peer victimization. This may be a fruitful area of inqury, as there is considerable evidence that youth and adults with ADHD have a higher tendency to be both perpetrators and victims than their typically developing counterparts (Wiener & Mak, 2008; Wymbs, Dawson, Suhr, Bunford, & Gidycz, 2017). Furthermore, some literature indicates that characteristics related to ED, such as anger, aggression, and behavioral self-regulation (Hanish et al., 2004), emotional lability and reactivity (Rosen, Milich, & Harris, 2012), and negative affectivity

(Fogleman, Walerius, Rosen, & Leaberry, 2016) are potent risk factors for the development and maintenance of chronic peer victimization in children and adolescents, including children with ADHD (Fogleman et al., 2016). Given these findings obtained with characteristics related to ED and with children, and the finding that chronic peer victimization becomes increasingly stable over time (Scholte, Engels, Overbeek, De Kemp, & Haselager, 2007), there is reason to believe that ED, in association with ADHD, confers risk for peer victimization among adolescents. Future research studies would benefit from a focus on these associations.

Also relevant here is the association between ADHD and other commonly co-occurring psychiatric disorders and between ED and these same disorders. Anxiety disorders, bipolar disorder, depression, ODD, and conduct disorder are among the disorders that have a relatively high prevalence, and frequently co-occur with ADHD (see Becker & Fogleman, Chapter 9, this volume) and are associated with various manifestations of ED. Although it is more common for children with ADHD and comorbid psychopathologies than for children with ADHD alone to exhibit ED (Factor, Reyes, & Rosen, 2014) and there is within-ADHD group comorbidity-related heterogeneity in ED (Karalunas et al., 2014), there have only been two studies to date where the relationship between ED and a comorbid psychiatric disorder was explicitly examined (i.e., the comorbid psychiatric disorder or symptoms were not simply included as a covariate) in adolescents with ADHD, and both focused on depression as the co-occurring disorder (with both controlling for ODD symptoms in data analyses). In one of these studies (with a clinical sample diagnosed with ADHD; Bunford, Evans, Becker, et al., 2015), the negative association between ADHD and social skills was mediated by ED. This indirect effect was relevant for youth with nonclinical and subclinical depression but not for adolescents with clinical depression. In the other study with a community sample (i.e., nondiagnosed ADHD sample; Seymour, Chronis-Tuscano, Iwamoto, Kurdziel, & MacPherson, 2014), some participants were children, whereas others were young adolescents at the time of enrollment; however, because all were followed for 3 years and even the youngest reached young adolescence by the time of the third year, I include this study among ones conducted with adolescents with ADHD. Here, findings indicated that ED measured during the second year of the study mediated the relationship between first-year ADHD symptoms (dimensionally) and third-year depression symptoms, accounting for first-year depression symptoms.

In terms of implications of the first study, it may be that depression moderated the mediational effect, because there are characteristics of depression that overshadow the negative effects of ED on social skills in youth with ADHD. Indeed, depression has been shown to exacerbate social problems among youth with ADHD (Becker, Langberg, Evans, Girio-Herrera, & Vaughn, 2015; Daviss, 2008), and its presence necessitates more intensive interventions (McQuade, Hoza, Murray-Close, Waschbusch, & Owens, 2011). Relatedly, though following a slightly different conceptualization, it may be that the "overshadowing" by depression is not a result of the effect of depression being so strong that an effect of ED cannot be detected. Rather, the overshadowing may be a result of some overlap between symptoms of depression (i.e., a mood disorder) and ED (i.e., deficits in regulating emotions). Accordingly, there is some evidence for a "nonspecific ED factor" that is common across externalizing and internalizing disorders (Silk et al., 2003). Youth with a depressive disorder exhibit poor emotional understanding, low self-efficacy to regulate emotions, and difficulties coping with and expressing anger (Zeman, Cassano, Perry-Parrish, & Stegall, 2006). It may be that the more severe the depression, the greater the overlap between ED and depression and thus the overshadowing at clinical but not at the nonclinical or subclinical levels. In combination with the results of the first study, the implications of the second study are that over time, there may be a bidirectional or reciprocal effect between ED and depression, when occurring in the context of ADHD (and that is why there is evidence both for depression as a moderator of the ADHD–ED relationship and for ED as a mediator of the ADHD–depression relationship), where, depending on study design or research question, ED first confers risk for depression (as indicated in the younger [M_{age} = 11.00; SD = 0.81 years with range of 9–12] sample of Seymour et al., 2014), but then depression confers risk for ED or modulates its effect on outcomes (as indicated in the older [M_{age} = 12.15; SD = 0.95 years with range of 10–14] sample of Bunford, Evans, Becker, et al., 2015).

Regardless of which (if either and not both) interpretation is correct, considerably more research is needed on the relation between ED and disorders commonly comorbid with ADHD in adolescents with ADHD. For example, adolescence is a core risk phase for the development of anxiety symptoms and syndromes, ranging from transient mild symptoms to full-blown anxiety disorders (Beesdo, Knappe, & Pine, 2011). Similarly, the incidence of depression rises sharply after puberty (Thapar, Collishaw, Pine, & Thapar, 2012). ED, in combination with these comorbidities, may complicate the clinical picture and prognosis.

Subtype-Based Differences

Another phenomenon that is highly relevant to any discussion of the association of ADHD with ED is that of ADHD subtype-based differences in ED. According to some conceptualizations, ED may vary as a function of ADHD subtype. For example, in Barkley's (1997) comprehensive neuropsychological model of ADHD, all individuals with ADHD exhibit a primary deficit in inhibition, and those with the hyperactive–impulsive (HI) and combined subtypes but not those with the inattentive subtype (IA) also exhibit secondary deficits in the self-regulation of affect, motivation, and arousal (i.e., ED). Similarly, Sonuga-Barke (2002) argues that HI symptoms reflect deficits in "hot" executive functions (consistent with ED), whereas IA symptoms reflect deficits in "cool" functions (see Bunford, Brandt, et al., 2015, for a review). The implication of these conceptualizations is that the association between ADHD and ED is relevant for the HI and combined subtypes but not the IA subtype, and this is exactly what Barkley explicitly argued in a more recent theoretical article (Barkley, 2010).

Although some empirical findings support this conceptualization, others do not. While Maedgen and Carlson (2000) found that *children* with ADHD-C, but not children with ADHD-IA, exhibit ED, our group (Bunford et al., 2018) found no differences between subtypes in a sample of young adolescents with ADHD. In considering ADHD symptoms dimensionally, Seymour et al. (2014) found that both HI and IA symptoms in the first year of the study had an indirect effect on third-year depression through second-year ED, yet IA was a less robust predictor than HI of second-year ED. There are several plausible explanations of these differences in results. For example, there may be third variables, such as age and measurement modality, that explain the discrepant results across studies. The findings of Maedgen and Carlson (2000) indicate a subtype difference with data obtained with 8- to 11-year-old children; those of Seymour et al. (2014) indicate some but less convincing evidence for a bona fide subtype difference with data obtained with 9- to 12- and 11- to 14-year-old young adolescents, and our findings suggest a lack of subtype difference with data collected from 12- to 16-year-old adolescents. Given that changes in context, expectations, and maturation are associated with differences in the manifestation of ADHD symptoms in childhood versus adolescence (Langberg et al., 2008; Wolraich et al., 2005), it may be that ED also manifests differently across development (i.e., from childhood through young adolescence into middle adolescence) in youth with ADHD where in childhood it is more differentiated across subtypes, with this differentiation decreasing over development and time.

Another reason for the discrepancy across results, as we argued earlier (Bunford et al., 2018), may be that different situations elicit ED in different subtypes. Specifically, the laboratory task employed by Maedgen and Carlson (2000) might elicit ED but not in a manner that is representative of the multiple contexts of a youth's day. When a greater number of situations is sampled, such as with a rating scale (which is how we and Seymour and colleagues [2014] measured ED), ED may be detectable in more than one subtype. It may also be that although there are distinct etiological contributions to and behavioral manifestation of ED across subtypes (Nigg, 2010), the phenomenological experience of ED captured by a rating scale is comparable or the same. Regardless of the reasons behind inconsistencies in the literature, it is a serious limitation in this area of research that most authors of empirical studies focused on ED, in association with ADHD, fail to examine subtype-based differences. The findings of a recent meta-analysis, for example, indicate that 61 of the 77 included studies did not address the ED and ADHD-subtype question whatsoever (Graziano & Garcia, 2016).

Etiological and Maintaining Factors

Understanding what causes something—or at least partially accounts for its emergence—allows for understanding of the degree to which it is malleable (e.g., changeable via prevention or treatment) and of potentially less versus more useful approaches to intervention. Thus, although largely speculative given the state of the science, a discussion of the etiological and maintaining factors related to ED in association with ADHD is warranted. Although much is known about etiological and maintaining factors of ED, when it occurs in the context of certain disorders, little is known about these factors specifically in the case of ADHD. Although it is certainly a reasonable hypothesis that some of the etiological contributors and maintaining factors of ED overlap across disorders, the differences in the way in which it manifests across these indicate that there are at least some differences in what causes and what sustains it.

The ensuing discussion will rely on both the (meager) empirical evidence on the etiology of ED in ADHD and also on theory on its development and maintenance in borderline personality disorder (BPD). I argue, in essence, that there is a biological vulnerability among youth with ADHD to develop difficulties with emotion regulation, and this interacts with environmental influences to produce differences in the emotion regulation phenotype. To describe relevant environmental influences, I chose to rely on the theory on ED in BPD not only because of its clarity and elegance but also because of connectedness and similarities between ADHD and BPD. Specifically, approximately half of children with ADHD continue to exhibit clinically significant symptoms in adulthood, accompanied by psychiatric comorbidities, with BPD encountered more often than expected by chance (Bernardi et al., 2012). One explanatory hypothesis about this greater-than-chance co-occurrence is that ADHD and BPD are distinct disorders sharing common genetic and environmental risk factors (Prada et al., 2014). Similarities between adult ADHD and BPD include neuroanatomical and neurophysiological concomitants, personality traits, and features such as behavioral and emotional dysregulation, impulsivity, irritability, and impaired stress tolerance (Nigg, 2005; Prada et al., 2014). Next, I summarize two studies focused on the etiology of ED in ADHD, then discuss theoretical models on the development and maintenance of ED in BPD. Acknowledging the probability of shared and unique etiological and maintaining factors of ED across disorders, I conclude this section by focusing on the constructs of equifinality and multifinality.

Regarding biological vulnerability for ED, some data indicate that there is not only a common genetic liability for ED and ADHD (Merwood et al., 2014) but also that the cosegregation of ED and ADHD in families may be a result of genetic or of environmental (familial) risk factors. Nevertheless, the pattern of inheritance of ED and ADHD suggests that ED may be a familial subtype of ADHD (Surman et al., 2011).

Regarding environmental influences, the characteristics of certain social settings (e.g., family, parent–child, peer relationships) may contribute to the development and maintenance of ED in youth with ADHD. In conceptual models of BPD and, by extension, ED as a core feature of BPD (Linehan, 1993), the role of the social environment and a transactional process between the individual and his or her environment has been underscored in explaining the development and maintenance of ED. Accordingly, most individuals who develop BPD, at some point or throughout development, are surrounded by an emotionally invalidating environment, wherein their attempts to communicate about their emotions are met by erratic, extreme, or inappropriate responses by others. Combined with a biological vulnerability, individuals exposed to such invalidating environments develop an emotional vulnerability characterized by heightened sensitivity to affective stimuli, a tendency to experience emotions as extreme and intense, and difficulty with timely return to emotional baseline. Several social interactions or processes can be conceptualized as invalidating, as long as they are characterized by presence of interactions that are critical, conflictual, and negative, and absence of interactions that are empathic and supportive (Fruzzetti et al., 2005). For an extended discussion and examples of the role of an invalidating environment, see Bunford, Evans, and Wymbs (2015) and Fruzzetti et al. (2005). Suffice to say, a child who has a predisposition to developing ED and experiences consistently invalidating responses to his or her emotions is at heightened risk for developing ED. Such a predisposition may be the common genetic liability for ED and ADHD. In addition, the family environments of children with ADHD have been described as conflicted and stressful, and the parents of children with ADHD report more conflict and stress, less marital satisfaction, aversive and demanding parent–child interactions, poor parenting practices, and less authoritative parenting beliefs, than the parents of typically developing children (Johnston & Mash, 2001; see Wiener, Chapter 6, this volume). As such, the family, parent–child, and sibling relationships in the families of children with ADHD may be particularly prone to exhibit dynamics redolent of an emotionally invalidating environment. For example, parents who are in conflicted relationships with other family members and stressed may be more likely to invalidate, either intentionally or unintentionally, than parents without these conflicts or stressors. In response, children with ADHD and ED may exhibit dysregulated behaviors, and parents may respond in an increasingly more negative (including invalidating) manner, resulting in a cycle of increasing dysregulation matched with increasing invalidation.

Despite the plausibility of this conceptualization, no research has focused on the degree to which these family (or, broadly, social) characteristics are present in the lives of children with ADHD and, if present, whether they are related to the development and maintenance of ED. It will be fruitful for the authors of future studies to examine these questions, as they may have considerable implications for prevention and treatment.

As noted, although it is reasonable to assume that there are shared biological and environmental risk and maintaining factors of ED across disorders with which it is associated, there are sufficient differences in the manifestations of ED to suggest that there are also differences in these mechanisms. Indeed, diversity in process and outcome are among the hallmarks of the developmental psychopathology perspective. Developmental psychopathologists argue that there are multiple contributors to adaptive or maladaptive outcomes in any given individual, that the factors and their relative contributions vary among individuals, and that there are myriad pathways to any particular manifestation of adaptive or disordered behavior (Cicchetti & Rogosch, 1996). The pertinent principle of equifinality indicates that, in any open system, a diversity of pathways, including chance events or what biologists refer to as *nonlinear epigenesis,* may lead to the same outcome. In other words, in any open system, the same end state may be reached from a variety of different initial conditions and through different processes (Cicchetti & Rogosch, 1996). The principle of multifinality indicates that any one component may function differently depending on the organization of the system in which it operates. As such, the effect of any one component may vary in different systems. Actual effects depend on the conditions set by additional components. Likewise, individuals may begin on the same major pathway and, as a function of subsequent events, exhibit very different patterns of adaptation or maladaptation (Cicchetti & Rogosch, 1996).

Accordingly, there are likely multiple contributors to the development of ED in ADHD, including in any given youth, and these contributing factors and their relative influence probably varies across youth. It is further likely that youth who begin on the same major "ED pathway" ultimately exhibit very different manifestations ED (e.g., no ED, negative ED, positive ED). Disentangling various "ED resilience and risk profiles" in youth with ADHD will doubtlessly be one of the next key research tasks. Importantly, ability to characterize resilience and risk factors, both ED and such factors, has to be appropriately and rigorously measurable. Yet there is little guidance in the literature on best practices for measuring ED in ADHD, and this is especially the case in adolescents (Bunford, Evans, et al., 2017).

Measurement Considerations

Measures of ED in children with ADHD have been evaluated at many levels of the measurement continuum (as conceptualized in the Research Domain Criteria [RDoC] matrix, the continuum ranges from the most micro-level analysis of genes to the most macro-level analysis of self-report on interviews or ratings scales, through the more micro levels of molecules, cells, and brain circuits and the more macro levels of physiology and behavior [behavioral observation or performance on laboratory tasks]; Morris & Cuthbert, 2012). Examples of ED measures or measurement levels examined among children with ADHD include genetic (Merwood et al., 2014; Surman et al., 2011), physiological (Bunford, Evans, et al., 2017; Musser et al., 2011; Musser, Galloway-Long, Frick, & Nigg, 2013), observational (Maedgen & Carlson, 2000; Melnick & Hinshaw, 2000), parent and self-report on rating scale (Seymour et al., 2012), and ecological momentary assessment (EMA; Rosen & Epstein, 2010; Rosen, Epstein, & Van Orden, 2013) methods.

Parallel assessment at different measurement levels and modalities is important for gaining information on which contexts the assessed characteristic does–does not occur (De Los Reyes et al., 2015), and is considered best practice in the assessment of mental health concerns (Youngstrom, Choukas-Bradley, Calhoun, & Jensen-Doss, 2015). Yet knowledge about ED in adolescents with ADHD is based exclusively on studies wherein ED was assessed via self-report on rating scales (Bunford, Evans, Becker, et al., 2015; Bunford et al., 2018; Seymour et al., 2014). Some have argued that due to increasing cognitive maturity and the largely internal nature of emotions, self-report may be a sufficient measurement method for ED in adolescence (Rohrbeck, Azar, & Wagner, 1991; Soto, John, Gosling, & Potter, 2008; Walden, Harris, & Catron, 2003). However, without additional measures (e.g., collateral report) of ED, this cannot be confirmed. Moreover, others have shown that youth with ADHD exhibit both a substantial response bias and a tendency to use a dichotomous and positively skewed response style when reporting on their emotion regulation (Rosen et al., 2013), challenging the view that self-report is sufficient and suggesting that additional, complementary measurement methods of ED should be evaluated and used in adolescents with ADHD.

In addition to measurement of ED proper, there is a similar need for assessment of hypothesized underlying mechanisms at many levels of the measurement continuum. Specifically, differences in the RDoC negative and positive valence and arousal/regulatory (e.g., resting state activity, heart rate variability; Bunford, Evans, et al., 2017) domain characteristics that likely correspond to differences in emotion regulation (as do cognitive systems [e.g., cognitive–effortful control] and social process systems [e.g., facial expression identification, theory of mind], though perhaps more distally).

Because aspects of both the negative and the positive valence domains are implicated in the etiology and maintenance of ED and ADHD, and because each domain comprises several constructs and some constructs comprise subconstructs, for purposes of feasibility and manageability, I use the negative valence domain frustrative nonreward construct (within the RDoC framework) to illustrate the intended main points and highlight pertinent considerations. First, *frustrative nonreward* is a series or set of reactions (accompanied by an internal state characterized by frustration) elicited in response to prevention or withdrawal of an expected reward, such as an inability to obtain a reward following repeated or sustained efforts (National Institute of Mental Health, 2011). As conveyed in this definition, it stands to reason that frustrative nonreward underlies certain expressions of negative ED. In addition, youth with ADHD have been shown to exhibit greater frustration in response to nonreward than do youth without ADHD (Douglas & Parry, 1994). Established measures of frustrative nonreward have been identified by the National Institute of Mental Health Negative Valence Domain Workshop Group at the level of molecules (e.g., GABA, dopamine, serotonin), circuits (amygdala, hypothalamus, locus coeruleus, orbitofrontal cortex, striatum, periaqueductal gray), behavior such as physical and relational aggression, and self-report on rating scales, each of which is to be measured in the context of an appropriate experimental paradigm, such as a Laboratory Aggression Paradigm or the Point Subtraction Aggression Paradigm (National Institute of Mental Health, 2011). In a multimethod and multi-informant framework, accounting for possibility of both equifinality and multifinality, one could consider any or all of the previously mentioned indices of frustrative nonreward and examine whether differences between individuals low versus high on ED and without versus with ADHD emerge, and furthermore, whether ED and ADHD have an additive/synergistic effect on such indices.

In the case of adolescents with ADHD, the following considerations may be key. First, adaptation for age appropriateness across development is likely more relevant as one progresses from left (more micro, e.g., genes) to right (more macro, e.g., observable behavior) on the measurement continuum (e.g., measurement of genes and molecules would involve similar procedures in children as measures in adolescents and in adults, but there may be different behavioral coding criteria during behavioral observation used with children vs. adolescents vs. adults due to variation in the way in which behavioral expression of frustrative nonreward manifests across development). Relatedly, such adaptation may be progressively more prudent beyond the level of brain circuits given marked changes in central and autonomic nervous system functioning from childhood into adulthood.

In addition, evidence suggests that it is crucially important to account for pubertal status in research with adolescents. Specifically, data obtained in animal studies indicate that sex hormones (estrogen, progesterone, and testosterone) are critically involved in myelination (Cooke & Woolley, 2005; Romeo & McEwen, 2004; Sá, Lukoyanova, & Madeira, 2009). In humans, there is an established relationship among sex hormones, white matter, and functional connectivity in the brain. Specifically, ovarian hormones (estradiol and progesterone) may enhance both corticocortical and subcorticocortical functional connectivity, whereas androgens (testosterone) may decrease subcorticocortical functional connectivity but increase functional connectivity between subcortical brain areas (Peper, van den Heuvel, Mandl, Pol, & van Honk, 2011). As such, especially when investigating possible underlying mechanisms of ED (e.g., frustrative nonreward), the contribution of sex hormones and pubertal status should be measured and taken into account.

Medication status, past or present, is also important to consider. Studies show that medication treatment alters brain chemistry and observable behaviors, and that such alteration is, in some cases, permanent. For example, in one study, while adults with childhood ADHD who had never been treated with methylphenidate showed decreased activation in the ventral striatum and the subgenual cingulate in response to emotional stimuli, these changes were not observed in males with childhood ADHD who had been (but were not, at the time of the study) treated with methylphenidate for at least 1 year (Schlochtermeier et al., 2011).

PREVENTION AND TREATMENT IMPLICATIONS

Considering everything that has been discussed, a key remaining issue is whether ED is malleable. ED can be prevalent and impairing among youth with ADHD but, if it is not malleable, then research efforts spent on it are valuable only to some basic extent and mainly on a conceptual level. However, if ED is a malleable characteristic, then better understanding what it is, its correlates, and what types of things cause and maintain it are all informative with regard to interventions. *Behavioral interventions* are changes made through a systematic process to develop or improve behaviors, cognitions, emotions, knowledge, and skills (Harrison, Bunford, Evans, & Owens, 2013, p. 557) and can take the form of prevention and treatment.

Regarding prevention, ED clearly appears to be a risk or vulnerability factor for functional impairment and negative outcomes, though it may be more relevant in certain outcomes compared to others (e.g., social vs. academic impairment), and in subpopulations, such as individuals with ADHD who experienced childhood maltreatment (Bunford, Wymbs, et al., 2017). Research is sorely needed on ED prevention techniques that are appropriate and effective for youth with ADHD, and on *when and for whom* ED prevention is warranted.

Regarding treatment, a large body of work indicates that ED—at least when it occurs in the context of some disorders—is malleable. For example, dialectical behavior therapy (DBT) has been shown to result in improvements on rating scale measures of ED in samples of adolescents and adults with BPD, bipolar disorder, and binge-eating disorder (e.g., Axelrod, Perepletchikova, Holtzman, & Sinha, 2011; Goldstein, Axelson, Birmaher, & Brent, 2007; Telch, Agras, & Linehan, 2001). However, there are currently no published treatment studies of youth (children or adolescents) with ADHD wherein ED was examined as an outcome variable. Nevertheless, the results of treatment studies with participants who exhibit characteristics that are highly relevant to ED, such as anger management problems, emotional lability, severe mood dysregulation disorder, and other emotional problems, are worthy of mention. These results generally indicate that treatments that purportedly improve ED are acceptable and feasible, and are associated with changes in ADHD symptoms and, in some cases, depression (see Bunford, Evans, & Wymbs, 2015, for extended discussion and review). Importantly, however, ED was either not specifically or not comprehensively measured in any of these studies, preventing us from knowing whether ED associated with ADHD is a malleable characteristic and therefore a useful treatment target.

The results of a small, unpublished clinical trial (Bunford, 2016) are encouraging in this regard. In that study, the Interpersonal Skills Group (ISG) intervention originally designed to improve the social functioning of teens, including those with ADHD (Evans et al., 2016), was modified to directly target ED and was tested in a randomized, crossover (i.e., waitlist-controlled) trial at a juvenile detention facility (ISG—Corrections Modified [ISG-CM]). ISG-CM was delivered in 13, 90-minute group sessions by a doctoral-level clinician with considerable prior experience in delivering manualized treatments, including the traditional ISG protocol, and an undergraduate student, in line with the delivery model of ISG employed in prior studies. Participants were 12 detained juvenile offender youth ages 14–18 years (100% male), six of whom had a clinical presentation consistent with ADHD (i.e., seven youth self-reported symptoms, duration, and impairment consistent with a diagnosis of ADHD and the parents of six of these reported symptoms on the Disruptive Behavior Disorders Rating Scale [Pelham, Gnagy, Greenslade, & Milich, 1992] that reached diagnostic threshold for ADHD [data from one youth's parent were missing]). Eight youth were randomly assigned to receive the ISG-CM intervention first, and eight youth were assigned to a waitlist control condition (then received the ISG-CM intervention). (A total of four youth discontinued due to unexpected discharge from the facility). Adolescents found the treatment highly satisfactory and also found each of the three treatment elements (i.e., psychoeducation, practice, and mindfulness mediation) likeable and beneficial/helpful. In line with expectations, the treatment, relative to no treatment, was associated with either an attenuation of an increase in or a decrease in self- and staff-rated verbal aggression, staff-rated aggression against property, and self-rated anger (measured on the Buss–Perry Aggression Questionnaire and conceptualized as an index of ED given its item content (e.g., "I flare up quickly but get over it quickly," "When frustrated, I let my irritation show," "I sometimes feel like a powder keg ready to explode," "I am an eventempered person,"), as well as staff-, teacher-, and self-rated ED. When in ISG-CM, relative to when not in ISG-CM, youth also exhibited an increase in daily behavior points (with greater points indicating better behavior and greater participation in activities at the detention facility), and those in treatment had fewer unsuccessful days in this domain than those not in treatment. As such, modified versions of ISG wherein ED is directly targeted (for another example, see Bunford & Evans, 2017) may be a promising approach to the psychosocial treatment of adolescents, including those with ED and ADHD.

Conclusion

In this chapter, I have argued that ED is an associated feature of ADHD, and that this association has considerable relevance in adolescence due to asynchronicity among biological/brain- and self-regulatory skills development, combined with a decreased role of environmental input into emotion regulation and an increased demand for adaptive emotion regulation skills. Another reason why the relationship between ED and ADHD is key in adolescence is related to the role of that relationship in functional impairments and negative outcomes, including ones that are related to unique transitions during the teenage years. Yet, compared to the literature on the association between ED and ADHD in children, there is little focus on that association in adolescents. It is prudent for the next generation of studies to address questions related to the effect of ED, *beyond* ADHD, on adolescent functional impairment and negative outcomes; on best practices for measuring ED in this age group and therefore the benefits and incremental utility of multimethod and multi-informant measures; etiological and maintaining factors, as well as underlying mechanisms of ED; whether ED is malleable in the context of ADHD; and when, for whom, and what aspects and techniques of intervention should be implemented.

References

Arain, M., Haque, M., Johal, L., Mathur, P., Nel, W., Rais, A., . . . Sharma, S. (2013). Maturation of the adolescent brain. *Neuropsychiatric Disease and Treatment, 9,* 449–461.

Axelrod, S. R., Perepletchikova, F., Holtzman, K., & Sinha, R. (2011). Emotion regulation and substance use frequency in women with substance dependence and borderline personality disorder receiving dialectical behavior therapy. *American Journal of Drug and Alcohol Abuse, 37*(1), 37–42.

Banks, S. J., Eddy, K. T., Angstadt, M., Nathan, P. J., & Phan, K. L. (2007). Amygdala–frontal connectivity during emotion regulation. *Social Cognitive and Affective Neuroscience, 2*(4), 303–312.

Barkley, R. A. (1997). Behavioral inhibition, sustained attention, and executive functions: Constructing a unifying theory of ADHD. *Psychological Bulletin, 121*(1), 65–94.

Barkley, R. A. (2010). Deficient emotional self-regulation: A core component of attention-deficit/hyperactivity disorder. *Journal of ADHD and Related Disorders, 1,* 5–37.

Barkley, R. A., Anastopoulos, A. D., Guevremont, D. C., & Fletcher, K. E. (1992). Adolescents with attention deficit hyperactivity disorder: Mother–adolescent interactions, family beliefs and conflicts, and maternal psychopathology. *Journal of Abnormal Child Psychology, 20*(3), 263–288.

Becker, S. P., Langberg, J. M., Evans, S. W., Girio-Herrera, E., & Vaughn, A. J. (2015). Differentiating anxiety and depression in relation to the social functioning of young adolescents with ADHD. *Journal of Clinical Child and Adolescent Psychology, 44*(6), 1015–1029.

Beesdo, K., Knappe, S., & Pine, D. S. (2011). Anxiety and anxiety disorders in children and adolescents: Developmental issues and implications for DSM-V. *Psychiatric Clinics of North America, 32*(3), 483–524.

Bernardi, S., Faraone, S. V., Cortese, S., Kerridge, B. T., Pallanti, S., Wang, S., & Blanco, C. (2012). The lifetime impact of attention deficit hyperactivity disorder: Results from the National Epidemiologic Survey on Alcohol and Related Conditions (NESARC). *Psychological Medicine, 42*(4), 875–887.

Bowlby, J. (1969). *Attachmemt and loss: Vol. 1. Attachment.* New York: Basic Books.

Bowlby, J. (1973). *Attachment and loss: Vol. 2. Separation, anxiety, and anger.* New York: Basic Books.

Bunford, N. (2016). *Interpersonal Skills Group—Corrections Modified for detained juvenile offenders with externalizing disorders: A controlled pilot clinical trial.* Columbus: Ohio University.

Bunford, N., Brandt, N. E., Golden, C., Dykstra, J. B., Suhr, J. A., & Owens, J. S. (2015). Attention-deficit/hyperactivity disorder symptoms mediate the association between deficits in executive functioning and social impairment in children. *Journal of Abnormal Child Psychology, 43*(1), 133–147.

Bunford, N., & Evans, S. W. (2017). Emotion regulation and social functioning in adolescence: Conceptualization and treatment. In J. R. Harrison, B. K. Schultz, & S. W. Evans (Eds.), *School mental health services for adolescents* (pp. 161–181). New York: Oxford University Press.

Bunford, N., Evans, S. W., Becker, S. P., & Langberg, J. M. (2015). Attention-deficit/hyperactivity disorder and social skills in youth: A moderated mediation model of emotion dysregulation and depression. *Journal of Abnormal Child Psychology, 43*(2), 283–296.

Bunford, N., Evans, S. W., & Langberg, J. M. (2018). Emotion dysregulation is associated with social impairment among young adolescents with ADHD. *Journal of Attention Disorders, 22*(1), 66–82.

Bunford, N., Evans, S. W., & Wymbs, F. (2015). ADHD and emotion dysregulation among children and adolescents. *Clinical Child and Family Psychology Review, 18*(3), 185–217.

Bunford, N., Evans, S. W., Zoccola, P. M., Owens, J. S., Flory, K., & Spiel, C. F. (2017). Correspondence between heart rate variability and emotion dysregulation in children, including children with ADHD. *Journal of Abnormal Child Psychology, 45*(7), 1325–1337.

Bunford, N., Wymbs, B. T., Dawson, A. E., & Shorey, R. C. (2017). Childhood maltreatment, emotional lability, and alcohol problems in young adults at-risk for ADHD: Testing moderation and moderated moderation. *Journal of Psychoactive Drugs, 49*(4), 316–325.

Bush, G., Valera, E. M., & Seidman, L. J. (2005). Functional neuroimaging of attention-deficit/hyperactivity disorder: A review and suggested future directions. *Biological Psychiatry, 57*(11), 1273–1284.

Canli, T., & Lesch, K.-P. (2007). Long story short: The serotonin transporter in emotion regulation and social cognition. *Nature Neuroscience, 10*(9), 1103–1109.

Casey, B. J., Jones, R. M., & Hare, T. A. (2008). The adolescent brain. *Annals of the New York Academy of Sciences, 1124*, 111–126.

Castellanos, F. X., Giedd, J. N., Berquin, P. C., Walter, J. M., Sharp, W., Tran, T., . . . Rapoport, J. L. (2001). Quantitative brain magnetic resonance imaging in girls with attention-deficit/hyperactivity disorder. *Archives of General Psychiatry, 58*(3), 289–295.

Castellanos, F. X., Giedd, J. N., Hamburger, S. D., Marsh, W. L., & Rapoport, J. L. (1996). Brain morphometry in Tourette's syndrome: The influence of comorbid attention-deficit/hyperactivity disorder. *Neurology, 47*, 1581–1583.

Cicchetti, D., & Rogosch, F. A. (1996). Equifinality and multifinality in developmental psychopathology. *Development and Psychopathology, 8*(4), 597–600.

Cole, P. M., Marin, S. E., & Dennis, T. A. (2004). Emotion regulation as a scientific construct: Methodological challenges for child development research. *Child Development, 75*(2), 317–333.

Cole, P. M., Michel, M. K., & Teti, L. O. D. (1994). The development of emotion regulation and dysregulation: A clinical perspective. *Monographs of the Society for Research in Child Development, 59*(2–3), 73–102.

Cooke, B. M., & Woolley, C. S. (2005). Gonadal hormone modulation of dendrites in the mammalian CNS. *Journal of Neurobiology, 64*(1), 34–46.

Coyne, J. C., & Downey, G. (1991). Social factors and psychopathology: Stress, social support, and coping processes. *Annual Review of Psychology, 42*, 401–425.

Daviss, W. B. (2008). A review of co-morbid depression in pediatric ADHD: Etiologies, phenomenology, and treatment. *Journal of Child and Adolescent Psychopharmacology, 18*(6), 565–571.

De Los Reyes, A., Augenstein, T. M., Wang, M., Thomas, S. A., Drabick, D. A. G., Burgers, D. E., & Rabinowitz, J. (2015). The validity of the multi-informant approach to assessing child and adolescent mental health. *Psychological Bulletin, 141*(4), 858–900.

Douglas, V. I., & Parry, P. A. (1994). Effects of reward and nonreward on frustration and attention in attention deficit disorder. *Journal of Abnormal Child Psychology, 22*(3), 281–302.

Edden, R. A. E., Crocetti, D., Zhu, H., Gilbert, D. L., & Mostofsky, S. H. (2012). Reduced GABA concentration in attention-deficit/hyperactivity disorder. *Archives of General Psychiatry, 69*(7), 750–753.

Evans, S. W., Langberg, J. M., Schultz, B. K., Vaughn, A., Altaye, M., Marshall, S. A., & Zoromski, A. K. (2016). Evaluation of a school-based treatment program for young adolescents with ADHD. *Journal of Consulting and Clinical Psychology, 84*(1), 15–30.

Factor, P. I., Reyes, R. A., & Rosen, P. J. (2014). Emotional impulsivity in children with ADHD associated with comorbid—not ADHD—symptomatology. *Journal of Psychopathology and Behavioral Assessment, 36*(4), 530–541.

Fischer, M., Barkley, R. A., Smallish, L., & Fletcher, K. (2007). Hyperactive children as young adults: Driving abilities, safe driving behavior, and adverse driving outcomes. *Accident Analysis and Prevention, 39*(1), 94–105.

Fogleman, N. D., Walerius, D. M., Rosen, P. J., & Leaberry, K. D. (2016). Peer

victimization linked to negative affect in children with and without ADHD. *Journal of Applied Developmental Psychology, 46,* 1–10.
Forssberg, H., Fernell, E., Waters, S., Waters, N., & Tedroff, J. (2006). Altered pattern of brain dopamine synthesis in male adolescents with attention deficit hyperactivity disorder. *Behavioral and Brain Functions, 2*(1), 1–10.
Fruzzetti, A. E., Shenk, C., & Hoffman, P. (2005). Family interaction and the development of borderline personality disorder: A transactional model. *Development and Psychopathology, 17,* 1007–1030.
Goldstein, T. R., Axelson, D. A., Birmaher, B., & Brent, D. A. (2007). Dialectical behavior therapy for adolescents with bipolar disorder: A 1-year open trial. *Journal of the American Academy of Child and Adolescent Psychiatry, 46*(7), 820–830.
Graziano, P., & Garcia, A. (2016). Attention-deficit hyperactivity disorder and children's emotion dysregulation: A meta-analysis. *Clinical Psychology Review, 46,* 106–123.
Hanish, L. D., Eisenberg, N., Fabes, R. A., Spinrad, T. L., Ryan, P., & Schmidt, S. (2004). The expression and regulation of negative emotions: Risk factors for young children's peer victimization. *Development and Psychopathology, 16*(2), 335–353.
Harrison, J. R., Bunford, N., Evans, S. W., & Owens, J. S. (2013). Educational accommodations for students with behavioral challenges: A systematic review of the literature. *Review of Educational Research, 83*(4), 551–597.
Henker, B., & Whalen, C. K. (1989). Hyperactivity and attention deficits. *American Psychologist, 44*(2), 216–223.
Herrmann, M. J., Schreppel, T., Biehl, S. C., Jacob, C., Heine, M., Boreatti-Hümmer, A., . . . Fallgatter, A. J. (2009). Emotional deficits in adult ADHD patients: An ERP study. *Social Cognitive and Affective Neuroscience, 4*(4), 340–345.
Hoy, E., Weiss, G., Minde, K., & Cohen, N. (1978). The hyperactive child at adolescence: Cognitive, emotional, and social functioning. *Journal of Abnormal Child Psychology, 6*(3), 311–324.
John, K. (2001). Measuring children's social functioning. *Child Psychology and Psychiatry Review, 6*(4), 181–189.
Johnson, P. A., Hurley, R. A., Benkelfat, C., Herpertz, S. C., & Taber, K. H. (2003). Understanding emotion regulation in borderline personality disorder: Contributions of neuroimaging. *Journal of Neuropsychiatry and Clinical Neurosciences, 15*(4), 397–402.
Johnston, C., & Mash, E. J. (2001). Families of children with attention-deficit/hyperactivity disorder: Review and recommendations for future research. *Clinical Child and Family Psychology Review, 4*(3), 183–207.
Karalunas, S. L., Fair, D., Musser, E. D., Aykes, K., Iyer, S. P., & Nigg, J. T. (2014). Subtyping attention-deficit/hyperactivity disorder using temperament dimensions: Toward biologically based nosologic criteria. *JAMA Psychiatry, 71*(9), 1015–1024.
Kent, L., Doerry, U., Hardy, E., Parmar, R., Gingell, K., Hawi, Z., & Craddock, N. (2002). Evidence that variation at the serotonin transporter gene influences susceptibility to attention deficit hyperactivity disorder (ADHD): Analysis and pooled analysis. *Molecular Psychiatry, 7*(8), 908–912.
Kopp, C. B. (1989). Regulation of distress and negative emotions: A developmental view. *Developmental Psychology, 25*(3), 343–354.
Krauel, K., Duzel, E., Hinrichs, H., Santel, S., Rellum, T., & Baving, L. (2007). Impact of emotional salience on episodic memory in attention-deficit/hyperactivity disorder: A functional magnetic resonance imaging study. *Biological Psychiatry, 61*(12), 1370–1379.
Landau, S., & Moore, L. A. (1991). Social skill deficits in children with attention-deficit hyperactivity disorder. *School Psychology Review, 20*(2), 235–251.
Langberg, J. M., Epstein, J. N., Altaye, M., Molina, B. S. G., Arnold, L. E., & Vitiello, B. (2008). The transition to middle school is associated with changes in the

developmental trajectory of ADHD symptomatology in young adolescents with ADHD. *Journal of Clinical Child and Adolescent Psychology, 37*(3), 651–663.

Laviolette, S. R. (2007). Dopamine modulation of emotional processing in cortical and subcortical neural circuits: Evidence for a final common pathway in schizophrenia? *Schizophrenia Bulletin, 33,* 971–981.

Linehan, M. M. (1993). Skills training manual for treating borderline personality disorder. Retrieved from *http://proxy.lib.sfu.ca/login?url=http://search.ebscohost.com/login.aspx?direct=true&db=psyh&an=1995-98090-000&site=ehost-live.*

Maedgen, J. W., & Carlson, C. L. (2000). Social functioning and emotional regulation in the attention deficit hyperactivity disorder subtypes. *Journal of Clinical Child Psychology, 29*(1), 30–42.

Mazefsky, C. A., Herrington, J., Siegel, M., Scarpa, A., Maddox, B. B., Scahill, L., & White, S. W. (2013). The role of emotion regulation in autism spectrum disorder. *Journal of the American Academy of Child and Adolescent Psychiatry, 52*(7), 679–688.

McQuade, J. D., Hoza, B., Murray-Close, D., Waschbusch, D. A., & Owens, J. S. (2011). Changes in self-perceptions in children with ADHD: A longitudinal study of depressive symptoms and attributional style. *Behavior Therapy, 42*(2), 170–182.

Melnick, S. M., & Hinshaw, S. P. (2000). Emotion regulation and parenting in AD/HD and comparison boys: Linkages with social behaviors and peer preference. *Journal of Abnormal Child Psychology, 28*(1), 73–86.

Merwood, A., Chen, W., Rijsdijk, F., Skirrow, C., Larsson, H., Thapar, A., & Asherson, P. (2014). Genetic associations between the symptoms of attention-deficit/hyperactivity disorder and emotional lability in child and adolescent twins. *Journal of the American Academy of Child and Adolescent Psychiatry, 53*(2), 209–220.

Mitchell, J. T., Van Voorhees, E. E., Dennis, M. F., McClernon, F. J., Calhoun, P. S., Kollins, S. H., & Beckham, J. C. (2012). Assessing the role of attention-deficit/hyperactivity disorder symptoms in smokers with and without posttraumatic stress disorder. *Nicotine and Tobacco Research, 14*(8), 986–992.

Molina, B. S. G., & Pelham, W. E. (2003). Childhood predictors of adolescent substance use in a longitudinal study of children with ADHD. *Journal of Abnormal Psychology, 112*(3), 497–507.

Morris, S. E., & Cuthbert, B. N. (2012). Research Domain Criteria: Cognitive systems, neural circuits, and dimensions of behavior. *Dialogues in Clinical Neuroscience, 14*(1), 29–37.

Musser, E. D., Backs, R. W., Schmitt, C. F., Ablow, J. C., Measelle, J. R., & Nigg, J. T. (2011). Emotion regulation via the autonomic nervous system in children with attention-deficit/hyperactivity disorder (ADHD). *Journal of Abnormal Child Psychology, 39*(6), 841–852.

Musser, E. D., Galloway-Long, H. S., Frick, P. J., & Nigg, J. T. (2013). Emotion regulation and heterogeneity in attention-deficit/hyperactivity disorder. *Journal of the American Academy of Child and Adolescent Psychiatry, 52*(2), 163–171.

National Institute of Mental Health. (2011). Positive valence systems: Workshop proceedings. Retrieved from *www.nimh.nih.gov/research-priorities/rdoc/positive-valence-systems-workshop-proceedings.shtml.*

Nigg, J. T. (2005). Neuropsychologic theory and findings in attention-deficit/hyperactivity disorder: The state of the field and salient challenges for the coming decade. *Biological Psychiatry, 57*(11), 1424–1435.

Nigg, J. T. (2010). Attention-deficit/hyperactivity disorder endophenotypes, structure, and etiological pathways. *Current Directions in Psychological Science, 19*(1), 24–29.

Okado, I., & Mueller, C. W. (2016). The relationship between child-reported positive affect and parent-reported emotional and behavioral problems in ADHD youth. *Journal of Child and Family Studies, 10,* 2954–2965.

Pelham, W., Gnagy, E. M., Greenslade, K. E., & Milich, R. (1992). Teacher ratings of DSM-III-R symptoms for the disruptive behavior disorders. *Journal of the American Academy of Child and Adolescent Psychiatry, 31*(2), 210–218.

Peper, J. S., van den Heuvel, M. P., Mandl, R. C. W., Pol, H. E. H., & van Honk, J. (2011). Sex steroids and connectivity in the human brain: A review of neuroimaging studies. *Psychoneuroendocrinology, 36*(8), 1101–1113.

Prada, P., Hasler, R., Baud, P., Bednarz, G., Ardu, S., Krejci, I., . . . Perroud, N. (2014). Distinguishing borderline personality disorder from adult attention deficit/hyperactivity disorder: A clinical and dimensional perspective. *Psychiatry Research, 217*(1–2), 107–114.

Rohrbeck, C. A., Azar, S. T., & Wagner, P. E. (1991). Child Self-Control Rating Scale: Validation of a child self-report measure. *Journal of Clinical Child Psychology, 20*, 179–183.

Romeo, R. D., & McEwen, B. S. (2004). Sex differences in steroid-induced synaptic plasticity. *Advances in Molecular and Cell Biology, 34*, 247–258.

Rosen, P. J., & Epstein, J. N. (2010). A pilot study of ecological momentary assessment of emotion dysregulation in children. *Journal of ADHD and Related Disorders, 1*(4), 39–52.

Rosen, P. J., Epstein, J. N., & Van Orden, G. (2013). I know it when I quantify it: Ecological momentary assessment and recurrence quantification analysis of emotion dysregulation in children with ADHD. *Attention Deficit and Hyperactivity Disorders, 5*(3), 283–294.

Rosen, P. J., Milich, R., & Harris, M. J. (2012). Dysregulated negative emotional reactivity as a predictor of chronic peer victimization in childhood. *Aggressive Behavior, 38*(5), 414–427.

Sá, S. I., Lukoyanova, E., & Madeira, M. D. (2009). Effects of estrogens and progesterone on the synaptic organization of the hypothalamic ventromedial nucleus. *Neuroscience, 162*(2), 307–316.

Schlochtermeier, L., Stoy, M., Schlagenhauf, F., Wrase, J., Park, S. Q., Friedel, E., . . . Ströhle, A. (2011). Childhood methylphenidate treatment of ADHD and response to affective stimuli. *European Neuropsychopharmacology, 21*(8), 646–654.

Scholte, R. H. J., Engels, R. C. M. E., Overbeek, G., De Kemp, R. A. T., & Haselager, G. J. T. (2007). Stability in bullying and victimization and its association with social adjustment in childhood and adolescence. *Journal of Abnormal Child Psychology, 35*(2), 217–228.

Ŝeibokaité, L., Endriulaitiené, A., Sullman, M. J., Markŝaitytė, R., & Žardeckaité-Matulaitiené, K. (2017). Difficulties in emotion regulation and risky driving among Lithuanian drivers. *Traffic Injury Prevention, 18*(7), 688–693.

Semrud-Clikeman, M., Steingard, R. J., Filipek, P., Biederman, J., Bekken, K., & Renshaw, P. F. (2000). Using MRI to examine brain–behavior relationships in males with attention deficit disorder with hyperactivity. *Journal of the American Academy of Child and Adolescent Psychiatry, 39*(4), 477–484.

Seymour, K. E., Chronis-Tuscano, A., Halldorsdottir, T., Stupica, B., Owens, K., & Sacks, T. (2012). Emotion regulation mediates the relationship between ADHD and depressive symptoms in youth. *Journal of Abnormal Child Psychology, 40*(4), 595–606.

Seymour, K. E., Chronis-Tuscano, A., Iwamoto, D. K., Kurdziel, G., & MacPherson, L. (2014). Emotion regulation mediates the association between ADHD and depressive symptoms in a community sample of youth. *Journal of Abnormal Child Psychology, 42*(4), 611–621.

Silk, J. S., Steinberg, L., & Morris, A. S. (2003). Adolescents' emotion regulation in daily life: Links to depressive symptoms and problem behavior. *Child Development, 74*(6), 1869–1880.

Sjöwall, D., Backman, A., & Thorell, L. B. (2015). Neuropsychological heterogeneity in preschool ADHD: Investigating the interplay between cognitive, affective and motivation-based forms of regulation. *Journal of Abnormal Child Psychology, 43*(4), 669–680.

Sonuga-Barke, E. J. S. (2002). Psychological heterogeneity in AD/HD—A dual pathway model of behaviour and cognition. *Behavioural Brain Research, 130,* 29–36.

Soto, C. J., John, O. P., Gosling, S. D., & Potter, J. (2008). The developmental psychometrics of big five self-reports: Acquiescence, factor structure, coherence, and differentiation from ages 10 to 20. *Journal of Personality and Social Psychology, 94*(4), 718–737.

Steinberg, L. (2005). Cognitive and affective development in adolescence. *Trends in Cognitive Sciences, 9*(2), 69–74.

Surman, C. B. H., Biederman, J., Spencer, T., Yorks, D., Miller, C. A., Petty, C. R., & Faraone, S. V. (2011). Deficient emotional self-regulation and adult attention deficit hyperactivity disorder: A family risk analysis. *American Journal of Psychiatry, 168*(6), 617–623.

Telch, C. F., Agras, W. S., & Linehan, M. M. (2001). Dialectical behavior therapy for binge eating disorder. *Journal of Consulting and Clinical Psychology, 69*(6), 1061–1065.

Thapar, A., Collishaw, S., Pine, D. S., & Thapar, A. K. (2012). Depression in adolescence. *Lancet, 379*(9820), 1056–1067.

Thayer, J. F., & Lane, R. D. (2000). A model of neurovisceral integration in emotion regulation and dysregulation. *Journal of Affective Disorders, 61*(3), 201–216.

Trógolo, M. A., Melchior, F., & Medrano, L. A. (2014). The role of difficulties in emotion regulation on driving behavior. *Journal of Behavior, Health and Social Issues, 6*(1), 107–117.

Vadalá, R., Giugni, E., Pichiecchio, A., Balottin, U., & Bastianello, S. (2011). Attention deficit hyperactivity disorder (ADHD): From a childhood neuropsychiatric disorder to an adult condition. *Functional Neurology, 26*(3), 117–119.

Volkow, N. D., Wang, G.-J., Newcorn, J., Telang, F., Solanto, M. V., Fowler, J. S., . . . Swanson, J. M. (2007). Depressed dopamine activity in caudate and preliminary evidence of limbic involvement in adults with attention-deficit/hyperactivity disorder. *Archives of General Psychiatry, 64*(8), 932–940.

Walden, T. A., Harris, V. S., & Catron, T. F. (2003). How I feel: A self-report measure of emotional arousal and regulation for children. *Psychological Assessment, 15*(3), 399–412.

Wiener, J., & Mak, M. (2008). Peer victimization in children with attention-deficit/hyperactivity disorder. *Psychology in the Schools, 46,* 116–131.

Williams, L. M., Hermens, D. F., Palmer, D., Kohn, M., Clarke, S., Keage, H., . . . Gordon, E. (2008). Misinterpreting emotional expressions in attention-deficit/hyperactivity disorder: Evidence for a neural marker and stimulant effects. *Biological Psychiatry, 63*(10), 917–926.

Wolraich, M. L., Wibbelsman, C. J., Brown, T. E., Evans, S. W., Gotlieb, E. M., Knight, J. R., . . . Wilens, T. (2005). Attention-deficit/hyperactivity disorder among adolescents: A review of the diagnosis, treatment, and clinical implications. *Pediatrics, 115*(6), 1734–1746.

Wymbs, B. T., Dawson, A. E., Suhr, J. A., Bunford, N., & Gidycz, C. A. (2017). ADHD symptoms as risk factors for intimate partner violence perpetration and victimization. *Journal of Interpersonal Violence, 32*(5), 659–681.

Youngstrom, E. A., Choukas-Bradley, S., Calhoun, C. D., & Jensen-Doss, A. (2015). Clinical guide to the evidence-based assessment approach to diagnosis and treatment. *Cognitive and Behavioral Practice, 22*(1), 20–35.

Zeman, J., Cassano, M., Perry-Parrish, C., & Stegall, S. (2006). Emotion regulation in children and adolescents. *Journal of Developmental and Behavioral Pediatrics, 27*(2), 155–168.

CHAPTER 6

The Ripple Effect of Adolescent ADHD

Family Relationships

Judith Wiener

> She helped me get [a] laptop. . . . She's done a lot for me . . . fighting for me, vouching for me, all that stuff.
>
> —Wiener and Daniels (2016, p. 9)

> My dad has involvement but he tries to be a little bit more accepting and try to . . . talk it a different way. My mom's like, "What are you going to do? You're never going to get anywhere . . . blah, blah, blah." My dad's more like . . . he kind of gives you more advice. . . . It's a little better listening to my dad.
>
> —Wiener and Daniels (2016, p. 9)

> Yea, when sometimes my mom's trying to tell me something and at the moment I think of it as like, she's nagging me. But really, when I actually think about it, she's just trying to help me in any way she can. Being a good mom.
>
> —Haydicky, Wiener, and Shecter (2017, p. 1029)

Family relationships contribute to the healthy development of adolescents (Lila, van Aken, Musitu, & Buelga, 2006) in spite of teens' increasing autonomy with regard to decision-making and values and the time they spend with close friends and romantic partners (Goossens, 2006). As attested to by the adolescents with attention-deficit/hyperactivity disorder

(ADHD) quoted above, family support is especially important for them because of their impairments in academic functioning (Evans, Van der Oord, & Rogers, Chapter 8, this volume) and peer relations (McQuade, Chapter 7, this volume); problems with executive functions manifesting in difficulties with organization, planning and time management (Doidge, Saoud, & Toplak, Chapter 4, this volume); and co-occurring oppositional behaviors and conduct problems, anxiety, and depression (Becker & Fogleman, Chapter 9, this volume). It may also be more challenging for parents to provide the support these teens need because of parenting stress, their own subclinical or clinical levels of ADHD symptoms, or other psychopathology such as anxiety and depression (Johnston & Chronis-Tuscano, 2015; Deault, 2010).

This chapter on families of adolescents with ADHD addresses the following five questions:

1. To what extent do parenting and adolescent behaviors influence each other?
2. Are the relationships (parent–adolescent, marital/co-parenting, sibling) in families of adolescents with ADHD less supportive and more conflictual than those of other adolescents and, if so, what are the adolescent, parent, and social factors that contribute to positive and negative relationships?
3. Do parents of adolescents with ADHD differ from other parents with regard to parenting cognitions (self-efficacy, attributions) and parenting stress and, if so, what are the predictors and implications of maladaptive cognitions and stress?
4. Is parental ADHD associated with problematic parenting practices, family relationships, adolescent behavioral outcomes, maladaptive cognitions, and parenting stress?
5. To what extent should parents be involved in interventions for adolescents with ADHD?

In order to provide a developmental context for the research on families of adolescents, for each of these questions I summarize the conclusions from previous reviews of the research on families of children with ADHD before describing the research on families of adolescents with ADHD and discussing the limitations and implications of that research. There are several contextual factors that influence family functioning of adolescents and their families including socioeconomic status (SES), parental marital and co-parenting relationships, and culture (Lila et al., 2006). Acculturation conflict, for example, is a key factor in the relationship between adolescents and their parents in immigrant families (e.g., Geva & Wiener, 2015). It is beyond the scope of this chapter to examine these contextual factors systematically, but I will mention them when they are relevant specifically to adolescents with ADHD. The conclusion provides a theoretical formulation and a discussion of implications for future research and clinical practice.

The Reciprocal Relationship between Parenting Practices and Adolescent Outcome

Summary of Child Research

There is considerable evidence that for youth with and without ADHD, parental rejection and coercive control that involves arbitrary discipline, frequent hostile verbal communication, and physical punishment are associated with negative outcomes. Johnston and Chronis-Tuscano (2015), in their recent review of research on children with ADHD, however, concluded that in early childhood, ADHD symptoms in children are "primary drivers of parenting difficulties such as overreactivity or inconsistency" (p. 194). They based their conclusions on research describing changes in parenting behaviors in parent–child dyads that manipulate child medication status, and on laboratory studies in which parents are more coercive in interactions with child actors who simulate symptoms of ADHD and other disruptive behaviors. Johnston and Chronis-Tuscano concluded that ineffective parenting and parent–child relationship difficulties are associated with conduct problems such as oppositional behaviors and aggression in children, and that this effect is more pronounced in children with ADHD. In her review, Deault (2010) found that childhood depressive symptoms were predicted by children's perceptions that their parents used more power-assertive discipline strategies, and by maternal depression and anxiety. Childhood anxiety symptoms were predicted by parent overprotectiveness, maternal anxiety, and low levels of positive parenting. These reviews raise questions about the relationship between parenting behavior and positive and negative outcomes in their adolescent children, and the degree to which adolescent characteristics affect parenting.

Research on Adolescents with ADHD

In adolescents, the negative outcomes of negative parenting (i.e., low parental warmth; parental rejection; inconsistent, coercive or timid discipline) include oppositional and defiant behaviors, callous and unemotional traits, delinquency and substance abuse, anxiety, and depression; these associations are particularly robust in adolescents with diagnosed ADHD or high levels of ADHD symptoms (Burke, Pardini, & Loeber, 2008; Chang, Chiu, Wu, & Gau, 2013; Gau & Chang, 2013; Graziano et al., 2016; Pires & Jenkins, 2007; Tandon, Tillman, Spitznagel, & Luby, 2014) and in low-income single-parent families (Hurtig et al., 2007). Positive parenting in studies of adolescents with ADHD involves dimensions such as parental warmth and caring, ongoing and frank communication between parents and teens, parental knowledge and monitoring of adolescent activities, and systematic and consistent parenting. These aspects of positive parenting are associated with a reduction of the above negative outcomes in adolescents with ADHD (Gianotta & Rydell, 2016; Pires & Jenkins, 2007; Pollak, Poni, Gershy, & Aran, 2017). With the exception of a study conducted in Taiwan, none of the studies showed links between parenting behaviors and severity of ADHD symptoms within samples of adolescents with ADHD. Gau and Chang (2013), who found that inattentive symptom severity in adolescent boys diagnosed with ADHD was associated with coercive parenting, suggested that Taiwanese mothers might interpret adolescent inattention as intentional and defiant, and be especially concerned about these symptoms due to the pressure for academic success in their culture.

As indicated by Johnston and Chronis-Tuscano (2015), in relation to younger children, it is likely that coercive, inconsistent, or authoritarian parenting does not cause adolescent problem behaviors; instead, parents may use these negative parenting strategies in response to their children's behaviors. Most of the studies reported earlier are not longitudinal or did not examine reciprocal effects. The results of a large longitudinal study by Burke et al. (2008), however, suggest that the relationship between the behaviors of adolescents with disruptive behavior disorders, 68.9% of whom were diagnosed with ADHD, and their parents' behaviors is bidirectional and transactional, especially in relation to oppositional defiant disorder (ODD) symptoms. In addition to parental timid discipline predicting ODD symptoms, ODD symptoms predicted increases in timid discipline, lower parental involvement, and poorer communication. There was no association, however, between parenting behaviors and severity of youth ADHD symptoms. The results of this study suggest that parents whose children are frequently oppositional and defiant often withdraw from parenting over time.

Discussion

There are several limitations of the research on parenting behaviors and adolescent outcomes in adolescents with ADHD. I was not able to identify research that examined potential links between parenting strategies and positive outcomes such as self-esteem, domain-specific (e.g., academic, social) self-concepts, quality of life, improved academic achievement, and friendships in adolescents with ADHD. In addition, in some studies, both parenting practices and adolescent behaviors were measured exclusively by parents (presumably primarily the mother but often not indicated) or adolescent report. This common method variance was a limitation of two (Burke et al., 2008; Pires & Jenkins, 2007) of the three longitudinal studies. In order to obviate this problem, Graziano et al. (2016) examined both parent report of parenting behaviors and observations of parents and teens interacting. The observational measure of parenting behavior was not associated with parent-rated teen behavioral outcomes. Few studies investigated contextual factors that influence parenting behaviors in parents of adolescents with ADHD. Although a lower proportion of families of children with ADHD are intact than families of typically developing children (Wymbs et al., 2008), none of these studies investigating parenting behaviors of parents of adolescents with ADHD compared intact versus nonintact families.

Family Relationships in Families of Adolescents with ADHD

Summary of Child Research

Literature reviews on family relationships of children with ADHD summarized results of observational studies examining the interactions between parents and children (mainly mothers and sons) with ADHD on laboratory tasks in which they were asked to play a game or solve a problem. As described by Johnston and Mash (2001), dyads of children with ADHD with conduct problems have the highest level of conflictual interactions; children with ADHD who are not diagnosed with conduct problems, however, also have higher levels of conflict with their parents than do typically developing children. A recent study suggests that these conflictual interactions might be associated with insecure attachment, which predicted variance in externalizing behaviors, social skills, and mood regulation in Israeli 11- to 12-year-old children (Al-Yagon, Forte, & Avarahami, 2017). Adults with ADHD have lower levels of marital satisfaction and are more likely to be divorced than other adults (Johnston & Chronis-Tuscano, 2015). Twin studies, however, suggest that parent genetic factors do not contribute to divorce rates among parents of children with ADHD (Schermerhorn et al., 2012). As indicated by Johnston and Chronis-Tuscano (2015), there are few studies of sibling relationships. It is unclear from these reviews whether the conflictual relationships between parents and children with ADHD continue or intensify when the children become teenagers, and whether these conflicts might be associated with insecure attachment. Research with families of adolescents may also provide information about intraparental and sibling relationships in families of adolescents with ADHD.

Research on Adolescents with ADHD

Passionate discussion and some level of conflict between adolescents and their parents in the context of a generally warm and supportive relationship are adaptive in terms of adolescent development; frequent and intense conflict, however, is maladaptive (e.g., Goossens, 2006). There is considerable evidence from research conducted in the United States, Canada, and Taiwan that families of adolescents with ADHD have higher levels of conflict than other families according to mother, father, and adolescent reports, and these findings apply to both male and female adolescents (Barkley, Anastopoulos, Guevremont, & Fletcher, 1992; Barkley, Fischer, Edelbrock, & Smallish, 1991; Chang et al., 2013; Gau & Chang, 2013; Markel & Wiener, 2014). Compared with dyads of parents and adolescents without ADHD, adolescents with ADHD and their parents were more likely to argue about issues related to school (e.g., getting up in the morning and getting to school on time, getting low grades and getting in trouble at school) according to parent reports, and to money and curfew according to both parent and adolescent reports (Markel & Wiener, 2014). The rates of self-reported and parent-reported hostile conflict were increased when the adolescent had comorbid ADHD and ODD (Barkley et al., 1991; Barkley, Anastopoulos, et al., 1992). Similarly, observations of adolescents and their mothers interacting in a situation where they were required to engage in problem solving to resolve their conflicts indicated that adolescents with comorbid ADHD and ODD and their mothers had more hostile interactions than dyads with adolescents with ADHD and those with typically developing teens (Fletcher, Fischer, Barkley, & Smallish, 1996). When attempting to resolve conflict, parent–adolescent interactions were not affected when adolescents with ADHD were taking methylphenidate (Pelham et al., 2017). In addition to adolescents' co-occurring oppositional behaviors, parent factors also contribute to conflict between adolescents with ADHD and their parents. Fathers of adolescents with ADHD who believed that the conflicts with their children were their sons' or daughters' responsibility, and that a conflictual relationship would be stable over time, reported higher levels of conflict (Markel & Wiener, 2014). Mothers' ADHD symptoms were associated with higher parent–adolescent conflict according to parent and adolescent reports, whereas fathers' ADHD symptoms were associated with lower levels of father–adolescent conflict (Babinski et al., 2016; Grimbos & Wiener, 2018). The high level of conflict in adolescents with ADHD and their parents is especially concerning, because increases in conflict over time during adolescence contributed to increases in antisocial behaviors in Swedish adolescents with hyperactive–impulsive symptoms (Giannotta & Rydell, 2016). Furthermore, parent–adolescent conflict is associated with co-occurring depression, peer victimization, and suicidal behavior in adolescents with ADHD (Daviss & Diler, 2014).

The high level of conflict between adolescents with ADHD and their parents is typically interpreted as being related to the adolescents' challenging behaviors, and current emotion regulation difficulties on the part of the teens and their parents. Research based on attachment theory, however, suggests that this conflict may be associated with attachment processes.

Secure attachment typically occurs in children who have had warm relationships with their parents and whose parents are consistently responsive to their needs. Insecure attachment is thought to result from interactions with parents who are not responsive to their children's needs. This may occur due to discontinuities in parenting or to parents trying to control their children by threatening to withdraw love or abandon them (Bowlby, 1977). Insecurely attached adolescents and adults may avoid relationships with others or may be preoccupied with relationship issues and intimacy. According to Allen (2008), due to their capacity to think abstractly and reflect on their attachment experiences, adolescents' conceptualization of their relationships with parents and peers develop from early to late adolescence. Because adolescents become increasingly competent to engage in daily activities, they strive for autonomy and evaluate their parents more objectively. In conflict situations with their parents, securely attached teens typically engage in the types of productive problem solving that allows them to preserve both their positive relationships with their families and their need for autonomy. Adolescents with an avoidant attachment pattern, on the other hand, less often engage in the problem solving needed to resolve conflicts and have higher levels of externalizing behaviors.

Attachment theory has been the basis of three studies with adolescents with ADHD or ADHD symptoms. Two of the three studies were conducted with samples of Israeli adolescents and both used exclusively self-report questionnaires. Scharf, Oshri, Eshkol, and Pilowsky (2014) found that in a community sample of more than 500 adolescents in grades 7–9, securely attached teens had lower levels of inattention than did teens who had avoidant and preoccupied attachment patterns. Furthermore, teens with a preoccupied attachment pattern had higher levels of both inattention and hyperactivity than did teens with secure or avoidant attachment. Al-Yagon (2016) found that Israeli adolescents with comorbid learning disabilities (LD) and ADHD had more insecure attachment patterns with mothers than did adolescents without ADHD. Attachment with fathers did not differentiate the groups. Although insecure attachment with mothers was associated with negative affect, loneliness, and externalizing problems in adolescents with LD who did not have comorbid ADHD, insecure attachment only predicted negative affect in adolescents with comorbid LD and ADHD. In a retrospective study with participants recruited from adoption databases in five countries (Belgium, Canada, Chile, The Netherlands, and Romania), Roskam et al. (2014) examined the predictive role of early attachment deprivation on level of adolescent ADHD symptoms measured by adoptive parent report in a large sample of 11- to 16-year-old adolescents adopted from over 30 countries prior to the age of 7. Before their adoption, most of these children lived in institutional settings. After controlling for variables such as adolescent age and gender, length of time in the adoptive family, country of origin and adoption, and SES, older age at adoption predicted higher adoptive parent-rated adolescent ADHD symptoms but not adolescent internalizing and externalizing problems.

Parental marital/coparenting satisfaction and status are important to consider when examining the family relationships of adolescents with ADHD. Children of single parents are 1.85 times more likely to have ADHD than are children living in two-parent families (see Russell, Ford, Williams, & Russell, 2016, for review). Parents of clinic-referred adolescents with ADHD in the United States were more likely to be divorced, and the length of marriage prior to divorce was shorter than that of parents of typically developing adolescents (Wymbs et al., 2008). Paternal antisocial behavior was a strong predictor of marriage dissolution in this sample. In addition, child and adolescent ODD and CD, but not child ADHD symptom severity, predicted marriage dissolution (Wymbs et al., 2008) or differentiated adolescents with ADHD in divorced and intact families (Heckel, Clarke, Barry, McCarthy, & Selikowitz, 2009). The one study I could find on sibling relationships of youth with ADHD (ages 6–18) showed that ADHD symptoms in one child or adolescent were associated with siblings experiencing less happiness in life. There was also more conflict between siblings when one child or teen had higher levels of ADHD symptoms (Peasgood et al., 2016).

Discussion

There are several limitations to the research on family relationships of adolescents with ADHD. There are higher levels of maladaptive parent–adolescent and marital conflict than in other families, and this conflict is associated with parent-reported adolescent ODD and depressive symptoms, teen suicidal behavior, parental ADHD, and paternal antisocial behavior. That a higher proportion of adolescents with ADHD live in families in which their biological parents are not living together is not surprising; this likely occurs because, compared to parents of typically developing children, parents of children with ADHD report higher levels of verbal hostility and conflict in their relationships and lower levels of marital satisfaction (e.g., Johnston & Behrenz, 1993). It is difficult to interpret the results of the attachment research. The studies suggest a relationship between insecure attachment and ADHD symptoms in adolescents, but it would be inappropriate to conclude that this relationship is causal. It is possible that ADHD symptoms in infants and young children may elicit inconsistent and rejecting styles of parenting and delay adoption. Furthermore, the complex attachment processes that are normative in adolescence may be exacerbated by ADHD symptoms. Given the association between avoidant attachment strategies in adolescence, parent–adolescent conflict, and externalizing behaviors such as conduct disorder and substance abuse (Allen, 2008), it would have been helpful if the studies investigating attachment and ADHD symptoms had measured oppositional and other externalizing problems. It is also possible that both genetic (including the shared genes between parents and children with ADHD) and prenatal factors influence perinatal and early childhood behavior which, as discussed earlier, may impact parenting. Only one study examined sibling well-being and relationships, but that study had a sample that was predominantly children and early adolescents and did not differentiate variables such as age differences, birth order, and whether the sibling had ADHD or another disability.

Parent Cognitions and Affect: Self-Efficacy, Attributions, and Stress

Parents' cognitions and affect, such as their beliefs about their competence as parents (parental self-efficacy or sense of competence), their attributions for their children's behaviors, and the degree to which they experience parenting stress, are important aspects of research on families of youth with ADHD. In accordance with Weiner's (1980) cognitive–emotion–action model, parents who believe that their children are able to control and thereby prevent their negative behaviors (i.e., have internal attributions) are more likely to have negative emotions (including parenting stress) and to use coercive discipline practices (e.g., Dix, Ruble, & Zambrano, 1989). *Parenting stress,* which refers to stress that occurs when parents perceive the demands of parenting to exceed their resources for dealing with these demands (Deater-Deckard, 2004), emanates from parents' perceptions that their children's behavior is very challenging (referred to as the *child or adolescent domain* of parenting stress), their perceptions that their relationships with their children are inadequate (*adolescent–parent relationship domain* [APR]), and their perceptions that they are inadequately supported as parents and experience guilt and social alienation due to the parent role (*parent domain*) (Sheras, Abidin, & Konold, 1998). Higher parental self-efficacy, adaptive attributions for their children's behavior, and lower parenting stress are associated with positive parenting practices and parent–child relationships (Abidin, 1992) and parents' ability to implement parenting interventions (Kazdin, 1995).

Summary of Child Research

Parents of children with ADHD have lower levels of parenting self-efficacy with regard to their general parenting abilities (Johnston & Mash, 2001; Johnston & Chronis-Tuscano, 2015) and their ability to support their children's learning (Rogers, Marton, Wiener, & Tannock, 2009) than do parents of children without ADHD. Furthermore, among parents of children with ADHD, parenting sense of competence is associated with parents' acquisition of effective parenting strategies (Johnston, Mah, & Regenbal,

2010). As reviewed by Johnston and Mash (2001), parents of children with ADHD are more likely than parents of children without ADHD to believe that their children's disruptive behaviors are uncontrollable and stable. Moreover, among mothers of children with ADHD, attributions for children's disruptive behavior as controllable, stable, and occurring in many contexts predicted maintenance of these behaviors (Johnston, Hommersen, & Seipp, 2009). In a meta-analysis, Theule, Wiener, Jenkins, and Tannock (2013) reported that parents of children with ADHD up to and including the age of 12 had considerably higher levels of parenting stress than did parents of typically developing children. Parenting stress was found to be associated with child inattentive and hyperactive–impulsive symptoms, child conduct and internalizing problems, parental depressive symptoms, and low marital quality. Theule et al. noted that, at the time of their review, no studies had investigated parenting stress in adolescents with ADHD.

Research on Adolescents with ADHD

The research on cognitions in parents of adolescents with ADHD is limited. Both mothers and fathers of adolescents with ADHD have lower parenting self-efficacy in relation to supporting their teens' learning than do parents of typically developing adolescents (Musabelliu, Rogers, & Wiener, 2018). In spite of higher levels of conflict between adolescents with ADHD and their parents than between typically developing adolescents and their parents, Markel and Wiener (2014) found no differences between parents of adolescents with and without ADHD in their attributions for those conflicts, and mothers' attributions for conflict were not associated with the number or intensity of conflicts they reported. Consistent with attribution theory, fathers of adolescents with ADHD who had internal and stable attributions for their children's conflicts reported that they had conflict over more issues.

A few studies of parenting stress in parents of adolescents with ADHD have been published since the Theule et al. (2013) meta-analysis I described earlier. In a 5-year longitudinal study of girls with ADHD (mean age 9.4 at the beginning of the study), Gordon and Hinshaw (2017) found that mothers of girls with ADHD reported more parenting stress than did mothers of girls without ADHD, and that among the girls with ADHD, maternal parent domain stress assessed during childhood predicted mother-reported internalizing and externalizing behaviors in adolescence. In addition, higher maternal stress with regard to the girls' behavior and the mothers' relationship with the girls (a combination of adolescent domain and APR domain stress), measured when the girls were adolescents, was associated with increases in youth-reported depressive symptoms and mother-reported externalizing symptoms.

Wiener, Biondic, Grimbos, and Herbert (2016) found that both mothers and fathers of adolescents with ADHD experienced higher stress in the adolescent and APR domains than do parents of adolescents without ADHD, and mothers also experienced higher stress in the parent domain. Mothers and fathers whose teens with ADHD had clinical levels of ODD behaviors according to parent report experienced higher levels of parenting stress in the adolescent and APR domains than did other parents of adolescents with ADHD and parents of typically developing adolescents. When adolescents were classified as having clinical levels of ODD according to teacher report, however, there were no between-group differences in their parents' levels of parenting stress. Mothers' reports of their own ADHD symptoms accounted for variance in parenting stress in the adolescent and parent domains over and above adolescent ADHD status, whereas fathers' reports of their ADHD symptoms accounted for variance in APR domain stress over and above adolescent ADHD status. Mothers' ADHD symptoms were also associated with higher levels of stress, whereas fathers' ADHD symptoms were associated with lower levels of stress. Biondic and Wiener (2019) sought to clarify whether parent ADHD symptoms or depressive symptoms, which are highly comorbid in adults with ADHD (Barkley, 2015a), predicted parenting stress. Both their own ADHD and depressive symptoms predicted maternal parenting stress in the adolescent and APR domains, and depressive symptoms predicted maternal parent domain stress. Fathers' parent domain stress was predicted by their own depressive symptoms and mothers' ADHD and depressive symptoms.

Discussion

Due to the limited number of studies on parenting self-efficacy and attributions of parents of adolescents with ADHD, there are few conclusions that can be drawn. Future research should determine whether parents of adolescents with ADHD have low parenting self-efficacy and identify potential predictors of parenting self-efficacy, such as adolescent conduct problems and parental psychopathology. It is important to understand parents' attributions for the behaviors of their teens with ADHD because of the association between maladaptive attributions and coercive discipline practices.

Both mothers and fathers of adolescents with ADHD experience higher levels of parenting stress than do parents of typically developing adolescents, and their stress is associated with adolescent externalizing and internalizing behaviors as perceived by the parents, as well as increases in girls' self-reported depressive symptoms from childhood to adolescence (longitudinal studies of boys with ADHD have not been conducted). There are several possible interpretations of the Wiener et al. (2016) finding that parent-reported, but not teacher reported, ODD is associated with parenting stress. First, when parent ratings are used, there is common source bias for ratings of adolescent ODD and parenting stress; some parents may experience even mildly elevated levels of oppositional behaviors as stressful. Second, as discussed by Wiener et al., adolescents typically have several teachers who often teach more than 100 students and may thus be less familiar with adolescent behaviors than parents. Moreover, adolescents may behave differently in the structured environment of the school, where they may try harder to regulate their emotions than at home. This is important, because a diagnosis of ODD does not require that behaviors occur in more than one setting (American Psychiatric Association, 2013). In addition, there are other possible adolescent behaviors that may contribute to parenting stress that have not been investigated. For example, screen time is associated with more sleep disturbances and internalizing and externalizing behavior problems in community samples of adolescents (e.g., Parent, Sanders, & Forehand, 2016), and adolescents with ADHD engage in higher amounts of video gaming (e.g., Walther, Morgenstern, & Hanewinkel, 2012) and have more sleep problems (e.g., Gau & Chiang, 2009) than do typically developing adolescents (see Mulraney, Sciberras, & Becker, Chapter 10, this volume). This might contribute to parenting stress, because the teens may be reluctant to get up in the morning and go to school, which was one of the sources of parent–adolescent conflict reported by Markel and Wiener (2014).

Parental ADHD predicted higher levels of parenting stress for mothers and lower levels for fathers. This might be due to the different roles that mothers and fathers play with regard to care giving. As discussed by Wiener et al. (2016), mothers are typically involved in all aspects of caregiving; consequently, mothers' ADHD symptoms may be impairing in terms of their role in monitoring their adolescents' activities and scaffolding their teens' planning and organizing of schoolwork and activities. Fathers, on the other hand, are typically involved in recreational activities with adolescents, which may be less affected by the functional impairment associated with adolescents' ADHD symptoms. The finding that mothers' self-reported depressive symptoms were associated with their parenting stress and mothers' ADHD and depression were associated with fathers' parent domain stress is also consistent with this interpretation about caregiving roles, in that fathers may experience stress when they need to take on the day-to-day parenting role when their co-parent is unable to do so due to the functional impairment associated with ADHD and depression.

PARENTAL ADHD

Summary of Child Research

As described earlier, parental ADHD has been examined in relation to parenting behaviors, parent–child relationships, parenting stress, and child and adolescent outcomes. Mothers who have elevated ADHD symptoms or diagnosed ADHD have challenges with monitoring their children's behavior, planning and organizing their children's activities, and problem solving (Johnston, Mash, Miller, & Ninowski, 2012). They also use inconsistent discipline practices and are less responsive to their children's needs than are mothers without ADHD.

Johnston et al. (2012) proposed a model of the mechanisms driving the association between parental ADHD symptoms, parenting behaviors, and child outcome. They hypothesized that ADHD core deficits, including cool executive functions (working memory, inhibitory control, planning), hot executive functions (motivation, delay aversion, sensitivity to reward and punishment), and self-regulation of behavior and emotion, lead to parenting impairments. These impairments are conceptualized as being interrelated and include problematic parenting cognitions and affect (low parental sense of competence, maladaptive attributions for child behavior, high parenting stress), inadequate control behaviors (monitoring of child behavior, planning and problem solving, unclear guidance), and low levels of emotional responsiveness (hostile or overreactive discipline, warmth and sensitivity, rejection). According to the model, inadequate control behaviors and low levels of emotional responsiveness are directly associated with parental ADHD core deficits, but these relations could be partially mediated by parental cognitions and stress. Child ADHD symptoms and externalizing problems are posited to increase as a result of inadequate parental control behaviors and low levels of emotional responsiveness. Johnston et al. also suggested some potential moderators of the relationships, including parent gender and ADHD subtype, child age and gender, child temperament, and genetic risk. The question that I address below is whether research on families of adolescents with ADHD supports the Johnston et al. model or suggests the need for modifications to the model.

Research on Adolescents with ADHD

In a longitudinal study of adolescents ages 11–14, Mazursky-Horowitz et al. (2015) found that mothers with high levels of ADHD symptoms were more distressed by their children's emotional expression, responded more harshly, and were less sensitive to their children's emotional needs. Furthermore, mothers' deficits in self-regulation of emotion mediated the relationship between their ADHD symptoms and responses to their teens' emotions. This study supports the component of the Johnston et al. (2012) model that posits self-regulation of emotion is an important mechanism that drives the negative parenting responses of mothers with high levels of ADHD symptoms. According to the similarity–fit hypothesis, positive emotions and relationships are more likely to occur when the two individuals have similar characteristics, whereas the similarity–misfit hypothesis suggests that emotions and relationships are more likely to be negative when the two individuals have similar characteristics (Johnston et al., 2012; Psychogiou, Daley, Thompson, & Sonuga-Barke, 2007, 2008). Mothers' ADHD symptoms are associated with more conflict and higher parenting stress in relation to the behavior of their teens with ADHD, whereas fathers' ADHD symptoms are associated with less conflict and lower parenting stress in terms of their relationships with their teens with ADHD (Grimbos & Wiener, 2018; Wiener et al., 2016). These studies support the similarity–misfit hypothesis in relation to mothers and the similarity–fit hypothesis in relation to fathers, as well as the position of Johnston et al. (2012) that parent gender may be a potential moderator due to the differential roles parents play in the home.

Discussion

Although generally supportive of the Johnston et al. (2012) model, the minimal research on parental ADHD symptoms and the functioning of families of adolescents with ADHD highlights the central role of the adolescent–parent relationship, which is not explicitly articulated in the model. In addition to fewer conflicts, a positive adolescent–parent relationship involves both parents and teens feeling that they are accepted and emotionally supported (Lila et al., 2006). *Social perspective taking,* the ability to understand the other person's perspective and use that understanding in problem solving to work out a solution that meets the needs of both parties, is associated with positive relationships (Yeates, Schultz, & Selman, 1991). Both children (Marton, Wiener, Rogers, & Moore, 2009) and adolescents (Timmermanis, Haydicky, Shecter, & Wiener, 2016) with ADHD, however, experience challenges with social perspective taking. The data are mixed with regard to adults with ADHD; some studies suggest ongoing problems with social cognition, including facial recognition of emotions, empathy, and social perspective taking in these adults, whereas others find no differences in social cognition between adults with and without ADHD (see Bora & Pantelis, 2016, for review). It is therefore unclear whether fathers with ADHD typically have developed the requisite social perspective-taking skills to be sensitive to their teens' needs.

Interventions

Summary of Child Research

Behavioral parent training (BPT), which is also referred to as *behavioral management training,* is efficacious for preschool and school-age children (see Pelham & Fabiano, 2008, for review); several of these programs have been evaluated and are used widely. The core components of these programs are psychoeducation about ADHD and the antecedent–behavior–consequence (ABC) model, and teaching parents to acquire and use specific strategies such as setting aside quality play time with their children, using effective methods for making requests and praising compliance, planned ignoring and development of incentive systems; and using time-out effectively. Although BPT is an efficacious treatment for families of children with ADHD, parental psychopathology, including maternal depression and ADHD, have been found to limit treatment effectiveness (Chronis, Chacko, Fabiano, Wymbs, & Pelham, 2004). The main question I address in this section is whether directing interventions, such as BPT, primarily at parents, is associated with enhanced outcome in adolescents with ADHD or whether adding a parent component to treatments directed at the adolescents themselves is helpful.

Research on Adolescents with ADHD

It is not as clear whether BPT is helpful for families of adolescents with ADHD. The adolescents participating in the studies by Barkley and his colleagues that investigated BPT for parents of adolescents with ADHD had comorbid ODD or CD, and the investigators compared BPT to other forms of treatment, including structural family therapy, problem-solving communication training (PSCT) alone and in combination with BPT (Barkley, Guevremont, Anastopoulos, & Fletcher, 1992; Barkley, Edwards, Laneri, Fletcher, & Metevia, 2001). The aim of these intervention studies was typically to reduce parent–teen conflict. There were modest reductions in parent–teen conflicts and adolescent internalizing and externalizing symptoms in a small proportion of the treatment samples for all of these therapies.

One of the components of BPT interventions is psychoeducation about ADHD, which has been evaluated as a treatment on its own. Following a 10-week, 2-hours per week course on the nature of ADHD, managing challenging adolescent behaviors, and advocating for their children, parents of adolescents with ADHD reported enhanced communication and reductions in conflict with their teens (McCleary & Ridley, 1999). In addition to psychoeducation, Gisladottir and Svavarsdottir (2017) engaged 145 parents of 65 adolescents in Iceland in a therapeutic conversation that focused on parents' strengths, beliefs, and emotions about parenting, boundary setting, and parenting behaviors. They were taught to use reflective listening and motivational interviewing with their adolescent children. Parents (both primary and secondary caregivers) reported higher quality of life postintervention.

In contrast to interventions aimed mainly at parents of adolescents with ADHD, there is some evidence that adding an intervention for parents as a supplement to treatments for teens may enhance the potency of treatment. For example, Sibley et al. (2013) investigated the effectiveness of a summer treatment program in which adolescents received 300 hours of therapy focusing on academic and social skills, and parents received 15 hours of BPT. A reliable decrease in parent–adolescent conflict was found in 70–85% of the families. Similarly, parent involvement in individual cognitive-behavioral therapy (CBT; see Sprich & Burbridge, Chapter 16, this volume) with adolescents was associated with relatively substantial gains (Antshel, Faraone, & Gordon, 2014). This treatment consisted of three core modules (psychoeducation, teaching skills to reduce distractibility, and cognitive restructuring) and optional modules on reducing procrastination, improving communication skills, and reducing anger/frustration. Parents were present during the psychoeducation and reducing distractibility sessions, but the therapy was directed at teens. Adolescent gains were evident in school attendance, parent-reported externalizing symptoms, and adolescent and teacher reported inattention. Adolescents with comorbid ODD–CD benefited less than teens with comorbid anxiety and depression or with ADHD and no comorbid disorder. The teens also required lower doses of medication to maintain their level of functioning.

Mindfulness treatments (see Davis & Mitchell, Chapter 17, this volume) that include a parent component have also been shown to be promising with adolescents with ADHD (Haydicky, Schecter, Wiener, & Ducharme, 2015; van de Weijer-Bergsma, Formsma, de Bruin, & Bogels, 2012). In the Haydicky et al. evaluation of MYmind, which used a mixed-methods design, data were collected from 20 adolescents ages 13–18 at four time points, 8 weeks apart—baseline, pretreatment, posttreatment, and follow-up. As no treatment was provided during the baseline period, participants were their own controls for the effect of treatment. Parents and adolescents received treatment simultaneously in different rooms with different therapists. In addition to mindfulness, MYmind involved psychoeducation and CBT. Parents reported reductions in adolescent inattentive symptoms, conduct problems, and peer relations difficulties, and reductions in their own parenting stress between pretreatment and posttreatment that exceeded those between baseline and pretreatment. These changes were maintained at follow-up. Although there were no significant reductions in adolescent self-reported anxiety and depressive symptoms between pre- and posttreatment, these symptoms were reduced significantly during the follow-up period, perhaps because these teens continued with meditation practice. In the qualitative component of the study with five of the families, Haydicky et al. (2017) reported that the treatment was associated with an improved parent–adolescent relationship, because both the teens and parents used some of the mindfulness strategies during conflicts to regulate their emotions. They claimed that they found it easier to empathize with each other, to engage in social perspective taking, and as a result, resolve their conflicts. Although intriguing, this preliminary finding needs to be investigated in future research with larger samples to test these treatment mechanisms empirically.

Addressing the academic impairment of adolescents with ADHD has been a priority in several recent intervention studies, with most involving provision of small-group instruction to the teens in organization and homework recording and management (see Langberg, Smith, & Green, Chapter 15, this volume). Sibley et al. (2016) added parent–teen behavior therapy and motivational interviewing to the teaching of organizational, time management, and planning (OTP) skills in a randomized controlled trial of the Supporting Teens' Autonomy Daily (STAND) program with 128 adolescents with ADHD and their parents (see Sibley, Chapter 14, this volume). Adolescents and their families were randomly assigned to receive STAND or treatment as usual. The program consists of 10 manualized family therapy sessions in which families select modules that pertain to organizing academic and nonacademic activities and homework based on the teens' needs. Parent-rated improvements in the treatment group relative to the control group were observed for ADHD symptoms, OTP skills, disruptive behavior, homework recording and contracting, parent implementation of home privileges, and parenting stress. The reduction in ADHD symptoms and parenting stress and gains in OTP skills were maintained at 6-month follow-up. Furthermore, using video conferencing in the implementation of the STAND program did not jeopardize treatment integrity or family satisfaction with the program (Sibley, Comer, & Gonzalez, 2017).

Discussion

The Sibley et al. (2016) study investigating the combination of training in OTP skills, parent–teen behavior therapy, and motivational interviewing was the only published randomized controlled trial of interventions with adolescents and their families that I could find. This study provided strong evidence in favor of this combined intervention. It is difficult, however, to ascertain whether BPT or psychoeducation alone produce reliable changes in adolescent or parent functioning, because none of the studies of these interventions included a no-treatment control group, and the effect sizes were modest. There are several reasons why BPT appears to be less efficacious with adolescents than with younger children. Although children with ADHD interact with peers, they typically do so in the presence of adults, such as parents and teachers. Most adolescents, however, have more autonomy and spend time interacting with peers online or face-to-face without adult monitoring (Lila et al., 2006). Consequently, there are many contexts in which parent-manipulated contingencies may not be effective with adolescents, and it may be important to involve the teens directly in treatment. In addition, treatments that involve adolescents with ODD–CD and parents communicating with each other (e.g., PSCT, structural family therapy) may be problematic in some cases, because the conflict between parents and adolescents may be long-standing and so intense that it interferes with the treatment process.

Although some of the treatments involving adolescents and their parents are promising, the absence of a no-treatment control group or baseline treatment-as-usual period in some of the studies (Antshel et al., 2014; Sibley et al., 2013), or a control condition in which teens receive treatment but parents are not involved in the randomized controlled trial or quasi-experimental studies makes it difficult to draw conclusions about the efficacy of inclusion of parents in treatments for adolescents with ADHD. Parent and adolescent responses in the qualitative study that was part of the mixed-methods evaluation of MYmind (Haydicky et al., 2017), however, suggest that including parents in treatment may be helpful, because parents and teens are able to communicate more effectively in part as a result of acquiring a common set of terms with which to share their experiences. In the MYmind treatment, parents were involved not only to help their adolescent children but also to learn skills for managing their own emotions. In spite of the data suggesting that parental involvement in treatment may be helpful, intervention studies to date suggest that a substantial amount of the treatment must be directed at the teens themselves.

Conclusion and Implications

Adolescents with ADHD are at risk for many negative outcomes, including co-occurring externalizing and internalizing behavior problems, and disorders such as ODD, CD (see Becker & Fogleman, Chapter 9, this volume), substance abuse (see Kennedy, McKone, & Molina, Chapter 11, this volume), sleep problems (see Mulraney, Sciberras, & Becker, Chapter 10, this volume), academic failure (see Evans, Van der Oord, & Rogers, Chapter 8, this volume), and peer rejection and victimization (see McQuade, Chapter 7, this volume). These impairments and comorbid disorders, at least in part, are considered to have a biological basis (Barkley, 2015b). Nevertheless, as established in this review of the research, family factors contribute to the development of these negative outcomes and may also contribute to positive outcomes; in the right environment, these at-risk teens may be resilient. The mechanisms for this are still not entirely clear due to limited research, but there is some evidence for pathways that need to be verified by future research. Johnston and Chronis-Tuscano (2015) proposed a model depicting their understanding of the development of children with ADHD and their families. Parent–child relationships are central to the model. Parent and child characteristics, as well as other family (e.g., marital/co-parenting relationship, sibling relationships) and social (e.g., school, community, cultural) factors are predictive of the quality of the parent–child relationship, and the quality of the parent–child relationship is associated with adaptive and maladaptive parenting, which predicts child outcome.

Figure 6.1 is a modification of the Johnston and Chronis-Tuscano (2015) model that pertains to current understanding of the development of adolescents with ADHD in the context of their families. Solid arrows represent relationships that are supported by more than one research study, whereas dashed arrows represent potential relationships that currently have limited support. In this model, the parent–adolescent relationship is depicted as having a major impact on parenting processes and adolescent outcome. Key aspects of a positive adolescent–parent relationship include communication based on reciprocal empathy and perspective taking, low levels of conflict, family cohesion, and secure attachment. Conversely, high levels of conflict, which occur due to inability to understand the other's perspective and communicate appropriately, low family cohesion, and insecure attachment are characteristics of a negative parent–adolescent relationship.

As I described earlier, there is considerable research supporting the reciprocal link illustrated in Figure 6.1 between a negative parent–adolescent relationship and maladaptive authoritarian and permissive parenting that includes parental rejection, low levels of knowledge and monitoring of adolescent activities, and inconsistent and coercive discipline. Furthermore, the link between these maladaptive parenting processes and the development of adolescent risky behaviors, as well as internalizing and externalizing behavior problems/disorders, has been demonstrated in several studies. The research also suggests that conduct problems are associated with higher levels of parenting stress and parent–adolescent conflict. Adaptive parenting practices such as warmth and caring, responsiveness, knowledge and monitoring, consistency, support for OTP, and expecting compliance to reasonable requests, on the other hand, have been shown to be associated with lower levels of adolescent negative outcomes. There is a paucity of research investigating whether positive parenting is associated with positive outcomes such as adolescent self-esteem, accurate domain-specific self-appraisals (e.g., self-perceptions of academic and social competence), quality of life, development of close friendships and romantic relationships, and achievement in academics and other areas of adolescent interests.

Research supports the position illustrated in the model that parenting stress and parental attributions for adolescent behavior (specifically fathers' beliefs that conflicts are their children's responsibility and likely to be stable) are important contributors to the parent–adolescent relationship. Maternal ADHD is associated with higher levels of stress and conflict, whereas paternal ADHD is associated with lower levels of conflict with their teens with ADHD, likely because of the different roles fathers play in the family. Furthermore, maternal ADHD and depressive symptoms exacerbate paternal parenting stress. It is not clear, however, whether

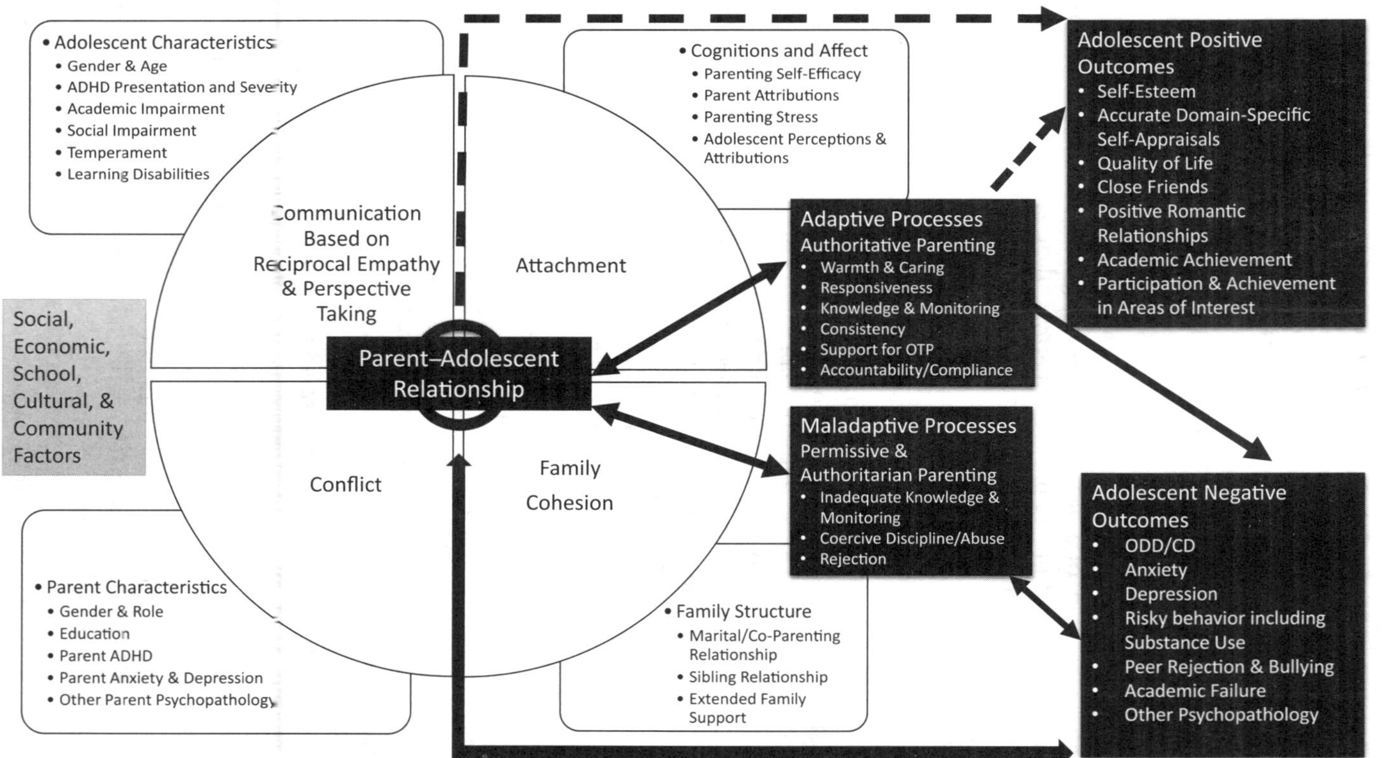

FIGURE 6.1. Family relationships of adolescents with ADHD.

parents of more than one child or teen with ADHD experience higher levels of parenting stress. Low SES and nonintact families are risk factors for both challenging parent–adolescent relationships and negative adolescent outcomes.

In addition to the paucity of research on family factors affecting positive outcomes in adolescents with ADHD, there are several aspects of the model that require more research to establish their validity. In most studies, adolescent gender and age are included in the description of the samples, but studies have not explicitly reported on gender differences or investigated whether parent–adolescent relationships vary with adolescent age. Similarly, most studies include only mothers or do not identify whether parent participants are male or female. Variables such as parent age and education are seldom examined. Although there are cultural differences in family functioning in relation to children with various disabilities and disorders (see Geva & Wiener, 2015, for a review), and the research I have reviewed suggests that there might be cultural differences in relation to parental attributions for their teens' ADHD symptoms and impairment (Gau & Chang, 2013), there is insufficient research on adolescents with ADHD to draw any conclusions in this regard. Similarly, I was not able to find published studies that investigated the impact of extended family support on parent well-being and adolescent functioning, and I could find only one study on each of parental self-efficacy and sibling relationships.

Given the limitations of the research on interventions that are directed at parents of adolescents with ADHD or that include parent involvement as a supplement to adolescent treatments such as social skills training, CBT and mindfulness, it is currently inappropriate to give specific recommendations for treatment for adolescents with ADHD that includes their families. The CBT treatment evaluated in the Antshel et al. (2014) study, the STAND intervention evaluated in the Sibley et al. (2016) study, and the mindfulness-based CBT program developed by Bogels and her colleagues (2008) and evaluated by Haydicky et al. (2015, 2017; van de Weijer-Bergsma et al., 2012) are promising interventions that should be evaluated in future studies in randomized controlled trials in which treatment with adolescents alone and treatment with a parent supplement are compared with each other and with no treatment. The degree and type of parent involvement also needs to be considered. The research does not provide information as to whether outcomes are better when parents participate actively in sessions with teens, merely observe the sessions so that they are aware of the strategies their children are learning and can facilitate generalization, or receive similar treatment in a separate room. There is also no research indicating whether these treatments are more efficacious when the teens are receiving appropriate medication for their ADHD symptoms. Furthermore, depending on the focus of the intervention, in these studies, it is important to consider multiple outcomes, including reduction in adolescent oppositional and conduct problems, anxiety, and depressive symptoms, and improvement in academic performance and social skills and social relationships. It is also helpful to examine parent outcomes, such as reductions in maladaptive parental cognitions and parenting stress, and to determine whether these parent variables contribute to changes in adolescent behaviors. In addition to examining changes in frequency and intensity of conflict, it may also be appropriate to examine whether treatment is associated with positive aspects of parent–adolescent relationships, such as enhanced communication and collaboration, concern for the others' well-being, and appreciation of each other.

I began this chapter with some quotations that illustrate the views of adolescents with ADHD who participated in qualitative studies about their relationships with their parents (Haydicky et al., 2017; Wiener & Daniels, 2016). I also conclude this chapter with the perceptions of these teens. When interviewed, several of the adolescents communicated that they wanted their parents to decrease involvement in their daily lives and schoolwork gradually, and asked that parents respect their autonomy. Conversely, they said that they wanted their parents to hold them accountable for doing their schoolwork and other responsibilities. The teens claimed that it would be helpful if their parents understood their perspective, encouraged them with regard to career goals, and kept them engaged. They strongly expressed the feeling that their parents should be aware that they cannot always control their behaviors, and that sometimes they make mistakes and engage in risk taking due to their problems with self-regulation. Some of the adolescents who participated in a mindfulness intervention claimed that the intervention, among other things, enhanced their understanding of their parents' perspective; they communicated that it must be stressful to parent a child with ADHD and expressed their appreciation.

References

Abidin, R. R. (1992). The determinants of parenting behavior. *Journal of Clinical Child Psychology, 21,* 407–412.

Allen, J. (2008). The attachment system in adolescence. In J. Cassidy & P. R. Shaver (Eds.), *Handbook of attachment: Theory, research and clinical applications* (2nd ed., pp. 419–435). New York: Guilford Press.

Al-Yagon, M. (2016). Perceived close relationships with parents, teachers, and peers: Predictors of social, emotional, and behavioral features in adolescents with LD or comorbid LD and ADHD. *Journal of Learning Disabilities, 49,* 597–615.

Al-Yagon, M., Forte, D., & Avrahami, L. (2017, September 1). Executive functions and attachment relationships in children with ADHD: Links to externalizing/internalizing problems, social skills, and negative mood regulation. *Journal of Attention Disorders.* Retrieved from *www.researchgate.net/publication/319878922_Executive_Functions_and_Attachment_Relationships_in_Children_With_ADHD_Links_to_ExternalizingInternalizing_Problems_Social_Skills_and_Negative_Mood_Regulation.*

American Psychiatric Association. (2013). *Diagnostic and statistical manual of mental disorders* (5th ed.). Arlington, VA: Author.

Antshel, K. M., Faraone, S. V., & Gordon, M. (2014). Cognitive behavioral treatment outcomes in adolescent ADHD. *Journal of Attention Disorders, 18,* 483–495.

Babinski, D. E., Pelham, W. E., Jr., Molina, B. S. G., Gnagy, E. M., Waschbusch, D. A., Wymbs, B. T., . . . Kuriyan, A. B. (2016). Maternal ADHD, parenting, and psychopathology among mothers of adolescents with ADHD. *Journal of Attention Disorders, 20,* 458–468.

Barkley, R. A. (2015a). Comorbid psychiatric disorders and psychological maladjustment in adults with ADHD. In R. A. Barkley (Ed.), *Attention-deficit hyperactivity disorder: A handbook for diagnosis and treatment* (4th ed., pp. 343–355). New York: Guilford Press.

Barkley, R. A. (2015b). Etiologies of ADHD. In R. A. Barkley (Ed.), *Attention-deficit hyperactivity disorder: A handbook for diagnosis and treatment* (4th ed., pp. 356–390). New York: Guilford Press.

Barkley, R. A., Anastopoulos, A. D., Guevremont, D. C., & Fletcher, K. E. (1992). Adolescents with attention deficit hyperactivity disorder: Mother–adolescent interactions, family beliefs and conflicts, and maternal psychopathology. *Journal of Abnormal Child Psychology, 20,* 263–288.

Barkley, R. A., Edwards, G., Laneri, M., Fletcher, K., & Metevia, L. (2001). The efficacy of problem-solving communication training alone, behavior management training alone, and their combination for parent–adolescent conflict in teenagers with ADHD and ODD. *Journal of Consulting and Clinical Psychology, 69,* 926–941.

Barkley, R. A., Fischer, M., Edelbrock, C., & Smallish, L. (1991). The adolescent outcome of hyperactive children diagnosed by research criteria—III. Mother–child interactions, family conflicts and maternal psychopathology. *Journal of Child Psychology and Psychiatry, 32,* 233–255.

Barkley, R. A., Guevremont, D. C., Anastopoulos, A. D., & Fletcher, K. E. (1992). A comparison of three family therapy programs for treating family conflicts in adolescents with attention-deficit hyperactivity disorder. *Journal of Consulting and Clinical Psychology, 60,* 450–462.

Biondic, D., & Wiener, J. (2019). Parental psychopathology and parenting stress in parents of adolescents with attention-deficit/hyperactivity disorder (ADHD). *Journal of Child and Family Studies.* Retrieved from *https://link.springer.com/article/10.1007/s10826-019-01430-8.*

Bogels, S., Hoogstad, B., van Dun, L., de Schutter, S., & Restifo, K. (2008). Mindfulness training for adolescents with externalizing disorders and their parents. *Behavioral and Cognitive Psychotherapy, 36,* 193–209.

Bora, E., & Pantelis, C. (2016). Meta-analysis of social cognition in attention-deficit/hyperactivity disorder (ADHD): Comparison with healthy controls and autistic spectrum disorder. *Psychological Medicine, 46*(4), 699–716.

Bowlby, J. (1977). The making and breaking of affectional bonds: I. Aetiology and psychopathology in the light of attachment theory. *British Journal of Psychiatry, 130,* 201–210.

Burke, J. D., Pardini, D. A., & Loeber, R. (2008). Reciprocal relationships between parenting behavior and disruptive psychopathology from childhood through adolescence. *Journal of Abnormal Child Psychology, 36,* 679–692.

Chang, L., Chiu, Y., Wu, Y., & Gau, S. S. (2013). Father's parenting and father–child relationship among children and adolescents with attention-deficit/hyperactivity disorder. *Comprehensive Psychiatry, 54*(2), 128–140.

Chronis, A. M., Chacko, A., Fabiano, G. A., Wymbs, B. T., & Pelham, W. E., Jr. (2004).

Enhancements to the behavioral parent training paradigm for families of children with ADHD: Review and future directions. *Clinical Child and Family Psychology Review, 7,* 1–27.

Daviss, W. B., & Diler, R. S. (2014). Suicidal behaviors in adolescents with ADHD: Associations with depressive and other comorbidity, parent–child conflict, trauma exposure, and impairment. *Journal of Attention Disorders, 18,* 680–690.

Deater-Deckard, K. (2004). Parenting stress and child adjustment: Some old hypotheses and new questions. *Clinical Psychology: Science and Practice, 5,* 314–332.

Deault, L. C. (2010). A systematic review of parenting in relation to the development of comorbidities and functional impairments in children with attention-deficit/hyperactivity disorder (ADHD). *Child Psychiatry and Human Development, 41*(2), 168–192.

Dix, T., Ruble, D. N., & Zambrano, R. J. (1989). Mothers' implicit theories of discipline: Child effects, parent effects, and the attribution process. *Child Development, 60,* 1373–1391.

Fletcher, K. E., Fischer, M., Barkley, R. A., & Smallish, L. (1996). A sequential analysis of the mother–adolescent interactions of ADHD, ADHD/ODD, and normal teenagers during neutral and conflict discussions. *Journal of Abnormal Child Psychology, 24,* 271–297.

Gau, S. S., & Chang, J. P. (2013). Maternal parenting styles and mother–child relationship among adolescents with and without persistent attention-deficit/hyperactivity disorder. *Research in Developmental Disabilities, 34,* 1581–1594.

Gau, S. S., & Chiang, H. L. (2009). Sleep problems and disorders among adolescents with persistent and subthreshold attention-deficit/hyperactivity disorders. *Journal of Sleep and Sleep Disorders Research, 32*(5), 671–679.

Geva, E., & Wiener, J. (2015). *Psychological assessment of culturally and linguistically diverse children and adolescents: A practitioner's guide.* New York: Springer.

Giannotta, F., & Rydell, A. M. (2016). The prospective links between hyperactive/impulsive, inattentive, and oppositional-defiant behaviors in childhood and antisocial behavior in adolescence: The moderating influence of gender and the parent–child relationship quality. *Child Psychiatry and Human Development, 47,* 857–870.

Gisladottir, M., & Svavarsdottir, E. K. (2017). The effectiveness of therapeutic conversation intervention for caregivers of adolescents with ADHD: A quasi-experimental design. *Journal of Psychiatric and Mental Health Nursing, 24,* 15–27.

Goossens, L. (2006). The many faces of adolescent autonomy: Parent–adolescent conflict, behavioral decision-making, and emotional distancing. In S. Jackson & L. Goossens (Eds.), *Handbook of adolescent development* (pp. 135–153). New York: Psychology Press.

Gordon, C. T., & Hinshaw, S. P. (2017). Parenting stress and youth symptoms among girls with and without attention-deficit/hyperactivity disorder. *Parenting, 17,* 11–29.

Graziano, P. A., Fabiano, G., Willoughby, M. T., Waschbusch, D., Morris, K., Schatz, N., & Vujnovic, R. (2016). Callous–unemotional traits among adolescents with attention-deficit/hyperactivity disorder (ADHD): Associations with parenting. *Child Psychiatry and Human Development, 48,* 1–14.

Grimbos, T., & Wiener, J. (2018). Testing the similarity fit/misfit hypothesis in adolescents and parents with ADHD. *Journal of Attention Disorders, 22*(13), 1224–1234.

Haydicky, J., Shecter, C., Wiener, J., & Ducharme, J. M. (2015). Evaluation of MBCT for adolescents with ADHD and their parents: Impact on individual and family functioning. *Journal of Child and Family Studies, 24,* 76–94.

Haydicky, J., Wiener, J., & Shecter, C. (2017). Mechanisms of action in concurrent parent–child mindfulness training: A qualitative exploration. *Mindfulness, 8*(4), 1018–1035.

Heckel, L., Clarke, A., Barry, R., McCarthy, R., & Selikowitz, M. (2009). The relationship between divorce and the psychological well-being of children with ADHD: Differences in age, gender, and subtype. *Emotional and Behavioural Difficulties, 14*(1), 49–68.

Hurtig, T., Ebeling, H., Taanila, A., Miettunen, J., Smalley, S., McGough, J., . . . Moilanen, I. (2007). ADHD and comorbid disorders in relation to family environment and symptom severity. *European Child and Adolescent Psychiatry, 16*(6), 362–369.

Johnston, C., & Behrenz, K. (1993). Childrearing discussions in families of nonproblem children and ADHD children with higher and lower levels of aggressive–defiant behavior. *Canadian Journal of School Psychology, 9,* 53–65.

Johnston, C., & Chronis-Tuscano, A. (2015). Families and ADHD. In R. A. Barkley (Ed.), *Attention-deficit hyperactivity disorder: A handbook for diagnosis and treatment* (4th ed., pp. 191–209). New York: Guilford Press.

Johnston, C., Hommersen, P., & Seipp, C. M. (2009). Maternal attributions and child oppositional behavior: A longitudinal study of boys with and without attention-deficit/hyperactivity disorder. *Journal of Consulting and Clinical Psychology, 77*(1), 189–195.

Johnston, C., Mah, J., & Regambal, M. (2010). Parenting cognitions and treatment beliefs as predictors of experience using behavioral parenting strategies in families of children with attention-deficit/hyperactivity disorder. *Behavior Therapy, 41,* 491–504.

Johnston, C., & Mash, E. J. (2001). Families of children with attention-deficit/hyperactivity disorder: Review and recommendations for future research. *Clinical Child and Family Psychology Review, 4,* 183–207.

Johnston, C., Mash, E. J., Miller, N., & Ninowski, J. E. (2012). Parenting in adults with attention-deficit/hyperactivity disorder (ADHD). *Clinical Psychology Review, 32,* 215–228.

Kazdin, A. E. (1995). Child, parent, and family dysfunction as predictors of outcome in cognitive-behavioral treatment of antisocial children. *Behaviour Research and Therapy, 33,* 271–281.

Langberg, J. M., Evans, S. W., Schultz, B. K., Becker, S. P., Altaye, M., & Girio-Herrera, E. (2016). Trajectories and predictors of response to the Challenging Horizons Program for adolescents with ADHD. *Behavior Therapy, 47,* 339–354.

Lila, M., van Aken, M., Musitu, G., & Buelga, S. (2006). Families and adolescents. In S. Jackson & L. Goossens (Eds.), *Handbook of adolescent development* (pp. 154–174). Hove, UK: Psychology Press.

Markel, C., & Wiener, J. (2014). Attribution processes in parent–adolescent conflict in families of adolescents with and without ADHD. *Canadian Journal of Behavioural Science, 46,* 40–48.

Marton, I., Wiener, J., Rogers, M., Moore, C., & Tannock, R. (2009). Empathy and social perspective taking in children with attention-deficit/hyperactivity disorder. *Journal of Abnormal Child Psychology, 37,* 107–118.

Mazursky-Horowitz, H., Felton, J. W., MacPherson, L., Ehrlich, K. B., Cassidy, J., Lejuez, C. W., & Chronis-Tuscano, A. (2015). Maternal emotion regulation mediates the association between adult attention-deficit/hyperactivity disorder symptoms and parenting. *Journal of Abnormal Child Psychology, 43*(1), 121–131.

McCleary, L., & Ridley, T. (1999). Parenting adolescents with ADHD: Evaluation of a psychoeducation group. *Patient Education and Counseling, 38,* 3–10.

Musabelliu, G., Rogers, M., & Wiener, J. (2018). Parental involvement in the learning of adolescents with and without ADHD. *School Psychology International, 39*(3), 234–250.

Parent, J., Sanders, W., & Forehand, R. (2016). Youth screen time and behavioral health problems: The role of sleep duration and disturbances. *Journal of Developmental and Behavioral Pediatrics, 37*(4), 277–284.

Peasgood, T., Bhardwaj, A., Biggs, K., Brazier, J. E., Coghill, D., Cooper, C. L., . . . Nadkarni, A. (2016). The impact of ADHD on the health and well-being of ADHD children and their siblings. *European Child and Adolescent Psychiatry, 25,* 1217–1231.

Pelham, W. E., Jr., & Fabiano, G. A. (2008). Evidence-based psychosocial treatments for attention-deficit/hyperactivity disorder. *Journal of Clinical Child and Adolescent Psychology, 37*(1), 184–214.

Pelham, W. E., Jr., Meichenbaum, D. L., Smith, B. H., Sibley, M. H., Gnagy, E. M., & Bukstein, O. (2017). Acute effects of MPH on the parent–teen interactions of adolescents with ADHD. *Journal of Attention Disorders, 21,* 158–167.

Pires, P., & Jenkins, J. M. (2007). A growth curve analysis of the joint influences of parenting affect, child characteristics and deviant peers on adolescent illicit drug use. *Journal of Youth and Adolescence, 36,* 169–183.

Pollak, Y., Poni, B., Gershy, N., & Aran, A. (2017, August 1). The role of parental monitoring in mediating the link between adolescent ADHD symptoms and risk-taking behavior. *Journal of Attention Disorders.* [Epub ahead of print]

Psychogiou, L., Daley, D. M., Thompson, M. J., & Sonuga-Barke, E. J. (2007). Testing the interactive effect of parent and child ADHD on parenting in mothers and fathers: A further test of the similarity–fit hypothesis. *British Journal of Developmental Psychology, 425,* 419–433.

Psychogiou, L., Daley, D. M., Thompson, M. J., & Sonuga-Barke, E. J. (2008). Do maternal attention-deficit/hyperactivity disorder symptoms exacerbate or ameliorate the negative effect of child attention-deficit/hyperactivity disorder symptoms on parenting? *Development and Psychopathology, 20,* 121–137.

Rogers, M. A., Wiener, J., Marton, I., & Tannock, R. (2009). Parental involvement in children's learning: Comparing parents of children with and without attention-deficit/hyperactivity disorder (ADHD). *Journal of School Psychology, 47,* 167–185.

Roskam, I., Stievenart, M., Tessier, R., Muntean, A., Escobar, M. J., Santelices, M. P., . . . Pierrehumbert, B. (2014). Another way of thinking about ADHD: The predictive role of early attachment deprivation in adolescents' level of symptoms. *Social Psychiatry and Psychiatric Epidemiology, 49,* 133–144.

Russell, A. E., Ford, T., Williams, R., & Russell, G. (2016). The association between socioeconomic disadvantage and attention deficit/hyperactivity disorder (ADHD): A systematic review. *Child Psychiatry and Human Development, 47*(3), 440–458.

Scharf, M., Oshri, A., Eshkol, V., & Pilowsky, T. (2014). Adolescents' ADHD symptoms and adjustment: The role of attachment and rejection sensitivity. *American Journal of Orthopsychiatry, 84,* 209–217.

Schermerhorn, A. C., D'Onofrio, B. M., Slutske, W. S., Emery, R. E., Turkheimer, E., Harden, K. P., . . . Martin, N. G. (2012). Offspring ADHD as a risk factor for parental marital problems: Controls for genetic and environmental confounds. *Twin Research and Human Genetics, 15,* 700–713.

Sheras, P. L., Abidin, R. R., & Konold, T. R. (1998). *Stress Index for Parents of Adolescents.* Odessa, FL: Psychological Assessment Resources.

Sibley, M. H., Comer, J. S., & Gonzalez, J. (2017). Delivering parent–teen therapy for ADHD through videoconferencing: A preliminary investigation. *Journal of Psychopathology and Behavioral Assessment, 39*(3), 467–485.

Sibley, M. H., Graziano, P. A., Kuriyan, A. B., Coxe, S., Pelham, W. E., Rodriguez, L., . . . Ward, A. (2016). Parent–teen behavior therapy + motivational interviewing for adolescents with ADHD. *Journal of Consulting and Clinical Psychology, 84,* 699–712.

Sibley, M. H., Ross, J. M., Gnagy, E. M., Dixon, L. J., Conn, B., & Pelham, W. E., Jr. (2013). An intensive summer treatment program for ADHD reduces parent–adolescent conflict. *Journal of Psychopathology and Behavioral Assessment, 35,* 10–19.

Tandon, M., Tillman, R., Spitznagel, E., & Luby, J. (2014). Parental warmth and risks of substance use in children with attention-deficit/hyperactivity disorder. *Addiction Research and Theory, 22,* 239–250.

Theule, J., Wiener, J., Jenkins, J., & Tannock, R. (2013). Parenting stress in families of children with ADHD: A meta-analysis. *Journal of Emotional and Behavioral Disorders, 21*(1), 3–17.

Timmermanis, V. K., Haydicky, J., Shecter, C., & Wiener, J. (2016, February). *Maybe she isn't nagging me?: Social perspective taking of adolescents with ADHD.* Symposium presented at the National Association of School Psychologists Convention, New Orleans, LA.

van de Weijer-Bergsma, E., Formsma, A. R., de Bruin, E. I., & Bogels, S. M. (2012). The effectiveness of mindfulness training on behavioral problems and attentional functioning in adolescents with ADHD. *Journal of Child and Family Studies, 21,* 775–787.

Walther, B., Morgenstern, M., & Hanewinkel, R. (2012). Co-occurrence of addictive behaviours: Personality factors related to substance use, gambling and computer gaming. *European Addiction Research, 18*(4), 167–174.

Weiner, B. (1980). A cognitive (attribution)–emotion–action model of motivated behavior: An analysis of judgements of help-giving. *Journal of Personality and Social Psychology, 39,* 186–200.

Wiener, J., Biondic, D., Grimbos, T., & Herbert, M. (2016). Parenting stress of parents of adolescents with attention-deficit hyperactivity disorder. *Journal of Abnormal Child Psychology, 44*(3), 561–574.

Wiener, J., & Daniels, L. (2016). School experiences of adolescents with attention-deficit hyperactivity disorder. *Journal of Learning Disabilities, 49*(6), 567–581.

Wymbs, B. T., Pelham, W. E., Jr., Molina, B. S. G., Gnagy, E. M., Wilson, T. K., & Greenhouse, J. B. (2008). Rate and predictors of divorce among parents of youths with ADHD. *Journal of Consulting and Clinical Psychology, 76*(5), 735–744.

Yeates, K., Schultz, L., & Selman, R. L. (1991). The development of interpersonal negotiation strategies in thought and action: A social–cognitive link to behavioral adjustment and social status. *Merrill–Palmer Quarterly, 37*(3), 369–405.

CHAPTER 7

Peer Functioning in Adolescents with ADHD

Julia D. McQuade

Spurred by hormonal and cognitive maturation, adolescence is a time of increased interest in and contact with peers (Nelson, Leibenluft, McClure, & Pine, 2005). During adolescence, youth become more concerned with, and motivated by, peer acceptance; peers begin to have a more powerful influence on behavior, and new interests in romantic and sexual relationships develop (Forbes & Dahl, 2010; Nelson et al., 2005). Adolescents also must navigate new relationship dynamics: Social groups shift from primarily single-sex to mixed-sex, peer relationships can become romantic or sexual in nature, and new social spheres develop as youth often transition to larger school systems (Grover, Nangle, Serwik, & Zeff, 2007; Petersen & Hamburg, 1986). The social shifts during adolescence have been described as "a reorganization of social behavior" that serves to support critical developmental milestones including individuation from family, relationship intimacy, identity formation, and the development of adult social behaviors (e.g., sexual or romantic; Forbes & Dahl, 2010).

It is not hard to imagine that youth with attention-deficit/hyperactivity disorder (ADHD) would struggle with the shifting social dynamics of adolescence. The social impairments of children with ADHD are well established (see Hoza, 2007; McQuade & Hoza, 2015), and DSM-5 outlines social impairments as a key domain affected by the symptoms of the disorder (American Psychiatric Association, 2013). Failure to pay attention and difficulty staying on task are likely to limit encoding of social cues and create challenges in responding appropriately to peers. Excessive talking, interrupting, and failure to wait one's turn are likely to annoy peers and to limit give-and-take exchanges. Restlessness and fidgeting during a social interaction also may give the impression of an individual who is disinterested or impatient. Indeed, in childhood, youth with ADHD are often described as intrusive, annoying, and disruptive during peer interactions (e.g., Pelham & Bender, 1982). They have difficulty encoding and understanding social information (e.g., Matthys, Cuperus, & van Engeland, 1999) and fail to adjust their social behaviors to changing social demands (e.g., Landau & Milich, 1988). These social challenges are poorly tolerated by peers and result in dislike within minutes of a new social interaction (Erhardt & Hinshaw, 1994; Pelham & Bender, 1982). In fact, between 50 and 80% of children with ADHD are estimated to be rejected (i.e., actively disliked) by their broader peer group (Hoza, 2007). Children with ADHD also tend to have fewer, less stable, and poorer quality friendships (Normand et al., 2013) and gravitate toward peers with similar behavioral problems (e.g., Blachman & Hinshaw, 2002).

Initial evidence suggests that these early social impairments place youth with ADHD on a negative developmental trajectory that increases risk for social, psychological, and functional impairments during adolescence. For instance, within a sample of females with and without ADHD, Mikami and Hinshaw (2006) found that childhood peer rejection was associated with greater externalizing problems, internalizing problems, and eating pathology, and with poorer academic achievement in adolescence (ages 11–18 years). Mrug and colleagues (2012) similarly found that in the Multimodal Treatment of ADHD (MTA) sample, which included children with ADHD and a local normative comparison group, childhood peer rejection predicted greater cigarette smoking, delinquency, and anxiety in early adolescence (mean age of 14 years) and more global impairment in both early and later adolescence (mean ages of 14 and 16 years, respectively). Both studies found these negative effects of peer rejection above and beyond the effects of a childhood ADHD diagnosis, suggesting further exacerbation of later impairments when childhood peer problems are present.

Research also suggests there may be cascading effects of social impairments as youth with ADHD transition from childhood into adolescence. In the MTA sample, Murray-Close and colleagues (2010) found that children with ADHD (mean age of 10 years) had poorer social skills, more aggression, and more peer rejection than youth without the disorder, and these early social impairments persisted into early and later adolescence (mean ages of 14 and 16 years, respectively). In addition, there was evidence of "spillover effects" across social impairment areas. For instance, childhood peer rejection and aggression were associated with poorer social skills in early adolescence, which, in turn, was associated with greater peer rejection and aggression in later adolescence. These results suggest there may be compounding effects of early social challenges as youth with ADHD move across development and into adolescence. Early social challenges may limit preparation for the shifting social dynamics of adolescence, making youth with ADHD poorly equipped to handle these developmental transitions.

Unfortunately, research investigating the social impairments of adolescents with ADHD has been relatively limited and has often focused on broad characterizations of social impairment (e.g., global ratings of social problems). However, available evidence clearly suggests that the social challenges of youth with ADHD persist into adolescence and may begin to manifest in novel ways. Impairments in peer relationships continue, including group-level peer rejection, a lack of dyadic friendships, and heightened risk for peer victimization (i.e., bullying). Social impairments also manifest in negative or ineffective social behaviors and social skills, which may take place during face-to-face interactions and on social media platforms. Evidence from the adult ADHD literature suggests that impairments in romantic relationships and risky sexual behavior also may begin to emerge during adolescence. This chapter reviews what is currently known about the social impairments of adolescents with ADHD and the implications for treatment.

PEER RELATIONSHIPS

Peer Acceptance and Rejection

One important indicator of social functioning in childhood and adolescence is the extent to which the broader peer group accepts (i.e., likes) versus rejects (i.e., dislikes) a child. Peer rejection is one of the most pervasive and intractable social impairments of children with ADHD (Hoza, 2007) and is a critical marker of risk for later maladjustment (Mikami & Hinshaw, 2006; Mrug et al., 2012). Peer rejection may have particularly negative implications during adolescence, when youth become more independent from parents and lean on peers for social support (Forbes & Dahl, 2010). Though limited, research suggests that the global peer rejection experienced by children with ADHD (Hoza, 2007) persists into adolescence (de Boer & Pijl, 2016; Sibley, Evans, & Serpell, 2010; Vitulano et al., 2014). For instance, peers are more likely to nominate early adolescents with ADHD (ages 12–14 years) as individuals they would "rather not like to hang out with" and are less likely to nominate adolescents with ADHD as individuals they would "like to hang out with" relative to adolescents without ADHD (de Boer & Pijl, 2016). Similarly, adolescents with ADHD are rated by their parents and teachers as more rejected by their peers than are adolescents without the disorder (Bagwell, Molina, Pelham, & Hoza, 2001; Hinshaw, Owens, Sami, & Fargeon, 2006).

Dyadic Friendships

Adolescents with ADHD also continue to demonstrate impairments in their mutual friendships. Healthy friendships may be particularly critical in adolescence, as these relationships provide opportunities to develop intimacy, sensitivity toward another's needs, and negotiation skills; these skills then form the foundation for successful adult relationships (Berndt, 2004). Mutual friendships in childhood also may buffer youth with ADHD from the development of later social problems (Becker, Fite, Luebbe, Stoppelbein, & Greening, 2013; Cardoos & Hinshaw, 2011).

Parent and teacher reports indicate that adolescents with ADHD (ages 13–18 years) have fewer close friends than do adolescents without ADHD (Bagwell et al., 2001). As in childhood (Whalen & Henker, 1985), adolescents with ADHD also may continue to gravitate toward deviant peers. Bagwell and colleagues (2001) found that 45% of parents of adolescents with ADHD reported that their adolescents' friends were a bad influence on their child, as compared to 28% of parents of adolescents without ADHD. Marshal, Molina, and Pelham (2003) also found that adolescents with ADHD (ages 13–18 years) were more likely to affiliate with deviant peers (e.g., those who use more substances) relative to adolescents without ADHD; deviant peer affiliation also was associated with subsequent increased risk for substance use, and this effect was particularly strong for adolescents with ADHD. These results suggest that adolescents with ADHD are not only drawn to deviant peers, but they may also be highly susceptible to their negative influence (also see Kennedy, McKone, & Molina, Chapter 11, this volume). Adolescents with high levels of ADHD symptoms (ages 12–15 years) also have reported spending more time socializing with peers and drinking alcohol and smoking cigarettes, and less time with family relative to adolescents who are low in ADHD symptomatology (Whalen, Jamner, Henker, Delfino, & Lozano, 2002). This may suggest that adolescents with ADHD are less well monitored by parents, which could provide more opportunities to participate in deviant behaviors with peers. Some evidence also suggests that deviant peer affiliation is particularly likely among adolescents with ADHD with a comorbid diagnosis of conduct disorder (Bagwell et al., 2001).

Interestingly, adolescents and young adults with ADHD may not perceive as many impairments in their friendships as adult raters do (e.g., teachers). Specifically, adolescents with and without ADHD do not differ in self-reported friendship quality (McNamara, Willoughby, Chalmers, & YLC-CURE, 2005; Al-Yagon, 2016), negativity within friendships (Rokeach & Wiener, 2017), friendship satisfaction (Moyá, Stringaris, Asherson, Sandberg, & Taylor, 2014), or number of friends (Bagwell et al., 2001). In fact, one study actually found that adolescents with ADHD and their close friend (ages 11–17 years) both reported more positive friendship quality than did adolescent friend pairs in which neither person had ADHD (Glass, Flory, & Hankin, 2012). It is possible that over time, youth with ADHD begin to find friends who are more tolerant of their social interaction style and behaviors, and they may therefore experience less dyadic relationship challenges. If adolescents with ADHD are befriending deviant peers, then it is also possible that these deviant peers admire the negative behaviors that youth with ADHD display. However, other research has found that older adolescents with ADHD (ages 16–18 years) report lower perceptions of social support in their friendships than do younger adolescents with ADHD (ages 13–15 years), which may suggest that some aspects of friendship quality do decline across development (Rokeach & Wiener, 2017).

It is also possible that the relative lack of self-reported friendship impairments in adolescents with ADHD reflects a positive illusory bias. A subset of adolescents with ADHD display a positive illusory bias and overestimate their social functioning relative to external indicators (e.g., teacher ratings; Bourchtein, Langberg, Owens, Evans, & Perera, 2017; Hoza, Murray-Close, Arnold, Hinshaw, & Hechtman, 2010). This overestimation of social functioning may stem from self-defensive motivations or from difficulties accurately perceiving social feedback (e.g., McQuade, Mendoza, Larsen, & Breaux, 2017), which may also explain why adolescents with ADHD fail to report friendship challenges (but see Jiang & Johnston, 2017, for potential methodological explanations for this bias).

Peer Victimization

Adolescence is also a time of increased peer victimization or bullying (Pellegrini & Long, 2002). Research suggests that adolescents with ADHD are at heightened risk for peer victimization (Becker, Mehari, Langberg, & Evans, 2017; Sciberras, Ohan, & Anderson, 2012; Unnever & Cornell, 2003). In fact, Becker and colleagues (2017) found that in an early adolescent sample of 11- to 15-year-olds with ADHD, over half of the participants reported one or more peer victimization experiences, occurring at least once per week. These victimization experiences were more likely to take relational forms in which harm was inflicted by manipulating social status (e.g., gossip, systematic exclusion) rather than physical forms in which the harm involved a physical assault. However, this study did not include a comparison sample of adolescents without ADHD, precluding comparisons of victimization rates in adolescents with and without ADHD. Nevertheless, as in the broader developmental literature (e.g., Reijntjes, Kamphuis, Prinzie, & Telch, 2010), peer victimization was found to be associated with negative outcomes for adolescents with ADHD, predicting greater anxiety for boys and girls and greater depression and lower self-esteem for boys (Becker et al., 2017).

SOCIAL SKILLS AND SOCIAL BEHAVIORS

Adolescents with ADHD may display a number of social skills deficits and social behavior problems that contribute to their impaired social relationships. Of serious concern are findings from the MTA sample that youth with a childhood diagnosis of ADHD continue to demonstrate impaired social skills (e.g., assertiveness, cooperation) in adolescence (mean age of 16), even when accounting for the effects of intensive behavioral and/or pharmacological childhood treatment (Molina et al., 2009). Aggressive behavior also may be moderately stable over time, with girls with childhood ADHD demonstrating higher rates of aggressive behavior than those without the disorder when assessed in both childhood (ages 6–12 years) and adolescence (ages 11–18 years; Mikami, Lee, Hinshaw, & Mullin, 2008). However, other evidence suggests that young adolescents with ADHD may show modest improvements in aggression and prosocial skills. Kofler, Larsen, Sarver, and Tolan (2015) followed youth with and without clinical elevations in ADHD symptoms from sixth to eighth grade and found that those with clinical elevations in ADHD symptomatology demonstrated a reduction in aggressive behavior and an increase in prosocial behavior over time. However, these developmental changes did not correspond to a complete normalization of behavior, as even in eighth-grade adolescents with elevated ADHD symptoms continued to be higher in aggression and lower in prosocial behavior than those with low ADHD symptoms.

Initial evidence also suggests that adolescents with ADHD may have challenges with social information processing and problem solving. For instance, Sibley and colleagues (2010) presented a series of social vignettes to young adolescents with and without ADHD (mean age of 12 years) and assessed their social understanding and judgments. Adolescents with ADHD had more difficulty encoding and understanding cause-and-effect relationships and provided more ineffective social solutions than did those without ADHD. Similarly, Mikami and colleagues (2008) found that adolescent girls (ages 11–18 years) with childhood ADHD provided more ineffective solutions to hypothetical social situations than did girls without a history of the disorder. Interestingly, in both studies, there were no ADHD group differences in aggressive cognitions (e.g., inferring hostile intent in peers; Mikami et al., 2008; Sibley et al., 2010); in addition, Mikami and colleagues (2008) found that aggressive cognitions were not associated with aggressive behavior in adolescent girls with ADHD, which suggests that biased hostile thinking may not be driving their aggressive behavior.

Initial evidence suggests that the social behaviors of adolescents with ADHD also may differ in single-sex versus mixed-sex groups. In one study, the social behaviors of early adolescent boys and girls with ADHD (mean age of 13 years) were coded during single-sex and mixed-sex recreational group activities (e.g., Ultimate Frisbee) that occurred during a summer treatment program (STP). Adolescent girls with ADHD were less assertive and had poorer self-management and compliance when participating in mixed-sex relative to single-sex groups. However, boys with ADHD had more appropriate and less inappropriate social behavior in mixed-sex groups relative to single-sex groups (Babinski, Sibley, Ross, & Pelham, 2013). These results may suggest that adolescent girls with ADHD have a particularly difficult time navigating mixed-sex group dynamics. However, because there was not a comparison group, it is unclear whether these gender differences in social behaviors are atypical. At the same time, this is one of the only studies to use observational methods to characterize the social behaviors of adolescents with ADHD. In addition, results suggest that it is important to consider how the social behaviors and performance of adolescents with ADHD differs across contexts (e.g., one-on-one vs. groups, friends vs. new acquaintances, single-sex vs. mixed-sex dyads).

Challenges in Social Media Contexts

Social challenges also may manifest in online venues during adolescence. In a nationally representative U.S. sample, 89% of adolescents (ages 13–17 years) reported using one or more popular social media sites such as Facebook or Twitter. In addition, 88% of adolescents reported having or having access to a cell phone or smartphone, with a reported average of 30 texts sent and received per day (Lenhart, 2015). Although these technological venues offer adolescents new ways to connect with peers, they also can create new social challenges as impulsive social missteps can be public, saved, and shared with others. Unfortunately, there is no research investigating texting behaviors in adolescents with ADHD and very little work examining social media usage in well-characterized ADHD samples.

Mikami, Szwedo, Ahmad, Samuels, and Hinshaw (2015) have conducted the most comprehensive and rigorous study of the social media impairments of individuals with ADHD. Using a sample of females with and without childhood ADHD, the authors found that young adult women (ages 17–24 years) with a history of childhood ADHD reported a greater preference for online social communication and a greater tendency to use online methods to interact with strangers relative to women without childhood ADHD. At the same time, women with childhood ADHD had fewer friends on Facebook, and coding of their Facebook pages indicated less closeness and support from Facebook friends. Several of these childhood ADHD effects were also mediated by face-to-face peer problems during childhood and adolescence (e.g., less acceptance and more rejection by the peers). Mikami and colleagues speculate that peer problems earlier in development may deprive girls with ADHD of important opportunities to practice and develop social skills; this may make girls with ADHD ill-equipped to navigate online social interactions, leading to poorer quality online social relationships. Yet because face-to-face interactions have been challenging, girls with ADHD also may gravitate toward online social venues, perceiving them as potentially easier than face-to-face exchanges. Indeed, other evidence suggests that in adulthood, ADHD symptomatology may be associated with more self-reported compulsive social media usage (Andreassen et al., 2016). However, it is unclear whether compulsive social media usage first emerges during adolescence, and whether this behavior is specifically linked to a diagnosis of ADHD.

Limited evidence also suggests that adolescents with ADHD may be at increased risk for engaging in and experiencing cyberbullying (e.g., bullying through e-mail, instant messaging, social media, the Web, or text interactions; Heiman, Olenik-Shemesh, & Eden, 2015; Yen et al., 2014). For instance, Heiman and colleagues (2015) reported that 18.7% of Israeli adolescent students with ADHD (ages 12–16 years) reported a history of cybervictimization relative to 12.6% of students without ADHD. In addition, 16.7% of adolescents with ADHD reported perpetrating cyberbullying as compared to 11.0% of students without ADHD. As with in-person peer victimization, in partially ADHD samples, cybervictimization is associated with increases in depression and suicidality (Yen et al., 2014) and with greater loneliness, lower social support, and lower perceived social self-efficacy (Heiman et al., 2015). However, these studies were conducted in Taiwan (Yen et al., 2014) and in Israel (Heiman et al., 2015) and may not generalize to other cultural contexts. They also relied on self-report measures, which may inflate correlates with adjustment outcomes due to shared method variance.

ROMANTIC AND SEXUAL RELATIONSHIPS

Romantic Relationships

Research in adult samples suggests that the social impairments of adolescents with ADHD also may extend to romantic relationship challenges. It is unclear whether individuals with ADHD have more (Barkley, Fischer, Smallish, & Fletcher, 2006) or fewer romantic relationships (Babinski et al., 2011); however, within romantic relationships, impairments clearly exist. Specifically, the romantic relationships of adults with ADHD are characterized by less relationship satisfaction (Ben-Naim, Marom, Krashin, Gifter, & Arad, 2017; Canu, Tabor, Michael, Bazzini, & Elmore, 2014; Moyá et al., 2014), lower levels of intimacy (Ben-Naim et al., 2017), and more negative behaviors during conflict (Canu et al., 2014; Moyá et al., 2014). For instance, Canu and colleagues (2014) coded the interaction style of young adult romantic couples (ages 17–33 years) with and without a partner with ADHD while discussing areas of conflict. Couples that included a partner with the combined presentation of ADHD displayed greater negativity, criticism, complaints, and rejection, and less positivity than couples that included a partner with the inattentive presentation of ADHD or when neither partner had ADHD.

Subtype differences in interactions with potential romantic partners also have been found in heterosexual college males with and without ADHD (ages 17–22 years; Canu & Carlson, 2003). Males with the predominantly inattentive presentation of ADHD were coded as more passive and withdrawn during an interaction with an unfamiliar female confederate and were rated by female coders as less appealing as a romantic partner relative to males with the combined presentation of ADHD or males without ADHD. Males with the combined presentation generally did not differ from males without ADHD in coded behavior during the interaction with the unfamiliar female, although on self-report measures they reported increased sexual drive, earlier initiation of dating experiences (e.g., age of first date), and lower likelihood of being a virgin relative to males with predominantly inattentive ADHD or without ADHD.

The romantic relationships of individuals with ADHD also may be characterized by aggression and victimization. For instance, young adult males with a history of childhood ADHD (ages 18–25 years) were five times more likely than males without a history of ADHD to report engaging in violent behaviors toward their partner in the last year (e.g., throwing things at the partner, hitting the partner with something hard; Wymbs et al., 2012). Females with childhood ADHD also reported increased risk for experiencing victimization within romantic relationships, with approximately 30% of young adult women with a history of ADHD (ages 17–24 years) reporting experiences of intimate partner violence, relative to only 6% of comparison women (Guendelman, Ahmad, Meza, Owens, & Hinshaw, 2016).

Unfortunately, researchers have not examined the social behaviors or qualities of romantic relationships in adolescents with ADHD. However, it is likely that the problematic relationship dynamics identified in adult samples first begin to emerge in early romantic relationships (see Collins, Welsh, & Furman, 2009). Peer rejection and a lack of friendships in adolescence (e.g., Bagwell et al., 2011) also may limit opportunities to develop intimate relationships and the social skills needed for effective communication and conflict resolution in later romantic relationships. Problems with social problem solving (e.g., Sibley et al., 2010) also may leave youth with ADHD ill-equipped to handle the emotionally loaded and sometimes complex disagreements that can occur between romantic partners.

Sexual Behaviors

Linked to romantic relationships are sexual experiences, which often first begin in adolescence. Although early sexual experiences provide opportunities for the development of sexual identity and intimacy, there also are risks associated with sexual behavior (e.g., unplanned pregnancy, sexually transmitted diseases). Individuals with ADHD appear particularly likely to engage in risky sexual behaviors (Barkley et al., 2006; Flory, Molina, Pelham, Gnagy, & Smith, 2006; Hechtman et al., 2016; Sarver, McCart, Sheidow, & Letourneau, 2014). For instance, in a sample of adolescents involved in the juvenile justice system (ages 12–17 years), ADHD symptoms were associated with a greater total number of risky sexual behaviors (e.g., early sexual debut, multiple partners, casual sex, inconsistent condom use; Sarver et al., 2014). In a community sample of Russian adolescents (ages 12–17 years), higher levels of inattentive symptoms (but not hyperactive–impulsive symptoms) also predicted engagement in risky sexual behavior (having unprotected sex, more than one sexual partner, intoxication during last intercourse, failure to use a condom during last intercourse, or history of partner pregnancy; Isaksson, Stickley, Koposov, & Ruchkin, 2018). Young adults with a childhood diagnosis of ADHD also report engaging in more casual sex, having more partner pregnancies, more sexual partners, and an earlier initiation of sexual activity and intercourse than adults without a history of ADHD (Flory et al., 2006; Hechtman et al., 2016). Barkley and colleagues (2006) reported that 17% of young adults (mean age of 21 years) with a history of childhood hyperactivity reported contracting a sexually transmitted disease (compared to 4% of community controls), and 25% reported rarely or never using birth control (compared to 10% of controls). In a large Taiwanese sample of adolescents with and without ADHD (ages 12–17 years), those with ADHD were approximately three times more likely to acquire a sexually transmitted disease (HIV, syphilis, genital warts, gonorrhea, chlamydial infection, or trichomoniasis) when followed between 2 and 11 years (Chen et al., 2018). Comorbid conduct disorder or substance use also may account for, or exacerbate, engagement in risky sexual behavior in those with ADHD (Chen et al., 2018; Sarver et al., 2014), though others find that ADHD symptomatology remains a unique risk factor even when accounting for comorbidity and substance use (Flory et al., 2006; Isaksson et al., 2018).

Treatment of Social Impairments

There has been limited research investigating how best to treat the peer problems of adolescents with ADHD. However, studies from child samples suggest that traditional evidence-based treatments (e.g., behavior modification and/or stimulant medication) may not be sufficient. For instance, Hoza and colleagues (2005) reported that in the MTA, randomization to intensive behavioral modification (including participation in an STP with social skills training) and/or carefully titrated stimulant medication failed to normalize the peer functioning of children with ADHD; in addition, these treatments were generally not superior to community care on peer-assessed social outcomes. A similar rigorous investigation of the effects of behavior modification and medication on the social functioning of adolescents with ADHD has not been conducted. However, researchers have examined changes in social functioning following participation in an adolescent STP, which involved short-term intensive behavioral modification and sports-based social skills training (Sibley et al., 2011; Sibley, Smith, Evans, Pelham, & Gnagy, 2012). Sibley and colleagues (2012) reported that approximately 81% of adolescents with ADHD (ages 11–16 years) participating in the STP were rated by parents as at least somewhat improved in social skills; however, only 28% of parents rated social skills as *much improved* or very much *improved,* which suggests that social gains were relatively modest. Smith and colleagues (1998) also reported that in the context of an STP, adolescents with ADHD (ages 12–17 years) demonstrated a reduction in counselor-coded behaviors associated with peer dislike (e.g., defiance, teasing peers, impulsivity) when taking a low dose of methylphenidate (10 mg) relative to when on a placebo pill. Further reductions in aversive social behaviors generally were not observed when medication dose was increased to 20 mg or to 30 mg, and there was some evidence of increased social withdrawal at higher doses. Unfortunately, these studies did not examine whether social improvement generalized to contexts outside of the STP or are reflected in more objective measures of social functioning, such as peer nominations of liking and friendship. Given results from child studies (e.g., Hoza et al., 2005), it is unlikely that behavior therapy and/or medication are sufficient to address the range of social impairments that adolescents with ADHD display.

Other researchers have developed skills-based treatments to try to address the social skills and social cognition deficits of adolescents with ADHD. Social skills training typically involves teaching children specific social skills (e.g., cooperation) in a structured setting, with opportunities to practice the skills with either the clinician or other group members. At least in child samples, there is limited evidence to suggest that social skills training, either alone or when embedded within intensive behavior modification, is effective in addressing the social impairments of youth with ADHD (de Boo & Prins, 2007; Hoza et al., 2005; Quinn, Kavale, Mathur, Rutherford, & Forness, 1999). Though limited, evidence from adolescent ADHD samples supports this more general conclusion. For instance, Sadler, Evans, Schultz, and Zoromski (2011) designed a short-term, school-based social skills group for adolescents with ADHD (ages 13–17 years) that focused on improving understanding of cause-and-effect relationships and self-monitoring skills. In the treatment, adolescents identified personal social goals (e.g., "Being seen as funny"), then discussed with a staff member their success in meeting their goals during weekly semistructured activities and free time with other group participants. Discussions focused on a comparison of the adolescent's and a staff member's perception of the adolescent's behavior and on identifying specific steps to improve subsequent social performance. Unfortunately, only 33% of adolescents displayed mastery of the intervention (i.e., rated by staff members as displaying behavior consistent with their personal goal over multiple consecutive sessions). Those who mastered the intervention were rated by parents as showing greater reductions in social impairment, but they did not show improvement in social skills relative to those who did not master the intervention.

In a more intensive, long-term intervention, the Challenging Horizons Program (CHP) was designed to improve both academic and social skills in sixth through eighth graders with ADHD (Schultz, Evans, Langberg, & Shoemann, 2017). CHP, a yearlong afterschool psychosocial treatment, focuses on teaching adolescents homework organization (see Langberg, Smith, & Green, Chapter 15, this volume) and social problem-solving skills. As part of the program, adolescents participate in interpersonal skills groups and have opportunities to practice social skills during recreational activities. Schultz and colleagues reported that participation in the CHP, as well as compliance with the CHP, was not associated with improvements in parent-rated social skills related to communication, cooperation, assertion, empathy, or engagement; however, CHP participation did predict improved self-control social skills, and greater treatment compliance predicted improved self-control and responsibility social skills. The limited effects on social functioning are discouraging, particularly given the length of program (i.e., twice weekly for one full school year) and the multiple opportunities for generalization of skills through peer interaction.

Other researchers have speculated that the treatments reviewed earlier may be ineffective because they focus exclusively on the adolescents' impairments. For instance, Hoza (2007) has argued that even if youth with ADHD show improvement in social behaviors or skills, this is unlikely to translate into improved social relationships, because peers have already developed a negative bias toward the child. Hoza therefore suggested that interventions need to address peer group attitudes in order to see real changes in the social functioning of youth with ADHD. Recent research suggests that this approach holds promise, at least for children. Specifically, in the context of an STP, Mikami and colleagues (2013) randomly assigned children with and without ADHD (ages 6–9 years) to a classroom employing traditional contingency management strategies or to a classroom in which the teacher had been trained to promote social inclusion. Teachers in the socially inclusive classroom modeled warm interactions with each child, publicly highlighted each child's individual strengths, promoted inclusion through explicit classroom rules and cooperative activities, and privately (rather than publicly) reviewed point losses related to a token economy system. The researchers found that at the end of the 2-week intervention, children with ADHD were rated by peers as less disliked and had more reciprocated friendships and more positive peer ratings when in the socially inclusive classroom relative to the traditional contingency management classroom. Importantly, children with ADHD did not differ in behavior problems in the two classrooms, suggesting that the positive peer effects were likely a result of the classroom environment and not the individual child. Though preliminary, these results suggest that classroom culture may play a critical role in either promoting or mitigating peer challenges for youth with ADHD. This likely continues into adolescence; however, the multiple teachers in middle and high school and the larger school systems may make addressing peer climate more challenging. Adolescents also may be more strongly influenced by peers' than by adults' behaviors (Forbes & Dahl, 2010). That said, researchers have been successful in reducing other negative social behaviors (e.g., bullying) in high school students using universal schoolwide interventions that change peer culture through teacher-based lessons and individual online trainings (e.g., Kärnä et al., 2011). Similar approaches may be able to also promote social inclusion.

Another consideration in treating the social impairments of adolescents with ADHD is whether group-based treatment is advisable. On the one hand, the group format of the STP and of many social skills training groups offers real-time opportunities to practice social skills with clinician feedback. This may be a critical factor in order to see generalization of effects to other peer contexts. At the same time, researchers have observed peer contagion in group-based social interventions, in which children may begin to model the negative social behaviors of other group members. One particularly concerning form of peer contagion is *deviancy training,* in which antisocial behaviors are promoted through positive peer attention and modeling (see Gifford-Smith, Dodge, Dishion, & McCord, 2005). This may be particularly likely to occur in adolescents with ADHD, who have been shown to gravitate toward more antisocial peers (e.g., Bagwell et al., 2011). Although opportunities to practice social interactions are likely critical to any effective social intervention, clinicians need to be aware of these potential iatrogenic effects.

Parents also may be able to play a role in reducing social impairments in adolescents with ADHD. Preliminary evidence from child research suggests that parents can be effectively coached to facilitate positive social experiences for children with ADHD (e.g., Mikami, Lerner, Griggs, McGrath, & Calhoun, 2010). Similar approaches with parents of adolescents with ADHD may be feasible, with a focus on teaching parents how to promote opportunities for affiliation with prosocial peers (e.g., targeted extracurricular activities) and to decrease opportunities for risky social behaviors (e.g., substance use). Parents also may require explicit clinician coaching in how to speak with their adolescent about responsible social media usage, safe sex practices, and healthy romantic relationships (e.g., free from aggression and victimization). It may be hard for parents to engage in these conversations, but doing so may be highly critical for adolescents with ADHD who are at risk for challenges in these areas.

CONCLUSION

Peer problems, a common, enduring, and often intractable impairment of youth with ADHD, frequently persists into adolescence. Not only are adolescents less accepted and more rejected by their larger peer group, but they also are less likely to have mutual friendships (e.g., Bagwell et al., 2001). Even when adolescents with ADHD do have friends, these friendships may be characterized by engagement in more deviant social behavior and substance use (e.g., Marshal et al., 2003). Adolescents with ADHD also continue to display noxious social behaviors such as aggression and have difficulty with social skills and social problem solving (e.g., Mikami et al., 2008; Sibley et al., 2010). In addition, youth with ADHD may be poorly equipped to handle the onset of romantic and sexual relationships; they may fail to develop effective skills to negotiate conflict with romantic partners (Canu & Carlson, 2003) and are more likely to engage in risky sexual behaviors (e.g., Flory et al., 2006).

The cause of the continued social problems in adolescents with ADHD is likely multifaceted. Researchers have argued that youth with ADHD have a social performance deficit that limits their ability to respond appropriately in social situations (de Boo & Prins, 2007). This may stem from the symptoms of ADHD, the underlying neuropsychological impairments, challenges with emotion regulation, or a combination of these factors (e.g., Bunford, Evans, Becker, & Langberg, 2015; Kofler et al., 2011; McQuade, Penzel, Silk, & Lee, 2017). Peer problems during childhood also are likely to further exacerbate any performance-based deficits of adolescents with ADHD, limiting opportunities to develop the foundational social skills needed for the more mature and intimate relationships that emerge in adolescence. Other factors that may contribute to or exacerbate the social problems of adolescents with ADHD should also be examined, such as co-occurring mental health symptoms (e.g., Bagwell et al., 2001; Becker, Langberg, Evans, Girio-Herrera, & Vaughn, 2015), particularly as factors contributing to social impairments among adolescents with ADHD may themselves be important treatment targets with downstream effects. In addition, a minority of adolescents with ADHD are socially well adjusted, which may protect against impairments in other areas of functioning (e.g., Dvorsky, Langberg, Evans, & Becker, 2018). Researchers also need to examine why some adolescents with ADHD remain socially well adjusted and whether this subset of youth traverses a distinct developmental trajectory.

Additional research characterizing how social impairments unfold and shift across development in youth with ADHD is sorely needed. There is also a lack of research characterizing the specific social behavior challenges that emerge in adolescence, particularly in the context of online social exchanges, mixed-sex groups, and with potential or current romantic partners. With a few notable exceptions, few longitudinal studies have examined predictors and consequences of poor social functioning in adolescents with ADHD and potential transactional and bidirectional effects of risk factors. Such work is likely to provide additional treatment targets and help researchers and clinicians refine available treatments in order to better address the social impairments of this population.

References

Al-Yagon, M. (2016). Perceived close relationships with parents, teachers, and peers: Predictors of social, emotional, and behavioral features in adolescents with LD or comorbid LD and ADHD. *Journal of Learning Disabilities, 49,* 597–615.

American Psychiatric Association. (2013). *Diagnostic and statistical manual of mental disorders* (5th ed.). Arlington, VA: Author.

Andreassen, C. S., Billieux, J., Griffiths, M. D., Kuss, D. J., Demetrovics, Z., Mazzoni, E., & Pallesen, S. (2016). The relationship between addictive use of social media and video games and symptoms of psychiatric disorders: A large-scale cross-sectional study. *Psychology of Addictive Behaviors, 30,* 252–262.

Babinski, D. E., Pelham, W. J., Molina, B. G., Gnagy, E. M., Waschbusch, D. A., Yu, J., . . . Karch, K. M. (2011). Late adolescent and young adult outcomes of girls diagnosed with ADHD in childhood: An exploratory investigation. *Journal of Attention Disorders, 15,* 204–214.

Babinski, D. E., Sibley, M. H., Ross, J. M., & Pelham, W. E. (2013). The effects of single versus mixed gender treatment for adolescent girls with ADHD. *Journal of Clinical Child and Adolescent Psychology, 42,* 243–250.

Bagwell, C. L., Molina, B. G., Pelham, W. E., & Hoza, B. (2001). Attention-deficit hyperactivity disorder and problems in peer relations: Predictions from childhood to adolescence. *Journal of the American Academy of Child and Adolescent Psychiatry, 40,* 1285–1292.

Barkley, R. A., Fischer, M., Smallish, L., & Fletcher, K. (2006). Young adult outcome of hyperactive children: Adaptive functioning in major life activities. *Journal of the American Academy of Child and Adolescent Psychiatry, 45,* 192–202.

Becker, S. P., Fite, P. J., Luebbe, A. M., Stoppelbein, L., & Greening, L. (2013). Friendship intimacy exchange buffers the relation between ADHD symptoms and later social problems among children attending an after-school care program. *Journal of Psychopathology and Behavioral Assessment, 35,* 142–152.

Becker, S. P., Langberg, J. M., Evans, S. W., Girio-Herrera, E., & Vaughn, A. J. (2015). Differentiating anxiety and depression in relation to the social functioning of young adolescents with ADHD. *Journal of Clinical Child and Adolescent Psychology, 44,* 1015–1029.

Becker, S. P., Mehari, K. R., Langberg, J. M., & Evans, S. W. (2017). Rates of peer victimization in young adolescents with ADHD and associations with internalizing symptoms and selfesteem. *European Child and Adolescent Psychiatry, 26,* 201–214.

Ben-Naim, S., Marom, I., Krashin, M., Gifter, B., & Arad, K. (2017). Life with a partner with ADHD: The moderating role of intimacy. *Journal of Child And Family Studies, 26,* 1365–1373.

Berndt, T. J. (2004). Children's friendships: Shifts over a half-century in perspectives on their development and their effects. *Merrill–Palmer Quarterly, 50,* 206–223.

Blachman, D. R., & Hinshaw, S. P. (2002). Patterns of friendship among girls with and without attention-deficit/hyperactivity disorder. *Journal of Abnormal Child Psychology, 30,* 625–640.

Bourchtein, E., Langberg, J. M., Owens, J. S., Evans, S. W., & Perera, R. A. (2017). Is the positive illusory bias common in young adolescents with ADHD?: A fresh look at prevalence and stability using latent profile and transition analyses. *Journal of Abnormal Child Psychology, 45,* 1063–1075.

Bunford, N., Evans, S. W., Becker, S. P., & Langberg, J. M. (2015). Attention-deficit/hyperactivity disorder and social skills in youth: A moderated mediation model of emotion dysregulation and depression. *Journal of Abnormal Child Psychology, 43,* 283–296.

Canu, W. H., & Carlson, C. L. (2003). Differences in heterosocial behavior and outcomes of ADHD-symptomatic subtypes in a college sample. *Journal of Attention Disorders, 6,* 123–133.

Canu, W. H., Tabor, L. S., Michael, K. D., Bazzini, D. G., & Elmore, A. L. (2014). Young adult romantic couples' conflict resolution and satisfaction varies with partner's attention-deficit/hyperactivity disorder type. *Journal of Marital And Family Therapy, 40,* 509–524.

Cardoos, S. L., & Hinshaw, S. P. (2011). Friendship as protection from peer victimization for girls with and without ADHD. *Journal of Abnormal Child Psychology, 39,* 1035–1045.

Chen, M., Hsu, J., Huang, K., Bai, Y., Ko, N., Su, T., . . . Chen, T. (2018). Sexually transmitted infection among adolescents and young adults with attention-deficit/hyperactivity disorder: A nationwide longitudinal study. *Journal of the American Academy of Child and Adolescent Psychiatry, 57,* 48–53.

Collins, W. A., Welsh, D. P., & Furman, W. (2009). Adolescent romantic relationships. *Annual Review of Psychology, 60,* 631–652.

de Boer, A., & Pijl, S. J. (2016). The acceptance and rejection of peers with ADHD and ASD in general secondary education. *Journal of Educational Research, 109,* 325–332.

de Boo, G. M., & Prins, P. M. (2007). Social incompetence in children with ADHD: Possible moderators and mediators in social-skills training. *Clinical Psychology Review, 27,* 78–97.

Dvorsky, M. R., Langberg, J. M., Evans, S. W., & Becker, S. P. (2018). The protective effects of social factors on the academic functioning of adolescents with ADHD. *Journal of Clinical Child and Adolescent Psychology, 47*(5), 713–726.

Erhardt, D., & Hinshaw, S. P. (1994). Initial sociometric impressions of attention-deficit hyperactivity disorder and comparison boys: Predictions from social behaviors and from nonbehavioral variables. *Journal of Consulting and Clinical Psychology, 62,* 833–842.

Flory, K., Molina, B. G., Pelham, W. J., Gnagy, E., & Smith, B. (2006). Childhood ADHD predicts risky sexual behavior in young adulthood. *Journal of Clinical Child and Adolescent Psychology, 35,* 571–577.

Forbes, E. E., & Dahl, R. E. (2010). Pubertal development and behavior: Hormonal activation of social and motivational tendencies. *Brain and Cognition, 72,* 66–72.

Gifford-Smith, M., Dodge, K. A., Dishion, T. J., & McCord, J. (2005). Peer influence in children and adolescents: Crossing the bridge from developmental to intervention science. *Journal of Abnormal Child Psychology, 33,* 255–265.

Glass, K., Flory, K., & Hankin, B. L. (2012). Symptoms of ADHD and close friendships in adolescence. *Journal of Attention Disorders, 16,* 406–417.

Grover, R. L., Nangle, D. W., Serwik, A., & Zeff, K. R. (2007). Girl friend, boy friend, girlfriend, boyfriend: Broadening our understanding of heterosocial competence. *Journal of Clinical Child and Adolescent Psychology, 36,* 491–502.

Guendelman, M. D., Ahmad, S., Meza, J. I., Owens, E. B., & Hinshaw, S. P. (2016). Childhood attention-deficit/hyperactivity disorder predicts intimate partner victimization in young women. *Journal of Abnormal Child Psychology, 44,* 155–166.

Hechtman, L., Swanson, J. M., Sibley, M. H., Stehli, A., Owens, E. B., Mitchell, J. T., . . . Nichols, J. Q. (2016). Functional adult outcomes 16 years after childhood diagnosis of attention-deficit/hyperactivity disorder: MTA results. *Journal of the American Academy of Child and Adolescent Psychiatry, 55,* 945–952.

Heiman, T., Olenik-Shemesh, D., & Eden, S. (2015). Cyberbullying involvement among students with ADHD: Relation to loneliness, self-efficacy and social support. *European Journal of Special Needs Education, 30,* 15–29.

Hinshaw, S. P., Owens, E. B., Sami, N., & Fargeon, S. (2006). Prospective follow-up of girls with attention-deficit/hyperactivity disorder into adolescence: Evidence for continuing cross-domain impairment. *Journal of Consulting and Clinical Psychology, 74,* 489–499.

Hoza, B. (2007). Peer functioning in children with ADHD. *Journal of Pediatric Psychology, 32,* 655–663.

Hoza, B., Gerdes, A. C., Mrug, S., Hinshaw, S. P., Bukowski, W. M., Gold, J. A., . . . Wigal, T. (2005). Peer-assessed outcomes in the multimodal treatment study of children with attention deficit hyperactivity disorder. *Journal of Clinical Child and Adolescent Psychology, 34,* 74–86.

Hoza, B., Murray-Close, D., Arnold, L. E., Hinshaw, S. P., & Hechtman, L. (2010). Time-dependent changes in positively biased self-perceptions of children with attention-deficit/hyperactivity disorder: A developmental psychopathology perspective. *Development and Psychopathology, 22,* 375–390.

Isaksson, J., Stickley, A., Koposov, R., & Ruchin, V. (2018). The danger of being inattentive—ADHD symptoms and risky sexual behavior in Russian adolescents. *European Psychiatry, 47,* 42–48.

Jiang, Y., & Johnston, C. (2017). Controlled social interaction tasks to measure self-perceptions: No evidence of positive illusions in boys with ADHD. *Journal of Abnormal Child Psychology, 45,* 1051–1062.

Kärnä, A., Voeten, M., Little, T. D., Poskiparta, E., Alanen, E., & Salmivalli, C. (2011). Going to scale: A nonrandomized nationwide trial of the KiVa antibullying program for grades 1–9. *Journal of Consulting and Clinical Psychology, 79,* 796–805.

Kofler, M. J., Larsen, R., Sarver, D. E., & Tolan, P. H. (2015). Developmental trajectories of aggression, prosocial behavior, and social–cognitive problem solving in emerging adolescents with clinically elevated attention-deficit/hyperactivity disorder symptoms. *Journal of Abnormal Psychology, 124,* 1027–1042.

Kofler, M. J., Rapport, M. D., Bolden, J., Sarver, D. E., Raiker, J. S., & Alderson, R. M. (2011). Working memory deficits and social problems in children with ADHD. *Journal of Abnormal Child Psychology, 39,* 805–817.

Landau, S., & Milich, R. (1988). Social communication patterns of attention-deficit-disordered boys. *Journal of Abnormal Child Psychology, 16,* 69–81.

Lenhart, A. (2015). Teen, social media and technology overview. Retrieved from *www.pewinternet.org/2015/04/09/teens-social-media-technology-2015.*

Marshal, M. P., Molina, B. G., & Pelham, W. J. (2003). Childhood ADHD and adolescent substance use: An examination of deviant peer group affiliation as a risk factor. *Psychology of Addictive Behaviors, 17,* 293–302.

Matthys, W., Cuperus, J. M., & Van Engeland, H. (1999). Deficient social problem-solving in boys with ODD/CD, with ADHD, and with both disorders. *Journal of the American Academy of Child and Adolescent Psychiatry, 38,* 311–321.

McNamara, J. K., Willoughby, T., Chalmers, H., & & YLC-CURA. (2005). Psychosocial status of adolescents with learning disabilities with and without comorbid attention deficit hyperactivity disorder. *Learning Disabilities Research and Practice, 20,* 234–244.

McQuade, J. D., & Hoza, B. (2015). Peer relationships of children with ADHD. In R. A. Barkley (Ed.), *Attention-deficit hyperactivity disorder: A handbook for diagnosis and treatment* (pp. 210–222). New York: Guilford Press.

McQuade, J. D., Mendoza, S. A., Larsen, K. L., & Breaux, R. P. (2017). The nature of social positive illusory bias: Reflection of social impairment, self-protective motivation, or poor executive functioning? *Journal of Abnormal Child Psychology, 45,* 289–300.

McQuade, J. D., Penzel, T. E., Silk, J. S., & Lee, K. H. (2017). Parasympathetic nervous system reactivity moderates associations between children's executive functioning and social and academic competence. *Journal of Abnormal Child Psychology, 45*(7), 1355–1367.

Mikami, A. Y., Griggs, M. S., Lerner, M. D., Emeh, C. C., Reuland, M. M., Jack, A., & Anthony, M. R. (2013). A randomized trial of a classroom intervention to increase peers' social inclusion of children with attention-deficit/hyperactivity disorder. *Journal of Consulting and Clinical Psychology, 81,* 100–112.

Mikami, A. Y., & Hinshaw, S. P. (2006). Resilient adolescent adjustment among girls: Buffers of childhood peer rejection and attention-deficit/hyperactivity disorder. *Journal of Abnormal Child Psychology, 34,* 825–839.

Mikami, A. Y., Lee, S. S., Hinshaw, S. P., & Mullin, B. C. (2008). Relationships between social information processing and aggression among adolescent girls with and without ADHD. *Journal of Youth and Adolescence, 37,* 761–771.

Mikami, A. Y., Lerner, M. D., Griggs, M. S., McGrath, A., & Calhoun, C. D. (2010). Parental influence on children with attention-deficit/hyperactivity disorder: II. Results of a pilot intervention training parents as friendship coaches for children. *Journal of Abnormal Child Psychology, 38,* 737–749.

Mikami, A. Y., Szwedo, D. E., Ahmad, S. I., Samuels, A. S., & Hinshaw, S. P. (2015). Online social communication patterns among emerging adult women with histories of childhood attention-deficit/hyperactivity disorder. *Journal of Abnormal Psychology, 124,* 576–588.

Molina, B. G., Hinshaw, S. P., Swanson, J. M., Arnold, L. E., Vitiello, B., Jensen, P. S., . . . Houck, P. R. (2009). The MTA at 8 years: Prospective follow-up of children treated for combined-type ADHD in a multisite study. *Journal of the American Academy of Child and Adolescent Psychiatry, 48,* 484–500.

Moyá, J., Stringaris, A. K., Asherson, P., Sandberg, S., & Taylor, E. (2014). The impact of persisting hyperactivity on social relationships: A community-based, controlled 20-year follow-up study. *Journal of Attention Disorders, 18,* 52–60.

Mrug, S., Molina, B. G., Hoza, B., Gerdes, A. C., Hinshaw, S. P., Hechtman, L., & Arnold, L. E. (2012). Peer rejection and friendships in children with attention-deficit/hyperactivity disorder: Contributions to long-term outcomes. *Journal of Abnormal Child Psychology, 40,* 1013–1026.

Murray-Close, D., Hoza, B., Hinshaw, S. P., Arnold, L. E., Swanson, J., Jensen, P. S., . . . Wells, K. (2010). Developmental processes in peer problems of children with attention-deficit/hyperactivity disorder in the Multimodal Treatment Study of Children with ADHD: Developmental cascades and vicious cycles. *Development and Psychopathology, 22,* 785–802.

Nelson, E. E., Leibenluft, E., McClure, E., & Pine, D. S. (2005). The social re-orientation of adolescence: A neuroscience perspective on the process and its relation to psychopathology. *Psychological Medicine, 35,* 163–174.

Normand, S., Schneider, B. H., Lee, M. D., Maisonneuve, M., Chupetlovska-Anastasova, A., Kuehn, S. M., & Robaey, P. (2013). Continuities and changes in the friendships of children with and without ADHD: A longitudinal, observational study. *Journal of Abnormal Child Psychology, 41*(7), 1161–1175.

Pelham, W. E., & Bender, M. E. (1982). Peer relationships in hyperactive children: Description and treatment. *Advances in Learning and Behavioral Disabilities, 1,* 365–436.

Pellegrini, A. D., & Long, J. D. (2002). A longitudinal study of bullying, dominance, and victimization during the transition from primary school through secondary school. *British Journal of Developmental Psychology, 20,* 259–280.

Petersen, A. C., & Hamburg, B. A. (1986). Adolescence: A developmental approach to problems and psychopathology. *Behavior Therapy, 17,* 480–499.

Quinn, M., Kavale, K. A., Mathur, S. R., Rutherford, R. J., & Forness, S. R. (1999). A meta-analysis of social skill interventions for students with emotional or behavioral disorders. *Journal of Emotional and Behavioral Disorders, 7,* 54–64.

Reijntjes, A., Kamphuis, J. H., Prinzie, P., & Telch, M. J. (2010). Peer victimization and internalizing problems in children: A meta-analysis of longitudinal studies. *Child Abuse and Neglect, 34,* 244–252.

Rokeach, A., & Wiener, J. (2017, October 1). Friendship quality in adolescents with ADHD. *Journal of Attention Disorders.* [Epub ahead of print]

Sadler, J. M., Evans, S. W., Schultz, B. K., & Zoromski, A. K. (2011). Potential mechanisms of action in the treatment of social impairment and disorganization in adolescents with ADHD. *School Mental Health, 3,* 156–168.

Sarver, D. E., McCart, M. R., Sheidow, A. J., & Letourneau, E. J. (2014). ADHD and risky sexual behavior in adolescents: Conduct problems and substance use as mediators of risk. *Journal of Child Psychology and Psychiatry, 55,* 1345–1353.

Schultz, B. K., Evans, S. W., Langberg, J. M., & Schoemann, A. M. (2017). Outcomes for adolescents who comply with long-term psychosocial treatment for ADHD. *Journal of Consulting and Clinical Psychology, 85,* 250–261.

Sciberras, E., Ohan, J., & Anderson, V. (2012). Bullying and peer victimisation in adolescent girls with attention-deficit/hyperactivity disorder. *Child Psychiatry and Human Development, 43,* 254–270.

Sibley, M. H., Evans, S. W., & Serpell, Z. N. (2010). Social cognition and interpersonal impairment in young adolescents with ADHD. *Journal of Psychopathology and Behavioral Assessment, 32,* 193–202.

Sibley, M. H., Pelham, W. E., Evans, S. W., Gnagy, E. M., Ross, J. M., & Greiner, A. R. (2011). An evaluation of a summer treatment program for adolescents with ADHD. *Cognitive and Behavioral Practice, 18,* 530–544.

Sibley, M. H., Smith, B. H., Evans, S. W., Pelham, W. E., & Gnagy, E. M. (2012). Treatment response to an intensive summer treatment program for adolescents with ADHD. *Journal of Attention Disorders, 16,* 443–448.

Smith, B. H., Pelham, W. E., Evans, S., Gnagy, E., Molina, B., Bukstein, O., . . . Willoughby, M. (1998). Dosage effects of methylphenidate on the social behavior of adolescents diagnosed with attention deficit hyperactivity disorder. *Experimental and Clinical Psychopharmacology, 6,* 187–204.

Unnever, J. D., & Cornell, D. G. (2003). Bullying, self-control, and ADHD. *Journal of Interpersonal Violence, 18,* 129–147.

Vitulano, M. L., Fite, P. J., Hopko, D. R., Lochman, J., Wells, K., & Asif, I. (2014). Evaluation of underlying mechanisms in the link between childhood ADHD symptoms and risk for early initiation of substance use. *Psychology of Addictive Behaviors, 28,* 816–827.

Whalen, C. K., & Henker, B. (1985). The social worlds of hyperactive (ADHD) children. *Clinical Psychology Review, 5,* 447–478.

Whalen, C. K., Jamner, L. D., Henker, B., Delfino, R. J., & Lozano, J. M. (2002). The ADHD spectrum and everyday life: Experience sampling of adolescent moods, activities, smoking, and drinking. *Child Development, 73,* 209–227.

Wymbs, B., Molina, B., Pelham, W., Cheong, J., Gnagy, E., Belendiuk, K., . . . Waschbusch, D. (2012). Risk of intimate partner violence among young adult males with childhood ADHD. *Journal of Attention Disorders, 16,* 373–383.

Yen, C., Chou, W., Liu, T., Ko, C., Yang, P., & Hu, H. (2014). Cyberbullying among male adolescents with attention-deficit/hyperactivity disorder: Prevalence, correlates, and association with poor mental health status. *Research in Developmental Disabilities, 35,* 3543–3553.

CHAPTER 8

Academic Functioning and Interventions for Adolescents with ADHD

Steven W. Evans
Saskia Van der Oord
Emma E. Rogers

For many years, parents were told that their children with attention-deficit/hyperactivity disorder (ADHD) would outgrow the disorder when they began adolescence. Research eventually revealed what parents have known for decades—that the vast majority of adolescents with ADHD do not outgrow the impairment associated with ADHD when they enter puberty (see Larsson, Chapter 2, this volume). Problems establishing and maintaining friendships and succeeding in school remain and can contribute to many other serious problems during adolescence (e.g., substance use, driving accidents, school dropout). School-related impairment for adolescents with ADHD has received considerable attention and has been a common target of treatment development (Kent et al., 2011). The demands of academic environments pull for skills and abilities that are limited according to the symptom profiles of adolescents with ADHD. For example, difficulties attending to details, completing tasks, organizing, remembering assignments, talking excessively, and interrupting others are behaviors that will lead to academic failure and discipline problems in school. In fact, research has indicated strong associations between teacher ratings of the two ADHD symptom factors (i.e., inattention and hyperactivity/impulsivity) and impairment in academic progress, classroom functioning, relationships with teachers, and relationships with peers (Zoromski, Owens, Evans, & Brady, 2015). For adolescents, the inattentive symptoms appear to be most associated with teacher-reported interpersonal and academic impairment (Zoromski et al., 2015).

Reports indicate that 9.3% of high school-age students are reported by their parents to have a diagnosis of ADHD (Akinbami, Liu, Pastor, & Reuben, 2011); thus, there is likely to be an average of two to three students with the disorder in every classroom. These students present unique challenges to teachers. They are more likely than their peers to have significant academic impairment in math and reading (Frazier, Youngstrom, Glutting, & Watkins, 2007), as well as writing (Molitor et al., 2016). In addition, adolescents with ADHD are much less likely than their peers to turn in completed homework, submitting only 64% of assigned homework compared to 83% among peers without ADHD (Kent et al., 2011). High school students with ADHD also have significantly lower grade point averages, more absences, more placements in remedial courses, and receive more failing grades, and are more likely to drop out of school than high school students without ADHD (Kent et al., 2011). As might be expected from the nature of these problems, they are much less likely to attend college, graduate from college, and maintain employment than young adults without ADHD (Barkley, Murphy, & Fischer, 2008; Kuriyan et al., 2013). In addition to these hardships experienced during adolescence, evidence indicates that these problems during high school are associated with poor outcomes as adults. In particular, problems with school functioning, including academic and behavior problems (e.g., failing grades, disciplinary sanctions), predict worse post-high school education outcomes. High school functioning and parent education, but not diagnosis, accounted for all differences in postsecondary education outcomes between those with and without ADHD (Kuriyan et al., 2013). These findings show that high school functioning is critically important to long-term education and employment. Given these problems, it is not surprising that adults with ADHD report reduced financial independence and greater financial reliance on the welfare system and parents than their peers without ADHD (Altszuler et al., 2016).

The problems experienced at school by adolescents with ADHD often co-occur with other problems characteristic of this age group, such as using alcohol and illicit substances (Molina, Pelham, Gnagy, Thompson & Marshal, 2007), spending time with peers who engage in deviant behaviors (Marshal, Molina, & Pelham, 2003), driving accidents (Barkley, Murphy, & Kwasnik, 1996), and experiencing conflict with their parents (Johnston & Mash, 2001) (in this volume, see Wiener, Chapter 6; McQuade, Chapter 7; Becker & Fogleman, Chapter 9; Mulraney, Sciberras, & Becker, Chapter 10; Kennedy, McKone, & Molina, Chapter 11; Garner, Chapter 12). Similar to alcohol and substance abuse and related deviant behaviors, academic impairments are life-changing problems with negative consequences far beyond adolescence. As a result of the seriousness of these problems, considerable research has focused on trying to understand why academic problems occur and how we can help adolescents with ADHD improve their functioning at school. In the remainder of this chapter, we focus on these two areas of research.

UNDERSTANDING SCHOOL IMPAIRMENT

In order to best understand the nature of impairment associated with ADHD, investigators have taken a developmental psychopathology approach to theory and research. Much of the early research focused on underlying cognitive mechanisms that may account for the symptoms and impairment. Using experimental tasks, researchers examined cognitive elements of inattention, along with activation, motivation and inhibition, to try to explain the problems of youth with ADHD (e.g., Sergeant, 2000). This work has a long history (e.g., Douglas, 1999; Quay, 1997) that predates the relatively recent approaches characterized by Research Domain Criteria (RDoC; Morris & Cuthbert, 2012). These cognitive constructs related to ADHD have evolved and are being examined in relation to emotional characteristics and neuroimaging studies using large datasets that allow us to address research questions that could not have been considered previously (e.g., Baroni & Castellanos, 2015).

Some of this work has led to the development of etiological models of ADHD. One such comprehensive model, the ontogenic process model, traces the core etiology to trait impulsivity conferred by reductions in mesolimbic dopamine functioning (Beauchaine, Shader, & Hinshaw, 2016). Similar in some ways to earlier models (Quay, 1997), trait impulsivity can be observed as a preference for immediate rewards over larger, long-term rewards. As a result, individuals with ADHD are more driven by immediate reinforcement and need more frequent and stronger reinforcers than do typically developing individuals to learn and perform optimally in daily life (sometimes called *motivation deficits*; Luman, Oosterlaan, & Sergeant, 2005). The most familiar model of ADHD, initially proposed by Barkley (1997), described a large set of cognitive deficits that comprise an executive dysfunction model of the disorder. Executive functions allow individuals to regulate their behavior, thoughts, and emotions, and thereby enable self-control (Baddeley, 2007; Dovis, Van der Oord, Wiers, & Prins, 2012). Barkley proposed a primary executive functioning deficit, which he labeled *behavioral inhibition,* to be central to ADHD symptomatology. This behavioral inhibition exerts direct control on behavior and facilitates opportunities for four other executive functions to impact behavior (working memory, self-regulation of affect–motivation–arousal, internalizing speech, and reconstitution); each of these includes many other, related cognitive functions. Following the work of Barkley, others have also proposed deficits of executive functions to be central to ADHD (e.g., Rapport, Chung, Shore, & Isaacs, 2001; Nigg, 2006). However, the focus of this work has shifted to working memory deficits as being central in ADHD symptomatology (Rapport et al., 2001), as meta-analyses show this to be the most impaired executive function associated with ADHD (Martinussen, Hayden, Hogg-Johnson, & Tannock, 2005; Wilcutt, Doyle, Nigg, Faraone, & Pennington, 2005). As in the ontogenic model, in which inattention is thought to be impaired due to a preference for immediate over larger, long-term reinforcers, inattention is not primary in these executive function models but is thought to be impaired as a result of executive functioning processes.

Executive functioning and activation or motivation deficits compromise one's ability to succeed with schoolwork. For example, as students progress into middle school and high school, reinforcement for academic work is more intermittent than it is in elementary school. Thus, students with trait impulsivity may be easily distracted by other activities, such as gaming or playing on their mobile phone, in which immediate reinforcement is common (Dovis et al., 2012). Furthermore, problems with working memory may contribute to a surface-level approach to learning in which the individual with ADHD reads quickly and listens shallowly, without thinking about what is being read or said. This disorganized and surface-level approach to learning becomes increasingly incompatible with success in middle school and high school, as students are expected to function more independently than during their younger years. These chronic academic problems and the potential resulting disengagement from school contribute to the attractiveness of activities that provide more frequent and immediate reinforcement such as delinquency, skipping school, and drug use. According to the ontogenic process model, engagement in these tempting alternatives to academics interacts with trait impulsivity to determine risk for additional comorbid clinical problems such as oppositional behavior, delinquency, and substance use.

Of course, this path from trait impulsivity and working memory deficits to school dropout and substance use is not absolute. There is considerable evidence that the developmental constructs of multifinality and equifinality are constantly at work along with gene–environment interactions and even epigenetics (e.g., Bhat, Joober, & Sengupta, 2017). As investigators have identified various risk and protective factors, the complexities of these issues become increasingly apparent. For example, the relationship between socioeconomic status (SES) and ADHD is such that children in low-SES families are roughly twice as likely to have ADHD as children in high-SES families (Russell, Ford, Williams, & Russell, 2016). SES may be a marker for other causal mechanisms related to pre- and postnatal environmental risk factors (e.g., prematurity, maternal smoking, health care).

Similarly, the path from ADHD to substance use includes functional indicators that increase risk, such as social impairment, poor grades, and delinquency, as well as some protective factors, including parents' knowledge and monitoring of their child's friends and activities (Molina et al., 2012). In addition to having implications for substance use, aspects of social functioning can serve as a protective factor against future academic impairment (Dvorsky, Langberg, Evans, & Becker, 2018). Between 32 (self-report) and 60% (parent report) of adolescents with ADHD exhibit social impairment, and there are risk factors (e.g., negative parenting, depression) and protective factors (e.g., participation in extracurricular activities, parent involvement) for social impairment in adolescents with ADHD (Ray, Evans, & Langberg, 2017). Furthermore, these risk and protective factors are not static, as changes occur in the environment and the child across development from early adolescence just prior to puberty to the verge of adulthood. It is clear from this brief survey of risk and protective factors that many characteristics of the person and environment interact over time in a manner that changes with development, thus creating an incredibly complex puzzle.

One of the largest contextual changes for young adolescents is the transition from elementary school to middle school (Langberg et al., 2008). Particularly dramatic is the change from having one teacher who acts in a pseudoparenting role to having many teachers with whom students often have very minimal relationships. The elementary school student always knows whom to ask if he or she has problems or questions, and the teacher knows the relative strengths and weaknesses of the students and can proactively help students be successful. This changes to multiple teachers, who each teach over 100 students per day and cannot know the students as well as elementary teachers do, so their ability to help a struggling student is less. Furthermore, students are required to learn the differences in rules and expectations across classrooms and the preferences and communication styles across teachers, and adjust their behavior accordingly from one period to the next each day. In addition, social opportunities and challenges increase, as there are many more peers with whom to interact. As a result, the social drama, bullying, and pettiness of early adolescence can tax the social competence of any young adolescent, especially those with ADHD, who may already have limitations in these areas (e.g., Becker, Mehari, Langberg, & Evans, 2017). The onset of puberty and romantic relationships further adds confusion to an already complicated social experience. Moreover, social activities that are increasingly less monitored by adults require greater self-reliance than ever before in making decisions about what activities adolescents will or will not engage in (e.g., delinquency, bullying, cheating, substance use). What one wears, who he or she sits with at lunch, sexting, and the constantly changing parameters for what characterizes the "in-crowd" make it challenging for the young adolescent to prioritize academic success. All of this occurs at a time when many young adolescents experience an increased relationship strain and possibly distancing from their parents. Thus, the increased expectations and challenges occur at the same time that the foundation of the parent–child relationship may be changing. At a minimum, for some, these developmental challenges are distracting, and for others they may lead to deflated self-esteem and even depression (Becker, Langberg, Evans, Girio-Herrera, & Vaughn, 2015).

Many of these new realities of adolescence persist into the high school years, although for many, there is some relief from the importance of conforming and the acceptability of differences, as they enter the phase of late adolescence in which conforming to the group becomes less important and building and exploring one's own identity becomes more important (Christie & Viner, 2005). However, expectations for students to independently manage their responsibilities continue to increase as adolescents wrestle with the developmental challenges of autonomy and self-reliance. As they approach the end of high school, the freedom and pressure to decide what to do after high school presents itself. For some youth, especially many with ADHD, the connection between what one does each day at school and what opportunities will be available in a year or two after high school does not seem real. The failure to make these connections can compromise motivation, lead to unrealistic goals, and result in an adolescent ill-prepared to graduate.

These changes provide opportunities to increase risk or enhance resilience throughout the years of adolescence. The complexity of this myriad of factors can make it difficult for parents and other adults to know how to help adolescents be successful throughout this developmental period. Developing effective treatments to address these issues can be much more difficult than the relative simplicity of the well-supported behavioral treatments for young children, such as the Daily Report Card (DRC) and classroom point systems. Nevertheless, progress has been made on treatment approaches to improve school functioning for adolescents with ADHD.

Intervening to Address School Impairment

Services most frequently provided to adolescents with ADHD at school in the United States are through special education or Section 504 and include providing extended time on tests, small-group instruction, prompting, and other services often referred to as *accommodations* (Murray et al., 2014; Spiel, Evans, & Langberg, 2014). Unfortunately, a review of frequently provided services revealed that little to no evidence supports their benefit (Harrison, Bunford, Evans, & Owens, 2013). The only exception is reading tests aloud to students with ADHD, for which there is evidence of a differential boost (Spiel et al., 2016). These findings indicate that a large portion of the services listed on individualized education programs or 504 plans for adolescents with ADHD are unlikely to improve their competencies and help them independently meet age-appropriate expectations at school.

When reviewing school-based services for adolescents with ADHD, it becomes apparent that there are at least two purposes for services, and rarely does one service achieve both purposes. One common purpose is to quickly *eliminate a problem* related to a student's impairment. For example, some adolescents with ADHD rarely complete their homework and often lose their materials for class. One common solution is to eliminate this demand for the student. Consistent with the purpose of eliminating this expectation, this change immediately solves the problem. The student's grades are likely to improve, as the student is no longer penalized for failing to complete homework and losing the materials. A second example involves taking notes in class. When a student has trouble attending to class and taking notes, in line with reducing expectations, teachers sometimes provide the student with the teacher's notes or notes from another student. However, this approach does not foster self-reliance, as it does not help the adolescent learn to take notes independently. The second purpose for school-based services is to *enhance the competencies* of the student so that he or she can independently meet age-appropriate expectations. With regard to the problem of taking notes, the solution might be to teach the adolescent how to take notes, which is a strategy that has been shown to be effective for adolescents with ADHD (Evans, Pelham, & Grudberg, 1995). Taking the time to teach the student how to take notes could enable the student to independently meet this age-appropriate expectation. As noted earlier, the examples provided for each purpose do not achieve the other purpose. In other words, removing the expectation for completing homework, managing materials, or taking notes does nothing to enhance the student's ability to independently meet age-appropriate expectations. Similarly, teaching a student to independently take notes does not immediately solve the problem. The student will need repeated practice, coaching, and performance feedback over time before being proficient at taking notes. This approach takes more of adults' time than the other approaches, and the student may continue to do poorly for a while after initiating instruction and training.

Recognition of these two approaches has been addressed in a treatment model developed by Evans, Owens, Mautone, DuPaul, and Power (2014) called the life course model of care. The model prescribes treatment approaches based on the likelihood that the treatment will help the adolescent independently demonstrate behavior consistent with age-appropriate expectations. Treatments most likely to achieve that goal are prioritized ahead of those less likely to achieve the goal. Based on this principle, the authors recommend that behavioral and training interventions should be the first priority. When successful, these treatments can help youth independently achieve age-appropriate expectations. In the life course model, the second priority for treatment is medication. If medication effectively eliminates problem behavior or helps to facilitate a student exhibiting adaptive behaviors, then age-appropriate expectations may remain in place and be achieved. The reason that medication follows (rather than precedes) behavioral or training interventions is because the benefits of medication are typically restricted to the time that the student is taking the medication. Thus, unlike the behavioral or training interventions, the need for medication may not diminish. As a result, with medication, the student is not meeting age-appropriate expectations as independently as with successful psychosocial interventions. Finally, the life course model indicates that reducing expectations should be a last resort. As described earlier, services or accommodations that involve reducing expectations do not help students independently meet age-appropriate expectations, although there are some situations in which accommodations could be used in conjunction with training interventions to facilitate overall improvement. For example, a teacher could provide a student with notes from a peer for a few weeks, while teaching the student to independently take notes. After achieving a level of competency, the teacher could discontinue providing the student with notes from a peer and require reliance on the student's new note-taking skills.

Developmental Treatment Considerations

During adolescence, several environmental and developmental changes that take place can make many of the problems of the adolescent with ADHD worse. As noted earlier, adolescence is a period with a developmental need for independence and autonomy, less management by parents and teachers, a less structured school environment than elementary school, and an increasing role of peers in the life of the adolescent (Christie & Viner, 2005). Several studies indicate increased problems with planning and organization in middle school and high school as compared to elementary school (Boyer, Geurts, & Van der Oord, 2018; Langberg, Becker, Epstein, Vaughn, & Girio-Herrera, 2013; Toplak, Bucciarelli, Jain, & Tannock, 2009). Also, increasing deficits in motivation are often present in adolescence, including a lack of motivation for school tasks, diminished motivation for treatment (Carlson, Booth, Shin, & Canu, 2002; Johnson, Mellor, & Brann, 2008; Morsink et al., 2017), and an increasing preference for risky activities that give immediate reinforcement for behavior (e.g., substance abuse, drunk driving, unprotected sex; Sarver, McCart, Sheidow, & Letourneau, 2014). Overall, as society expects adolescents to become increasingly self-reliant, teens with ADHD often fail to keep pace with this expectation and may further disengage from school and positive peer groups.

Given these developmental and contextual changes experienced during adolescence, well-established treatments for children (behaviorally focused parent or teacher training) can be difficult to implement with adolescents. Behavior management interventions are much more complicated to implement, as the structure of secondary schools make classroom behavioral interventions challenging. Students have numerous teachers, and secondary school teachers have many more students than do elementary classroom teachers. As a result, behavioral classroom interventions such as the DRC may not be feasible to consistently implement for many adolescents (Evans & Youngstrom, 2006). One of the prerequisites for successful implementation of many behavioral approaches is that adults can monitor students' behavior, which is often not possible in secondary school. Similar challenges exist in the home, as many adolescents may spend time at home alone on a regular basis. In addition, when spending time with their friends, adolescents are often not monitored by adults. These changes in the environment make the implementation of well-established behavioral interventions difficult.

There are also changes in youth that limit the effectiveness of behavioral interventions. One such challenge is difficulty identifying rewards and punishments that are adequately salient to change behavior. Stickers and other trinkets that worked for children are not adequate for many adolescents, as they often prefer more expensive items. One common approach involves using more costly material rewards, but as these are more expensive than those used for children, rewards are less likely to be immediate and more likely to require sustained changes in behavior and may not be possible for many families. Given their core deficit of trait impulsivity, delayed rewards are much less salient for adolescents with ADHD than they might be for adolescents without the disorder. Making privileges contingent is a less costly example of rewards and punishments to modify targeted behaviors. Although we are not aware of research on this topic, we have seen examples of some of the difficulties of this approach with adolescents. First, many adolescents become expert at detecting and challenging details of the contingencies, even when they helped make the plan, often resulting in frustration or exhaustion of parents. This can lead parents to completely abandon the behavioral plan. Also, contingent privileges sometimes involve regulating access to social activities (e.g., staying out late, using the car). When adolescents do not achieve these privileges or if they lose them, they are often faced with the potentially humiliating experience of explaining their unavailability to friends. Instead of risking these humiliating experiences, we have seen adolescents respond to a behavioral system by simply quit caring about the contingent privileges. They tell their parents that they do not want to stay out late or have friends over. Sometimes these statements may not be true, but simply are a strategy to disrupt their parents' motivation to adhere to the agreement. Other times, this is a coping response to feeling humiliated by these "childish systems." If an adolescent does quit caring about social activities, parents are faced with the same problems they had before they started the behavioral intervention (e.g., an adolescent who does not complete schoolwork or who gets into trouble), and now they also have a child who is becoming socially isolated and apathetic about social and recreational events. This can lead parents to abandon the behavioral interventions. As a result of these marked environmental and developmental changes in adolescence, well-established behavioral treatments that are regularly provided for children with ADHD (e.g., behaviorally focused parent or teacher training) may not be as effective or practical for adolescents.

These challenges have led some researchers to develop and evaluate other forms of treatment for adolescents. Some have continued with a behavioral approach, but with added aspects of motivational interviewing and parent–teen negotiating (e.g., Fabiano et al., 2016; Sibley et al., 2016) (see Chapter 14). Others have adapted cognitive behavioral approaches to address some of the impairment associated with adolescents with ADHD (Sprich, Safren, Finkelstein, Remmert, & Hammerness, 2016; Vidal et al., 2015; also see Sprich & Burbridge, Chapter 16, this volume). Because adolescents with ADHD are at risk for developing comorbid disorders (Yoshimasu et al., 2012) such as depression, depressive self-statements and cognitive distortions about themselves or their capacities for changing their behavior (e.g., "I can never organize my binder. I am just useless") have been targeted with cognitive restructuring techniques in some interventions (Boyer, Geurts, Prins, & Van der Oord, 2015; Sprich, Burbridge, Lerner, & Safren, 2015; Vidal et al., 2015). Finally, some work has focused on interventions to improve social and academic functioning (Evans et al., 2016; Langberg, Epstein, Becker, Girio-Herrera, & Vaughn, 2012). Given the importance of social and academic functioning at school and its relationship to adolescents' future, many of these treatments developed for adolescents have included a specific focus on these important outcomes (e.g., Boyer et al., 2015; Evans et al., 2016). However, some treatments have primarily only considered the effects of treatment in terms of reducing ratings of ADHD symptoms and/or global indices of functioning (e.g., Sprich et al., 2016; Vidal et al., 2015) without adequately considering functioning. In one innovative treatment approach, Fabiano and colleagues (2016) developed a behavioral family intervention focused specifically on improving the driving behavior of adolescents (see Garner, Chapter 12, this volume). As other treatments are covered in other chapters, we only consider treatments in the next section that target school functioning specifically.

The psychosocial treatments developed for youth with ADHD tend to fall into one of three categories, although some are combinations. Many of the well-established treatments for children with ADHD are behavioral interventions. In other words, change is achieved by manipulating the contingencies in the environment targeted for behavior change. Distinct from a behavioral approach is a cognitive-behavioral treatment (CBT) approach that incorporates behavioral approaches with cognitive techniques such as monitoring and modifying self-statements and cognitive restructuring. The third approach taken for adolescents with ADHD is a training approach that involves two main elements, including instruction and repeated practice with coaching and feedback, but does not include the manipulation of contingencies in the targeted environments. Two elements of training interventions that have been identified as critical to outcomes are the amount of practice with feedback and the degree with which the skills practiced are directly useful in daily living (Evans, Owens, Wymbs, & Ray, 2018). After reviewing the short history of treatment development for adolescents with ADHD, we will focus on some of the interventions that have been developed and evaluated to address impairment at school.

Treatment Development for Adolescents with ADHD

The earliest psychosocial treatment studies for adolescents with ADHD include two behavioral–family therapy studies conducted by Barkley and associates (Barkley, Guevremont, Anastopoulos, & Fletcher, 1992; Barkley, Edwards, Laneri, Fletcher, & Metevia, 2001) and an evaluation of a training intervention focused on note taking in class (Evans et al., 1995). The family therapy approach was a modified version of a behavioral–family systems approach developed by Robin and Foster (1989), and these early family therapy studies did not include a measure of functioning at school. The note-taking study examined whether middle school students with ADHD could learn to independently take notes in a lecture format history class in an analogue classroom. Students were trained and provided with regular feedback over 12 class sessions followed by a 5-week evaluation. During the evaluation, both taking notes in class and having notes in study hall were experimentally manipulated so that effects of each could be evaluated independently and assessed in combination. Students who took notes in class had significantly higher observed on-task behavior than those who did not take notes. Also, having notes in study hall independently and in combination with taking notes resulted in significantly higher scores on assignments than either only taking or only having notes. This was an early example of the potential role of training interventions to target impairment at school for adolescents with ADHD.

During the first decade of the 2000s, much of the published intervention development work for adolescents with ADHD focused on developing the Challenging Horizons Program (CHP). Initially, the CHP was a treatment development laboratory in the context of an afterschool program that operated three afternoons per week in collaboration with a public middle school. Many interventions were developed and piloted in the context of the program. Academic interventions were developed that targeted problems related to disorganized materials, lack of tracking assignments, note taking from text, and interpersonal skills. A series of pilot studies were conducted both to develop the procedures and evaluate patterns of responding (Evans, Axelrod, & Langberg, 2004; Evans, Schultz, DeMars, & Davis, 2011; Evans, Serpell, Schultz, & Pastor, 2007) and to examine a variation of the program for high school students (Evans, Schultz, & DeMars, 2014). During a recent formal evaluation of the CHP, the afterschool program was provided twice per week for 2 hours and 15 minutes per session over the course of a school year at middle schools. A mentoring version of the CHP was provided as an alternative treatment and included biweekly meetings with a school professional who focused primarily on training organization and study skills from the CHP curriculum. The third condition in the trial was a community care control group. The randomized trial (N = 326) of the CHP revealed medium to large effects for parent ratings of homework and organization, as well as grade point average. The most unique finding from this research was that differences in outcomes between the afterschool program condition and control group were larger 1 year after treatment than they were immediately posttreatment. This long-term benefit was found with both the intent-to-treat analyses (Evans et al., 2016) and the completers' analyses (Schultz, Evans, Langberg, & Schoemann, 2017) and is unique among medication or psychosocial treatment studies of youth with ADHD. It may be that a training approach prepares some of the participants to continue effectively using the target skills beyond the extensive practice and coaching that they receive.

The results of the large trial we have described indicated little benefit for the mentoring version of the CHP. Previous studies with the mentoring version revealed that meaningful benefits may not be achieved until after 2 years of implementation (Evans et al., 2007), and this may explain the negligible results in the large trial that only included 1 year of intervention. Another school-based intervention for adolescents shares some similarities with the CHP mentoring services. The Homework, Organization, and Planning Skills (HOPS) intervention adds a system of rewards to the CHP mentoring program and includes greater parent involvement. This 11-week, 16-session intervention provided by school personnel focuses on organization and planning strategies similar to those in the CHP (see Langberg, Smith, & Green, Chapter 15, this volume). Langberg, Epstein, Becker, Girio-Herrera, and Vaughn (2012) reported gains in parent-rated indices of organization and homework, and there was a main effect for the group on grade point average. In a large trial with middle school-age students, investigators contrasted HOPS with homework supervision sessions including a point system and a waitlist condition. Moderate to large effects were found when comparing many of the parent ratings of organization and homework completion and some of the teacher ratings between HOPS and the waitlist condition (Langberg et al., 2018). The supervised homework condition yielded similar effects but with fewer gains than HOPS compared to waitlist. There were no significant differences between the two treatment conditions on grades. Moderation analyses indicated that for participants with more severe problems, HOPS was more beneficial than the homework supervision. The homework supervision condition in this study was an enhanced version of what is often provided in a small-group study hall in middle and high schools for students with ADHD. Many middle school and high school students with ADHD attend a small-group study hall, and educators prompt them to stay on task and coordinate their assignments with their teachers (this is sometimes called a *pestering intervention*). The major difference between the homework supervision condition in the HOPS study and its typical implementation in schools is that there was a behavioral point system in the study that is usually not present in schools. Although a pestering intervention can help students complete assignments, it does not facilitate independence, as the students often become dependent on the study hall instructor telling them what to do and keeping them on task.

Another program with similarities to the CHP mentoring condition is a version of CHP for high schools. This version includes mentoring sessions provided by school staff and focused on training organization and study skills. In a pilot study of this intervention for high school students (ages 13–17) with ADHD, only a few small benefits in grades and parent-rated symptoms and impairment were reported (Evans, Schultz, & DeMars, 2014). The investigators reported that in spite of consistent supervision of school staff members who provided the sessions, there was considerable variability in the number of sessions provided. Post hoc probit dose–response regression analyses revealed large dosage effects for family and school impairment. Based on these analyses, the investigators recommended that sessions occur at least twice weekly to produce meaningful gains. A large randomized trial is currently under way to evaluate this modified version of the CHP with high school students (Evans & DuPaul, Principal Investigators).

Although these studies suggest that CHP and HOPS may be useful approaches to reduce the academic impairment of adolescents with ADHD, the treatment research for adolescents is still in relatively early stages. Many questions about implementation remain, and additional research is needed to understand how characteristics of students may be associated with response to these interventions (for related studies, see Langberg et al., 2013, 2016). In contrast to services typically provided to adolescents with ADHD, as described earlier, these interventions are aligned with the goal of increasing the competencies of adolescents so that they can independently meet age-appropriate expectations.

In the CHP and the HOPS, the skills trained are highly relevant to the daily functioning of the adolescents, and there is frequent practice with feedback. There are training interventions that focus on skills less relevant to daily school functioning but are designed to address underlying cognitive deficiencies that may cause impairment. The most common of these are computerized cognitive training programs. Although most studies of these interventions do not measure school-related outcomes (e.g., Bink, Van Nieuwenhuizen, Popma, Bongers, & van Boxtel, 2015; Bikic, Østergaard Christensen, Leckman, Bilenberg, & Dalsgaard, 2017), the study by Steeger and colleagues (2016) did. They evaluated the effect of Cogmed working memory training (Klingberg et al., 2005) alone and when paired with a five-session parent training program in a sample of 91 young adolescents (ages 11–15 years) with ADHD. They found no benefits for either treatment, or the combination, on ratings of symptoms or measures of functioning at school or at home. The lack of effects for the parent training may have been due to the small number of sessions. Furthermore, these findings are similar to the results of other cognitive training studies that often report gains on the computer task assessing the cognitive function trained (e.g., working memory) but mostly null findings with cognitive training programs such as these on clinically relevant outcomes or symptoms in daily life (Dovis, van der Oord, Wiers, & Prins, 2015; Evans et al., 2018). Although the number of training repetitions are high (mostly 20–25 sessions in a short time span of 4 to 5 weeks), the skills being taught are not relevant to daily activities and may account for the lack of findings.

Sibley (2016) developed a clinic-based behavioral–family treatment for adolescents with ADHD targeting home and school functioning. The Supporting Teens' Academic Needs Daily (STAND) therapy approach includes engagement, skills development, and mobilizing modules (see Sibley, Chapter 14, this volume). Specifically, a combination of motivational interviewing (MI) techniques (e.g., change talk, affirmations) and behavior therapy is implemented to achieve change. Therapists teach adolescents methods for recording assignments, study skills, and techniques for staying organized. The adolescents' use and practice of these skills are facilitated by parent–teen contracts that lead to parents providing behavioral contingencies at home based on the adolescent's use of the targeted skills. Thus, the parent–adolescent behavioral contract specifies the contingencies to be manipulated at home to modify behavior. MI is used to enhance family engagement and work toward specific goals. Sibley and colleagues (2016) reported the results of a randomized trial with STAND that included 128 participants ages 11–15 years with ADHD (67 in the STAND group and 61 in the no-treatment control group). Families in the treatment condition attended an average of 8.34 out of 10 sessions lasting 50 minutes and demonstrated statistically significant benefits compared to those in the control condition on parent-rated organization, disruptive behavior,

ADHD symptoms, observed amount of homework assignments recorded, and parent stress from baseline to posttreatment. The authors noted a lack of benefit for the treatment group on grade point average and other academic performance measures (e.g., teacher ratings of organization and work completion) and hypothesized that treatment may have needed to be longer to achieve this benefit. The lack of an effect with teacher ratings is a common result across many studies of adolescents with ADHD (Evans et al., 2016; Langberg et al., 2012) and is often attributed to the complexities associated with secondary school teacher ratings (i.e., teachers have over 100 students and only see them for 1 hour per day; student behavior varies widely across classrooms). Research on teacher ratings in secondary schools raises questions about the reliability and validity of these measures (Evans, Allen, Moore, & Strauss, 2005; Molina, Pelham, Blumenthal, & Galiszewski, 1998), and their lack of sensitivity to change is evident in a growing number of studies. The authors reported some benefits for STAND at follow-up; however, they were smaller and included fewer variables than posttreatment differences.

Individual clinic-based therapy has also been the focus of intervention development for adolescents with ADHD, as school-based treatment may be difficult to implement in some countries due to policy and mental health service provision model limitations. Boyer and colleagues (2015) developed an intervention called Plan My Life (PML) that included eight individual sessions with the adolescent and two with his or her parents. PML focused on enhancing organizational skills, such as the use of a diary and note taking in young adolescents (ages 12–16 years) with ADHD. During every session an organizational skill was discussed and practiced. Clinicians monitored for negative thoughts about the skills taught and helped adolescents revise these self-statements. MI techniques were used throughout the treatment by therapists trained and supervised in MI. Parent sessions were focused on the balance between control and letting go, parenting goals, and communication with the adolescent. In their study, PML was compared to a solution-focused treatment (SFT) that was included to control for nonspecific treatment effects (Boyer, Geurts, et al., 2015). There were 159 participants randomized to one of the two treatment conditions, and there were no significant group × treatment interactions for any of the outcomes across five domains at posttreatment or follow-up (Boyer, Geurts, et al., 2016). However, moderation analyses suggested that the PML intervention was more effective than SFT for a subgroup of adolescents with comorbid anxiety (Boyer, Doove, et al., 2016). Although the skills trained in PML were certainly useful in daily activities, the effects of this intervention may have been limited by the relatively few opportunities for practice with performance feedback. Other, similar treatments have reported small gains for symptom reduction and no benefits for school-related impairment (Sprich et al., 2016; Vidal et al., 2015).

Conclusions

Due to developmental and contextual differences between children and adolescents with ADHD, adolescents face many unique challenges that necessitate treatment approaches that are different than best practices for children. Their cognitive development and pursuit of autonomy and self-reliance, coupled with the dramatic increase in time spent without adult supervision, limit the effectiveness of standard behavioral approaches. The importance of relationships with peers increases, and these become more complex as, through their peer groups, adolescents are exposed to romantic relationships, drugs and alcohol, delinquent behaviors, and disengagement from school. Although this chapter has focused on school-related impairment, the diverse challenges of adolescence, coupled with the problems associated with ADHD, provide a complex set of difficulties for these youth.

The complexity of impairment associated with adolescents with ADHD requires new approaches to treatment. Most of the treatment development work is fairly recent, and relative successes and failures are to be expected. Training and behavioral approaches supplemented by cognitive therapy techniques and MI are the common threads through the treatments developed with the intention of helping adolescents independently meet age-appropriate expectations at school. Both school- and clinic-based approaches have been undertaken. Although there are advantages to providing treatment in the schools for adolescents with ADHD, unfortunately, to date, school-based treatments for these adolescents have only been tested and implemented in the United States. School mental health development has been slower to evolve in Europe, although recent efforts are moving it forward (Kovess et al., 2015). Development and evaluation research on the CHP has been conducted for almost 20 years, and the school functioning outcomes appear to be the strongest to date. The CHP is not compatible with a clinic-based delivery model; however, it has been integrated into middle school classrooms and implemented by school staff. This integrated model of the CHP is more feasible than an afterschool program for potential dissemination. Future developmental work is needed and could potentially benefit from integrating the strengths of the different types of treatments.

In summary, although ADHD in adolescence is highly impairing, and adolescence is a transitional phase with multiple risks, such as school dropout and comorbidity, up to a few years ago, there were very few psychosocial treatment studies for adolescents with ADHD. These psychological treatments are much needed; although in controlled settings stimulant medication improves functioning on important academic outcomes (Evans et al., 2001), these benefits are often reduced and may be limited to certain domains (i.e., math) in similar studies in more naturalistic settings (Pelham et al., 2017; Kortekaas-Rijlaarsdam, Luman, Sonuga-Barke, & Oosterlaan, 2019). Moreover, psychosocial treatments appear to be more effective than medications for some key behaviors for academic success (Langberg et al., 2010). Thus, although medications may certainly be helpful for addressing the treatment needs of adolescents with ADHD (Sibley, Kuriyan, Evans, Waxmonsky, & Smith, 2014), for adolescents with ADHD there is a clear need for effective treatments that can reduce impairment at school and the serious problems in adulthood that may follow from this.

References

Akinbami, L. J., Liu, X., Pastor, P. N., & Reuben, C. A. (2011). *Attention deficit hyperactivity disorder among children aged 5–17 years in the United States, 1998–2009* (NCHS Data Brief No. 70). Hyattsville, MD: National Center for Health Statistics.

Altszuler, A. R., Page, T. F., Gnagy, E. M., Coxe, S., Arrieta, A., Molina, B. S., & Pelham, W. E., Jr. (2016). Financial dependence of young adults with childhood ADHD. *Journal of Abnormal Child Psychology, 44*, 1217–1229.

Baddeley, A. D. (2007). *Working memory, thought and action.* Oxford, UK: Oxford University Press.

Barkley, R. A. (1997). Behavioral inhibition, sustained attention, and executive functions: Constructing a unifying theory of ADHD. *Psychological Bulletin, 121*, 65–94.

Barkley, R. A., Edwards, G., Laneri, M., Fletcher, K., & Metevia, L. (2001). The efficacy of problem-solving communication training alone, behavior management training alone, and their combination for parent–adolescent conflict in teenagers with ADHD and ODD. *Journal of Consulting and Clinical Psychology, 69*, 926–941.

Barkley, R. A., Guevremont, D., Anastopoulos, A. D., & Fletcher, K. (1992). A comparison of three family therapy programs for treating family conflicts in adolescents with attention-deficit hyperactivity disorder. *Journal of Consulting and Clinical Psychology, 60*, 450–462.

Barkley, R. A., Murphy, K. R., & Fischer, M. (2008). *ADHD in adults: What the science tells us.* New York: Guilford Press.

Barkley, R. A., Murphy, K. R., & Kwasnik, D. (1996). Motor vehicle driving competencies and risks in teens and young adults with attention deficit hyperactivity disorder. *Pediatrics, 98*, 1089–1095.

Baroni, A., & Castellanos, F. X. (2015). Neuroanatomic and cognitive abnormalities in attention-deficit/hyperactivity disorder in the era of "high definition" neuroimaging. *Current Opinion in Neurobiology, 30*, 1–8.

Beauchaine, T. P., Shader, T. M., & Hinshaw, S. P. (2016). An ontogenic processes model of externalizing psychopathology. In T. Beauchaine & S. Hinshaw (Eds.), *The Oxford handbook of externalizing spectrum disorders* (pp. 485–502). New York: Oxford University Press.

Becker, S. P., Langberg, J. M., Evans, S. W., Girio-Herrera, E., & Vaughn, A. J. (2015). Differentiating anxiety and depression in relation to the social functioning of young adolescents with ADHD. *Journal of Clinical Child and Adolescent Psychology, 44*, 1015–1029.

Becker, S. P., Mehari, K. R., Langberg, J. M., & Evans, S. W. (2017). Rates of peer victimization in young adolescents with ADHD and associations with internalizing symptoms and self-esteem. *European Child and Adolescent Psychiatry, 26,* 201–214.

Bhat, V., Joober, R., & Sengupta, S. M. (2017). How environmental factors can get under the skin: Epigenetics in attention-deficit/hyperactivity disorder. *Journal of the American Academy of Child and Adolescent Psychiatry, 56,* 278–280.

Bikic, A., Østergaard Christensen, T., Leckman, J. F., Bilenberg, N., & Dalsgaard, S. (2017). A double-blind randomized pilot trial comparing computerized cognitive exercises to Tetris in adolescents with attention-deficit/hyperactivity disorder. *Nordic Journal of Psychiatry, 71,* 7455–464.

Bink, M., Van Nieuwenhuizen, C., Popma, A., Bongers, I. L., & van Boxtel, G. J. (2015). Behavioral effects of neurofeedback in adolescents with ADHD: A randomized controlled trial. *European Child and Adolescent Psychiatry, 24,* 1038–1052.

Boyer, B., Doove, L., Geurts, H., Prins, P., Van Mechelen, I., & Van der Oord, S. (2016). Qualitative treatment–subgroup interactions in a randomized clinical trial of treatments for adolescents with ADHD: Exploring what cognitive-behavioral treatment works for whom. *PLOS ONE, 11,* 1–23.

Boyer, B., Geurts, H., Prins, P., & Van der Oord, S. (2015). Two novel CBTs for adolescents with ADHD: The value of planning skills. *European Child and Adolescent Psychiatry, 24,* 1075–1090.

Boyer, B., Geurts, H., Prins, P., & Van der Oord, S. (2016). One-year follow-up of two CBTs for adolescents with ADHD. *European Child and Adolescent Psychiatry, 25,* 333–337.

Boyer, B., Geurts, H., & Van der Oord, S. (2018). Planning skills of adolescents with ADHD. *Journal of Attention Disorders, 22,* 46–57.

Carlson, C. L., Booth, J. E., Shin, M., & Canu, W. H. (2002) Parent-, teacher-, and self-rated motivational styles in ADHD subtypes. *Journal of Learning Disabilities, 35,* 104–113.

Christie, D., & Viner, R. (2005). Adolescent development. *British Medical Journal, 330,* 301–304.

Douglas, V. I. (1999). Cognitive control processes in attention deficit/hyperactivity disorder. In H. C. Quay & A. E. Hogan (Eds.), *Handbook of disruptive behavior disorders* (pp. 105–138). Boston: Springer.

Dovis, S., Van der Oord, S., Wiers, R., & Prins, P. (2012). Can motivation normalize working memory and task persistence in children with attention-deficit/hyperactivity disorder?: The effects of money and computer-gaming. *Journal of Abnormal Child Psychology, 40,* 669–681.

Dovis, S., Van der Oord, S., Wiers, R., & Prins, P. (2015). Improving executive functioning in children with ADHD: Training multiple executive functions within the context of a computer game: A randomized double-blind placebo controlled trial. *PLOS ONE, 10,* e0121651.

Dvorsky, M. R., Langberg, J. M., Evans, S. W., & Becker, S. P. (2018). The protective effects of social factors on the academic functioning of adolescents with ADHD. *Journal of Clinical Child and Adolescent Psychology, 47*(5), 713–726.

Evans, S. W., Allen, J., Moore, S., & Strauss, V. (2005). Measuring symptoms and functioning of youth with ADHD in middle schools. *Journal of Abnormal Child Psychology, 33,* 695–706.

Evans, S. W., Axelrod, J., & Langberg, J. M. (2004). Efficacy of a school-based treatment program for middle school youth with ADHD: Pilot data. *Behavior Modification, 28,* 528–547.

Evans, S. W., Langberg, J. M., Schultz, B. K., Vaughn, A., Altaye, M., Marshall, S. A., & Zoromski, A. K. (2016). Evaluation of a school-based treatment program for young adolescents with ADHD. *Journal of Consulting and Clinical Psychology, 84,* 15–30.

Evans, S. W., Owens, J. S., Mautone, J. A., DuPaul, G. J., & Power, T. J. (2014). Toward a comprehensive, life course model of care for youth with ADHD. In M. Weist, N. Lever, C. Bradshaw, & J. Owens (Eds.), *Handbook of school mental health* (2nd ed., pp. 413–426). New York: Springer.

Evans, S. W., Owens, J. S., Wymbs, B. T., & Ray, A. R. (2018). Evidence-based psychosocial treatments for children and adolescents with attention-deficit/hyperactivity disorder. *Journal of Clinical Child and Adolescent Psychology, 47*(2), 157–198.

Evans, S. W., Pelham, W., & Grudberg, M. V. (1995). The efficacy of notetaking to improve behavior and comprehension with ADHD adolescents. *Exceptionality, 5,* 1–17.

Evans, S. W., Pelham, W. E., Smith, B. H., Bukstein, O., Gnagy, E. M., Greiner, A. R., . . . Baron-Myak, C. (2001). Dose–response effects of methylphenidate on ecologically valid measures of academic performance and classroom behavior in adolescents with ADHD. *Experimental and Clinical Psychopharmacology, 9,* 163–175.

Evans, S. W., Schultz, B. K., & DeMars, C. E. (2014). High school-based treatment for adolescents with attention-deficit/hyperactivity disorder: Results from a pilot study examining outcomes and dosage. *School Psychology Review, 43,* 185–202.

Evans, S. W., Schultz, B. K., DeMars, C. E., & Davis, H. (2011). Effectiveness of the Challenging Horizons After-School Program for young adolescents with ADHD. *Behavior Therapy, 42,* 462–474.

Evans, S. W., Serpell, Z. N., Schultz, B., & Pastor, D. (2007). Cumulative benefits of secondary school-based treatment of students with ADHD. *School Psychology Review, 36,* 256–273.

Evans, S. W., & Youngstrom, E. (2006). Evidence based assessment of attention-deficit hyperactivity disorder: Measuring outcomes. *Journal of the American Academy of Child and Adolescent Psychiatry, 45,* 1132–1137.

Fabiano, G. A., Schatz, N. K., Morris, K. L., Willoughby, M. T., Vujnovic, R. K., Hulme, K. F., . . . Pelham, W. E. (2016). Efficacy of a family-focused intervention for young drivers with attention-deficit hyperactivity disorder. *Journal of Consulting and Clinical Psychology, 84,* 1078–1093.

Frazier, T. W., Youngstrom, E. A., Glutting, J. J., & Watkins, M. W. (2007). ADHD and achievement: Meta-analysis of the child, adolescent, and adult literatures and a concomitant study with college students. *Journal of Learning Disabilities, 40,* 49–65.

Harrison, J. R., Bunford, N., Evans, S. W., & Owens, J. S. (2013). Educational accommodations for students with behavioral challenges: A systematic review of the literature. *Review of Educational Research, 83,* 551–597.

Johnson, E., Mellor, D., & Brann, P. (2008). Differences in dropout between diagnoses in child and adolescent mental health services. *Clinical Child Psychology and Psychiatry, 13,* 530–555.

Johnston, C., & Mash, E. J. (2001). Families of children with attention-deficit/hyperactivity disorder: Review and recommendations for future research. *Clinical Child and Family Psychology Review, 4,* 183–207.

Kent, K. M., Pelham, W. E., Molina, B. S. G., Sibley, M. H., Waschbusch, D. A., Yu, J., . . . Karch, K. M. (2011). The academic experience of male high school students with ADHD. *Journal of Abnormal Child Psychology, 39,* 451–462.

Klingberg, T., Fernell, E., Olesen, P. J., Johnson, M., Gustafsson, P., Dahlstrom, K., & Westerberg, H. (2005). Computerized training of working memory in children with ADHD—A randomized, controlled trial. *Journal of the American Academy of Child and Adolescent Psychiatry, 44,* 177–186.

Kortekaas-Rijlaarsdam, A. F., Luman, M., Sonuga-Barke, E., & Oosterlaan, J. (2019). Does methylphenidate improve academic performance?: A systematic review and meta-analysis. *European Child and Adolescent Psychology, 28*(2), 155–164.

Kovess, V., Carta, M. G., Pez, O., Bitfoi, A., Koc, C., Goelitz, D., . . . Otten, R. (2015). The School Children Mental Health in Europe (SCMHE) Project: Design and first results. *Clinical Practice and Epidemiology in Mental Health, 11*(Suppl. 1), 113–123.

Kuriyan, A. B., Pelham, W. E., Molina, B. S., Waschbusch, D. A., Gnagy, E. M., Sibley, M. H., . . . Kent, K. M. (2013). Young adult educational and vocational outcomes of children diagnosed with ADHD. *Journal of Abnormal Child Psychology, 41*, 27–41.

Langberg, J. M., Arnold, L. E., Flowers, A. M., Epstein, J. N., Altaye, M., Hinshaw, S. P., . . . Hechtman, L. (2010). Parent reported homework problems in the MTA study: Evidence for sustained improvement in behavioral treatment *Journal of Clinical Child and Adolescent Psychology, 39*, 220–233.

Langberg, J. M., Becker, S. P., Epstein, J. N., Vaughn, A. J., & Girio-Herrera, E. (2013). Predictors of response and mechanisms of change in an organizational skills intervention for students with ADHD. *Journal of Child and Family Studies, 22*, 1000–1012.

Langberg, J., Dvorsky, M., Molitor, S., Bourchtein, E., Eddy, L., Smith, Z., . . . Eadeh, H. (2018). Overcoming the research-to-practice gap: A randomized trial with two brief homework and organization interventions for students with ADHD as implemented by school mental health providers. *Journal of Consulting and Clinical Psychology, 86*, 39–55.

Langberg, J. M., Epstein, J. N., Altaye, M., Molina, B. S. G., Arnold, L. E., & Vitiello, B. (2008). The transition to middle school is associated with changes in the developmental trajectory of ADHD symptomatology in young adolescents with ADHD. *Journal of Clinical Child and Adolescent Psychology, 37*(3), 651–663.

Langberg, J. M., Epstein, J. N., Becker, S. P., Girio-Herrera, E., & Vaughn, A. J. (2012). Evaluation of the Homework, Organization, and Planning Skills (HOPS) intervention for middle school students with attention deficit hyperactivity disorder as implemented by school mental health providers. *School Psychology Review, 41*, 342–364.

Langberg, J. M., Evans, S. W., Schultz, B. K., Becker, S. P., Altaye, M., & Girio-Herrera, E. (2016). Trajectories and predictors of response to the Challenging Horizons Program for adolescents with ADHD. *Behavior Therapy, 47*, 339–354.

Luman, M., Oosterlaan, J., & Sergeant, J. A. (2005). The impact of reinforcement contingencies on AD/HD: A review and theoretical appraisal. *Clinical Psychology Review, 25*, 183–213.

Marshal, M. P., Molina, B. S., & Pelham, W. E., Jr. (2003). Childhood ADHD and adolescent substance use: An examination of deviant peer group affiliation as a risk factor. *Psychology of Addictive Behaviors, 17*, 293–302.

Martinussen, R., Hayden, J., Hogg-Johnson, S., & Tannock, R. (2005). A meta-analysis of working memory impairments in children with attention-deficit/hyperactivity disorder. *Journal of the American Academy of Child and Adolescent Psychiatry, 44*, 377–384.

Molina, B. S., Pelham, W. E., Blumenthal, J., & Galiszewski, E. (1998). Agreement among teachers' behavior ratings of adolescents with a childhood history of attention deficit hyperactivity disorder. *Journal of Clinical Child Psychology, 27*, 330–339.

Molina, B. S. G., Pelham, W. E., Cheong, J., Marshal, M. P., Gnagy, E. M., & Curran, P. J. (2012). Childhood attention-deficit/hyperactivity disorder (ADHD) and growth in adolescent alcohol use: The roles of funcitonal impairments, ADHD symptom persistence, and parental knowledge. *Journal of Abnormal Psychology, 121*(4), 922–935.

Molina, B. S., Pelham, W. E., Gnagy, E. M., Thompson, A. L., & Marshal, M. P. (2007). Attention-deficit/hyperactivity disorder risk for heavy drinking and alcohol use disorder is age specific. *Alcoholism: Clinical and Experimental Research, 31*, 643–654.

Molitor, S. J., Langberg, J. M., Bourchtein, E., Eddy, L. D., Dvorsky, M. R., & Evans, S. W. (2016). Writing abilities longitudinally predict academic outcomes of adolescents with ADHD. *School Psychology Quarterly, 31*, 393–404.

Morris, S. E., & Cuthbert, B. N. (2012). Research Domain Criteria: Cognitive systems, neural circuits, and dimensions of behavior. *Dialogues in Clinical Neuroscience, 14*, 29–37.

Morsink, S., Sonuga-Barke, E., Mies, G., Glory, N., Lemiere, J., Van der Oord, S., & Danckaerts, M. (2017). What motivates individuals with ADHD?: A qualitative analysis from the adolescent's point of view. *European Child and Adolescent Psychiatry, 26*, 923–932.

Murray, D. W., Molina, B. S. G., Glew, K., Houck, P., Greiner, A., Fong, D., . . . Jensen, P. S. (2014). Prevalence and characteristics of school services for high school students with attention-deficit/hyperactivity disorder. *School Mental Health, 6*, 264–278.

Nigg, J. T. (2006). *What causes ADHD?: Understanding what goes wrong and why.* New York: Guilford Press.

Pelham, W. E., Smith, B. H., Evans, S. W., Bukstein, O., Gnagy, E. M., Greiner, A. R., & Sibley, M. H. (2017). The effectiveness of short-and long-acting stimulant medications for adolescents with ADHD in a naturalistic secondary school setting. *Journal of Attention Disorders, 21*, 40–45.

Quay, H. C. (1997). Inhibition and attention deficit hyperactivity disorder. *Journal of Abnormal Child Psychology, 25*, 7–13.

Rapport, M., Chung, K. M., Shore, G., & Isaacs, P. (2001). A conceptual model of of child psychopathology: Implications for understanding attention deficit hyperactivity disorder and treatment efficacy. *Journal of Clinical Child Psychology, 30*, 48–58.

Ray, A. R., Evans, S. W., & Langberg, J. M. (2017). Factors associated with healthy and impaired social functioning in young adolescents with ADHD. *Journal of Abnormal Child Psychology, 45*, 883–897.

Robin, A. L., & Foster, S. L. (1989). *Negotiating parent–adolescent conflict: A behavioral–family systems approach.* New York: Guilford Press.

Russell, A. E., Ford, T., Williams, R., & Russell, G. (2016). The association between socioeconomic disadvantage and attention deficit/hyperactivity disorder (ADHD): A systematic review. *Child Psychiatry and Human Development, 47*, 440–458.

Sarver, D. E., McCart, M. R., Sheidow, A. J., & Letourneau, E. J. (2014). ADHD and risky sexual behavior in adolescents: Conduct problems and substance use as mediators of risk. *Journal of Child Psychology and Psychiatry, 55*, 1345–1353.

Schultz, B. K., Evans, S. W., Langberg, J. M., & Schoemann, A. M. (2017). Outcomes for adolescents who comply with long-term psychosocial treatment for ADHD. *Journal of Consulting and Clinical Psychology, 85*, 250–261.

Sergeant, J. (2000). The cognitive-energetic model: An empirical approach to attention-deficit hyperactivity disorder. *Neuroscience and Biobehavioral Reviews, 24*, 7–12.

Sibley, M. H. (2016). *Parent–teen therapy for executive function deficits and ADHD: Building skills and motivation.* New York: Guilford Press.

Sibley, M. H., Graziano, P. A., Kuriyan, A. B., Coxe, S., Pelham, W. E., Rodriguez, L., . . . Ward, A. (2016). Parent–teen behavior therapy + motivational interviewing for adolescents with ADHD. *Journal of Consulting and Clinical Psychology, 84,* 699–712.

Sibley, M. H., Kuriyan, A. B., Evans, S. W., Waxmonsky, J. G., & Smith, B. H. (2014). Pharmacological and psychosocial treatments for adolescents with ADHD: An updated systematic review of the literature. *Clinical Psychology Review, 34,* 218–232.

Spiel, C. F., Evans, S. W., & Langberg, J. M. (2014). Evaluating the content of Individualized Education Programs and 504 Plans of young adolescents with attention deficit/hyperactivity disorder. *School Psychology Quarterly, 29,* 452–468.

Spiel, C. F., Mixon, C. S., Holdaway, A. S., Evans, S. W., Harrison, J. R., Zoromski, A. K., & Yost, J. S. (2016). Is reading tests aloud an accommodation for youth with or at risk for ADHD? *Remedial and Special Education, 37,* 101–112.

Sprich, S. E., Burbridge, J., Lerner, J. A., & Safren, S. A. (2015). Cognitive-behavioral therapy for ADHD in adolescents: Clinical considerations and a case series. *Cognitive and Behavioral Practice, 22,* 116–126.

Sprich, S. E., Safren, S. A., Finkelstein, D., Remmert, J. E., & Hammerness, P. (2016). A randomized controlled trial of cognitive behavioral therapy for ADHD in medication treated adolescents. *Journal of Child Psychology and Psychiatry, 57,* 1218–1226.

Steeger, C. M., Gondoli, D. M., Gibson, B. S., & Morrissey, R. A. (2016). Combined cognitive and parent training interventions for adolescents with ADHD and their mothers: A randomized controlled trial. *Child Neuropsychology, 22,* 394–419.

Toplak, M. E., Bucciarelli, S. M., Jain, U., & Tannock, R. (2009). Executive functions: Performance-based measures and the Behavior Rating Inventory of Executive Function (BRIEF) in adolescents with attention deficit/hyperactivity disorder (ADHD). *Child Neuropsychology, 15,* 53–72.

Vidal, R., Castells, J., Richarte, V., Palomar, G., García, M., Nicolau, R., . . . Ramos-Quiroga, J. A. (2015). Group therapy for adolescents with attention-deficit/hyperactivity disorder: A randomized controlled trial. *Journal of the American Academy of Child and Adolescent Psychiatry, 54,* 275–282.

Wilcutt, E. G., Doyle, A. E., Nigg, J. T., Faraone, S. V., & Pennington, B. F. (2005). Validity of the executive functioning theory of attention-deficit/hyperactivity disorder: A meta-analytic review. *Biological Psychiatry, 1,* 1336–1346.

Yoshimasu, K., Barbaresi, W. J., Colligan, R. C., Voigt, R. G., Killian, J. M., Weaver, A. L., & Katusik, S. K. (2012). Childhood ADHD is strongly associated with a broad range of psychiatric disorders during adolescence: A population-based birth cohort study. *Journal of Child Psychology and Psychiatry, 53,* 1036–1043.

Zoromski, A., Owens, J. S., Evans, S. W., & Brady, C. (2015). Identifying ADHD symptoms most associated with impairment in early childhood, middle childhood, and adolescence using teacher report. *Journal of Abnormal Child Psychology, 43,* 1243–1255.

CHAPTER 9

Psychiatric Co-Occurrence (Comorbidity) in Adolescents with ADHD

Stephen P. Becker
Nicholas D. Fogleman

"The norm rather than the exception." This phrase is familiar to anyone who has read articles on psychiatric comorbidity, or co-occurrence, whether broadly (e.g., Rhee, Lahey, & Waldman, 2015; Sonuga-Barke, 1998; Widiger & Samuel, 2005) or in the area of attention-deficit/hyperactivity disorder (ADHD) specifically (e.g., Becker, Luebbe, & Langberg, 2012; Kutcher et al., 2004). This phrase is typically used to emphasize the high rates of psychiatric co-occurrence (comorbidity) and to underscore the importance of examining its causes, course, correlates, and consequences. At times, this phrase is used to draw attention to ongoing issues and controversies with categorical models of psychopathology. Indeed, as we are writing this chapter, the broader fields of psychiatry and clinical psychology continue to grapple with how best to conceptualize and classify psychopathology, whether in a categorical model, consistent with the *Diagnostic and Statistical Manual of Mental Disorders* (DSM-5; American Psychiatric Association, 2013) or in a dimensional model, consistent with a developmental psychopathology approach (Beauchaine, 2003; Drabick & Kendall, 2010; Forbes, Tackett, Markon, & Krueger, 2016) and hierarchical models of psychopathology (Kotov et al., 2017; Lahey, Krueger,

Rathouz, Waldman, & Zald, 2017). These debates and discussions are not the focus of this chapter, yet they provide an important backdrop for the study of co-occurrence in adolescents with ADHD, both historically and into the forseeable future. For instance, there are long-standing concerns with the term *comorbidity* (including the implication of independent disease processes and the reification of diagnostic entities) (Kaplan, Crawford, Cantell, Kooistra, & Dewey, 2006; Lilienfeld, Waldman, & Israel, 1994) and, as such, we intentionally prioritize using the term *co-occurrence*. In this chapter, we primarily review externalizing and internalizing psychopathologies that frequently co-occur with ADHD, including prevalence, risk factors and developmental processes, and functional correlates and consequences of co-occurrence. Given the focus of this chapter and the volume of studies in these areas, we necessarily limit our review to key studies specifically relevant to the developmental period of adolescence. As will become clear below, surprisingly few studies have examined co-occurring psychopathologies specifically in adolescents with ADHD. As ADHD has historically been conceptualized as an externalizing disorder, more studies have examined the co-occurrence of ADHD with other externalizing disorders/behaviors (*homotypic co-occurrence*), though there is substantial attention being devoted to the co-occurrence of ADHD with internalizing disorders/behaviors (*heterotypic co-occurrence*). In addition, we take care throughout to use terminology that reflects whether a study examined co-occurrence categorically (e.g., disorder, diagnosis) or dimensionally (e.g., symptoms). We then summarize existing knowledge regarding understudied and emerging co-occurring psychopathologies such as eating disorders, autism spectrum disorder (ASD), self-harm and suicide, and sluggish cognitive tempo (SCT). We do not review co-occurring sleep or substance use problems, as these topics are covered in other chapters in this text (Mulraney, Sciberras, & Becker, Chapter 10, and Kennedy, McKone, & Molina, Chapter 11, respectively); given space constraints, this chapter does not focus on learning, tic, elimination, or personality disorders or psychoses. Finally, we conclude by commenting on implications of psychiatric co-occurrence for intervention with adolescents with ADHD and review studies examining the role of co-occurring psychopathology in medication and psychosocial treatment.

A Bird's-Eye View of Rates of Psychiatric Co-Occurrence in Adolescents with ADHD

Findings from studies that include children and adolescents together indicate that other mental health disorders co-occur with ADHD at much higher levels than would be expected by chance. Very high rates of co-occurrence have also been reported in epidemiological studies. For instance, in a nationally representative sample of U.S. adolescents (ages 13–18 years), 92% of adolescents with ADHD met *lifetime* criteria for at least one other major class of disorders (i.e., disruptive, mood, anxiety, and/or substance use disorder) (Merikangas et al., 2010). In a birth cohort of 379 youth with ADHD and 758 age- and sex-matched comparison youth, ADHD was associated with a more than fourfold increased risk of having any psychiatric disorder diagnosis by age 19 (Yoshimasu et al., 2012). More specifically, approximately 60% of the ADHD group had at least one co-occurring disorder diagnosis, compared to 19% of the comparison group (Yoshimasu et al., 2012). Across samples of clinic-referred youth with ADHD spanning childhood and adolescence, 52–73% have at least one co-occurring psychiatric disorder, and 22–30% meet criteria for two or more co-occurring disorders (Elia, Ambrosini, & Berrettini, 2008; Jensen & Steinhausen, 2015; Klassen, Miller, & Fine, 2004; Reale et al., 2017).

Some researchers have reported general rates of psychiatric co-occurrence with ADHD in adolescents specifically. In a population-based birth cohort study, childhood ADHD was associated with a significantly increased risk of most disorders in adolescence, with ADHD strongly associated with both co-occurring internalizing–externalizing disorders (odds ratio = 10.6) or externalizing-only disorders (odds ratio = 10.0) (Yoshimasu et al., 2012). In a multiclinic observational study of youth in Italy, almost three-fourths (73.2%) of the adolescent sample (ages 12–17 years) had at least one co-occurring condition (including anxiety/mood disorders, oppositional defiant disorder [ODD] and conduct disorder [CD], learning disorders, sleep disorders, intellectual disability, language disorders, tic disorders, and ASD). In a subsample of adolescents (ages 16–18 years) from the Northern Finland 1986 Birth Cohort study, 46.7% of adolescents with ADHD had at least one co-occurring diagnosis, and 20% had two or more co-occurring diagnoses (Hurtig et al., 2007). This study also indicated that having a co-occurring diagnosis in adolescence was associated with a range of family environment variables, including living in a nonintact family, families with lower income, maternal life dissatisfaction, and parental stress and psychological distress (Hurtig et al., 2007). Another study that examined rates of co-occurring disorders among adolescents (ages 11–17 years) diagnosed with childhood ADHD found that 81% of adolescents who continued to meet criteria for ADHD in adolescence had at least one co-occurring psychiatric disorder, compared to 70% of adolescents who no longer met full criteria for ADHD and 35% of comparison adolescents (Gau, Ni, et al., 2010). This study indicates that adolescents with persistent ADHD are especially likely to have a co-occurring condition; it also demonstrates that even adolescents who no longer meet full criteria for ADHD are still at far higher risk for meeting criteria for a co-occurring psychiatric disorder than are adolescents with no history of ADHD.

Co-Occurring Externalizing Psychopathologies

Prevalence

As in childhood, co-occurring externalizing psychopathologies frequently co-occur with ADHD in adolescents, with studies examining rates of co-occurrence across diverse geographic locations. A study of 38 adolescents with ADHD in Turkey (ages 12–18 years) found rates of ODD and CD to be 71.1 and 7.9%, respectively (Yüce, Zoroglu, Ceylan, Kandemir, & Karabekiroglu, 2013), though the small sample size precludes drawing strong conclusions regarding these rates. A school-based study of adolescents (ages 12–14 years) in Brazil found rates of ODD and CD to be 21.7 and 26.1%, respectively (Rohde et al., 1999). In a general population study of Finnish adolescents (ages 16–18 years) with a lifetime diagnosis of ADHD, 43.1% met criteria for an externalizing disorder (31.6% with CD and 13.8% with ODD), with ADHD conferring an approximate 17-fold risk increase relative to adolescents without ADHD (Smalley et al., 2007). A large population-based study in the United States found evidence for concurrent ADHD and ODD in adolescence, even when correcting for other co-occurring conditions (odds ratios = 6.6 and 56.3 for boys and girls, respectively) (Costello, Mustillo, Erkanli, Keeler, & Angold, 2003). This study also found that ADHD modestly but significantly predicts subsequent ODD (Costello et al., 2003). Adolescent females (ages 11–18 years) with a childhood history of ADHD also have higher rates of externalizing behaviors, defined categorically or dimensionally, compared to adolescent females without an ADHD history (Hinshaw, Owens, Sami, & Fargeon, 2006).

Other studies indicate that children diagnosed with ADHD are at increased risk for having an externalizing disorder in adolescence. For example, youth with ADHD (ages 6–18 years) are far more likely than youth without ADHD to have a comorbid externalizing disorder diagnosis 4–5 years later in midadolescence (Biederman, Faraone, Milberger, Guite, et al., 1996; Biederman et al., 2006; Monuteaux, Faraone, Gross, & Biederman, 2007). In a seminal study, Barkley, Fischer, Edelbrock, and Smallish (1990) examined rates of ODD and CD in controls and children identified as hyperactive in childhood (ages 4–12 years) who completed a follow-up assessment 8 years later into adolescence. Using DSM-III-R criteria, 59 and 44% of the hyperactive children met criteria in adolescence for ODD and CD, respectively, with rates much higher than those found in the comparison sample (12 and 2%, respectively). When children in the Multimodal Treatment of ADHD (MTA) study were prospectively followed into adolescence (M_{age} = 16.6 years), adolescents with a childhood history of ADHD combined type had significantly higher rates of ODD and CD (17.7 and 8.1%, respectively) compared to adolescents from a local normative comparison group (LNCG; 2.6 and 2.1%, respectively), and the childhood ADHD sample also had significantly higher dimensionally assessed externalizing behavior scores than the LNCG group (Molina et al., 2009). In a sample of adolescents (ages 11–16 years) diagnosed with ADHD in childhood (50% continued to meet full criteria for ADHD in adolescence), 70% met criteria for ODD, and 33% met criteria for CD, with rates far higher relative to comparison adolescents (12 and 2%, respectively) (Gau, Lin, et al., 2010). In addition, adolescents with persistent ADHD were more likely to have ODD than were adolescents without persistent ADHD (Gau, Ni, et al., 2010). Similarly, late adolescents with a diagnosis of ADHD have a higher lifetime prevalence rate of having a disruptive behavior disorder (45%) compared to adolescents with subthreshold ADHD (24%), though it is worth noting that even adolescents with subthreshold ADHD had a higher rate of having a disruptive behavior disorder than adolescents who never met criteria for ADHD (10%) (Roy, Oldehinkel, Verhulst, Ormel, & Hartman, 2014). Thus, although rates across studies vary widely (18–70%), studies are consistent in documenting significantly higher rates of externalizing disorders among adolescents diagnosed with ADHD in childhood.

Risk Factors and Developmental Processes

Substantial research has focused on the possible developmental progression of ADHD, ODD, and CD, with mixed findings reported across studies. A community-based study of children (ages 6–10 years) with ADHD did not find ODD to be a precursor to CD in adolescence (ages 11–15 years), though negative parenting practices and maternal psychopathology predicted the persistence of ODD into adolescence (August, Realmuto, Joyce, & Hektner, 1999). In a sample of clinic-referred children with ADHD, Mannuzza, Klein, Abikoff, and Moulton (2004) also did not find ODD behaviors in childhood (M_{age} = 8.3 years) to predict having a CD diagnosis by late adolescence (M_{age} = 18 years), though childhood CD behaviors did. Yet other studies suggest that ADHD is a developmental precursor to externalizing behavior problems. For example, among children diagnosed with ADHD, greater ADHD symptom severity in childhood (as well as longer methylphenidate treatment duration, which may reflect ADHD severity) predicted ODD/CD in adolescence (Gau, Ni, et al., 2010). In a study of clinic-referred boys (ages 7–12 years at initial assessment), ADHD predicted future ODD, and ODD in turn predicted future CD, as well as anxiety and depression, pointing to the potentially important role of childhood ADHD as a starting point in the developmental sequence of both externalizing and internalizing psychopathology in adolescence (Burke, Loeber, Lahey, & Rathouz, 2005). Other researchers similarly have found that adolescents with ADHD and a co-occurring externalizing disorder are more likely to have bipolar disorder compared to adolescents with ADHD without a co-occurring externalizing disorder (Connor & Doerfler, 2008). Given the heterogeneity in findings across studies, there may be two subtypes of ADHD + ODD in childhood—one that is likely to lead to CD in adolescence and another that does not (Biederman, Faraone, Milberger, Jetton, et al., 1996). Environmental risk factors (e.g., family coercion and power struggles, deviant peer group affiliations, neighborhood violence) likely play a key role in the expression of impulsivity and may lead to the development of conduct problems in youth with ADHD (Beauchaine, Hinshaw, & Pang, 2010), though more studies are needed to directly test this possibility using longitudinal designs and methods that capture individual, family, and community context factors. Finally, whereas most studies have examined ADHD as a developmental precursor to externalizing behaviors, there are studies that challenge this assumption. In a birth cohort of 2,600 twins in Sweden that spanned ages 8–20, externalizing behaviors in middle childhood influenced ADHD symptoms in early adolescence, and ADHD symptoms in adolescence in turn influenced externalizing behaviors in early adulthood (Kuja-Halkola, Lichtenstein, D'Onofrio, & Larsson, 2015). Furthermore, the increased correlation between externalizing and ADHD behaviors from childhood to early adulthood was largely due to new genetic factors, supporting a developmentally dynamic process that includes bidirectional and time-varying etiological factors in understanding the co-occurrence of ADHD and externalizing dimensions (Kuja-Halkola et al., 2015).

In a prospective study of boys (ages 5–17 years) with ADHD, social problems predicted increased conduct problems 4 years later, when the mean sample was in midadolescence (Greene, Biederman, Faraone, Sienna, & Garcia-Jetton, 1997). Among girls with and without ADHD, lower self-perceived scholastic competence, but not peer rejection, in childhood was associated with increased externalizing behaviors in adolescence (Mikami & Hinshaw, 2006). In another study of girls with ADHD followed into adolescence/early adulthood (ages 11–22 years), a number of variables (e.g., socioeconomic status [SES], parental ADHD, family conflict) were examined as possible predictors of lifetime CD, with only paternal history of antisocial personality disorder (ASPD) significantly associated with increased risk of girls with ADHD developing CD throughout the follow-up period (Monuteaux et al., 2007). However, in additional analyses that separated girls with childhood-onset CD (onset < 12 years) and adolescent-onset CD (onset ≥ 12 years), girls with childhood-onset CD had greater levels of parental ASPD, whereas girls with adolescent-onset CD had greater family conflict (Monuteaux et al., 2007).

Functional Correlates and Consequences

A study of adolescents (ages 12–17 years) with and without ADHD found that adolescents with co-occurring ODD had more family conflicts, unreasonable beliefs about parent–teen relationships, and greater observed negative interactions during a neutral discussion task (planning a vacation with unlimited funds), and mothers of these adolescents also reported greater personal distress and less marital satisfaction (Barkley, Anastopoulos, Guevremont, & Fletcher, 1992; Fletcher, Fischer, Barkley, & Smallish, 1996). In considering academics, although group sizes were small, one study found a trend for adolescents with ADHD + CD to have less placement in a regular classroom than adolescents with ADHD + ODD or ADHD without an externalizing disorder, whereas no group differences were found for adolescents who were placed in special education or had repeated a grade (Connor & Doerfler, 2008). Data from the U.S. National Comorbidity Survey Replication Adolescent Supplement (NCS-A) indicated not only strong direct effects of ADHD on educational outcomes, but also that indirect effects of ADHD on educational outcomes (i.e., below-average grades, repeating a grade, suspension) were primarily through temporally secondary co-occurring disruptive behavior disorders (Kessler et al., 2014).

CD in early adolescence is a strong predictor of substance use disorders by 18 years of age (Elkins, McGue, & Iacono, 2007; see also Kennedy et al., Chapter 11, this volume). Lifetime CD is also associated with a range of other functional outcomes, including placement in special classes; lower math achievement; more arrests; and sexual behaviors, including intercourse before age 16, a lifetime history of three or more sexual partners, and a lifetime history of pregnancy (Monuteaux et al., 2007). In addition, although longitudinal research indicates that all boys with ADHD are at increased risk for delinquency in adolescence and young adulthood, those with a co-occurring CD diagnosis in childhood are at higher risk for delinquent offending (Sibley et al., 2011). It is important to consider whether social functioning in part accounts for these associations. For example, ODD symptoms are associated with poorer social skills and lower social acceptance in young adolescents with ADHD (Becker, Langberg, Evans, Girio-Herrera, & Vaughn, 2015), and peer problems and peer affiliations, as well as family environment factors, have a prominent role in developmental models of externalizing and antisocial behaviors in adolescence (Deater-Deckard, 2001; Patterson, Debaryshe, & Ramsey, 1989). To further advance our understanding of the co-occurrence of conduct problems and ADHD in adolescence, we need studies that integrate neurodevelopmental models of peer influences (Albert, Chein, & Steinberg, 2013) with neurobiological models of ADHD that point to altered reward–cognitive control integration (Castellanos, Sonuga-Barke, Milham, & Tannock,

2006; Nigg & Casey, 2005) that may shed light on which youth with ADHD are most likely at risk for engaging in conduct problems and risk-taking behaviors.

Co-Occurring Internalizing Psychopathologies

Prevalence

Most, but not all, studies indicate that adolescents with ADHD are more likely to meet criteria for an internalizing disorder diagnosis than adolescents without ADHD. Part of the mixed findings may be due to studies either collapsing across internalizing disorders or examining more specific internalizing disorder diagnoses. In the 8-year follow-up study of children in the MTA study, adolescents with a childhood history of ADHD combined type/presentation had significantly higher rates of having an anxiety/depression diagnosis (10.4%) compared to adolescents from the LNCG group (5.2%), though analyses with dimensional internalizing scores found greater depressive symptoms in the ADHD group but no differences in anxiety symptoms (Molina et al., 2009). Among Finnish adolescents (ages 16–18 years) with a lifetime diagnosis of ADHD, 26.6% met criteria for an anxiety disorder (with rates highest for specific phobia and posttraumatic stress disorder [PTSD]) and 22.2% met criteria for a mood disorder (primarily major depression), with ADHD conferring a 2.4- and 2.9-fold risk increase for anxiety and mood disorders, respectively, relative to adolescents without ADHD (Smalley et al., 2007). In a follow-up study of children diagnosed with ADHD, 24% met criteria for a mood disorder, and 38% met criteria for an anxiety disorder in adolescence, compared to rates of 7.5 and 25%, respectively, in comparison adolescents (Gau, Lin, et al., 2010). Although rates of having an anxiety disorder diagnosis were not statistically significant between adolescents with and without a childhood history of ADHD, adolescents with a history of ADHD did have significantly higher rates of specific phobia than did adolescents without a history of ADHD (26 and 14%, respectively) (Gau, Lin, et al., 2010). Additional analyses indicated that youth, especially girls, who continued to meet full criteria for ADHD in adolescence were particularly likely to meet criteria for a specific phobia in adolescence (Gau, Ni, et al., 2010). Using data from the Great Smoky Mountains Study (GSMS), a large population-based community study, there was significant concurrent co-occurrence between ADHD and having an anxiety disorder, but not between ADHD and having a depressive disorder (Costello et al., 2003). Bauermeister et al. (2007), using a larger age span (ages 4–17 years), similarly found that there was not an increased association between ADHD and any depressive disorder in either a clinic or a community sample after adjusting for the presence of other disorders. Yet longitudinal evidence indicates that childhood ADHD is associated with significantly increased risk of depression and depressive symptoms in adolescence (Biederman, Ball, et al., 2008; Biederman, Faraone, Milberger, Guite, et al., 1996; Biederman et al., 2006), as well as early adulthood (Meinzer et al., 2013, 2016). In contrast, Bagwell, Molina, Kashdan, Pelham, and Hoza (2006) did not find differences in rates of anxiety or mood disorders in adolescents (ages 13–18 years) with and without a childhood history of ADHD. Still other studies provide mixed findings, with adolescent females with a childhood history of ADHD having more internalizing psychopathology when measured dimensionally but not categorically (Hinshaw et al., 2006). Overall, findings across studies indicate that adolescents with ADHD have greater internalizing psychopathology than do adolescents without ADHD, with results generally consistent when internalizing psychopathology is measured either categorically or dimensionally.

Risk Factors and Developmental Processes

Rates of depression increase across adolescence, especially for females (Avenevoli, Swendsen, He, Burstein, & Merikangas, 2015). There appears to be large genetic overlap between ADHD and depressive symptoms in youth (Cole, Ball, Martin, Scourfield, & McGuffin, 2009). Reward responsivity, emotion dysregulation, and poorer/conflictual parent–child relationships have been proposed as mechanisms linking ADHD and depression (Meinzer, Pettit, & Viswesvaran, 2014). These domains are frequently implicated in disruptive behavior disorders, and youth with ADHD + ODD and/or ADHD + CD are at greater risk for mood disorders (including both major depression and bipolar disorder) in adolescence (Biederman, Petty, et al., 2008; Chen et al., 2013; Roy et al., 2014). Relatedly, there is some evidence from an all-female sample that childhood conduct problems are associated with increased internalizing symptoms in adolescence (Lee & Hinshaw, 2006). Similarly, in a clinic-referred sample of children with ADHD (93.7% boys), externalizing disorder symptoms in childhood predicted anxiety and mood disorders in adolescence (Bagwell et al., 2006).

It has also been suggested that the impairments in socioemotional and academic functioning experienced by children with ADHD may lead to depression. In partial support of this demoralization model (Meinzer et al., 2014), there is evidence that peer problems (but not academic problems) mediate the association between childhood attention problems and adolescent depressive symptoms (Humphreys et al., 2013). Similarly, Rinsky and Hinshaw (2011) found that adolescent social problems mediate the associate between childhood executive functioning deficits and adolescent internalizing–externalizing comorbidity in girls with ADHD, and among a predominantly male sample, Bagwell et al. (2006) demonstrated that social problems in childhood predict the presence of anxiety and mood disorders in adolescence. However, in a sample of 320 young adolescents (ages 10–14 years at baseline) with ADHD, both social and academic impairment at baseline predicted depressive symptoms 18 months later, and the association between social impairment and depressive symptoms was partially mediated by parent–adolescent conflict (Eadeh et al., 2017). Finally, in a prospective sample of girls with and without ADHD, Mikami and Hinshaw (2006) found higher academic competence in childhood to be associated with fewer internalizing symptoms in adolescence. Studies are needed that evaluate possible additive (and multiplicative) effects of social and academic problems on co-occurring internalizing problems. It is also important to consider the extent to which internalizing symptoms, and specific anxiety and depression dimensions, relate to social and peer functioning. A cross-sectional study of 310 young adolescents (ages 10–14 years) with ADHD found that having a co-occurring depression diagnosis is more clearly associated than having an anxiety diagnosis with poorer peer functioning, but analyses examining specific dimensions of depression and anxiety found that both anhedonia and social anxiety relate to poorer social functioning across parent and adolescent reports (Becker et al., 2015).

Emerging evidence also points to emotion regulation as an important domain for understanding the link between ADHD and depression. In an initial cross-sectional study of young adolescents (ages 10–14 years) with and without ADHD, poorer emotion regulation accounted for the association between ADHD and depressive symptoms (Seymour et al., 2012). Building on this finding, in a diverse community sample, the prospective association between ADHD symptoms in early adolescents (ages 10–13 years) and depressive symptoms 2 years later was mediated by emotion regulation difficulties, with hyperactive–impulsive symptoms more strongly predictive than inattentive symptoms of emotion regulation difficulties (Seymour, Chronis-Tuscano, Iwamoto, Kurdziel, & MacPherson, 2014).

A large body of literature demonstrates that cognitive variables (e.g., rumination, locus of control) are implicated in the development of depression (Garber & Horowitz, 2002). Taking a developmental perspective, Ostrander and Herman (2006) found that less effective parent management (an environmental variable) accounted for the association between ADHD and depressive symptoms in younger children (under age 8), whereas both parent management and a stronger external locus of control (a cognitive variable) accounted for this association in adolescents (age 10 years and older). Findings from this study, albeit cross-sectional, point to the increasing importance of cognitive variables as children with ADHD transition to adolescence. Still, environmental domains are also likely important, with environmental adversities including interpersonal trauma, parent–child conflict, and negative life events found to be associated with lifetime depression in adolescents with ADHD (Daviss, Diler, & Birmaher, 2009). In line with a vulnerability–stress model, cognitive and environmental factors likely interact to increase risk for depressive symptoms in youth with ADHD.

Although there is some longitudinal evidence that academic problems help explain the association between attention problems and depressive symptoms in school-age children (Herman, Lambert, Ialongo, & Ostrander, 2007), few studies have examined this possibility in adolescents. One longitudinal study of male youth did not find poorer school functioning (i.e., grade retention, placement in special classes, or need for in-school educational support) to be associated with the persistence of major depression (Biederman, Mick, & Faraone, 1998). However, the study relied on broad, parent-report measures of school functioning; additional studies using a multimethod, multi-informant design are needed to more thoroughly understand the possible influence of academic difficulties on internalizing psychopathology in adolescents with ADHD.

To date, most studies examining predictors of internalizing symptoms in youth with ADHD have focused on child-, family-, and peer-level factors; there is a need for studies examining school- and community-level domains. Stickley, Koposov, Koyanagi, Inoue, and Ruchkin (2019) recently examined community violence exposure in a representative sample of 505 Russian adolescents (ages 12–17 years). Using multivariate logistic regression analyses, the investigators found that adolescents with elevated ADHD symptoms who were directly victimized by community violence were at elevated risk for depressive symptoms, with the association between violence exposure and depression accounted for in part by posttraumatic stress symptoms (Stickley et al., 2019).

Functional Correlates and Consequences

Very few studies have examined functional correlates and consequences of internalizing symptoms in adolescents with ADHD specifically. Among adolescent/young adult females with ADHD, having a depression diagnosis was not associated with poorer academic or social functioning (Biederman, Ball, et al., 2008). However, in the same study, having a depression diagnosis was associated with significantly increased odds of having had intercourse and having been pregnant (Biederman, Ball, et al., 2008). Clearly, much more work is needed to understand the contribution and impact of co-occurring internalizing symptoms across functional outcomes in adolescents with ADHD.

There is ongoing interest in the extent to which internalizing symptoms, and anxiety specifically, may in some instances attenuate negative behaviors associated with ADHD. Most notably, anxiety may buffer the association between ADHD and externalizing behaviors such as impulsivity, aggression, and delinquency. Mixed findings have been reported in the literature examining this possibility in samples spanning childhood and adolescence (Becker, Luebbe, Stoppelbein, Greening, & Fite, 2012;

Danforth, Doerfler, & Connor, 2019; Falk, Lee, & Chorpita, 2017), but very few studies have examined the possible attenuating role of anxiety in adolescents specifically. In a 10-year longitudinal study of normative youth, Murray et al. (2018) found no evidence that ADHD and anxiety symptoms interacted in predicting either reactive or proactive aggression, with consistent results across the school-age and adolescent time points. In considering the impact of anxiety on attention, Vloet, Konrad, Herpertz-Dahlmann, Polier, and Günther (2010) found that youth (ages 8–15 years) with ADHD and a co-occurring anxiety disorder diagnosis performed better on tasks of sustained and selective attention than did youth with ADHD only, though the groups did not differ on a task of alertness or response inhibition. This buffering effect appears to be specific to anxiety, as another study did not find that adolescents with ADHD and a co-occurring depressive disorder differed from adolescents with ADHD only in attentional functioning (Günther, Konrad, De Brito, Herpertz-Dahlmann, & Vloet, 2011). Sauder, Beauchaine, Gatzke-Kopp, Shannon, and Aylward (2012) conducted an innovative study examining interactive effects of heterotypic externalizing and internalizing symptoms on neuroanatomy in a sample of 35 adolescent boys (ages 12–16 years) oversampled for externalizing disorders (11 boys with ADHD and 13 with ADHD + CD). Significant interactions of parent-reported hyperactivity–impulsivity and internalizing symptoms were found in relation to the gray-matter volumes in the left putamen and left hippocampus, and bilaterally in the anterior cingulate cortex (ACC), with internalizing symptoms associated with smaller reductions in gray matter. The authors concluded that there may be "neuroprotective effects of anxiety among children with externalizing behavior disorders" (Sauder et al., 2012, p. 350), providing important preliminary neuroanatomical support for a potentially dampening effect of trait anxiety on youth externalizing behaviors. However, it is important to note that anxiety still poses overall risk for increased impairment in adolescence. For instance, in a prospective study of young children (ages 4–6 years) with ADHD, baseline anxiety symptoms (and CD symptoms) uniquely predicted poorer functioning in adolescence (ages 15–18 years) (Lahey et al., 2016). Additional work is needed to determine whether, and under what circumstances, co-occurring anxiety symptoms (and specific anxiety dimensions) increase or decrease risk for impairment and various functional outcomes.

Understudied and Emerging Co-Occurrences

Eating Disorders

In a follow-up study of children diagnosed with ADHD, Gau, Lin, et al. (2010) found that 3.2% of the children had an eating disorder in adolescence, compared to 0% of comparison adolescents, though this difference was not statistically significant. In a 5-year longitudinal study of females with and without ADHD (ages 6–18 years at the initial assessment), females with ADHD were at marginally higher risk than controls to meet criteria for a lifetime eating disorder; however, group differences were not observed for 12-month prevalence of eating disorders at the assessment conducted in midadolescence (M_{age} = 16.7 years) (Biederman et al., 2006). There is some evidence that adolescent females with ADHD combined type/presentation (ADHD-C), but not ADHD predominantly inattentive type/presentation (ADHD-I), have more eating disorder symptoms compared to adolescent females without ADHD (Hinshaw et al., 2006). Additional analyses from the same sample found that girls with ADHD-C in childhood had more bulimia nervosa symptoms and body image dissatisfaction in adolescence than did comparison girls (Mikami et al., 2010). Similar results were found when examining bulimia nervosa symptoms in the MTA study sample (Mikami et al., 2010), and both studies found impulsivity symptoms to be the best predictor of adolescent eating pathology (Mikami et al., 2010; Mikami, Hinshaw, Patterson, & Lee, 2008). Other possible mechanisms warranting additional research attention include peer rejection, punitive parenting behaviors, and emotion dysregulation (Mikami et al., 2008).

Sluggish Cognitive Tempo

SCT refers to a set of behavioral symptoms characterized by excessive daydreaming, mental confusion and fogginess, staring, lethargy, and slowed behavior/thinking (Becker & Barkley, 2018). SCT symptoms are distinct from, yet strongly associated with, both ADHD-I behaviors and internalizing symptoms (Becker et al., 2016). Very few studies have examined SCT in adolescence specifically (Becker et al., 2016). Yet extant research indicates that SCT symptoms may increase as children transition to adolescence (Leopold et al., 2016), and SCT is independently associated with poorer functioning in adolescence, including poorer academic functioning (Langberg, Becker, & Dvorsky, 2014), higher internalizing symptoms (Becker & Langberg, 2013; Smith & Langberg, 2017), and suicidal ideation (Becker, Holdaway, & Luebbe, 2018). In a sample of 51 adolescents (ages 13–18 years) with ASD, SCT was associated with greater autism symptomatology, in addition to internalizing symptoms and metacognitive deficits (Duncan, Tamm, Birnschein, & Becker, 2018). Furthermore, the only longitudinal study of SCT to extend into adolescence found that childhood SCT symptoms predicted higher internalizing symptoms, more shyness, and lower reading achievement in adolescence in a population-based sample of twins (Becker, Burns, Leopold, Olson, & Willcutt, 2018). In addition, when controlling for ADHD-I symptoms, childhood SCT symptoms were associated with *fewer* externalizing behaviors in adolescence (Becker, Burns, et al., 2018). These findings point to the need for additional studies examining SCT in adolescence, particularly in relation to developmentally salient domains such as romantic relations, risk taking, substance use, eating pathology, and self-harm, particularly since extant findings suggest that SCT may increase risk for internalizing problems, yet perhaps buffer against the development of externalizing behavior problems (Becker & Willcutt, 2019). Studies are often needed to examine whether SCT is differentially related to adjustment or long-term outcomes in adolescents with and without ADHD.

Autism Spectrum Disorder

Prior to the publication of DSM-5 (American Psychiatric Association, 2013), ADHD and ASD could not formally be co-diagnosed and, as such, the literature remains rather limited. ADHD and ASD share high phenotypic (Sinzig, Walter, & Doepfner, 2009), neuroanatomical (Brieber et al., 2007), and genetic overlap (for a review, see Antshel, Zhang-James, Wagner, Ledesma, & Faraone, 2016), and dual diagnoses appear necessary to examine co-occurring profiles (Gargaro, Rinehart, Bradshaw, Tonge, & Sheppard, 2011) and to identify effective treatment interventions (Yoshida & Uchiyama, 2004). Indeed, recent studies have demonstrated high rates of co-occurrence of ASD among adolescents with ADHD. In a study of 14,825 children and adolescents (ages 4–17 years), ASD co-occurred in 12.4%, with a median age of 8 for co-occurring diagnoses and higher prevalence rates among males (13.3%) than females (9.2%) (Jensen & Steinhausen, 2015). In another study, using data from the National Survey of Children's Health (ages 2–17 years), nearly 20% of children diagnosed with ASD had initially been diagnosed with ADHD, and children who received a diagnosis of ADHD prior to ASD were diagnosed with ASD approximately 3 years later (Miodovnik, Harstad, Sideridis, & Huntington, 2015). Interestingly, in a sample of 17,173 participants (ages 0–84 years), Hartman, Geurts, Franke, Buitelaar, and Rommelse (2016) demonstrated that co-occurring ADHD and ASD symptoms are highest during the adolescent years, leading the authors to recommend adolescence as a critical developmental period for co-occurring ADHD and ASD assessment, second only to early childhood. Overall, adolescents with co-occurring ADHD and ASD demonstrate greater impairment and severity of clinical symptoms (Sprenger et al., 2013). For instance, children and adolescents with ADHD + ASD exhibit more tantrum behaviors, conduct problems, and internalizing symptoms than do children with ADHD or ASD alone (Goldin, Matson, Tureck, Cervantes, & Jang, 2013; Jang et al., 2013). Furthermore, in a study by Ashwood et al. (2015), children and adolescents (ages 7–16 years) with ADHD + ASD demonstrated the greatest impairments in their adaptive functioning relative to children with ADHD or ASD alone. However, longitudinal studies have yet to examine the predictors and course of these co-occurring impairments. Further attention is greatly needed in this area, especially given the high rates of co-occurring symptoms in adolescence and the lack of developmentally informed studies examining co-occurrence of ADHD and ASD across adolescence, and associations with functional correlates and consequences.

Self-Harm and Suicide

Adolescents with ADHD report more deliberate self-harm and suicidal ideation than do adolescents without ADHD (Hurtig, Taanila, Moilanen, Nordstrom, & Ebeling, 2012). In a prospective study of girls in adolescence and early adulthood (ages 11–23), higher rates of suicidal ideation were found in adolescent girls with ADHD (68%) compared to adolescent girls without ADHD (43%) (Biederman, Ball, et al., 2008). Children with ADHD are also at much higher risk of attempting suicide by age 18 (18.4% of youth with ADHD compared to 5.7% of comparison youth), with maternal depression in young childhood predicting increased risk of suicidal ideation and female sex predicting increased risk for suicide attempt by age 18 (Chronis-Tuscano et al., 2010). Both depressive symptoms and conduct problems, and their interactions, may be important in elucidating the pathways linking ADHD to suicidal ideation and behaviors in adolescence (Cho et al., 2008; Kessler et al., 2014). For example, both childhood and concurrent emotional and behavioral problems are associated with suicidal and/or self-harm behaviors in adolescents with ADHD (Hurtig et al., 2012). Similarly, in an all-female sample, Swanson, Owens, and Hinshaw (2014) found that impulsivity and co-occurring externalizing behaviors in adolescence (M_{age} = 14.2 years) partially mediate the association between childhood ADHD (M_{age} = 9.1 years) and nonsuicidal self-injury in young adulthood (M_{age} = 19.6 years), whereas co-occurring internalizing symptoms partially mediated the association between childhood ADHD and suicide attempts in young adulthood. In contrast, in a sample of adolescent twins who endorsed suicidal ideation (probands), their co-twins, and matched controls, inattention, but not impulsivity or brooding, significantly increased likelihood of suicidal ideation in the probands compared to co-twins and controls (Sarkisian, Van Hulle, & Hill Goldsmith, 2019). When controlling for having a diagnosis of ADHD, inattention and brooding were both associated with increased risk for suicidal ideation (Sarkisian et al., 2019). In addition, environmental factors are important to include in models seeking to understand the link between ADHD and suicidal behaviors, with parent–child conflict, interpersonal trauma exposure, and social impairment identified as correlates of lifetime suicidal behaviors in adolescents with ADHD (Daviss & Diler, 2014). Much of the research examining suicidal ideation and behaviors in youth diagnosed with ADHD has examined the role of co-occurring disorders, and it will be important to also examine cognitive styles (e.g., brooding) and environmental factors, as well as other units of analysis, such as physiology and brain circuits and molecules (Cha et al., 2018), to better understand the prevalence and developmental course of suicidal thoughts and behaviors in youth with ADHD. It would likewise be advantageous to test more directly the prominent theories of suicide, such as the interpersonal model of suicide (Van Orden et al., 2010), in adolescents with ADHD.

Key Directions for Future Research

There are many directions for future research examining psychiatric co-occurrence in adolescents with ADHD, only a few of which we discuss here given space constraints. In short, given the research reviewed earlier, the question is less about *whether* adolescents with ADHD experience higher rates of psychiatric co-occurrence, but rather *why* and *when*.

Studies are needed that examine the development of co-occurring psychopathologies with ADHD across units of analysis. The development and interrelations of ADHD and co-occurring psychopathologies are clearly complex (Daviss, 2008; Jarrett & Ollendick, 2008). For example, in a review, Danforth, Connor, and Doerfler (2016) found that substantial genetic risk, neurodevelopmental impairment, executive functions (especially verbal working memory), and parent–child bidirectional influences contributed to the covariation of ADHD and conduct problems. Likewise, the prefrontal cortex (PFC) may be an important mechanism of comorbidity among disorders (Macdonald, Goines, Novacek, & Walker, 2016). Executive functioning weaknesses are well-documented in both externalizing and internalizing disorders, and may be a transdiagnostic risk factor for psychopathology (Caspi et al., 2014; Goschke, 2014). The PFC has a long period of developmental maturation that is delayed in ADHD (Shaw et al., 2007), which may make it more susceptible to environmental factors (e.g., drugs, stress, social experiences, and hormones) that can alter the course of the psychopathology (Macdonald et al., 2016). Studies that test integrated models, ideally in laboratory and longitudinal designs, are needed to test increasingly nuanced models of the developmental psychopathology of ADHD and co-occurring psychopathologies. Main effect models are not sufficient for understanding the interrelations between ADHD and other psychopathologies, as multiple neurobiological vulnerabilities interact to affect behavioral presentations (Beauchaine & Thayer, 2015).

Likewise, ADHD, as well as co-occurring psychopathologies, are heterogeneous, and more person-centered analyses (e.g., latent class analysis) would be informative for identifying and examining diverse phenotypes (Jarrett & Ollendick, 2008; Meinzer et al., 2014; for an example, see Hudziak et al., 1998). There is also a need for studies that examine resilience in youth with ADHD (Dvorsky & Langberg, 2016). As detailed earlier, many children with ADHD experience co-occurring symptoms in adolescence, but certainly not all do. Among children with ADHD in early childhood (ages 4–6 years), between 24 and 47% were classified as well-adjusted in terms of ODD and CD and depression and anxiety symptoms, respectively, across two consecutive years in early adolescence (Lee, Lahey, Owens, & Hinshaw, 2008). It is crucial for our field to balance identifying factors that portend risk for the development of co-occurring psychopathology in youth with ADHD, as well as factors that are protective in buffering against negative outcomes. As noted by Mikami and Hinshaw (2006), there is also a need for additional research on mechanisms underlying protective effects and whether models of risk and resilience are similar for youth with and without ADHD.

Greater attention to the influence of sex on the course of co-occurring symptoms is another important area for future research. Some landmark longitudinal studies of ADHD have included only (or almost entirely) females (Biederman et al., 2006; Hinshaw et al., 2006) or males (Biederman, Faraone, Milberger, Curtis, et al., 1996; Sibley et al., 2011), precluding an examination of sex differences. Among children with ADHD in childhood, girls are more likely to have a co-occurring internalizing-only diagnosis in adolescence, whereas boys are more likely to have a co-occurring externalizing-only diagnosis (Yoshimasu et al., 2012). In addition, in a study that combined samples of males and females, Monuteaux, Mick, Faraone, and Biederman (2010) found evidence of greater stability of co-occurring psychopathology from childhood to adolescence in females than in males. Monuteaux et al. concluded that studies should more explicitly examine whether sex moderates the associations of ADHD in relation to risk factors and functional outcomes. In line with this possibility, among boys and girls with ADHD in early childhood (ages 4–6 years), girls had poorer parent- and interviewer-reported functioning compared to boys in adolescence (ages 15–18 years) (Lahey et al., 2016).

There is a need for more research examining co-occurring internalizing–externalizing psychopathologies. Internalizing and externalizing psychopathologies frequently co-occur, including in samples of youth with ADHD (Rutter, Kim-Cohen, & Maughan, 2006). For example, Yoshimasu et al. (2012) found that 20% of youth with ADHD had both an internalizing and an externalizing disorder diagnosis by age 19, compared to just 4% of age- and sex-matched comparison youth. Studies that examine externalizing *or* internalizing psychopathologies in isolation among adolescents with ADHD are likely not looking at a complete picture. Neuman et al. (2001) used latent class analysis in a population-based sample of adolescent females and found one class to be characterized by both elevated ODD symptoms and anxiety–depressive symptoms. In addition, in a recent meta-analysis, Caye et al. (2016) found co-occurring CD and major depressive disorder to be predictors of the persistence of ADHD from childhood to adulthood. Advances in neuroscience increasingly point to the importance of using transdiagnostic approaches to psychopathology. For example, anhedonia and irritability share common neural substrates with trait impulsivity that likely lead to heterotypic co-occurrence of externalizing and internalizing psychopathology (Zisner & Beauchaine, 2016).

Building from the need to better understand heterotypic co-occurrence, it must be acknowledged that the categorical DSM system of psychiatric diagnosis does not carve nature at its joints (Hyman, 2010; Kozak & Cuthbert, 2016). As such, it has been argued that "DSM disorders were a good place to start developing our understanding of the nature of psychopathology, but they are not a good place to stop" (Forbes et al., 2016, p. 976). This argument certainly extends to our understanding of psychiatric co-occurrence, as reliance on DSM categories likely obscures developmental pathways of co-occurrence. Descriptive research is highly informative, but it is insufficient for understanding the complexities of psychiatric co-occurrence with ADHD. It would be advantageous for researchers to move beyond DSM categories and to incorporate ontogenic trait approaches (e.g., externalizing liability of trait impulsivity) that utilize multiple levels of analysis (e.g., genetic vulnerability, neural/hormonal substrate, vulnerability trait, behavioral symptoms, environmental risks) (Beauchaine & McNulty, 2013). There is a particular need for the next generation of research examining psychiatric co-occurrence with ADHD to incorporate variables across multiple units of analysis and to ground such research in dimensional, hierarchical models of psychopathology (Forbes et al., 2016; Kotov et al., 2017; Lahey et al., 2017). As just one example, automatic nervous system (ANS) dysregulation (e.g., heart rate variability, respiratory sinus arrhythmia) is associated with most forms of psychopathology (Beauchaine, 2015; Beauchaine & Thayer, 2015), yet most studies have examined ANS dysregulation in specific disorders despite the likelihood that such dysregulation partially relates to an overall psychopathology liability (Hankin et al., 2016). Evaluating biology × environment interactions will advance our understanding of the development of co-occurring psychopathologies and continuities (Beauchaine & Cicchetti, 2016). It may be especially fruitful to investigate the interrelations of stressful life events, neurodevelopmental processes (including ANS dysregulation, hypothalamus–pituitary–adrenal [HPA] axis functioning, and brain development), and the onset and course of psychopathology symptoms that co-occur with ADHD, particularly as achievement domain stress (e.g., academic, extracurricular) becomes more prominent in adolescence specifically (Hankin et al., 2016). We concur with others about "important next questions about psychopathology that can only be addressed through a new generation of multiple levels of analysis research that identifies etiological and pathophysiological mechanisms, and specifies how environmental adversities interact with such mechanisms to promote concurrent comorbidity and heterotypic continuity" (Beauchaine & Cicchetti, 2016, p. 893). Studies in this vein will likewise be well suited to test developmental cascades relevant to understanding psychiatric co-occurrence in youth with ADHD (Masten & Cicchetti, 2010).

Considering Co-Occurrence in Intervention

Public costs for adolescents with ADHD are estimated to exceed $40,000 per adolescent over a 6-year period, and to double when co-occurring CD is present (Jones & Foster, 2009). It is thus of significant importance to evaluate the role of co-occurring psychopathology in pharmacological and psychosocial treatment.

Several studies have examined whether pharmacotherapy predicts risk for the development of co-occurring psychopathologies in youth with ADHD (see Brinkman, Froehlich, & Epstein, Chapter 18, this volume). In a retrospective study of 75 adolescents (ages 11–18 years), delayed ADHD pharmacotherapy was a strong predictor of major depression onset (Daviss, Birmaher, Diler, & Mintz, 2008), and in a prospective study of boys (ages 6–18 years) with ADHD, boys who were treated with psychostimulants were significantly less likely to have developed comorbid depressive or anxiety disorders or disruptive behavior 10 years later (Biederman, Monuteaux, Spencer, Wilens, & Faraone, 2009). Drawing from a national health insurance database, Lee et al. (2016) found that longer methylphenidate treatment had protective effect on youth with ADHD developing a depressive disorder, whereas length of atomoxetine treatment was not associated with the likelihood of developing depression. Additional studies are necessary to replicate and extend these findings, including possible mechanisms by which stimulant medication may be protective against the development of later co-occurring disorders and the role of factors that make it more likely for a child to receive pharmacological treatment (particularly when it is well monitored over time). There is additional evidence to suggest that adolescents with ADHD and major depression may be more resistant to antidepressant medications. Chen et al. (2016) demonstrated that adolescents with co-occurring ADHD and depression have an increased risk of treatment resistance to antidepressants at a 1-year follow-up relative to adolescents with major depression only. However, findings also revealed that regular ADHD treatment may reverse and decrease the risk of ADHD-related treatment resistance to antidepressants.

Co-occurring externalizing and internalizing disorders are also important to consider in psychosocial treatments. In an intensive summer treatment program involving 34 adolescents (M_{age} = 13.88), Sibley, Smith, Evans, Pelham, and Gnagy (2012) provided evidence that adolescents with ADHD and higher rates of oppositional and defiant behaviors demonstrated poorer response to treatment, such that they were less likely to improve social skills, cooperativeness, and frustration tolerance. In a more recent study by Sibley et al. (2016), 128 ethnically diverse teenagers (ages 11–15) with ADHD enrolled in a parent–teen skills-based therapy (see Sibley, Chapter 14, this volume); although initial results indicated that adolescent disruptive behavior at home improved relative to the treatment-as-usual condition, similar effects were not observed at follow-up, leading the authors to posit that this finding may have been related to reduced oversight and contingency management by parents.

This is not to say that treatments for adolescents with ADHD and co-occurring externalizing disorders are not effective. Other researchers have not found co-occurring externalizing problems to predict academic intervention response in adolescents with ADHD (Breaux et al., 2019; Langberg, Becker, Epstein, Vaughn, & Girio-Herrera, 2013). Furthermore, a meta-analysis of randomized controlled trials investigating psychosocial treatments in children and adolescents with ADHD suggested that behavioral interventions decrease co-occurring conduct problems (Daley et al., 2014). Additionally, in an afterschool program including 326 middle school adolescents (grades 6–8), there was a significant effect of treatment on decreasing both hyperactive–impulsive and oppositional defiant behaviors postintervention and at follow-up (Evans et al., 2016) (see Chapter 8). When comparing psychosocial treatments, in a study by Barkley, Guevremont, Anastopoulos, and Fletcher (1992), 61 adolescents (ages 12–18 years) with ADHD were enrolled in either behavior parent training, problem-solving and communication training, or structural family therapy; each treatment resulted in significant reductions in externalizing symptoms. Furthermore, in a sample of adolescents (ages 12–19 years) with ADHD assigned to either problem-solving communication therapy alone or a combination of behavior management training and problem-solving communication therapy, adolescents with ADHD + ODD were reported as having decreased parent–child conflict; however, only one-fourth of participants across both treatments demonstrated clinically significant improvements (Barkley, Edwards, Laneri, Fletcher, & Metevia, 2001).

Cognitive-behavioral therapy (CBT) appears to be a possibly effective treatment for addressing co-occurring internalizing disorders in adolescents with ADHD (Jarrett & Ollendick, 2012) (see Sprich & Burbridge, Chapter 16, this volume). In a CBT intervention consisting of psychoeducation and training in executive functioning, a total of 68 adolescents with ADHD and co-occurring anxiety demonstrated significant improvements across inattentive symptoms, academic performance, school attendance, and self-esteem; however, it is important to note that many adolescents did not normalize functioning (Antshel, Faraone, & Gordon, 2012). Additionally, in a study by Boyer, Geurts, Prins, and Van der Oord (2015) that consisted of two short-term CBTs, both treatments reduced co-occurring symptoms of internalizing and externalizing disorders from pre- to posttreatment, yet adolescents with co-occurring anxiety or depressive disorders benefited more from both CBT treatments relative to adolescents with ODD and CD. This is consistent with findings by Antshel and colleagues (2012), who demonstrated that according to parents and teachers, adolescents with comorbid anxiety/depression benefited more from CBT, whereas adolescents with comorbid ODD benefited less from CBT.

Not all studies have consistently found CBT to reduce symptoms of ADHD and co-occurring internalizing psychopathology. In a pilot study composed of a small sample of five boys (ages 9–12 years) diagnosed with co-occurring ADHD, ODD, and anxiety, results of a family-based CBT intervention (8 weeks) found that parents and adolescents reported high levels of satisfaction, yet there were no reductions in symptom domains post-treatment (Costin, Vance, Barnett, O'Shea, & Luk, 2002). Additional evidence suggests that ADHD diagnoses may moderate poorer immediate treatment response and remission rates in CBT among children with an anxiety disorder (Walczak, Ollendick, Ryan, & Esbjørn, 2018). Furthermore, in a 12-session group CBT intervention with 59 youth with ADHD (ages 15–21 years), anxiety symptoms were not significantly different between pre- and posttreatment; however, the authors note that this finding may have been related to low baseline scores for anxiety, as well as failure to include youth with co-occurring anxiety disorders (Vidal et al., 2015). Overall, although co-occurring ADHD and anxiety appear more treatment resistant relative to anxiety alone (Walczak et al., 2018), there are no studies of adolescence examining whether ADHD is more resistant to treatment in the presence of anxiety relative to ADHD alone.

There is preliminary evidence that dialectical behavioral therapy (DBT, a variation of CBT designed to improve mindfulness, interpersonal effectiveness, emotion regulation, and distress tolerance) is associated with fewer ADHD symptoms and improved quality of life among college students (Fleming, McMahon, Moran, Peterson, & Dreessen, 2015). Moreover, in a review that included studies of children and adolescents (i.e., ages 3–20 years), psychoeducation was associated with reduced internalizing symptoms, improvement in non-core ADHD symptoms, and behavior management across home and school settings (Montoya, Colom, & Ferrin, 2011). Some evidence for mindfulness programs suggests these treatments may also be effective at reducing co-occurring anxiety and depression in adults, but this have received scant examination in adolescents with ADHD (Zylowska et al., 2008; see Davis & Mitchell, Chapter 17, this volume). There is also evidence that combining medication and psychosocial treatments improves both symptoms of ADHD and co-occurring disorders. Reale et al. (2017) demonstrated that children and adolescents with ADHD and co-occurring disorders showed greater improvement when treated with medication alone or combined interventions, relative to psychosocial treatment, though combined treatment was particularly effective for adolescents with ADHD and co-occurring ODD. The investigators also found that children and adolescents with ADHD and co-occurring disorders were more likely to receive combined treatment, whereas children and adolescents with ADHD without co-occurring disorders were less likely to receive any treatment.

It is worth noting that studies frequently use certain psychopathologies as exclusion criteria, particularly youth with intellectual and developmental disorders or neurological problems (e.g., epilepsy). This is consistent with exclusion criteria by Sprich, Safren, Finkelstein, Remmert, and Hammerness (2016), who also excluded adolescents with active suicidal ideation, CD, and substance abuse/dependence. Moreover, bipolar disorder is commonly ruled out in many studies, which means that we do not know how adolescents with ADHD and co-occurring bipolar disorder respond to intervention. Evidence in a sample of children and adolescents ages 6–17 years suggests that ADHD and bipolar disorder are two distinct disorders, and medication treatments for bipolar disorder do not improve ADHD symptoms (Scheffer, Kowatch, Carmody, & Rush, 2005). Moreover, ADHD medication, in addition to medication for bipolar disorder, may be most effective for treating children with co-occurring ADHD and bipolar disorder (Scheffer et al., 2005). Given the frequency of co-occurring disorders among children with ADHD, future examination of co-occurring disorders with regard to treatment response is warranted. Some studies have provided evidence for treatments targeting specific deficits in emotion regulation among children with ADHD (Rosen et al., 2018); however, this treatment or other interventions focused on emotion regulation have yet to be translated into an adolescent-specific sample.

We encourage future researchers to assess specific domains of co-occurrence (e.g., specific anxiety and depression dimensions) and to report on whether co-occurring psychopathology was an exclusionary criterion, whether the intervention impacted co-occurring psychopathology (categorically and dimensionally, with particular attention to clinical significance), and whether co-occurring psychopathology predicted or moderated treatment effects. Until a larger body of research accumulates, it is difficult to draw firm conclusions regarding the role of co-occurring psychopathology for intervention response in adolescents with ADHD.

Conclusions

Adolescents with ADHD, like children with ADHD, are at elevated risk for a range of co-occurring psychopathologies that span externalizing and internalizing domains. These co-occurring psychopathologies contribute to the substantial heterogeneous characteristic of ADHD and add to the impairments experienced by adolescents with ADHD. To better understand and treat adolescents with ADHD, far more research is needed using carefully designed studies that can elucidate distinct developmental pathways and complex interactions. For example, ADHD severity, family conflict, peer rejection, and school problems appear to increase risk for co-occurring internalizing *and* externalizing psychopathologies, but we know little about factors that may increase (or decrease) risk for either internalizing *or* externalizing psychopathologies. For major advancements to be made in this regard, researchers need to examine multiple dimensions of psychopathology that cut across the internalizing and externalizing spectra, incorporate multiple informants and units of analysis, and include multiple time points across sensitive periods of development. It will also be important for studies to include typically developing adolescents and adolescents with a full range of ADHD symptomatology, such that researchers can evaluate whether adolescents with ADHD have similar or distinct pathways to other psychopathologies. Much important work has described and examined psychiatric co-occurrence in adolescents with ADHD, yet substantial work remains to build a body of theoretically driven research that can ultimately promote adaptation and resilience into and beyond the adolescent years for youth with ADHD.

References

Albert, D., Chein, J., & Steinberg, L. (2013). The teenage brain: Peer influences on adolescent decision making. *Current Directions in Psychological Science, 22,* 114–120.

American Psychiatric Association. (2013). *Diagnostic and statistical manual of mental disorders* (5th ed.). Arlington, VA: Author.

Antshel, K. M., Faraone, S. V., & Gordon, M. (2012). Cognitive behavioral treatment outcomes in Adolescent ADHD. *Journal of Attention Disorders, 18,* 483–495.

Antshel, K. M., Zhang-James, Y., Wagner, K. E., Ledesma, A., & Faraone, S. V. (2016). An update on the comorbidity of ADHD and ASD: A focus on clinical management. *Expert Review in Neurotherapeutics, 16,* 279–293.

Ashwood, K. L., Tye, C., Azadi, B., Cartwright, S., Asherson, P., & Bolton, P. (2015). Brief report: Adaptive functioning in children with ASD, ADHD and ASD + ADHD. *Journal of Autism and Developmental Disorders, 45,* 2235–2242.

August, G. J., Realmuto, G. M., Joyce, T., & Hektner, J. M. (1999). Persistence and desistance of oppositional defiant disorder in a community sample of children with ADHD. *Journal of the American Academy of Child and Adolescent Psychiatry, 38,* 1262–1270.

Avenevoli, S., Swendsen, J., He, J. P., Burstein, M., & Merikangas, K. R. (2015). Major depression in the national comorbidity survey-adolescent supplement: Prevalence, correlates, and treatment. *Journal of the American Academy of Child and Adolescent Psychiatry, 54,* 37–44.

Bagwell, C. L., Molina, B. S. G., Kashdan, T. B., Pelham, W. E., & Hoza, B. (2006). Anxiety and mood disorders in adolescents with childhood attention-deficit hyperactivity disorder. *Journal of Emtotional and Behavioral Disorders, 14,* 178–187.

Barkley, R. A., Anastopoulos, A. D., Guevremont, D. C., & Fletcher, K. E. (1992). Adolescents with attention deficit hyperactivity disorder: Mother–adolescent interactions, family beliefs and conflicts, and maternal psychopathology. *Journal of Abnormal Child Psychology, 20,* 263–288.

Barkley, R. A., Edwards, G., Laneri, M., Fletcher, K., & Metevia, L. (2001). The efficacy of problem-solving communication training alone, behavior management training alone, and their combination for parent–adolescent conflict in teenagers with ADHD and ODD. *Journal of Consulting and Clinical Psychology, 69,* 926–941.

Barkley, R. A., Fischer, M., Edelbrock, C. S., & Smallish, L. (1990). The adolescent outcome of hyperactive children diagnosed by research criteria: I. An 8-year prospective follow-up study. *Journal of the American Academy of Child and Adolescent Psychiatry, 29,* 546–557.

Barkley, R. A., Guevremont, D. C., Anastopoulos, A. D., & Fletcher, K. E. (1992). A comparison of 3 family-therapy programs for treating family conflicts in adolescents with attention-deficit/hyperactivity disorders. *Journal of Consulting and Clinical Psychology, 60,* 450–462.

Bauermeister, J. J., Shrout, P. E., Ramirez, R., Bravo, M., Alegria, M., Martinez-Taboas, A., . . . Canino, G. (2007). ADHD correlates, comorbidity, and impairment in community and treated samples of children and adolescents. *Journal of Abnormal Child Psychology, 35,* 883–898.

Beauchaine, T. P. (2003). Taxometrics and developmental psychopathology. *Development and Psychopathology, 15,* 501–527.

Beauchaine, T. P. (2015). Respiratory sinus arrhythmia: A transdiagnostic biomarker of emotion dysregulation and psychopathology. *Current Opinion in Psychology, 3,* 43–47.

Beauchaine, T. P., & Cicchetti, D. (2016). A new generation of comorbidity research in the era of neuroscience and research domain criteria. *Development and Psychopathology, 28,* 891–894.

Beauchaine, T. P., Hinshaw, S. P., & Pang, K. L. (2010). Comorbidity of attention-deficit/hyperactivity disorder and early-onset conduct disorder: Biological, environmental, and developmental mechanisms. *Clinical Psychology: Science and Practice, 17,* 327–336.

Beauchaine, T. P., & McNulty, T. (2013). Comorbidities and continuities as ontogenic processes: Toward a developmental spectrum model of externalizing psychopathology. *Development and Psychopathology, 25,* 1505–1528.

Beauchaine, T. P., & Thayer, J. F. (2015). Heart rate variability as a transdiagnostic biomarker of psychopathology. *International Journal of Psychophysiology, 98,* 338–350.

Becker, S. P., & Barkley, R. A. (2018). Sluggish cognitive tempo. In T. Banaschewski, D. Coghill, & A. Zuddas (Eds.), *Oxford textbook of attention deficit hyperactivity disorder* (pp. 147–153). Oxford, UK: Oxford University Press.

Becker, S. P., Burns, G. L., Leopold, D. R., Olson, R. K., & Willcutt, E. G. (2018). Differential impact of trait sluggish cognitive tempo and ADHD inattention in early childhood on adolescent functioning. *Journal of Child Psychology and Psychiatry, 59,* 1094–1104.

Becker, S. P., Holdaway, A. S., & Luebbe, A. M. (2018). Suicidal behaviors in college students: Frequency, sex differences, and mental health correlates including sluggish cognitive tempo. *Journal of Adolescent Health, 63,* 181–188.

Becker, S. P., & Langberg, J. M. (2013). Sluggish cognitive tempo among young adolescents with ADHD: Relations to mental health, academic, and social functioning. *Journal of Attention Disorders, 17,* 681–689.

Becker, S. P., Langberg, J. M., Evans, S. W., Girio-Herrera, E., & Vaughn, A. J. (2015). Differentiating anxiety and depression in relation to the social functioning of young adolescents with ADHD. *Journal of Clinical Child and Adolescent Psychology, 44,* 1015–1029.

Becker, S. P., Leopold, D. R., Burns, G. L., Jarrett, M. A., Langberg, J. M., Marshall, S. A., . . . Willcutt, E. G. (2016). The internal, external, and diagnostic validity of sluggish cognitive tempo: A meta-analysis and critical review. *Journal of the American Academy of Child and Adolescent Psychiatry, 55,* 163–178.

Becker, S. P., Luebbe, A. M., & Langberg, J. M. (2012). Co-occurring mental health problems and peer functioning among youth with attention-deficit/hyperactivity disorder: A review and recommendations for future research. *Clinical Child and Family Psychology Review, 15,* 279–302.

Becker, S. P., Luebbe, A. M., Stoppelbein, L., Greening, L., & Fite, P. J. (2012). Aggression among children with ADHD, anxiety, or co-occurring symptoms: Competing exacerbation and attenuation hypotheses. *Journal of Abnormal Child Psychology, 40,* 527–542.

Becker, S. P., & Willcutt, E. G. (2019). Advancing the study of sluggish cognitive tempo via DSM, RDoC, and hierarchical models of psychopathology. *European Child and Adolescent Psychiatry, 28,* 603–613.

Biederman, J., Ball, S. W., Monuteaux, M. C., Mick, E., Spencer, T. J., McCreary, M., . . . Faraone, S. V. (2008). New insights into the comorbidity between ADHD and major depression in adolescent and young adult females. *Journal of the American Academy of Child and Adolescent Psychiatry, 47,* 426–434.

Biederman, J., Faraone, S., Milberger, S., Curtis, S., Chen, L., Marrs, A., . . . Spencer, T. (1996). Predictors of persistence and remission of ADHD into adolescence: Results from a four-year prospective follow-up study. *Journal of the American Academy of Child and Adolescent Psychiatry, 35,* 343–351.

Biederman, J., Faraone, S., Milberger, S., Guite, J., Mick, E., Chen, L., . . . Perrin, J. (1996). A prospective 4-year follow-up study of attention-deficit hyperactivity and related disorders. *Archives of General Psychiatry, 53,* 437–446.

Biederman, J., Faraone, S. V., Milberger, S., Jetton, J. G., Chen, L., Mick, E., . . . Russell, R. L. (1996). Is childhood oppositional defiant disorder a precursor to adolescent conduct disorder?: Findings from a four-year follow-up study of children with ADHD. *Journal of the American Academy of Child and Adolescent Psychiatry, 35,* 1193–1204.

Biederman, J., Mick, E., & Faraone, S. V. (1998). Depression in attention deficit hyperactivity disorder (ADHD) children: "True" depression or demoralization? *Journal of Affective Disorders, 47,* 113–122.

Biederman, J., Monuteaux, M. C., Mick, E., Spencer, T., Wilens, T. E., Klein, K. L., . . . Faraone, S. V. (2006). Psychopathology in females with attention-deficit/hyperactivity disorder: A controlled, five-year prospective study. *Biological Psychiatry, 60,* 1098–1105.

Biederman, J., Monuteaux, M. C., Spencer, T., Wilens, T. E., & Faraone, S. V. (2009). Do stimulants protect against psychiatric disorders in youth with ADHD?: A 10-year follow-up study. *Pediatrics, 124,* 71–78.

Biederman, J., Petty, C. R., Monuteaux, M. C., Mick, E., Parcell, T., Westerberg, D., & Faraone, S. V. (2008). The longitudinal course of comorbid oppositional defiant disorder in girls with attention-deficit/hyperactivity disorder: Findings from a controlled 5-year prospective longitudinal follow-up study. *Journal of Developmental and Behavioral Pediatrics, 29,* 501–507.

Boyer, B. E., Geurts, H. M., Prins, P. J. M., & Van der Oord, S. (2015). Two novel CBTs for adolescents with ADHD: The value of planning skills. *European Child and Adolescent Psychiatry, 24,* 1075–1090.

Breaux, R. P., Langberg, J. M., Bourchtein, E., Eadeh, H. M., Molitor, S. J., & Smith, Z. R. (2019). Brief homework intervention for adolescents with ADHD: Trajectories and predictors of response. *School Psychology Quarterly, 34,* 201–211.

Brieber, S., Neufang, S., Bruning, N., Kamp-Becker, I., Remschmidt, H., Herpertz-Dahlmann, B., . . . Konrad, K. (2007). Structural brain abnormalities in adolescents with autism spectrum disorder and patients with attention deficit/hyperactivity disorder. *Journal of Child Psychology and Psychiatry, 48,* 1251–1258.

Burke, J. D., Loeber, R., Lahey, B. B., & Rathouz, P. J. (2005). Developmental transitions among affective and behavioral disorders in adolescent boys. *Journal of Child Psychology and Psychiatry, 46,* 1200–1210.

Caspi, A., Houts, R. M., Belsky, D. W., Goldman-Mellor, S. J., Harrington, H., Israel, S., . . . Moffitt, T. E. (2014). The p factor: One general psychopathology factor in the structure of psychiatric disorders? *Clinical Psychological Science, 2,* 119–137.

Castellanos, F. X., Sonuga-Barke, E. J., Milham, M. P., & Tannock, R. (2006). Characterizing cognition in ADHD: Beyond executive dysfunction. *Trends in Cognitive Sciences, 10,* 117–123.

Caye, A., Spadini, A. V., Karam, R. G., Grevet, E. H., Rovaris, D. L., Bau, C. H., . . . Kieling, C. (2016). Predictors of persistence of ADHD into adulthood: A systematic review of the literature and meta-analysis. *European Child and Adolescent Psychiatry, 25,* 1151–1159.

Cha, C. B., Franz, P. J., Guzman, M., Glenn, C. R., Kleiman, E. M., & Nock, M. K. (2018). Annual research review: Suicide among youth—epidemiology, (potential) etiology, and treatment. *Journal of Child Psychology and Psychiatry, 59,* 460–482.

Chen, M. H., Pan, T. L., Hsu, J. W., Huang, K. L., Su, T. P., Li, C. T., . . . Bai, Y. M. (2016). Attention-deficit hyperactivity disorder comorbidity and antidepressant resistance among patients with major depression: A nationwide longitudinal study. *European Neuropsychopharmacology, 26,* 1760–1767.

Chen, M. H., Su, T. P., Chen, Y. S., Hsu, J. W., Huang, K. L., Chang, W. H., . . . Bai, Y. M. (2013). Higher risk of developing mood disorders among adolescents with comorbidity of attention deficit hyperactivity disorder and disruptive behavior disorder: A nationwide prospective study. *Journal of Psychiatric Research, 47,* 1019–1023.

Cho, S. C., Kim, J. W., Choi, H. J., Kim, B. N., Shin, M. S., Lee, J. H., & Kim, E. H. (2008). Associations between symptoms of attention deficit hyperactivity disorder, depression, and suicide in Korean female adolescents. *Depression and Anxiety, 25,* E142–E146.

Chronis-Tuscano, A., Molina, B. S., Pelham, W. E., Applegate, B., Dahlke, A., Overmyer, M., & Lahey, B. B. (2010). Very early predictors of adolescent depression and suicide attempts in children with attention-deficit/hyperactivity disorder. *Archives of General Psychiatry, 67,* 1044–1051.

Cole, J., Ball, H. A., Martin, N. C., Scourfield, J., & McGuffin, P. (2009). Genetic overlap between measures of hyperactivity/inattention and mood in children and adolescents. *Journal of the American Academy of Child and Adolescent Psychiatry, 48,* 1094–1101.

Connor, D. F., & Doerfler, L. A. (2008). ADHD with comorbid oppositional defiant disorder or conduct disorder: Discrete or nondistinct disruptive behavior disorders? *Journal of Attention Disorders, 12,* 126–134.

Costello, E. J., Mustillo, S., Erkanli, A., Keeler, G., & Angold, A. (2003). Prevalence and development of psychiatric disorders in childhood and adolescence. *Archives of General Psychiatry, 60,* 837–844.

Costin, J., Vance, A., Barnett, R., O'Shea, M., & Luk, E. S. L. (2002). Attention deficit hyperactivity disorder and comorbid anxiety: Practitioner problems in treatment planning. *Child and Adolescent Mental Health, 7,* 16–24.

Daley, D., van der Oord, S., Ferrin, M., Danckaerts, M., Doepfner, M., Cortese, S., & Sonuga-Barke, E. J. S. (2014). Behavioral interventions in attention-deficit/hyperactivity disorder: A meta-analysis of randomized controlled trials across multiple outcome domains. *Journal of the American Academy of Child and Adolescent Psychiatry, 53,* 835–847.

Danforth, J. S., Connor, D. F., & Doerfler, L. A. (2016). The development of comorbid conduct problems in children with ADHD: An example of an integrative developmental psychopathology perspective. *Journal of Attention Disorders, 20,* 214–229.

Danforth, J. S., Doerfler, L. A., & Connor, D. F. (2019). Does anxiety modify the risk for, or severity of, conduct problems among children with co-occurring ADHD: Categorical and dimensional and analyses. *Journal of Attention Disorders, 23,* 797–808.

Daviss, W. B. (2008). A review of co-morbid depression in pediatric ADHD: Etiologies, phenomenology, and treatment. *Journal of Child and Adolescent Psychopharmacology, 18,* 565–571.

Daviss, W. B., Birmaher, B., Diler, R. S., & Mintz, J. (2008). Does pharmacotherapy for attention-deficit/hyperactivity disorder predict risk of later major depression? *Journal of Chld and Adolescent Psychopharmacology, 18,* 257–264.

Daviss, W. B., & Diler, R. S. (2014). Suicidal behaviors in adolescents with ADHD: Associations with depressive and other comorbidity, parent–child conflict, trauma exposure, and impairment. *Journal of Attention Disorders, 18,* 680–690.

Daviss, W. B., Diler, R. S., & Birmaher, B. (2009). Associations of lifetime depression with trauma exposure, other environmental adversities, and impairment in adolescents with ADHD. *Journal of Abnormal Child Psychology, 37,* 857–871.

Deater-Deckard, K. (2001). Annotation: Recent research examining the role of peer relationships in the development of psychopathology. *Journal of Child Psychology and Psychiatry, 42,* 565–579.

Drabick, D. A. G., & Kendall, P. C. (2010). Developmental psychopathology and the diagnosis of mental health problems among youth. *Clinical Psychology: Science and Practice, 17,* 272–280.

Duncan, A., Tamm, L., Birnschein, A. M., & Becker, S. P. (2018, November 14). Clinical correlates of sluggish cognitive tempo in adolescents with autism spectrum disorder. *Autism.* [Epub ahead of print]

Dvorsky, M. R., & Langberg, J. M. (2016). A review of factors that promote resilience in youth with ADHD and ADHD symptoms. *Clinical Child and Family Psychology Review, 19,* 368–391.

Eadeh, H. M., Bourchtein, E., Langberg, J. M., Eddy, L. D., Oddo, L., Molitor, S. J., & Evans, S. W. (2017). Longitudinal evaluation of the role of academic and social impairment and parent–adolescent conflict in the development of depression in adolescents with ADHD. *Journal of Child and Family Studies, 26,* 2374–2385.

Elia, J., Ambrosini, P., & Berrettini, W. (2008). ADHD characteristics: I. Concurrent co-morbidity patterns in children and adolescents. *Child and Adolescent Psychiatry and Mental Health, 2,* 15.

Elkins, I. J., McGue, M., & Iacono, W. G. (2007). Prospective effects of attention-deficit/hyperactivity disorder, conduct disorder, and sex on adolescent substance use and abuse. *Archives of General Psychiatry, 64,* 1145–1152.

Evans, S. W., Langberg, J. M., Schultz, B. K., Vaughn, A., Altaye, M., Marshall, S. A., & Zoromski, A. K. (2016). Evaluation of a school-based treatment program for young adolescents with ADHD. *Journal of Consulting and Clinical Psychology, 84,* 15–30.

Falk, A. E., Lee, S. S., & Chorpita, B. F. (2017). Differential association of youth attention-deficit/hyperactivity disorder and anxiety with delinquency and aggression. *Journal of Clinical Child and Adolescent Psychology, 46,* 653–660.

Fleming, A. P., McMahon, R. J., Moran, L. R., Peterson, A. P., & Dreessen, A. (2015). Pilot randomized controlled trial of dialectical behavior therapy group skills training for ADHD among college students. *Journal of Attention Disorders, 19,* 260–271.

Fletcher, K. E., Fischer, M., Barkley, R. A., & Smallish, L. (1996). A sequential analysis of the mother–adolescent interactions of ADHD, ADHD/ODD, and normal teenagers during neutral and conflict discussions. *Journal of Abnormal Child Psychology, 24,* 271–297.

Forbes, M. K., Tackett, J. L., Markon, K. E., & Krueger, R. F. (2016). Beyond comorbidity: Toward a dimensional and hierarchical approach to understanding psychopathology across the life span. *Development and Psychopathology, 28,* 971–986.

Garber, J., & Horowitz, J. L. (2002). Depression in children. In I. H. Gotlib & C. H. Hammen (Eds.), *Handbook of depression* (pp. 510–540). New York: Guilford Press.

Gargaro, B. A., Rinehart, N. J., Bradshaw, J. L., Tonge, B. J., & Sheppard, D. M. (2011). Autism and ADHD: How far have we come in the comorbidity debate? *Neuroscience and Biobehavioral Reviews, 35,* 1081–1088.

Gau, S. S., Lin, Y., Cheng, A. T., Chiu, Y., Tsai, W., & Soong, W. (2010). Psychopathology and symptom remission at adolescence among children with attention-deficit-hyperactivity disorder. *Australian and New Zealand Journal of Psychiatry, 44,* 323–332.

Gau, S. S., Ni, H., Shang, C., Soong, W., Wu, Y., Lin, L., & Chiu, Y. (2010). Psychiatric comorbidity among children and adolescents with and without persistent attention-deficit hyperactivity disorder. *Australian and New Zealand Journal of Psychiatry, 44,* 135–143.

Goldin, R. L., Matson, J. L., Tureck, K., Cervantes, P. E., & Jang, J. (2013). A comparison of tantrum behavior profiles in children with ASD, ADHD and comorbid ASD and ADHD. *Research in Developmental Disabilities, 34,* 2669–2675.

Goschke, T. (2014). Dysfunctions of decision-making and cognitive control as transdiagnostic mechanisms of mental disorders: Advances, gaps, and needs in current research. *International Journal of Methods in Psychiatric Research, 23,* 41–57.

Greene, R. W., Biederman, J., Faraone, S. V., Sienna, M., & Garcia-Jetton, J. (1997). Adolescent outcome of boys with attention-deficit/hyperactivity disorder and social disability: Results from a 4-year longitudinal follow-up study. *Journal of Consulting and Clinical Psychology, 65,* 758–767.

Günther, T., Konrad, K., De Brito, S. A., Herpertz-Dahlmann, B., & Vloet, T. D. (2011). Attentional functions in children and adolescents with ADHD, depressive disorders, and the comorbid condition. *Journal of Child Psychology and Psychiatry, 52,* 324–331.

Hankin, B. L., Snyder, H. R., Gulley, L. D., Schweizer, T. H., Bijttebier, P., Nelis, S., . . . Vasey, M. W. (2016). Understanding comorbidity among internalizing problems: Integrating latent structural models of psychopathology and risk mechanisms. *Development and Psychopathology, 28,* 987–1012.

Hartman, C. A., Geurts, H. M., Franke, B., Buitelaar, J. K., & Rommelse, N. N. J. (2016). Changing ASD-ADHD symptom co-occurrence across the lifespan with adolescence as crucial time window: Illustrating the need to go beyond childhood. *Neuroscience and Biobehavioral Reviews, 71,* 529–541.

Herman, K. C., Lambert, S. F., Ialongo, N. S., & Ostrander, R. (2007). Academic pathways between attention problems and depressive symptoms among urban African American children. *Journal of Abnormal Child Psychology, 35,* 265–274.

Hinshaw, S. P., Owens, E. B., Sami, N., & Fargeon, S. (2006). Prospective follow-up of girls with attention-deficit/hyperactivity disorder into adolescence: Evidence for continuing cross-domain impairment. *Journal of Consulting and Clinical Psychology, 74*, 489–499.

Hudziak, J. J., Heath, A. C., Madden, P. F., Reich, W., Bucholz, K. K., Slutske, W., . . . Todd, R. D. (1998). Latent class and factor analysis of DSM-IV ADHD: A twin study of female adolescents. *Journal of the American Academy of Child and Adolescent Psychiatry, 37*, 848–857.

Humphreys, K. L., Katz, S. J., Lee, S. S., Hammen, C., Brennan, P. A., & Najman, J. M. (2013). The association of ADHD and depression: Mediation by peer problems and parent–child difficulties in two complementary samples. *Journal of Abnormal Psychology, 122*, 854–867.

Hurtig, T., Ebeling, H., Taanila, A., Miettunen, J., Smalley, S., McGough, J., . . . Moilanen, I. (2007). ADHD and comorbid disorders in relation to family environment and symptom severity. *European Child and Adolescent Psychiatry, 16*, 362–369.

Hurtig, T., Taanila, A., Moilanen, I., Nordstrom, T., & Ebeling, H. (2012). Suicidal and self-harm behaviour associated with adolescent attention deficit hyperactivity disorder—A study in the Northern Finland Birth Cohort 1986. *Nordic Journal of Psychiatry, 66*, 320–328.

Hyman, S. E. (2010). The diagnosis of mental disorders: The problem of reification. *Annual Review of Clinical Psychology, 6*, 155–179.

Jang, J., Matson, J. L., Williams, L. W., Tureck, K., Goldin, R. L., & Cervantes, P. E. (2013). Rates of comorbid symptoms in children with ASD, ADHD, and comorbid ASD and ADHD. *Research in Developmental Disabilities, 34*, 2369–2378.

Jarrett, M. A., & Ollendick, T. H. (2008). A conceptual review of the comorbidity of attention-deficit/hyperactivity disorder and anxiety: Implications for future research and practice. *Clinical Psychology Review, 28*, 1266–1280.

Jarrett, M. A., & Ollendick, T. H. (2012). Treatment of comorbid attention-deficit/hyperactivity disorder and anxiety in children: A multiple baseline design analysis. *Journal of Consulting and Clinical Psychology, 80*, 239–244.

Jensen, C. M., & Steinhausen, H. C. (2015). Comorbid mental disorders in children and adolescents with attention-deficit/hyperactivity disorder in a large nationwide study. *ADHD Attention Deficit and Hyperactivity Disorders, 7*, 27–38.

Jones, D. E., & Foster, E. M. (2009). Service use patterns for adolescents with ADHD and comorbid conduct disorder. *Journal of Behavioral Health Services and Research, 36*, 436–449.

Kaplan, B., Crawford, S., Cantell, M., Kooistra, L., & Dewey, D. (2006). Comorbidity, co-occurrence, continuum: What's in a name? *Child: Care, Health and Development, 32*, 723–731.

Kessler, R. C., Adler, L. A., Berglund, P., Green, J. G., McLaughlin, K. A., Fayyad, J., . . . Zaslavsky, A. M. (2014). The effects of temporally secondary co-morbid mental disorders on the associations of DSM-IV ADHD with adverse outcomes in the US National Comorbidity Survey Replication Adolescent Supplement (NCS-A). *Psychological Medicine, 44*, 1779–1792.

Klassen, A. F., Miller, A., & Fine, S. (2004). Health-related quality of life in children and adolescents who have a diagnosis of attention-deficit/hyperactivity disorder. *Pediatrics, 114*, e541–e547.

Kotov, R., Krueger, R. F., Watson, D., Achenbach, T. M., Althoff, R. R., Bagby, R. M., . . . Zimmerman, M. (2017). The Hierarchical Taxonomy of Psychopathology (HiTOP): A dimensional alternative to traditional nosologies. *Journal of Abnormal Psychology, 126*, 454–477.

Kozak, M. J., & Cuthbert, B. N. (2016). The NIMH Research Domain Criteria initiative: Background, issues, and pragmatics. *Psychophysiology, 53,* 286–297.

Kuja-Halkola, R., Lichtenstein, P., D'Onofrio, B. M., & Larsson, H. (2015). Codevelopment of ADHD and externalizing behavior from childhood to adulthood. *Journal of Child Psychology and Psychiatry, 56,* 640–647.

Kutcher, S., Aman, M., Brooks, S. J., Buitelaar, J., van Daalen, E., Fegert, J., . . . Tyano, S. (2004). International consensus statement on attention-deficit/hyperactivity disorder (ADHD) and disruptive behaviour disorders (DBDs): Clinical implications and treatment practice suggestions. *European Neuropsychopharmacology, 14,* 11–28.

Lahey, B. B., Krueger, R. F., Rathouz, P. J., Waldman, I. D., & Zald, D. H. (2017). A hierarchical causal taxonomy of psychopathology across the life span. *Psychological Bulletin, 143,* 142–186.

Lahey, B. B., Lee, S. S., Sibley, M. H., Applegate, B., Molina, B. S. G., & Pelham, W. E. (2016). Predictors of adolescent outcomes among 4–6-year-old children with attention-deficit/hyperactivity disorder. *Journal of Abnormal Psychology, 125,* 168–181.

Langberg, J. M., Becker, S. P., & Dvorsky, M. R. (2014). The association between sluggish cognitive tempo and academic functioning in youth with attention-deficit/hyperactivity disorder (ADHD). *Journal of Abnormal Child Psychology, 42,* 91–103.

Langberg, J. M., Becker, S. P., Epstein, J. N., Vaughn, A. J., & Girio-Herrera, E. (2013). Predictors of response and mechanisms of change in an organizational skills intervention for students with ADHD. *Journal of Child and Family Studies, 22,* 1000–1012.

Lee, M. J., Yang, K. C., Shyu, Y. C., Yuan, S. S., Yang, C. J., Lee, S. Y., . . . Wang, L. J. (2016). Attention-deficit hyperactivity disorder, its treatment with medication and the probability of developing a depressive disorder: A nationwide population-based study in Taiwan. *Journal of Affective Disorders, 189,* 110–117.

Lee, S. S., & Hinshaw, S. P. (2006). Predictors of adolescent functioning in girls with attention deficit hyperactivity disorder (ADHD): The role of childhood ADHD, conduct problems, and peer status. *Journal of Clinical Child and Adolescent Psychology, 35,* 356–368.

Lee, S. S., Lahey, B. B., Owens, E. B., & Hinshaw, S. P. (2008). Few preschool boys and girls with ADHD are well-adjusted during adolescence. *Journal of Abnormal Child Psychology, 36,* 373–383.

Leopold, D. R., Christopher, M. E., Burns, G. L., Becker, S. P., Olson, R. K., & Willcutt, E. G. (2016). Attention-deficit/hyperactivity disorder and sluggish cognitive tempo throughout childhood: Temporal invariance and stability from preschool through ninth grade. *Journal of Child Psychology and Psychiatry, 57,* 1066–1074.

Lilienfeld, S. O., Waldman, I. D., & Israel, A. C. (1994). A critical examination of the use of the term and concept of comorbidity in psychopathology research. *Clinical Psychology: Science and Practice, 1,* 71–83.

Macdonald, A. N., Goines, K. B., Novacek, D. M., & Walker, E. F. (2016). Prefrontal mechanisms of comorbidity from a transdiagnostic and ontogenic perspective. *Development and Psychopathology, 28,* 1147–1175.

Mannuzza, S., Klein, R. G., Abikoff, H., & Moulton, J. L. (2004). Significance of childhood conduct problems to later development of conduct disorder among children with ADHD: A prospective follow-up study. *Journal of Abnormal Child Psychology, 32,* 565–573.

Masten, A. S., & Cicchetti, D. (2010). Developmental cascades. *Development and Psychopathology, 22,* 491–495.

Meinzer, M. C., Lewinsohn, P. M., Pettit, J. W., Seeley, J. R., Gau, J. M., Chronis-Tuscano, A., & Waxmonsky, J. G. (2013). Attention-deficit/hyperactivity disorder in adolescence predicts onset of major depressive disorder through early adulthood. *Depression and Anxiety, 30,* 546–553.

Meinzer, M. C., Pettit, J. W., & Viswesvaran, C. (2014). The co-occurrence of attention-deficit/hyperactivity disorder and unipolar depression in children and adolescents: A meta-analytic review. *Clinical Psychology Review, 34,* 595–607.

Meinzer, M. C., Pettit, J. W., Waxmonsky, J. G., Gnagy, E., Molina, B. S. G., & Pelham, W. E. (2016). Does childhood attention-deficit/hyperactivity disorder (ADHD) predict levels of depressive symptoms during emerging adulthood? *Journal of Abnormal Child Psychology, 44,* 787–797.

Merikangas, K. R., He, J. P., Burstein, M., Swanson, S. A., Avenevoli, S., Cui, L., . . . Swendsen, J. (2010). Lifetime prevalence of mental disorders in U.S. adolescents: Results from the National Comorbidity Survey Replication—Adolescent Supplement (NCS-A). *Journal of the American Academy of Child and Adolescent Psychiatry, 49,* 980–989.

Mikami, A. Y., & Hinshaw, S. P. (2006). Resilient adolescent adjustment among girls: Buffers of childhood peer rejection and attention-deficit/hyperactivity disorder. *Journal of Abnormal Child Psychology, 34,* 825–839.

Mikami, A. Y., Hinshaw, S. P., Arnold, L. E., Hoza, B., Hechtman, L., Newcorn, J. H., & Abikoff, H. B. (2010). Bulimia nervosa symptoms in the multimodal treatment study of children with ADHD. *International Journal of Eating Disorders, 43,* 248–259.

Mikami, A. Y., Hinshaw, S. P., Patterson, K. A., & Lee, J. C. (2008). Eating pathology among adolescent girls with attention-deficit/hyperactivity disorder. *Journal of Abnormal Psychology, 117,* 225–235.

Miodovnik, A., Harstad, E., Sideridis, G., & Huntington, N. (2015). Timing of the diagnosis of attention-deficit/hyperactivity disorder and autism spectrum disorder. *Pediatrics, 136,* e830–e837.

Molina, B. S., Hinshaw, S. P., Swanson, J. M., Arnold, L. E., Vitiello, B., Jensen, P. S., . . . Houck, P. R. (2009). The MTA at 8 years: Prospective follow-up of children treated for combined-type ADHD in a multisite study. *Journal of the American Academy of Child and Adolescent Psychiatry, 48,* 484–500.

Montoya, A., Colom, F., & Ferrin, M. (2011). Is psychoeducation for parents and teachers of children and adolescents with ADHD efficacious?: A systematic literature review. *European Psychiatry, 26,* 166–175.

Monuteaux, M. C., Faraone, S. V., Gross, L. M., & Biederman, J. (2007). Predictors, clinical characteristics, and outcome of conduct disorder in girls with attention-deficit/hyperactivity disorder: A longitudinal study. *Psychological Medicine, 37,* 1731–1741.

Monuteaux, M. C., Mick, E., Faraone, S. V., & Biederman, J. (2010). The influence of sex on the course and psychiatric correlates of ADHD from childhood to adolescence: A longitudinal study. *Journal of Child Psychology and Psychiatry, 51,* 233–241.

Murray, A. L., Booth, T., Obsuth, I., Zirk-Sadowski, J., Eisner, M., & Ribeaud, D. (2018). Testing the exacerbation and attenuation hypotheses of the role of anxiety in the relation between ADHD and reactive/proactive aggression: A 10-year longitudinal study. *Psychiatry Research, 269,* 585–592.

Neuman, R. J., Heath, A., Reich, W., Bucholz, K. K., Madden, P. A. F., Sun, L., . . . Hudziak, J. J. (2001). Latent class analysis of ADHD and comorbid symptoms in a population sample of adolescent female twins. *Journal of Child Psychology and Psychiatry, 42,* 933–942.

Nigg, J. T., & Casey, B. J. (2005). An integrative theory of attention-deficit/hyperactivity disorder based on the cognitive and affective neurosciences. *Development and Psychopathology, 17,* 785–806.

Ostrander, R., & Herman, K. C. (2006). Potential cognitive, parenting, and developmental mediators of the relationship between ADHD and depression. *Journal of Consulting and Clinical Psychology, 74,* 89–98.

Patterson, G. R., Debaryshe, B. D., & Ramsey, E. (1989). A developmental perspective on antisocial behavior. *American Psychologist, 44,* 329–335.

Reale, L., Bartoli, B., Cartabia, M., Zanetti, M., Costantino, M. A., Canevini, M. P., . . . Lombardy, A. G. (2017). Comorbidity prevalence and treatment outcome in children and adolescents with ADHD. *European Child and Adolescent Psychiatry, 26,* 1443–1457.

Rhee, S. H., Lahey, B. B., & Waldman, I. D. (2015). Comorbidity among dimensions of childhood psychopathology: Converging evidence from behavior genetics. *Child Development Perspectives, 9,* 26–31.

Rinsky, J. R., & Hinshaw, S. P. (2011). Linkages between childhood executive functioning and adolescent social functioning and psychopathology in girls with ADHD. *Child Neuropsychology, 17,* 368–390.

Rohde, L. A., Biederman, J., Busnello, E. A., Zimmermann, H., Schmitz, M., Martins, S., & Tramontina, S. (1999). ADHD in a school sample of Brazilian adolescents: A study of prevalence, comorbid conditions, and impairments. *Journal of the American Academy of Child and Adolescent Psychiatry, 38,* 716–722.

Rosen, P. J., Leaberry, K. D., Slaughter, K., Fogleman, N. D., Walerius, D. M., Loren, R. E. A., & Epstein, J. N. (2018). Managing Frustration for Children (MFC) group intervention for ADHD: An open trial of a novel group intervention for deficient emotion regulation. *Cognitive and Behavioral Practice.* [Epub ahead of print]

Roy, A., Oldehinkel, A. J., Verhulst, F. C., Ormel, J., & Hartman, C. A. (2014). Anxiety and disruptive behavior mediate pathways from attention-deficit/hyperactivity disorder to depression. *Journal of Clinical Psychiatry, 75,* e108–e113.

Rutter, M., Kim-Cohen, J., & Maughan, B. (2006). Continuities and discontinuities in psychopathology between childhood and adult life. *Journal of Child Psychology and Psychiatry, 47,* 276–295.

Sarkisian, K. L., Van Hulle, C. A., & Hill Goldsmith, H. (2019). Brooding, inattention, and impulsivity as predictors of adolescent suicidal ideation. *Journal of Abnormal Child Psychology, 47,* 333–344.

Sauder, C. L., Beauchaine, T. P., Gatzke-Kopp, L. M., Shannon, K. E., & Aylward, E. (2012). Neuroanatomical correlates of heterotypic comorbidity in externalizing male adolescents. *Journal of Clinical Child and Adolescent Psychology, 41,* 346–352.

Scheffer, R. E., Kowatch, R. A., Carmody, T., & Rush, A. J. (2005). Randomized, placebo-controlled trial of mixed amphetamine salts for symptoms of comorbid ADHD in pediatric bipolar disorder after mood stabilization with divalproex sodium. *American Journal of Psychiatry, 162,* 58–64.

Seymour, K. E., Chronis-Tuscano, A., Halldorsdottir, T., Stupica, B., Owens, K., & Sacks, T. (2012). Emotion regulation mediates the relationship between ADHD and depressive symptoms in youth. *Journal of Abnormal Child Psychology, 40,* 595–606.

Seymour, K. E., Chronis-Tuscano, A., Iwamoto, D. K., Kurdziel, G., & Macpherson, L. (2014). Emotion regulation mediates the association between ADHD and depressive symptoms in a community sample of youth. *Journal of Abnormal Child Psychology, 42,* 611–621.

Shaw, P., Eckstrand, K., Sharp, W., Blumenthal, J., Lerch, J. P., Greenstein, D., . . .

Rapoport, J. L. (2007). Attention-deficit/hyperactivity disorder is characterized by a delay in cortical maturation. *Proceedings of the National Academy of Sciences of the USA, 104,* 19649–19654.

Sibley, M. H., Graziano, P. A., Kuriyan, A. B., Coxe, S., Pelham, W. E., Rodriguez, L., . . . Ward, A. (2016). Parent–teen behavior therapy + motivational interviewing for adolescents with ADHD. *Journal of Consulting and Clinical Psychology, 84,* 699–712.

Sibley, M. H., Pelham, W. E., Molina, B. S., Gnagy, E. M., Waschbusch, D. A., Biswas, A., . . . Karch, K. M. (2011). The delinquency outcomes of boys with ADHD with and without comorbidity. *Journal of Abnormal Child Psychology, 39,* 21–32.

Sibley, M. H., Smith, B. H., Evans, S. W., Pelham, W. E., & Gnagy, E. M. (2012). Treatment response to an intensive summer treatment program for adolescents with ADHD. *Journal of Attention Disorders, 16,* 443–448.

Sinzig, J., Walter, D., & Doepfner, M. (2009). Attention deficit/hyperactivity disorder in children and adolescents with autism spectrum disorder: Symptom or syndrome? *Journal of Attention Disorders, 13,* 117–126.

Smalley, S. L., McGough, J. J., Moilanen, I. K., Loo, S. K., Taanila, A., Ebeling, H., . . . Jarvelin, M. R. (2007). Prevalence and psychiatric comorbidity of attention-deficit/hyperactivity disorder in an adolescent Finnish population. *Journal of the American Academy of Child and Adolescent Psychiatry, 46,* 1575–1583.

Smith, Z. R., & Langberg, J. M. (2017). Predicting academic impairment and internalizing psychopathology using a multidimensional framework of sluggish cognitive tempo with parent- and adolescent reports. *European Child and Adolescent Psychiatry, 26,* 1141–1150.

Sonuga-Barke, E. J. (1998). Categorical models of childhood disorder: A conceptual and empirical analysis. *Journal of Child Psychology and Psychiatry, 39,* 115–133.

Sprenger, L., Buhler, E., Poustka, L., Bach, C., Heinzel-Gutenbrunner, M., Kamp-Becker, I., & Bachmann, C. (2013). Impact of ADHD symptoms on autism spectrum disorder symptom severity. *Research in Developmental Disabilities, 34,* 3545–3552.

Sprich, S. E., Safren, S. A., Finkelstein, D., Remmert, J. E., & Hammerness, P. (2016). A randomized controlled trial of cognitive behavioral therapy for ADHD in medication-treated adolescents. *Journal of Child Psychology and Psychiatry, 57,* 1218–1226.

Stickley, A., Koposov, R., Koyanagi, A., Inoue, Y., & Ruchkin, V. (2019). ADHD and depressive symptoms in adolescents: The role of community violence exposure. *Social Psychiatry and Psychiatric Epidemiology, 54,* 683–691.

Swanson, E. N., Owens, E. B., & Hinshaw, S. P. (2014). Pathways to self-harmful behaviors in young women with and without ADHD: A longitudinal examination of mediating factors. *Journal of Child Psychology and Psychiatry, 55,* 505–515.

Van Orden, K. A., Witte, T. K., Cukrowicz, K. C., Braithwaite, S. R., Selby, E. A., & Joiner, T. E., Jr. (2010). The interpersonal theory of suicide. *Psychology Review, 117,* 575–600.

Vidal, R., Castells, J., Richarte, V., Palomar, G., Garcia, M., Nicolau, R., . . . Ramos-Quiroga, J. A. (2015). Group therapy for adolescents with attention-deficit/hyperactivity disorder: A randomized controlled trial. *Journal of the American Academy of Child and Adolescent Psychiatry, 54,* 275–282.

Vloet, T. D., Konrad, K., Herpertz-Dahlmann, B., Polier, G. G., & Günther, T. (2010). Impact of anxiety disorders on attentional functions in children with ADHD. *Journal of Affective Disorders, 124,* 283–290.

Walczak, M., Ollendick, T., Ryan, S., & Esbjørn, B. H. (2018). Does comorbidity predict poorer treatment outcome in pediatric anxiety disorders?: An updated 10-year review. *Clinical Psychology Review, 60,* 45–61.

Widiger, T. A., & Samuel, D. B. (2005). Diagnostic categories or dimensions?: A question for the *Diagnostic and statistical manual of mental disorders—fifth edition. Journal of Abnormal Psychology, 114,* 494–504.

Yoshida, Y., & Uchiyama, T. (2004). The clinical necessity for assessing attention deficit/hyperactivity disorder (AD/HD) symptoms in children with high-functioning pervasive developmental disorder (PDD). *European Child and Adolescent Psychiatry, 13,* 307–314.

Yoshimasu, K., Barbaresi, W. J., Colligan, R. C., Voigt, R. G., Killian, J. M., Weaver, A. L., & Katusic, S. K. (2012). Childhood ADHD is strongly associated with a broad range of psychiatric disorders during adolescence: A population-based birth cohort study. *Journal of Child Psychology and Psychiatry, 53,* 1036–1043.

Yüce, M., Zoroglu, S. S., Ceylan, M. F., Kandemir, H., & Karabekiroglu, K. (2013). Psychiatric comorbidity distribution and diversities in children and adolescents with attention deficit/hyperactivity disorder: A study from Turkey. *Neuropsychiatric Disease and Treatment, 9,* 1791–1799.

Zisner, A., & Beauchaine, T. P. (2016). Neural substrates of trait impulsivity, anhedonia, and irritability: Mechanisms of heterotypic comorbidity between externalizing disorders and unipolar depression. *Development and Psychopathology, 28,* 1177–1208.

Zylowska, L., Ackerman, D. L., Yang, M. H., Futrell, J. L., Horton, N. L., Hale, T. S., . . . Smalley, S. L. (2008). Mindfulness meditation training in adults and adolescents with ADHD: A feasibility study. *Journal of Attention Disorders, 11,* 737–746.

CHAPTER 10

Sleep Functioning in Adolescents with ADHD

Melissa Mulraney
Emma Sciberras
Stephen P. Becker

Sleep is a critical component of human life, and good sleep is essential to health. There has been long-standing interest in the sleep functioning of individuals with attention-deficit/hyperactivity disorder (ADHD), and there is now a large body of research investigating sleep problems in children with ADHD (Cortese, Faraone, Konofal, & Lecendreux, 2009; Kirov & Brand, 2014). However, there is a paucity of studies investigating sleep in adolescents with ADHD (Becker, 2019; Becker & Langberg, 2017). As we describe below, adolescence is a developmental period characterized by large alterations in sleep, neurobiology, and academic/social demands with the transition to high school. Thus, it cannot be assumed that what is known about sleep in children with ADHD will generalize to adolescents with ADHD. In this chapter, we (1) describe what is known about sleep functioning in adolescents with ADHD, (2) draw from research examining sleep in typically developing adolescents, as well as studies examining sleep in children and adults with ADHD, in considering key developmental factors and processes relevant to the study of sleep in adolescents with ADHD, and (3) offer considerations for assessing and treating sleep difficulties in adolescents with ADHD.

Structure and Systems Underlying Sleep and Changes in Adolescence

There are two types of human sleep: rapid-eye-movement (REM) sleep and non-rapid eye-movement (NREM) sleep. REM sleep is when dreaming primarily occurs, muscles are paralyzed, and individuals are easy to awaken (McCarley, 2007). NREM sleep comprises four progressively deeper sleep states. NREM sleep generally does not involve dreaming, and individuals have difficulty remembering their dreams if they do occur during NREM sleep periods (McCarley, 2007). During NREM sleep, muscles are not paralyzed, so individuals can move around, and it is during NREM sleep that night terrors, sleep-walking, and similar parasomnias occur (Kaufman & Milstein, 2013). Stages of NREM sleep are characterized by progressively increasing rates of delta waves on electroencephalographic (EEG) readings (McCarley, 2007) and as such are often referred to as slow-wave sleep.

The structure of sleep develops across the lifespan. In infancy, sleep cycles (cycling through REM and NREM sleep) typically last approximately 45 minutes (Stern, Parmelee, Akiyama, Schultz, & Wenner, 1969). The length of sleep cycles gradually increases through childhood, then rapidly changes during adolescence to reach adult lengths of approximately 90 minutes. Adolescence is a time that sees a large shift in the structure of sleep architecture. There is an approximately 40% reduction in the amount of slow-wave sleep accompanied by a decrease in REM sleep (in absolute terms, the proportion of total sleep time remains the same) through adolescence (Colrain & Baker, 2011). EEG studies show a decrease in time spent in delta sleep, as well as changes in total EEG power across all frequency bands during adolescence. These changes appear to correspond with maturation of the adolescent brain structure (Colrain & Baker, 2011). Magnetic resonance imaging (MRI) has shown that the increase in white matter and decrease in gray matter that is characteristic of adolescence begin in the dorsal parietal cortices and move anteriorly over the frontal cortex (Colrain & Baker, 2011). In a review of EEG studies, Colrain and Baker concluded that the decline in delta power follows the same time course and regionally dependent pattern of change as the decrease in gray-matter volume across adolescence, suggesting that these two processes are indeed linked.

In addition to sleep architecture, there are two major systems that control sleep: homeostatic pressure and the circadian rhythm (Borbély, 1982). *Homeostatic pressure* increases during periods of wakefulness and decreases during sleep, such that the longer a person has been awake, the greater his or her drive to go to sleep. If sleep quality is poor or sleep duration is insufficient, the homeostatic pressure does not adequately dissipate during sleep and likely results in sleepiness the following day. The homeostatic drive for sleep is developmentally sensitive and decreases with age: young children require naps after shorter periods of wakefulness than do older children (Owens et al., 2013). During adolescence, homeostatic pressure declines to levels below that seen in adulthood, meaning that adolescents often do not begin to feel tired until quite late in the night (Becker, Langberg, & Byars, 2015). Indeed, in finding sleep pressure to be lower among mature adolescents (Tanner stage 5) compared to prepubertal adolescents (Tanner stage 1), Taylor, Jenni, Acebo, and Carskadon (2005) concluded that "a developmental change of intrinsic sleep–wake regulation may provide physiologically mediated 'permission' for later bedtimes in older adolescents" (p. 239).

The *circadian rhythm* is the 24-hour body clock that regulates a number of bodily systems, such as arousal, sleep, appetite, and body temperature. The circadian rhythm is closely linked to genetic factors, particularly the *CLOCK* gene (Kissling et al., 2008). However, it is also impacted by environmental factors such as light and the timing of meals (Owens et al., 2013). The behavioral manifestation of an individual's circadian rhythm is referred to as his or her *chronotype* (Roenneberg et al., 2004). "Eveningness" is a chronotype characterized by a delayed sleep onset and a preference for activities in the evening, whereas "morningness" is a chronotype characterized by an advanced sleep period and a preference for rising early in the morning (Horne & Ostberg, 1976). These chronotypes are not all-or-nothing, but fall along a continuum, and most adults fall somewhere between an evening and a morning type. The circadian rhythm is also influenced by development, whereby children and elderly adults tend to be morning types, while that of adolescents typically shifts toward eveningness (Roenneberg et al., 2004). This can be of concern, as eveningness has been associated with a number of poor outcomes, such as internalizing symptoms (Giannotti, Cortesi, Sebastiani, & Ottaviano, 2002) and poor diet (Fleig & Randler, 2009). As outlined below, adolescence is also associated with significant environmental pressures (e.g., school start times) that mean the shift toward eveningness is not accompanied by the ability to sleep later. Thus, a large number of adolescents end up chronically sleep deprived and often experience a weekend phase delay where they attempt to recover the accumulated sleep debt by sleeping in late.

Sleep Problems in Adolescents

The American Academy of Sleep Medicine (2014) broadly categorizes sleep disorders into six domains: (1) insomnia, (2) sleep-related breathing disorders, (3) central disorders of hypersomnolence (e.g., narcolepsy), (4) circadian rhythm sleep–wake disorders, (5) parasomnias, and (6) sleep-related movement disorders (e.g., restless legs syndrome). During adolescence there is a change in the prevalence of sleep disorders, with a reduction of parasomnias and an increase in insomnia and delayed sleep phase disorder (Colrain

& Baker, 2011). It is probable that the shift in prevalence of particular sleep disorders is related to the biological, psychosocial, and contextual factors associated with sleep in the adolescent period. For example, the reduction in parasomnias such as sleepwalking and sleep terrors is likely related to the reduction in slow-wave sleep that occurs in adolescence. Furthermore, the increase in prevalence of delayed sleep phase disorder is likely a result of the decrease in homeostatic pressure and biological shift toward eveningness.

Prevalence and Types of Sleep Problems in Adolescents with ADHD

Epidemiological studies have consistently found a link between sleep problems and ADHD symptoms in large representative community samples of adolescents (for a review, see Lunsford-Avery, Krystal, & Kollins, 2016). Specifically, ADHD inattentive and hyperactive–impulsive symptoms are associated with insomnia (Hysing, Lundervold, Posserud, & Sivertsen, 2016), as well as delayed sleep phase and restless legs syndrome (Turkdogan, Bekiroglu, & Zaimoglu, 2011), though inattention is more strongly associated with insomnia and delayed sleep phase, whereas hyperactivity–impulsivity is more strongly associated with restless legs. In addition, inattentive symptoms, but not hyperactive–impulsive symptoms, are associated with sleep-disordered breathing (Johnson & Roth, 2006). These associations remained strong after researchers controlled for important confounds, including demographics, anxiety and depressive symptoms, medications, and electronic device use. However, these studies are all cross-sectional in nature, making causal and possible bidirectional relations unclear. It may be that adolescents with elevated ADHD symptoms are at increased risk for developing sleep problems, or that sleep problems contribute to—or exacerbate—ADHD symptoms. In line with this latter possibility, Becker, Epstein et al. (2019) recently conducted an experimental sleep restriction–extension protocol in 72 adolescents (ages 13–17 years) diagnosed with ADHD, comprising a phase stabilization week followed in randomized counterbalanced order by 1 week of sleep restriction (shifting bedtime to allow for 6.5 hours in bed) and 1 week of sleep extension (shifting bedtime to allow for 9.5 hours in bed). Forty-eight adolescents had complete actigraphy data and successfully completed the protocol (defined a priori as obtaining at least 1 hour more actigraphy-measured sleep during extension compared to restriction). Adolescents had more parent-reported inattentive symptoms, as well as more oppositional and sluggish cognitive tempo (SCT) symptoms, following restriction compared to extension. Although no effects were found on a continuous performance test, overall findings provide the first evidence that shortened sleep duration is a causal contributor to poorer daytime functioning in adolescents diagnosed with ADHD (Becker, Epstein, et al., 2019).

Surprisingly few naturalistic studies have examined sleep functioning in clinical samples of adolescents diagnosed with ADHD (for reviews, see Becker, 2019; Lunsford-Avery et al., 2016), though findings from extant studies generally align with findings from studies of children with ADHD and epidemiological samples of adolescents. Fisher et al. (2014) conducted a chart review of adolescent patients with ADHD (*N* = 218; ages 15–17) and found that 74% experienced self-reported sleep problems, most commonly difficulty initiating and maintaining sleep and experiencing nonrestorative sleep. The authors also found that girls with ADHD reported significantly more difficulties with sleep than did boys with ADHD, suggesting potentially important sex differences. In a sample of school-age children diagnosed with ADHD, Becker and colleagues (Becker, Cusick, Sidol, Epstein, & Tamm, 2018) also found more parent-reported sleep problems in girls (75%) than in boys (53%). However, given the paucity of research in this area and the lack of research on girls with ADHD, particularly in adolescence, it is clear that more work needs to be done in this area.

In contrast to Fisher et al. (2014), Langberg et al. (2017) reported mixed evidence in terms of high rates of sleep problems in a sample of 262 young adolescents (ages 10–15 years) carefully diagnosed with ADHD. Specifically, using the parent report, Children's Sleep Habits Questionnaire (CSHQ), 73% of the sample met established cutoff criteria for sleep problems (Owens, Spirito, & McGuinn, 2000), an overall prevalence rate remarkably similar to the rate of 74% in the Fisher et al. (2014) study. However, Langberg et al. (2017) found that less than 8% of adolescents with ADHD met their clinical threshold (defined as a mean item score of ≥ 2, indicating that the behaviors in that domain occur at least two to four times per week in a typical week) for any of the individual CSHQ subscales, with the exception of 28% meeting the threshold for daytime sleepiness. Similar findings emerged when examining adolescent self-reported sleep functioning: Approximately 7% reported problematic bedtime/sleep behavior, whereas 22% reported elevated daytime sleepiness (Langberg et al., 2017). It is important to note, however, that this study did not include a comparison group of adolescents without ADHD and the cutoffs for defining specific sleep problems were study-specific as opposed to established cutoff points in the literature. More recently, Becker, Langberg, and colleagues (2019) examined sleep and daytime sleepiness in a large sample of adolescents with (*n* = 162) and without (*n* = 140) ADHD. Controlling for a number of variables known to impact sleep (e.g., sex, pubertal development, medication use, comorbid psychiatric disorders), adolescents with ADHD had shorter diary and actigraphy school-night sleep duration, more adolescent- and parent-reported daytime sleepiness, and parent-reported difficulties with initiating and maintaining sleep than did adolescents without ADHD. Adolescents with ADHD were also more likely than comparison adolescents to report falling asleep in class and to have stayed up all night at least twice in the previous 2 weeks. Finally, 28% of adolescents with ADHD had clinically elevated parent-reported total sleep disturbance, compared to 5% of adolescents without ADHD (Becker, Langberg, et al., 2019). Despite these findings using a multimethod design, additional studies are clearly needed to describe rates of sleep problems in adolescents with ADHD, to identify specific domains of sleep that are commonly problematic in adolescents with ADHD, and to examine how rates of sleep problems change across adolescence.

In addition, the specific type of sleep problems experienced by adolescents with ADHD may vary according to ADHD subtype/presentation. In a sample of 325 adolescents with ADHD and 257 comparison youth in Taiwan, the adolescents with ADHD were more likely to experience sleep problems than the comparison youth, though the specific types of sleep problems differed across ADHD subgroups (Chiang et al., 2010). Adolescents with ADHD combined type or predominantly hyperactive–inattentive type were more likely to report parasomnias and nightmares than the comparison adolescents, and those with combined type were also more likely to experience circadian rhythm disturbances compared to the comparison group. Adolescents with ADHD predominantly inattentive type were more likely to experience hypersomnia than comparison adolescents (Chiang et al., 2010). However, until further studies are conducted, firm conclusions regarding any possible subtype/presentation differences in the sleep functioning of adolescents with ADHD would be premature.

Very few studies have used objective measures to examine sleep in adolescents with ADHD. Two studies (Moore et al., 2011; Mullin, Harvey, & Hinshaw, 2011) did not find actigraphy-measured total sleep time (TST) to be associated with a diagnosis of ADHD. Mullin et al. (2011) also found no differences between adolescents with ADHD and controls on actigraphy measured night wakings, sleep-onset latency, or sleep efficiency. It should be noted that both of these studies had small sample sizes (N = 14–16 adolescents with ADHD) and were likely underpowered to detect any differences. Mullin et al. did report a trend toward adolescents with ADHD having reduced TST (average of 7.07 hours) compared to healthy controls (average of 7.27 hours) despite having more weekend night data available (when sleep duration should be longer due to reduced restrictions on time in bed). As noted earlier, Becker, Langberg, et al. (2019) recently found adolescents with ADHD to have shorter actigraphy-measured schoolnight sleep duration than adolescents without ADHD, but other group differences in actigraphy-measured sleep were either nonsignificant or no longer significant when they controlled for other factors known to impact sleep. These findings are broadly consistent with actigraphy studies in children with ADHD. In a meta-analysis of objective sleep studies in children with ADHD, Cortese et al. (2009) reported that the majority of actigraphy studies do not reveal differences in most sleep parameters between children with ADHD and healthy controls. A small pilot study (ADHD n = 12, controls n = 12) used polysomnography (PSG) to investigate sleep in nonmedicated adolescent males (ages 10–16 years) (Prehn-Kristensen et al., 2011). This study found that, compared to controls, adolescents with ADHD had reduced latency to slow-wave sleep, increased sleep-onset latency, reduced sleep efficiency, and increased REM (all large Cohen's *d* effect sizes of ~3.0). Consistent with other studies using actigraphy (Moore et al., 2011; Mullin et al., 2011), there were no differences in TST as measured with PSG. Still, other studies with larger sample sizes are surely needed, including studies that can test possible age, sex, and ADHD subtype/presentation differences and whether the preliminary findings reported with male adolescents with ADHD generalize to female adolescents with ADHD.

In summary, epidemiological studies have demonstrated that there are robust associations between sleep problems and symptoms of inattention and hyperactivity–impulsivity, although the directionality of these relationships is unknown. Studies of adolescents with ADHD have generally not included a control sample or have utilized very small sample sizes. Thus, it is unknown whether sleep problems are more common in adolescents with ADHD than in the general population of adolescents. Regardless, it is imperative that more work be done in this area, particularly given that young people with ADHD are already at increased risk of poor long-term outcomes compared to their non-ADHD peers (Langberg & Becker, 2012) and sleep problems likely compound their existing difficulties.

Factors Associated with Sleep Problems in Adolescents with ADHD

A number of factors associated with poor sleep increase substantially during adolescence. There is limited evidence that applies directly to adolescents with ADHD, so we draw largely on the literature in this section as it pertains to the general population of adolescents. Furthermore, although a large number of factors have been associated with sleep problems in the general population of adolescents, we focus in this section on the biological (e.g., genetics), psychosocial (e.g., comorbid mental health problems), and contextual factors (e.g., electronic media use) that may be particularly salient to adolescents with ADHD.

Biological Contributions

Genetics

A link has been found between ADHD and the *CLOCK* gene, which regulates circadian rhythm. Specifically, ADHD is associated with a polymorphism that is implicated in disturbed sleep patterns and an evening chronotype (Kissling et al., 2008). The master clock is located in the suprachiasmatic nucleus (SCN) of the hypothalamus. SCN output regulates circadian rhythm in a number of hormones, including melatonin. ADHD has been associated with delayed dim light melatonin onset in both children (Van der Heijden, Smits, Someren, & Boudewijn Gunning, 2005) and adults (Van Veen, Kooij, Boonstra, Gordijn, & Van Someren, 2010). *Dim light melatonin onset* is the onset of melatonin secretion under dim light conditions and is thought to be the most accurate measure of circadian rhythm (Pandi-Perumal et al., 2007).

Neurobiology

Many of the neurological circuits involved in the regulation of arousal and sleep are the same as those involved in attention and have been implicated in ADHD (Owens et al., 2013); thus, a disruption in those circuits that leads to an individual developing ADHD will likely increase susceptibility to dysfunction in sleep and arousal. Furthermore, a recent pilot study of mazindol (a direct orexin-2 receptor agonist) found that it significantly improved ADHD symptoms in school-age children with ADHD (Konofal et al., 2014). This supports the hypothesis that the orexin system, which is involved in sleep–wake regulation and has been implicated in narcolepsy, may also be compromised in ADHD (Cortese, Konofal, & Lecendreux, 2008), though it remains to be seen whether this occurs similarly across development for individuals with ADHD.

Brain maturation is significantly delayed in young people with ADHD (Lunsford-Avery et al., 2016). As discussed earlier, the decline in slow-wave sleep that occurs during adolescence is linked to the maturation of grey and white matter. Consequently, the delay in neuromaturation observed in adolescents with ADHD may contribute to abnormal trajectories of slow-wave sleep (Lunsford-Avery et al., 2016). Furthermore, Kirov and Brand (2014) found that children with ADHD have less REM sleep than their same-age peers before the age of 10, but this reverses, so that adolescents with ADHD have significantly *more* REM sleep than their same-age peers.

Medication

Stimulant medication is the frontline treatment for ADHD, and one of the most commonly reported side effects of stimulant medication is sleep problems (Charach, Ickowicz, & Schachar, 2004). However, it is important to note that while medication can contribute to sleep problems in youth with ADHD, it is also clear that sleep problems in youth with ADHD are not wholly (or even primarily) attributable to medication use (Becker, Froehlich, & Epstein, 2016; Kidwell, Van Dyk, Lundahl, & Nelson, 2015; Weiss, Craig, Davies, Schibuk, & Stein, 2015), and that children with ADHD who are not on medication still experience higher rates of sleep problems than non-ADHD controls (Owens, Maxim, Nobile, McGuinn, & Msall, 2000). The majority of studies examining the impact of ADHD medications on sleep have been conducted in children. The few studies that have examined this in adolescents have reported mixed findings. Observational studies have reported both null (Becker, Langberg, & Evans, 2015; Gau & Chiang, 2009) and positive associations (Mick, Biederman, Jetton, & Faraone, 2000) between medication use and sleep problems. A double-blind, randomized, placebo-controlled, crossover, dose–response trial of mixed amphetamine salts versus dexmethylphenidate in adolescents with ADHD found a dose–response relationship between both medications and sleep problems (Santisteban, Stein, Bergmame, & Gruber, 2014). Specifically, higher doses were associated with longer sleep-onset latency and decreased total sleep time as measured by actigraphy. However, this study was brief (8 weeks), and findings in children with ADHD have demonstrated that sleep problems often arise in initial titration of medication and resolve over time after a stable dosage of medication is taken for some time (Stein, Weiss, & Hlavaty, 2012). It is not clear whether this would also be the case for adolescents with ADHD. An important factor to consider about the impact of ADHD medication on sleep in adolescents is the decrease in medication adherence during adolescence (see Brinkman, Froelich, & Epstein, Chapter 18, this volume). As management of the condition transitions from parents to adolescents, adherence to treatment often declines (McCarthy et al., 2012; Park & Kim, 2015), similar to what is often observed in other chronic illnesses (Gavin, Wamboldt, Sorokin, Levy, & Wamboldt, 1999; Tebbi, 1993).

In summary, there are a number of biological risk factors that increase risk for sleep problems in adolescents with ADHD; they are more likely to have a polymorphism on the *CLOCK* gene associated with a dysregulated circadian rhythm, there is significant overlap in the underlying neurobiology that regulates attention and arousal, and the use of ADHD medications is associated with difficulty sleeping. Further research is needed to understand the neurobiological overlap between sleep and ADHD, and how it develops across adolescence, and the role that ADHD medication plays in this in order to guide the development of treatments to normalize the underlying brain circuitry and thus effectively treat both ADHD and sleep problems.

Psychosocial Contributions

Comorbid Mental Health Problems

Comorbid internalizing and externalizing disorders are common among adolescents with ADHD (Smalley et al., 2007; see also Becker & Fogleman,

Chapter 9, this volume). During adolescence, the prevalence of internalizing disorders, particularly depression, increases (Cohen et al., 1993). There is strong evidence that sleep problems and internalizing problems are interrelated. Concurrently, sleep and internalizing problems are highly correlated both in typically developing adolescents and in those with ADHD (Becker, Langberg, & Byars, 2015). For example, in a sample of 5- to 13-year-old children with ADHD (M_{age} = 10.1, *SD* = 1.9 years), Lycett, Mensah, Hiscock, and Sciberras (2014) found that the presence of both an internalizing and externalizing disorder at baseline predicted persistent and transient sleep problems over the subsequent 12 months. In a sample of young adolescents (ages 10–14 years) diagnosed with ADHD, parent-reported sleep problems were associated with increases in depressive symptoms and externalizing symptoms 1 year later, even after researchers controlled for baseline symptoms, though sleep problems did not prospectively predict increases in anxiety (Becker, Langberg, & Evans, 2015). It has been hypothesized that sleep problems, anxiety, and depression have cascading effects on each other (Becker, Langberg, & Byars, 2015). For example, in typically developing youth, anxiety longitudinally increases risk for sleep problems, which in turn increases risk for depression (Johnson, Roth, & Breslau, 2006). Understanding the nature of these interrelationships in young people with ADHD is particularly pressing given that these people are at increased risk of experiencing both sleep problems and internalizing problems. If, indeed, there is a cascading relationship, intervening early will be important to stem the negative spiral and links to other deleterious outcomes. Research has yet to examine a number of other comorbidities, such as autism spectrum disorder and SCT symptoms, that are common in ADHD and may likely impact sleep in adolescents.

Family Factors

The family environment is an important consideration in understanding sleep in adolescents, and particularly in adolescents with ADHD (Becker, Langberg, & Byars, 2015). Families of adolescents with ADHD are characterized by high levels of parent–child conflict, disorganization, and a lack of structure compared to families of adolescents without ADHD (Deault, 2010). Parent–child conflict in childhood has been associated with sleep problems in early adolescence in typically developing children (Bell & Belsky, 2008; Kelly, Marks, & El-Sheikh, 2014), though this has yet to be specifically investigated in adolescents with ADHD. The disorganization and lack of structure in households of adolescents with ADHD may place them at particular risk of developing sleep problems. In non-ADHD samples, it has been demonstrated that adolescents with parent-set bedtimes (Short et al., 2011) and stricter household rules (Adam, Snell, & Pendry, 2007) have earlier bedtimes and obtain more sleep. Furthermore, those with parent-set bed times also experience less fatigue and improved daytime functioning (Short et al., 2011). It is likely that family functioning and adolescent sleep influence each other, whereby household disorganization and lack of structure contribute to adolescent delayed sleep and fatigue, which in turn contribute to parent–child conflict.

Academic, Social, and Cognitive Factors

Adolescents need to juggle increasing academic demands, shifting peer relationships, including for many the beginning of romantic relationships, extracurricular activities, including for some beginning part-time work, and learning to drive. In order to meet all of the expectations, many adolescents sacrifice sleep time (Becker, Langberg, & Byars, 2015), and this may be particularly salient for young people with ADHD given that disorganization and poor time management are core features of ADHD (American Psychiatric Association, 2013).

In healthy adolescents, poor sleep is associated with a range of neurocognitive impairments, including impaired executive function (Nilsson et al., 2005) and memory (Stickgold, 2013). Given that these areas are already impaired in many youth with ADHD (Shaw, Stringaris, Nigg, & Leibenluft, 2014; Willcutt, Doyle, Nigg, Faraone, & Pennington, 2005), it is likely that sleep problems will further exacerbate these impairments. For example, sleep problems in children with ADHD are related to working memory deficits (Sciberras, DePetro, Mensah, & Hiscock, 2015), and children with poor sleep and ADHD are more distractible than children with either disorder alone (Sawyer et al., 2009). However, studies to date that have investigated the relations between sleep and cognition in youth with ADHD have been cross-sectional, making directionality and causal contributions unknown. Lunsford-Avery et al. (2016) posit that the association between sleep and cognition may be bidirectional, whereby poor sleep impacts on cognition through its impact on brain plasticity, and neurocognitive deficits may lead to poor sleep habits due to increasing environmental demands restricting sleep (e.g., more time required to complete homework).

The increasing academic demands of secondary school likely impact on sleep in adolescents with ADHD. It has consistently been demonstrated that time spent on homework is negatively associated with sleep duration in typically developing youth (Becker, Langberg, & Byars, 2015). Many young people with ADHD struggle academically (DuPaul & Langberg, 2014; Zendarski, Sciberras, Mensah, & Hiscock, 2017) and, as a consequence, need to spend more time than their same-age peers completing homework tasks. Also, most homework difficulties occur in the late afternoon and evening hours leading to bedtime (Coghill et al., 2008), making homework difficulties particularly important to consider in models examining sleep in adolescents with ADHD.

Contextual Contributions

Electronic Devices and Media Use

The impact of electronic devices on sleep is an area of importance. A Norwegian population-based study of adolescents (N = 9,875, mean age 17 years) found that the majority of young people have multiple electronic devices in their bedroom and use multiple devices in the hour before bed (Hysing et al., 2015). Use of any electronic device was associated with sleep-onset latency of more than 60 minutes (odds ratios [ORs] 1.13–1.52) and a sleep deficit of more than 2 hours (ORs 1.12–1.53). Young people who used multiple devices in the hour before bed were at even higher risk of delayed sleep onset and a large sleep deficit (Hysing et al., 2015). It is likely that this is also the case for adolescents with ADHD. Baseline data from a randomized controlled trial (RCT) to treat sleep problems in children (ages 5–13) with ADHD indicated that 62% of children had at least one electronic device in the bedroom, and that 36% fell asleep using electronics (Sciberras, Song, Mulraney, Schuster, & Hiscock, 2017). Another study of 81 adolescents (ages 13–17 years) with ADHD found that 93% had a cell phone in their bedroom, 58% had a computer/laptop/tablet, 44% had a music player, and 41% had a television (Becker & Lienesch, 2018). Furthermore, 50–60% reported watching television or movies, texting, or being online with friends after 9:00 P.M., with duration across media types averaging 5.31 hours of nighttime media use (Becker & Lienesch, 2018). There are a number of ways that the use of electronic devices impacts sleep. Blue light emitted from screens inhibits the production of melatonin; thus, users are unable to fall asleep when desired (Owens & Adolescent Sleep Working Group, 2014). This may be particularly salient for individuals with ADHD, as studies have shown a delay in dim light melatonin onset in ADHD (Van der Heijden et al., 2005; Van Veen et al., 2010). Furthermore, the use electronics, whether socially or for entertainment, is often highly stimulating, and media use may directly displace sleep as the young person stays up later to continuing enjoying their use (Owens & Adolescent Sleep Working Group, 2014).

We are aware of only two studies that have examined electronic device or media use in relation to sleep among adolescents with ADHD specifically. Becker and Lienesch (2018) found that adolescents with ADHD who obtained less sleep than recommended also reported more nighttime media use. In addition, nighttime media use was associated with increased sleep problems across both adolescent and parent reports, as well as more adolescent-reported internalizing symptoms (Becker & Lienesch, 2018). Another study found that adolescents with ADHD spend more time using technology compared to adolescents without ADHD, and more parent- and adolescent-reported technology use was associated with more sleep–wake problems and less time in bed for adolescents with and without ADHD. However, parent-reported technology use was associated with teacher-reported daytime sleepiness only for adolescents with ADHD (Bourchtein et al., 2019). Despite the importance of these initial studies, it is important to note that both were limited by cross-sectional designs that cannot establish causality or temporal ordering of effects. More studies are needed, particularly ones that incorporate actigraphy and a longitudinal or experimental design, as this is a critical area for more research.

School Start Times

School start times vary significantly around the world and have demonstrable consequences relative to the amount of sleep adolescents obtain (Becker, Langberg, & Byars, 2015). In the United States, there is a high degree of variability in school start times, but they are typically earlier than most other countries in the world. The vast majority of U.S. high schools start before 8:30 A.M., with many beginning before 8:00 A.M. (Short et al., 2013). A survey of 14,000 U.S. adolescents found that only 8% of adolescents were obtaining the recommended 9 hours sleep, with 69% getting less than 7 hours (Eaton et al., 2010). In contrast, in Australia, where school start times are typically 8:30–9:00 A.M. (Olds, Maher, Blunden, & Matricciani, 2010; Short et al., 2013), adolescents have an average school night sleep duration of 9 hours (Olds et al., 2010). Changes to school start times have a discernable impact on sleep duration and associated outcomes in adolescents. Danner and Phillips (2008) reported that the year after school start times changed from 7:30 A.M. to 8:30 A.M. in some school districts in Kentucky, there was a corresponding increase in the average hours of sleep for adolescents living in those areas. The percentage of students obtaining at least 8 hours of sleep increased from 36 to 50%. Furthermore, there was a decrease of 17% in car crash rates for adolescent drivers. During the same time frame, in districts where school start times remained unchanged, car crashes increased by 8% for adolescent drivers. Although experimental evidence for the causal contribution of school start time to functioning remains lacking, these naturalistic findings are important and may be particularly relevant for adolescents with ADHD given their increased rates of both daytime sleepiness (Langberg et al., 2017) and poorer driving outcomes (Narad et al., 2018; see also Garner, Chapter 12, this volume).

Caffeine Use

Caffeine use is one factor that likely interacts with sleep and other factors in a number of unknown ways. Adolescents with a high caffeine intake are twice as likely to have difficulties sleeping and feel tired in the morning as adolescents with a low caffeine intake (Orbeta, Overpeck, Ramcharran, Kogan, & Ledsky, 2006). This can lead to higher levels of caffeine intake to compensate for daytime sleepiness (Owens & Adolescent Sleep Working Group, 2014). The impact of caffeine use in adolescents with ADHD is not known, nor do we know the impact of how it interacts with medication. It could have beneficial effects, allowing adolescents to concentrate better when completing their homework, thus resulting in more time available for sleep. But given what is known about the negative impact on sleep in community-based samples (Calamaro, Mason, & Ratcliffe, 2009), it is likely that caffeine use also exacerbates the difficulties adolescents with ADHD face when trying to sleep.

Transactional Relationships between Risk Factors and Sleep in Adolescents with ADHD

It is highly likely that a number of the factors we discussed earlier interact with each other to influence sleep and functioning, and that they have transactional relationships with sleep. However, to date, there is little research examining the interactions among biological, psychosocial, and contextual factors, and how these may develop and influence sleep in adolescents with ADHD (Becker, Langberg, & Byars, 2015). Most research has focused on one or two factors and how they interact with sleep over time. For example, Mulraney, Giallo, Lycett, Mensah, and Sciberras (2016) demonstrated that a bidirectional relationship existed between sleep problems and internalizing (but not externalizing) symptoms over a 12-month period in children ages 5–13 years with ADHD. As discussed earlier, it is likely that anxiety, sleep, and depression have a cascading relationship, whereby anxiety leads to sleep problems, which in turn contribute to the development of depression (Becker, Langberg, & Byars, 2015).

There is a clear need for longitudinal research that utilize a developmental psychopathology framework to tease apart the mechanisms through which various factors interact to influence the development and maintenance of sleep problems in adolescents with ADHD, as well as the consequences of sleep problems once they develop. Relatedly, very little is known about the *trajectories* of sleep problems among adolescents with ADHD and whether trajectories differ for adolescents with ADHD compared to their typically developing peers. Findings from such studies would be highly informative for early intervention and prevention.

Assessment and Treatment of Sleep Functioning in Adolescents with ADHD

Assessment

Sleep can be assessed using both subjective and objective methods. Subjective measures include clinical interviews, sleep diaries, and sleep questionnaires. Subjective measures are useful clinically (particularly for sleep problems that are behavioral in nature or that involve delayed sleep onset), or for large-scale epidemiological studies. In an interview, the clinician should inquire about sleep hygiene and common difficulties, including sleep onset latency, daytime sleepiness, night awakenings, sleep duration, and snoring. Useful, well validated questionnaires include the Pediatric Sleep Questionnaire (validated for children ages 2–18 years) (Chervin, Hedger, Dillon, & Pituch, 2000) and the Sleep Disturbance Scale for Children (ages 5–15 years) (Bruni et al., 1996). Both of these questionnaires include questions about sleep behavior and questions targeting sleep-related breathing disorders, parasomnias, and other clinical sleep problems (e.g., nightmares, narcolepsy, and enuresis) (Lewandowski, Toliver-Sokol, & Palermo, 2011). However, both of these are parent-report measures, and assessing self-reported sleep functioning becomes particularly important in adolescence, since parents may not directly observe several aspects of sleep functioning in adolescence (e.g., delayed sleep onset, night wakings, nighttime media use). Self-report questionnaires for use in adolescents with ADHD include the Sleep Habits Survey (SHS; Wolfson et al., 2003), the Adolescent Sleep Hygiene Scale (ASHS; LeBourgeois, Giannotti, Cortesi, Wolfson, & Harsh, 2005), the Adolescent Sleep–Wake Scale (ASWS; LeBourgeois et al., 2005), and the Pediatric Daytime Sleepiness Scale (PDSS; Drake et al., 2003). Objective measures offer distinct advantages but may be costly or difficult to administer (Sadeh, 2015). Objective measures commonly used in ADHD populations include actigraphy, PSG, the multiple sleep latency test (MLST), and dim light melatonin onset.

When assessing sleep problems in ADHD, there are a number of factors to consider. First, whether the young person is on medication and, if so, what the dosing schedule is and the likely impact on sleep. Second, there is some evidence that youth with ADHD experience significant night-to-night variability in their sleep (Becker, Sidol, Van Dyk, Epstein, & Beebe, 2017) which may need to be taken into consideration when selecting an appropriate sleep assessment measure. For instance, unless a breathing- or movement-related disorder is suspected, PSG may not be an ideal assessment tool. Actigraphy may prove to be more useful, as actigraphs are typically worn for at least a week and therefore capture the night-to-night variations and can also be used in tandem with sleep diaries to gain a fuller picture of contextual factors (e.g., activities immediately preceding bedtime) that can influence sleep functioning.

Treatment

There is very limited research on treatments for sleep problems in adolescents with ADHD. In terms of the pharmaceutical treatments, it is likely that findings from children and adults with ADHD will generalize to adolescents with ADHD. In terms of psychosocial treatments, given the unique challenges associated with the adolescent period, it is likely that treatments for other developmental stages will not translate to adolescents. As such, we focus on the literature concerning behavioral interventions for sleep problems in typically developing adolescents and suggest ways in which these treatments may need to be modified to be appropriate for adolescents with ADHD.

Pharmaceutical Treatment

Melatonin is perhaps the best-known medication to treat sleep problems in young people. Two double-blind, placebo-controlled randomized trials have demonstrated that melatonin significantly reduced sleep-onset latency compared to placebo and had few side effects in children with ADHD (Van der Heijden, Smits, Van Someren, Ridderinkhof, & Gunning, 2007; Weiss, Wasdell, Bomben, Rea, & Freeman, 2006). It seems likely that the results of these trials would generalize to adolescents. Weiss and colleagues' (2006) study included children ages 6–14, and a follow-up of Van der Heijden et al.'s (2007) cohort 3.7 years later (when the majority of participants were adolescents; mean age 12.39 years) found that 65% of young people were still taking melatonin daily (Hoebert, Van Der Heijden, Van Geijlswijk, & Smits, 2009). In 9% of cases, melatonin use was ceased due to resolution of sleep-onset problems; however, discontinuation of melatonin resulted in 92% of the young people experiencing a delay of sleep onset.

There is some limited evidence to suggest that other pharmaceutical agents may be beneficial for sleep in young people with ADHD. Two open-label studies (Prince, Wilens, Biederman, Spencer, & Wozniak, 1996; Wilens, Biederman, & Spencer, 1994) have demonstrated the safety of clonidine, an alpha-2 adrenergic agonist, and indicate that it may be efficacious in treating insomnia in children with ADHD. Modafinil is a wake-promoting agent used in the treatment of narcolepsy in adults. A review concluded that in addition to wake-promoting properties, modafinil has beneficial effects on attention, executive function, and learning in non-sleep-deprived adults (Battleday & Brem, 2015). Modafinil may therefore be useful in the treatment of excessively sleepy adolescents with ADHD, as it may help with both alertness and cognition. As discussed earlier, mazindol is an orexin-2 agonist that may be beneficial in the regulation of the sleep–wake cycle. An open-label pilot study of mazindol (1mg/day for 7 days) in 21 children with ADHD reported a large reduction in ADHD symptoms from baseline to the end of treatment, followed by a significant increase in ADHD symptoms once treatment ceased (Konofal et al., 2014).

Psychosocial Treatment

There is emerging research demonstrating efficacy of cognitive-behavioral therapy for insomnia (CBT-I) in adolescents with sleep problems (e.g.,

Blake, Sheeber, Youssef, Raniti, & Allen, 2017; Clarke et al., 2015; de Bruin, Bögels, Oort, & Meijer, 2015; Gradisar et al., 2011). For instance, an RCT demonstrated the efficacy of CBT-I plus bright light therapy for adolescents with delayed sleep phase disorder, with adolescents in the intervention group having reduced sleep-onset latency, less waking after sleep onset, increased total sleep time on school nights, and reduced daytime sleepiness and fatigue immediately postintervention (Gradisar et al., 2011). More recently, Harvey (2016) developed the Transdiagnostic Sleep and Circadian Intervention for Youth (TranS-C-Youth) for adolescents with sleep problems. The focus of TranS-C-Youth is to move the field toward a broader, transdiagnostic approach as opposed to treating a specific sleep problem (e.g., insomnia) or a specific psychiatric group (e.g., depression). An initial RCT revealed that, compared to psychoeducation, the TranS-C-Youth intervention was associated with greater improvements in several domains of sleep functioning (e.g., earlier endogenous circadian phase, less weeknight–weekend discrepancy in total sleep time, less daytime sleepiness), as well as improvements in parent-reported cognitive health (a composite domain that included thought and attention problems). However, the TranS-C-Youth intervention was not associated with more favorable youth self-report health outcomes (Harvey et al., 2018). Further work evaluating the TranS-C-Youth intervention, as well as other sleep interventions for adolescents, is needed (see Becker, 2019). It is also important to note that none of these interventions has been examined in adolescents with ADHD specifically.

In an RCT (*N* = 244), Hiscock et al. (2015) demonstrated the efficacy of a behavioral intervention for sleep in children (ages 5–13) with ADHD, with recent evidence supporting sustained impact on sleep and behavior 1 year later (Sciberras et al., 2019). The intervention comprises two face-to-face sessions with the parent and child held 2 weeks apart, with a follow-up phone call 2 weeks later. Session content included psychoeducation about normal sleep, sleep cycles, sleep cues, and sleep hygiene and a sleep management plan tailored to the individual child's sleep problem. There is overlap in the strategies employed in this intervention and in TranS-C-Youth. For example, both interventions recommend that a child with sleep-related anxiety utilize simple anxiety-reducing techniques such as imagery or a worry diary/box. Both interventions also recommend gradually and progressively shifting the bedtime earlier for young people experiencing a sleep phase delay. As such, it is likely that the Hiscock et al. (2015) intervention would be beneficial for adolescents with ADHD, although alterations to content would need to be made in order to make it more appropriate for adolescents. For example, the original intervention is largely parent driven; for it to be effective, the adolescent him- or herself would need to be the focus of the therapy.

Conclusions and Future Directions

It is encouraging that there has recently been substantial interest in examining sleep and treating problematic sleep in adolescents with ADHD. Nevertheless, our understanding of sleep in adolescents with ADHD remains very limited, as until recently most studies focused on sleep in school-age children with ADHD. Important directions for future research have been described in this chapter, as well as elsewhere (Becker & Langberg, 2017; Becker, Langberg, & Byars, 2015; Lunsford-Avery et al., 2016). We briefly note here the particularly pressing need for longitudinal studies that cover the adolescent period and use a multimethod design to examine the emergence and consequences of sleep problems in adolescents with ADHD. It is also important to determine whether adolescents with ADHD have different predictors and consequences of sleep problems compared to adolescents without ADHD. Research addressing these and other unanswered questions are important to informing prevention and intervention efforts best-suited to address sleep in adolescents with ADHD.

References

Adam, E. K., Snell, E. K., & Pendry, P. (2007). Sleep timing and quantity in ecological and family context: A nationally representative time-diary study. *Journal of Family Psychology, 21,* 4–19.

American Academy of Sleep Medicine. (2014). *International classification of sleep disorders* (3rd ed.). Darien, IL: Author.

American Psychiatric Association. (2013). *Diagnostic and statistical manual of mental disorders* (5th ed.). Arlington, VA: Author.

Battleday, R., & Brem, A.-K. (2015). Modafinil for cognitive neuroenhancement in healthy non-sleep-deprived subjects: A systematic review. *European Neuropsychopharmacology, 25,* 1865–1881.

Becker, S. P. (2019). The triple threat of sleep, adolescence, and ADHD. In H. Hiscock & E. Sciberras (Eds.), *Sleep and ADHD: An evidence-based guide to assessment and treatment* (pp. 257–294). Amsterdam: Elsevier.

Becker, S. P., Cusick, C. N., Sidol, C. A., Epstein, J. N., & Tamm, L. (2018). The impact of comorbid mental health symptoms and sex on sleep functioning in children with ADHD. *European Child and Adolescent Psychiatry, 27,* 353–365.

Becker, S. P., Epstein, J. N., Tamm, L., Tilford, A. A., Tischner, C. M., Isaacson, P. A., . . . Beebe, D. W. (2019). Shortened sleep duration causes sleepiness, inattention, and oppositionality in adolescents with attention-deficit/hyperactivity disorder: Findings from a crossover sleep restriction/extension study. *Journal of the American Academy of Child and Adolescent Psychiatry, 58*(4), 433–442.

Becker, S. P., Froehlich, T. E., & Epstein, J. N. (2016). Effects of methylphenidate on sleep functioning in children with attention-deficit/hyperactivity disorder. *Journal of Developmental and Behavioral Pediatrics, 37*(5), 395–404.

Becker, S. P., & Langberg, J. M. (2017). Difficult to bed and difficult to rise: Complex interplay among ADHD, sleep, and adolescence. *ADHD Report, 25*(1), 7–13, 16.

Becker, S. P., Langberg, J. M., & Byars, K. C. (2015). Advancing a biopsychosocial and contextual model of sleep in adolescence: A review and introduction to the special issue. *Journal of Youth and Adolescence, 44*(2), 239–270.

Becker, S. P., Langberg, J. M., Eadeh, H.-M., Isaacson, P. A., & Bourchtein, E. (2019, April 29). Sleep and daytime sleepiness in adolescents with and without ADHD: Differences across ratings, daily diary, and actigraphy. *Journal of Child Psychology and Psychiatry.* [Epub ahead of print]

Becker, S. P., Langberg, J. M., & Evans, S. W. (2015). Sleep problems predict comorbid externalizing behaviors and depression in young adolescents with attention-deficit/hyperactivity disorder. *European Child and Adolescent Psychiatry, 24*(8), 897–907.

Becker, S. P., & Lienesch, J. A. (2018). Nighttime media use in adolescents with ADHD: Links to sleep problems and internalizing symptoms. *Sleep Medicine, 51,* 171–178.

Becker, S. P., Sidol, C. A., Van Dyk, T. R., Epstein, J. N., & Beebe, D. W. (2017). Intraindividual variability of sleep/wake patterns in relation to child and adolescent functioning: A systematic review. *Sleep Medicine Reviews, 34,* 94–121.

Bell, B. G., & Belsky, J. (2008). Parents, parenting, and children's sleep problems: Exploring reciprocal effects. *British Journal of Developmental Psychology, 26*(4), 579–593.

Blake, M. J., Sheeber, L. B., Youssef, G. J., Raniti, M. B., & Allen, N. B. (2017). Systematic review and meta-analysis of adolescent cognitive-behavioral sleep interventions. *Clinical Child and Family Psychology Review, 20,* 227–249.

Borbély, A. A. (1982). A two process model of sleep regulation. *Human Neurobiology, 1*(3), 195–204.

Bourchtein, E., Langberg, J. M., Cusick, C. N., Breaux, R. P., Smith, Z. R., & Becker, S. P. (2019). Technology use and sleep in adolescents with and without attention-deficit/hyperactivity disorder. *Journal of Pediatric Psychology, 44*(5), 517–526.

Bruni, O., Ottaviano, S., Guidetti, V., Romoli, M., Innocenzi, M., Cortesi, F., & Giannotti, F. (1996). The Sleep Disturbance Scale for Children (SDSC): Construction and validation of an instrument to evaluate sleep disturbances in childhood and adolescence. *Journal of Sleep Research, 5*(4), 251–261.

Calamaro, C. J., Mason, T. B., & Ratcliffe, S. J. (2009). Adolescents living the 24/7 lifestyle: Effects of caffeine and technology on sleep duration and daytime functioning. *Pediatrics, 123*(6), e1005–e1010.

Charach, A., Ickowicz, A., & Schachar, R. (2004). Stimulant treatment over five years: Adherence, effectiveness, and adverse effects. *Journal of the American Academy of Child and Adolescent Psychiatry, 43*(5), 559–567.

Chervin, R. D., Hedger, K., Dillon, J. E., & Pituch, K. J. (2000). Pediatric Sleep Questionnaire (PSQ): Validity and reliability of scales for sleep-disordered breathing, snoring, sleepiness, and behavioral problems. *Sleep Medicine, 1*(1), 21–32.

Chiang, H. L., Gau, S. S. F., Ni, H. C., Chiu, Y. N., Shang, C. Y., Wu, Y. Y., . . . Soong, W. T. (2010). Association between symptoms and subtypes of attention-deficit hyperactivity disorder and sleep problems/disorders. *Journal of Sleep Research, 19*(4), 535–545.

Clarke, G., McGlinchey, E. L., Hein, K., Gullion, C. M., Dickerson, J. F., Leo, M. C., & Harvey, A. G. (2015). Cognitive-behavioral treatment of insomnia and depression in adolescents: A pilot randomized trial. *Behaviour Research and Therapy, 69,* 111–118.

Coghill, D., Soutullo, C., d'Aubuisson, C., Preuss, U., Lindback, T., Silverberg, M., & Buitelaar, J. (2008). Impact of attention-deficit/hyperactivity disorder on the patient and family: Results from a European survey. *Child and Adolescent Psychiatry and Mental Health, 2*(1), 31.

Cohen, P., Cohen, J., Kasen, S., Velez, C. N., Hartmark, C., Johnson, J., . . . Streuning, E. (1993). An epidemiological study of disorders in late childhood and adolescence—I. Age- and gender-specific prevalence. *Journal of Child Psychology and Psychiatry, 34*(6), 851–867.

Colrain, I. M., & Baker, F. C. (2011). Changes in sleep as a function of adolescent development. *Neuropsychology Review, 21*(1), 5–21.

Cortese, S., Faraone, S. V., Konofal, E., & Lecendreux, M. (2009). Sleep in children with attention-deficit/hyperactivity disorder: Meta-analysis of subjective and objective studies. *Journal of the American Academy of Child and Adolescent Psychiatry, 48*(9), 894–908.

Cortese, S., Konofal, E., & Lecendreux, M. (2008). Alertness and feeding behaviors in ADHD: Does the hypocretin/orexin system play a role? *Medical Hypotheses, 71*(5), 770–775.

Danner, F., & Phillips, B. (2008). Adolescent sleep, school start times, and teen motor vehicle crashes. *Journal of Clinical Sleep Medicine, 4*(6), 533–535.

de Bruin, E. J., Bögels, S. M., Oort, F. J., & Meijer, A. M. (2015). Efficacy of cognitive behavioral therapy for insomnia in adolescents: A randomized controlled trial with Internet therapy, group therapy and a waiting list condition. *Sleep, 38,* 1913–1926.

Deault, L. C. (2010). A systematic review of parenting in relation to the development of comorbidities and functional impairments in children with attention-deficit/hyperactivity disorder (ADHD). *Child Psychiatry and Human Development, 41,* 168–192.

Drake, C., Nickel, C., Burduvali, E., Roth, T., Jefferson, C., & Pietro, B. (2003). The Pediatric Daytime Sleepiness Scale (PDSS): Sleep habits and school outcomes in middle-school children. *Sleep, 26*(4), 455–458.

DuPaul, G. J., & Langberg, J. M. (2014). Educational impairments in children with ADHD. In R. A. Barkley (Ed.), *Attention-deficit/hyperactivity disorder: A handbook for diagnosis and treatment* (4th ed., pp. 169–190). New York: Guilford Press.

Eaton, D. K., McKnight-Eily, L. R., Lowry, R., Perry, G. S., Presley-Cantrell, L., & Croft, J. B. (2010). Prevalence of insufficient, borderline, and optimal hours of sleep among high school students—United States, 2007. *Journal of Adolescent Health, 46*(4), 399–401.

Fisher, B. C., Garges, D. M., Yoon, S. Y. R., Maguire, K., Zipay, D., & Gambino, M. (2014). Sex differences and the interaction of age and sleep issues in neuropsychological testing performance across the lifespan in an ADD/ADHD sample from the years 1989 to 2009. *Psychological Reports, 114*(2), 404–438.

Fleig, D., & Randler, C. (2009). Association between chronotype and diet in adolescents based on food logs. *Eating Behaviors, 10*(2), 115–118.

Gau, S. S.-F., & Chiang, H.-L. (2009). Sleep problems and disorders among adolescents with persistent and subthreshold attention-deficit/hyperactivity disorders. *Sleep, 32*(5), 671–679.

Gavin, L. A., Wamboldt, M. Z., Sorokin, N., Levy, S. Y., & Wamboldt, F. S. (1999). Treatment alliance and its association with family functioning, adherence, and medical outcome in adolescents with severe, chronic asthma. *Journal of Pediatric Psychology, 24,* 355–365.

Giannotti, F., Cortesi, F., Sebastiani, T., & Ottaviano, S. (2002). Circadian preference, sleep and daytime behaviour in adolescence. *Journal of Sleep Research, 11*(3), 191–199.

Gradisar, M., Dohnt, H., Gardner, G., Paine, S., Starkey, K., Menne, A., . . . Weaver, E. (2011). A randomized controlled trial of cognitive-behavior therapy plus bright light therapy for adolescent delayed sleep phase disorder. *Sleep, 34*(12), 1671–1680.

Harvey, A. G. (2016). A transdiagnostic intervention for youth sleep and circadian problems. *Cognitive and Behavioral Practice, 23*(3), 341–355.

Harvey, A. G., Hein, K., Dolsen, M. R., Dong, L., Rabe-Hesketh, S., Gumport, N. B., . . . Blum, D. J. (2018). Modifying the impact of eveningness chronotype ("night owls") in youth: A randomized controlled trial. *Journal of the American Academy of Child and Adolescent Psychiatry, 57,* 742–754.

Hiscock, H., Sciberras, E., Mensah, F., Gerner, B., Efron, D., Khano, S., & Oberklaid, F. (2015). Impact of a behavioural sleep intervention on symptoms and sleep in children with attention deficit hyperactivity disorder, and parental mental health: Randomised controlled trial. *British Medical Journal, 350,* h68.

Hoebert, M., Van Der Heijden, K. B., Van Geijlswijk, I. M., & Smits, M. G. (2009). Long-term follow-up of melatonin treatment in children with ADHD and chronic sleep onset insomnia. *Journal of Pineal Research, 47*(1), 1–7.

Horne, J. A., & Ostberg, O. (1976). A self-assessment questionnaire to determine morningness–eveningness in human circadian rhythms. *International Journal of Chronobiology, 4,* 97–110.

Hysing, M., Lundervold, A. J., Posserud, M.-B., & Sivertsen, B. (2016). Association between sleep problems and symptoms of attention deficit hyperactivity disorder in adolescence: Results from a large population-based study. *Behavioral Sleep Medicine, 14*(5), 550–564.

Hysing, M., Pallesen, S., Stormark, K. M., Jakobsen, R., Lundervold, A. J., & Sivertsen, B. (2015). Sleep and use of electronic devices in adolescence: Results from a large population-based study. *BMJ Open, 5,* Article e006748.

Johnson, E. O., & Roth, T. (2006). An epidemiologic study of sleep-disordered breathing symptoms among adolescents. *Sleep, 29,* 1135–1142.

Johnson, E. O., Roth, T., & Breslau, N. (2006). The association of insomnia with anxiety disorders and depression: Exploration of the direction of risk. *Journal of Psychiatric Research, 40*(8), 700–708.

Kaufman, D. M., & Milstein, M. J. (2013). Sleep disorders. In *Kaufman's clinical neurology for psychiatrists* (7th ed., pp. 365–396). London: Elsevier.

Kelly, R. J., Marks, B. T., & El-Sheikh, M. (2014). Longitudinal relations between parent–child conflict and children's adjustment: The role of children's sleep. *Journal of Abnormal Child Psychology, 42*(7), 1175–1185.

Kidwell, K. M., Van Dyk, T. R., Lundahl, A., & Nelson, T. D. (2015). Stimulant medications and sleep for youth with ADHD: A meta-analysis. *Pediatrics, 136*(6), 1144–1153.

Kirov, R., & Brand, S. (2014). Sleep problems and their effect in ADHD. *Expert Review of Neurotherapeutics, 14*(3), 287–299.

Kissling, C., Retz, W., Wiemann, S., Coogan, A. N., Clement, R. M., Hünnerkopf, R., . . . Thome, J. (2008). A polymorphism at the 3'-untranslated region of the *CLOCK* gene is associated with adult attention-deficit hyperactivity disorder. *American Journal of Medical Genetics B: Neuropsychiatric Genetics, 147*(3), 333–338.

Konofal, E., Zhao, W., Laouénan, C., Lecendreux, M., Kaguelidou, F., Benadjaoud, L., . . . Jacqz-Aigrain, E. (2014). Pilot Phase II study of mazindol in children with attention deficit/hyperactivity disorder. *Drug Design, Development and Therapy, 8,* 2321–2332.

Langberg, J. M., & Becker, S. P. (2012). Does long-term medication use improve the academic outcomes of youth with attention-deficit/hyperactivity disorder? *Clinical Child and Family Psychology Review, 15*(3), 215–233.

Langberg, J. M., Molitor, S. J., Oddo, L. E., Eadeh, H.-M., Dvorsky, M. R., & Becker, S. P. (2017, January 1). Prevalence, patterns, and predictors of sleep problems and daytime sleepiness in young adolescents with ADHD. *Journal of Attention Disorders.* [Epub ahead of print]

LeBourgeois, M. K., Giannotti, F., Cortesi, F., Wolfson, A. R., & Harsh, J. (2005). The relationship between reported sleep quality and sleep hygiene in Italian and American adolescents. *Pediatrics, 115*(10), 257.

Lewandowski, A. S., Toliver-Sokol, M., & Palermo, T. M. (2011). Evidence-based review of subjective pediatric sleep measures. *Journal of Pediatric Psychology, 36*(7), 780–793.

Lunsford-Avery, J. R., Krystal, A. D., & Kollins, S. H. (2016). Sleep disturbances in adolescents with ADHD: A systematic review and framework for future research. *Clinical Psychology Review, 50,* 159–174.

Lycett, K., Mensah, F. K., Hiscock, H., & Sciberras, E. (2014). A prospective study of sleep problems in children with ADHD. *Sleep Medicine, 15,* 1354–1361.

McCarley, R. W. (2007). Neurobiology of REM and NREM sleep. *Sleep Medicine, 8,* 302–330.

McCarthy, S., Wilton, L., Murray, M. L., Hodgkins, P., Asherson, P., & Wong, I. C. (2012). Persistence of pharmacological treatment into adulthood, in UK primary care, for ADHD patients who started treatment in childhood or adolescence. *BMC Psychiatry, 12,* 219.

Mick, E., Biederman, J., Jetton, J., & Faraone, S. V. (2000). Sleep disturbances associated with attention deficit hyperactivity disorder: The impact of psychiatric comorbidity and pharmacotherapy. *Journal of Child and Adolescent Psychopharmacology, 10,* 223–231.

Moore, M., Kirchner, H. L., Drotar, D., Johnson, N., Rosen, C., & Redline, S. (2011). Correlates of adolescent sleep time and variability in sleep time: The role of individual and health related characteristics. *Sleep Medicine, 12*(3), 239–245.

Mullin, B. C., Harvey, A. G., & Hinshaw, S. P. (2011). A preliminary study of sleep in adolescents with bipolar disorder, ADHD, and non-patient controls. *Bipolar Disorders, 13,* 425–432.

Mulraney, M., Giallo, R., Lycett, K., Mensah, F., & Sciberras, E. (2016). The bidirectional relationship between sleep problems and internalizing and externalizing problems in children with ADHD: A prospective cohort study. *Sleep Medicine, 17,* 45–51.

Narad, M. E., Garner, A. A., Antonini, T. N., Kingery, K. M., Tamm, L., Calhoun, H. R., & Epstein, J. N. (2018). Negative consequences of poor driving outcomes reported by adolescents with and without ADHD. *Journal of Attention Disorders, 22,* 1109–1112.

Nilsson, J. P., Söderström, M., Karlsson, A. U., Lekander, M., Åkerstedt, T., Lindroth, N. E., & Axelsson, J. (2005). Less effective executive functioning after one night's sleep deprivation. *Journal of Sleep Research, 14*(1), 1–6.

Olds, T., Maher, C., Blunden, S., & Matricciani, L. (2010). Normative data on the sleep habits of Australian children and adolescents. *Sleep, 33*(10), 1381–1388.

Orbeta, R. L., Overpeck, M. D., Ramcharran, D., Kogan, M. D., & Ledsky, R. (2006). High caffeine intake in adolescents: Associations with difficulty sleeping and feeling tired in the morning. *Journal of Adolescent Health, 38*(4), 451–453.

Owens, J., & Adoelscent Sleep Working Group. (2014). Insufficient sleep in adolescents and young adults: An update on causes and consequences. *Pediatrics, 134*(3), e921–e932.

Owens, J., Gruber, R., Brown, T., Corkum, P., Cortese, S., O'Brien, L., . . . Weiss, M. (2013). Future research directions in sleep and ADHD: Report of a consensus working group. *Journal of Attention Disorders, 17*(7), 550–564.

Owens, J. A., Maxim, R., Nobile, C., McGuinn, M., & Msall, M. (2000). Parental and self-report of sleep in children with attention-deficit/hyperactivity disorder. *Archives of Pediatrics and Adolescent Medicine, 154*(6), 549–555.

Owens, J. A., Spirito, A., & McGuinn, M. (2000). The Children's Sleep Habits Questionnaire (CSHQ): Psychometric properties of a survey instrument for school-aged children. *Sleep, 23,* 1043–1052.

Pandi-Perumal, S. R., Smits, M., Spence, W., Srinivasan, V., Cardinali, D. P., Lowe, A. D., & Kayumov, L. (2007). Dim light melatonin onset (DLMO): A tool for the analysis of circadian phase in human sleep and chronobiological disorders. *Progress in Neuro-Psychopharmacology and Biological Psychiatry, 31,* 1–11.

Park, J., & Kim, B. (2015, May 25). Comorbidity and factors affecting treatment non-persistence in ADHD. *Journal of Attention Disorders.* [Epub ahead of print]

Prehn-Kristensen, A., Göder, R., Fischer, J., Wilhelm, I., Seeck-Hirschner, M., Aldenhoff, J., & Baving, L. (2011). Reduced sleep-associated consolidation of declarative memory in attention-deficit/hyperactivity disorder. *Sleep Medicine, 12,* 672–679.

Prince, J. B., Wilens, T. E., Biederman, J., Spencer, T. J., & Wozniak, J. R. (1996). Clonidine for sleep disturbances associated with attention-deficit hyperactivity disorder: A systematic chart review of 62 cases. *Journal of the American Academy of Child and Adolescent Psychiatry, 35,* 599–605.

Roenneberg, T., Kuehnle, T., Pramstaller, P. P., Ricken, J., Havel, M., Guth, A., & Merrow, M. (2004). A marker for the end of adolescence. *Current Biology, 14*(24), R1038–R1039.

Sadeh, A. (2015). III. Sleep assessment methods. *Monographs of the Society for Research in Child Development, 80,* 33–48.

Santisteban, J., Stein, M., Bergmame, L., & Gruber, R. (2014). Effect of extended-release dexmethylphenidate and mixed amphetamine salts on sleep: A double-blind, randomized, crossover study in youth with attention-deficit hyperactivity disorder. *CNS Drugs, 28,* 825–833.

Sawyer, A. C., Clark, C. R., Keage, H. A., Moores, K. A., Clarke, S., Kohn, M. R., & Gordon, E. (2009). Cognitive and electroencephalographic disturbances in children with attention-deficit/hyperactivity disorder and sleep problems: New insights. *Psychiatry Research, 170,* 183–191.

Sciberras, E., DePetro, A., Mensah, F., & Hiscock, H. (2015). Association between sleep and working memory in children with ADHD: A cross-sectional study. *Sleep Medicine, 16,* 1192–1197.

Sciberras, E., Mulraney, M., Mensah, F., Oberklaid, F., Efron, D., & Hiscock, H. (2019, January 18). Sustained impact of a sleep intervention and moderators of treatment outcome for children with ADHD: A randomised controlled trial. *Psychological Medicine.* [Epub ahead of print]

Sciberras, E., Song, J. C., Mulraney, M., Schuster, T., & Hiscock, H. (2017). Sleep problems in children with attention-deficit hyperactivity disorder: Associations with parenting style and sleep hygiene. *European Child and Adolescent Psychiatry, 26,* 1129–1139.

Shaw, P., Stringaris, A., Nigg, J., & Leibenluft, E. (2014). Emotion dysregulation in attention deficit hyperactivity disorder. *American Journal of Psychiatry, 171,* 276–293.

Short, M. A., Gradisar, M., Lack, L. C., Wright, H. R., Dewald, J. F., Wolfson, A. R., & Carskadon, M. A. (2013). A cross-cultural comparison of sleep duration between US and Australian adolescents: The effect of school start time, parent-set bedtimes, and extracurricular load. *Health Education and Behavior, 40,* 323–330.

Short, M. A., Gradisar, M., Wright, H., Lack, L. C., Dohnt, H., & Carskadon, M. A. (2011). Time for bed: Parent-set bedtimes associated with improved sleep and daytime functioning in adolescents. *Sleep, 34,* 797–800.

Smalley, S. L., McGough, J. J., Moilanen, I. K., Loo, S. K., Taanila, A., Ebeling, H., . . . McCracken, J. T. (2007). Prevalence and psychiatric comorbidity of attention-deficit/hyperactivity disorder in an adolescent Finnish population. *Journal of the American Academy of Child and Adolescent Psychiatry, 46,* 1575–1583.

Stein, M. A., Weiss, M., & Hlavaty, L. (2012). ADHD treatments, sleep, and sleep problems: Complex associations. *Neurotherapeutics, 9,* 509–517.

Stern, E., Parmelee, A. H., Akiyama, Y., Schultz, M. A., & Wenner, W. H. (1969). Sleep cycle characteristics in infants. *Pediatrics, 43,* 65–70.

Stickgold, R. (2013). Parsing the role of sleep in memory processing. *Current Opinion in Neurobiology, 23,* 847–853.

Taylor, D. J., Jenni, O. G., Acebo, C., & Carskadon, M. A. (2005). Sleep tendency during extended wakefulness: Insights into adolescent sleep regulation and behavior. *Journal of Sleep Research, 14,* 239–244.

Tebbi, C. K. (1993). Treatment compliance in childhood and adolescence. *Cancer, 71*(Suppl. 10), 3441–3449.

Turkdogan, D., Bekiroglu, N., & Zaimoglu, S. (2011). A prevalence study of restless legs syndrome in Turkish children and adolescents. *Sleep Medicine, 12,* 315–321.

Van der Heijden, K. B., Smits, M. G., Van Someren, E. J., & Gunning, W. B. (2005). Idiopathic chronic sleep onset insomnia in attention-deficit/hyperactivity disorder: A circadian rhythm sleep disorder. *Chronobiology International, 22,* 559–570.

Van der Heijden, K. B., Smits, M. G., Van Someren, E. J., Ridderinkhof, K. R., & Gunning, W. B. (2007). Effect of melatonin on sleep, behavior, and cognition in ADHD and chronic sleep-onset insomnia. *Journal of the American Academy of Child and Adolescent Psychiatry, 46,* 233–241.

Van Veen, M. M., Kooij, J. S., Boonstra, A. M., Gordijn, M. C., & Van Someren, E. J. (2010). Delayed circadian rhythm in adults with attention-deficit/hyperactivity disorder and chronic sleep-onset insomnia. *Biological Psychiatry, 67,* 1091–1096.

Weiss, M. D., Craig, S. G., Davies, G., Schibuk, L., & Stein, M. (2015). New research on the complex interaction of sleep and ADHD. *Current Sleep Medicine Reports, 1,* 114–121.

Weiss, M. D., Wasdell, M. B., Bomben, M. M., Rea, K. J., & Freeman, R. D. (2006). Sleep hygiene and melatonin treatment for children and adolescents with ADHD and initial insomnia. *Journal of the American Academy of Child and Adolescent Psychiatry, 45,* 512–519.

Wilens, T. E., Biederman, J., & Spencer, T. (1994). Clonidine for sleep disturbances associated with attention-deficit hyperactivity disorder. *Journal of the American Academy of Child and Adolescent Psychiatry, 33,* 424–426.

Willcutt, E. G., Doyle, A. E., Nigg, J. T., Faraone, S. V., & Pennington, B. F. (2005). Validity of the executive function theory of attention-deficit/hyperactivity disorder: A meta-analytic review. *Biological Psychiatry, 57,* 1336–1346.

Wolfson, A. R., Carskadon, M. A., Acebo, C., Seifer, R., Fallone, G., Labyak, S. E., & Martin, J. L. (2003). Evidence for the validity of a Sleep Habits Survey for adolescents. *Sleep, 26*(2), 213–216.

Zendarski, N., Sciberras, E., Mensah, F., & Hiscock, H. (2017). Academic achievement and risk factors for adolescents with attention-deficit hyperactivity disorder in middle school and early high school. *Journal of Developmental and Behavioral Pediatrics, 38,* 358–368.

CHAPTER 11

Substance Use in Adolescents with ADHD

Traci M. Kennedy
Kirsten M. P. McKone
Brooke S. G. Molina

Adolescence is a transitional developmental period sandwiched between the dependence of childhood and the independence of adulthood. Characteristics of this developmental stage, such as heightened novelty seeking and risk taking (Spear, 2000), reflect developmental changes in neurobiology (Ernst, 2014; Steinberg, 2010) and dramatically increase risk for substance abuse and other potentially health-compromising behaviors. Substance use in adolescence is a developmental process (Masten, Faden, Zucker, & Spear, 2008; Palmer et al., 2009), typically starting with "gateway" substances that are legal in adulthood (i.e., cigarettes, alcohol) and increasing in frequency across adolescence (Johnston et al., 2017). Although adolescent substance use has declined in recent years, many adolescents currently use substances to the extent that it is sometimes more developmentally typical than atypical. Most teens have used at least one substance by 12th grade, with 61% reporting alcohol use and 48% reporting use of an illicit drug (Johnston et al., 2017). Substance use in adolescence is also influenced by social and contextual changes. Peers become the primary social influence in adolescents' lives, and teens spend considerably more time with them than with family or other adults (Barnes, Hoffman, Welte, Farrell, & Dintcheff, 2007). As such, most adolescent substance use is group-based (Chassin, Colder, Hussong, & Sher, 2013), and peer influence is a key factor in predicting an adolescent's own use of substances (Chassin & Barrera, 1997).

A rapidly expanding literature on attention-deficit/hyperactivity disorder (ADHD) and substance use began approximately 30 years ago, when several investigators began to report elevated substance use in samples with ADHD (e.g., Gittelman, Mannuzza, Shenker, & Bonagura, 1985; Hartsough & Lambert, 1987). Since then, studies have accumulated and have included increasingly sophisticated measurement of substance use outcomes, resulting in meta-analyses (e.g., Lee, Humphreys, Flory, Liu, & Glass, 2011) and theoretical reviews (e.g., Molina & Pelham, 2014). As we discuss in this chapter, the key symptoms of ADHD (e.g., impulsivity, inattention), along with its associated features (e.g., negative urgency, delay aversion, reward sensitivity), comorbidities (e.g., conduct disorder [CD]), and impairments (e.g., academic problems), are central to ADHD-related substance use vulnerability. These characteristics exacerbate the normative increases in risk taking, reward seeking, and susceptibility to peer influences that characterize adolescence and motivate substance use during this developmental period (Galvan, 2013). ADHD and substance use disorders (SUDs) also share etiology, including neurobiological underpinnings, as evidenced by family linkage, genetic, and neurobiological findings (e.g., Adisetiyo & Gray, 2017; Arcos-Burgos, Vèlez, Solomon, & Muenke, 2012; Biederman et al., 2008; Martel, Pierce, et al., 2009). Thus, the overlap between ADHD and SUDs runs deep. Finally, ADHD and SUDs are both developmental disorders that share a heightened period of vulnerability in adolescence and may exacerbate each other, making an understanding of their *codevelopment* across the teen years critical.

Defining and Measuring Adolescent Substance Use

To understand adolescent substance use, we first need to appreciate how it is defined and measured. In DSM-5, an SUD is continued use despite significant substance-related problems (American Psychiatric Association, 2013). However, because persistent and problematic substance use develops over time and requires ongoing access to restricted substances, many adolescents do not reach the level of diagnosable DSM disorder despite using substances at atypical levels that are prognostic of later disorder (Masten et al., 2008; McCarty, Ebel, Garrison, DiGiuseppe, Christakis, & Rivara, 2004). Thus, enhancing traditional dichotomous SUD diagnoses with developmentally sensitive dimensional metrics of substance use (e.g., frequency, quantity) more comprehensively characterizes SUD risk among adolescents, including adolescents with ADHD (Masten et al., 2008; Molina & Pelham, 2003).

Timing and course, including age of onset and trajectory of use, are key elements of adolescent substance use risk (Chassin, Sher, Hussong, & Curran, 2013; Derefinko et al., 2016). Moreover, because of the opportunistic and primarily social context of their substance use, adolescents' *patterns* of substance consumption need to be understood within a developmental context (Chassin et al., 2013). For example, although adolescents tend to drink alcohol less frequently than do adults, they may consume a higher volume of alcohol when they do drink (Chassin et al., 2013). Therefore, it is important to measure *heavy* substance use, such as binge drinking, which predicts worse outcomes than does moderate use (Chassin, Pitts, & Prost, 2002).

In this chapter we synthesize findings that draw on a range of these measurement approaches to provide a comprehensive understanding of adolescent substance use in the context of ADHD. First, we outline the unique risks for substance misuse faced by adolescents with ADHD against a backdrop of developmentally typical patterns of use. We then discuss mediating pathways that help to explain the link between adolescent ADHD and substance misuse. Treatment considerations follow, and we conclude by highlighting priorities for future research.

ADHD and Adolescent Substance Use

Theoretical, Genetic, and Biological Overlaps

ADHD is a pernicious risk factor for maladaptive substance use outcomes. The core symptoms of the disorder and associated characteristics (e.g., delay aversion, conduct problems) overlap with individual-difference factors that are known to confer risk for substance use (Chassin et al., 2013; Martel, Pierce, et al., 2009; see Molina & Pelham, 2014, for review). For example, temperament traits in early childhood that overlap with ADHD (e.g., self-control) indicate risk for the development of substance use problems later in life (e.g., Martel, Nigg, & von Eye, 2009; Martel, Pierce, et al., 2009; Moffitt et al., 2011). Consistent with this pattern, some have speculated that ADHD and SUDs represent two ends of a spectrum of interrelated externalizing disorders—an "externalizing phenotype"—such that ADHD in childhood may develop into CD in adolescence, then continue into an SUD and antisocial personality in adulthood (Arcos-Burgos et al., 2012; Beauchaine & McNulty, 2013).

Familial links between ADHD and substance use further position childhood ADHD as a risk factor for substance use problems. First, offspring of adults with SUDs tend to show higher rates of ADHD compared to offspring of parents without SUDs (Martel, Pierce, et al., 2009; Tarter, Kirisci, Habeych, Reynolds, & Vanyukov, 2004). The inverse is also true:

First-degree relatives (e.g., biological parents, siblings) of children with ADHD experience higher rates of SUDs (Biederman et al., 2008; Molina, Gnagy, Joseph, & Pelham, 2016; Skoglund, Chen, Franck, Lichtenstein, & Larsson, 2015). Evidence converges on a common genetic underpinning for ADHD and SUD that likely explains these familial patterns and appears to underlie the entire externalizing spectrum (Arcos-Burgos et al., 2012; Quinn et al., 2016). Furthermore, this common genetic liability accounts for *early-onset* substance use, highlighting the pronounced risk of ADHD for more severe, developmentally atypical substance use (Chang, Lichtenstein, & Larsson, 2012).

These genetic underpinnings likely give rise to proximal neurobiological markers of risk common to ADHD and substance use (see Adisetiyo & Gray, 2017, for review). For instance, altered functioning of dopaminergic circuits in the brain is correlated with ADHD symptoms; similarly, dysregulated dopamine functioning is involved in disrupted reward and reinforcement processes in the brain that are thought to underlie addiction (see Kollins & Adcock, 2014, for review). In a multisite study of over 2,000 young adolescents, participants with comorbid ADHD and CD and those with substance misuse showed the same abnormal patterns of activation in dopaminergic brain regions implicated in inhibitory control (Castellanos-Ryan et al., 2014). Other studies have likewise demonstrated altered functioning of brain regions involved in executive functioning and cognitive control in ADHD, such as the frontoparietal and corticostriatal–thalamocortical networks, that are also impaired in substance use (Adisetiyo & Gray, 2017). Thus, the same altered dopamine transmission throughout reward circuits of the brain may underlie both ADHD symptoms and risk for the development of SUDs.

Evidence for Problematic Substance Use among Adolescents with ADHD

Since the first studies in the 1980s (Hartsough & Lambert, 1987; Hechtman, Weiss, & Perlman, 1984; Mannuzza et al., 1991), a substantial body of literature has accumulated on substance use outcomes for children with ADHD. Initially concentrated in the United States, studies now include European samples as well. However, there is wide variability in sample sizes and types, from small clinical samples to large epidemiological registries of community-diagnosed youth, and approaches to substance use measurement vary widely as well. Studies that measure substance use developmentally are quite limited, as are studies of females with ADHD. Moreover, few studies can provide confident projections about risk of adolescent substance use extending past young adulthood. As a result, there are meaningful differences across studies' conclusions regarding substance use risk. Below we review the results of these studies by class of substance use, because there is some variability in risk as a function of substance type.

Nicotine

Across age and population (e.g., clinic- vs. community-recruited), increased risk for cigarette smoking is the most robust substance use outcome for adolescents with ADHD histories. Youth with ADHD have increased risk at all points along the developmental smoking continuum, from being more likely to try cigarettes to becoming nicotine-dependent, daily smokers who are likely to struggle with attempts to quit later in adulthood. A meta-analysis of prospective longitudinal studies examining the link between ADHD and substance use concluded that adolescents and young adults with childhood ADHD were twice as likely as individuals without ADHD to have ever used nicotine (Lee et al., 2011). This finding continues to be replicated (e.g., Rhodes et al., 2016; Sibley et al., 2014). For instance, among adolescents in the Pittsburgh ADHD Longitudinal Study (PALS), 63% with ADHD histories and 42% without had smoked a cigarette by mean age 16 (Rhodes et al., 2016). Youth with ADHD also tend to try smoking for the first time at younger ages than their peers (Groenman et al., 2013; Mitchell et al., 2019; Molina et al., 2018; Rhodes et al., 2016; see Kollins & Adcock, 2014, for review)—as early as ages 9–14 years (King, Iacono, & McGue, 2004; Molina, Flory, et al., 2007). Whereas some findings indicate that inattention symptoms appear uniquely linked to nicotine use (Burke, Loeber, & Lahey, 2001; Tercyak, Lerman, & Audrain, 2002), others implicate the hyperactivity–impulsivity dimension of ADHD (Chang et al., 2012). Impulsivity may prompt initial experimentation with cigarettes, but inattention and negative reinforcement may account for smoking escalation and maintenance at older ages.

Unlike most other forms of substance use, which typically increase throughout adolescence and early adulthood before declining in the mid- to late-20s, regular smoking often persists into the 30s and beyond (e.g., Pierce & Gilpin, 1996). Unfortunately, teens with ADHD, particularly those with the most severe symptom presentations, progress from smoking initiation to regular, habitual smoking more quickly than do their peers (Kollins & Adcock, 2014; Mitchell et al., 2019; Rhodes et al., 2016; Sibley et al., 2014). Subsequently, youth with ADHD go on to have higher rates of *daily* smoking (Milberger, Biederman, Faraone, Chen, & Jones, 1997; Molina & Pelham, 2003; Rhodes et al., 2016) and nicotine dependence as teens (Groenman et al., 2013; Kollins & Adcock, 2014; Mitchell et al., 2019). For instance, in the longitudinal follow-up of the children in the Multimodal Treatment of ADHD study (MTA), by mean age 17, 16.7% of adolescents with ADHD histories were daily smokers compared to 7.9% of adolescents without ADHD histories (Molina et al., 2013) and 2.5% of adolescents in the general population in 2016 (Johnston et al., 2017). In the same MTA study, nicotine dependence was also more likely for adolescents with ADHD histories (4.5%) compared to adolescents without ADHD (1.8%) (Molina et al., 2013). In their meta-analysis that pooled across 12 longitudinal studies with outcomes assessed in adolescence and young adulthood, Lee and colleagues (2011) convincingly showed that children with ADHD were nearly three times more likely than children without ADHD to ultimately develop nicotine dependence. Even among regular smokers, adolescents with ADHD tend to smoke at a higher frequency and more cigarettes than adolescent smokers without ADHD (Molina & Pelham, 2003; Kollins & Adcock, 2014; Sibley et al., 2014), although this finding does not appear to extend into young adulthood (Mitchell et al., 2019; Rhodes et al., 2016), suggesting a general pattern of precocious use in adolescents with ADHD. By adulthood, smokers without ADHD who begin their involvement at older ages may catch up in quantity and frequency. Finally, smokers with ADHD experience more intense craving and withdrawal symptoms during periods of abstinence (Rhodes et al., 2016) and have greater difficulty quitting as adolescents (Pagano, Delos-Reyes, Wasilow, Svala, & Kurtz, 2016) and adults than smokers without ADHD (Kollins & Adcock, 2014).

Vaping, in which an electronic device vaporizes liquids or solids into a mist that is inhaled, is a relatively new mode of substance consumption (Johnston et al., 2017). Current rates of vaping among 8th to 12th graders range from 6 to 13% nationally (Johnston et al., 2017). Data are lacking on rates and consequences of vaping among teens with ADHD, highlighting a need for future study.

Alcohol

Alcohol is legal, used widely by adults (Center for Behavioral Health Statistics and Quality [CBHSQ], 2016), and is often kept in homes, making it highly accessible to adolescents (Komro, Maldonado-Molina, Tobler, Bonds, & Muller, 2007). In fact, most adolescents have experimented with alcohol by the end of high school, with one-third of seniors reporting current use (Johnston et al., 2017). Perhaps because experimentation with alcohol is so developmentally typical, ADHD-specific risk related to alcohol consumption is less pronounced than that for other substances. In the general population, initiation of alcohol use typically occurs in mid- to late-adolescence (ages 15–18; DeWit, Adlaf, Offord, & Ogborne, 2000). At younger ages (9–15 years), youth with ADHD are more likely to have ever used alcohol than their peers (Molina, Pelham, et al., 2007; Molina, Flory, et al., 2007), but by late adolescence, when drinking alcohol is more typical, the group difference is absent (Lee et al., 2011; Molina & Pelham, 2003). Indeed, some prospective longitudinal studies report earlier onset of drinking (mean age 14) among youth with ADHD (Sibley et al., 2014), particularly those whose hyperactivity–impulsivity symptoms persist from childhood into adolescence (Chang et al., 2012). Other studies, however, have not documented ADHD risk for early use of alcohol (King et al., 2004), including one study that comprised primarily African American adolescents (Vitulano et al., 2014) who, as a group, tend to initiate alcohol use later than do European American adolescents (though they experience more alcohol-related problems when they do drink; Zapolski, Pedersen, McCarthy, & Smith, 2014). In the MTA, early substance use (including alcohol use) in adolescence predicted faster escalation to weekly binge drinking in early adulthood (Molina et al., 2018). Early onset of drinking was more common among teens with ADHD (52%) compared to teens without ADHD (43%).

More involved consumption in adolescence, such as heavy drinking,[1] is associated with especially high risk for later alcohol use disorder (AUD; Chassin et al., 2002; Hussong, Bauer, & Chassin, 2008). Heavy alcohol use typically escalates through adolescence and peaks in the early 20s (Chassin, Colder, et al., 2013). Because experimental, light alcohol use is common in adolescence, heavy drinking is more likely to distinguish teens with ADHD histories from those without (Molina, Pelham, et al., 2007), although relatively few studies report this outcome. In two studies, adolescents with ADHD histories reported more episodes of drunkenness and more alcohol-related problems than comparison participants, even at similar levels of overall alcohol use (Molina & Pelham, 2003; Quinn et al., 2016). In the follow-up of the MTA, ADHD probands were more likely than comparison peers to have used alcohol (more than five times or to the point of drunkenness) by mean age 15 (23 vs. 16%; Molina et al., 2013).

Of greatest concern, 2.5–6.4% of all adolescents will reach the level of AUD (CBHSQ, 2016; Palmer et al., 2009), and findings suggest a modestly elevated risk for adolescents with ADHD histories. Pooling across 11 studies that followed youth into adolescence and young adulthood, Lee and colleagues (2011) concluded that individuals with childhood ADHD were 1.7 times more likely to develop AUD. Similarly, a large (population-level) longitudinal cohort study in Denmark recently found elevated incidence rates of AUD by age 22 in individuals with ADHD (Ottosen, Petersen, Larsen, & Dalsgaard, 2016). However, differences in adolescent-onset AUD based on ADHD history appears specific to older versus younger adolescents/children. For example, older adolescents (ages 15–17 years) in the PALS

[1]Differences in body composition and metabolism in adolescents may require a modified operational definition of binge drinking in adolescents; young adolescents (ages 9–13) and girls (ages 9–17) require only three drinks in a 2-hour period to attain a comparable blood alcohol concentration to that exhibited in college students after four to five drinks in 2 hours (Donovan, 2009).

with ADHD had elevated rates of AUD compared to adolescents without ADHD, but group differences were not found among younger adolescents (ages 11–14 years; Molina, Pelham, et al., 2007), perhaps in part because of very low rates of AUD overall in early adolescence.

Marijuana

Marijuana is the second most commonly used substance in adolescence, after alcohol (Johnston et al., 2017; CBHSQ, 2016). Forty-five percent of 12th-grade students in the United States have used marijuana in their lifetime, with 22% reporting use in the past 30 days (Johnston et al., 2017). Like cigarette smoking, marijuana use is elevated among adolescents with ADHD histories, though this effect has also vacillated across studies (Lee et al., 2011). For example, adolescents with childhood ADHD in the PALS (mean age 15) were no more likely than comparison youth to have tried marijuana (Molina & Pelham, 2003), whereas youth with ADHD in the Minnesota Twin Study (mean age 15) were at increased risk (King et al., 2004). More recently, Sibley and colleagues (2014) found that once adolescents had tried marijuana, those with ADHD tended to use more frequently (with 10.6% endorsing daily marijuana use) and were more than twice as likely to develop cannabis use disorder. This pattern has been supported by other findings (Lee et al., 2011; Ottosen et al., 2016).

Early-age use of marijuana and ADHD has been investigated in a few studies. Molina and Pelham (2003) did not find a difference in age of first use by mean age 15 in an early examination in the PALS, nor did Sibley et al. (2014) in a similar-size sample of teens with ADHD diagnosed in preschool. However, more early marijuana users were found in the ADHD versus non-ADHD group (49 vs. 35%) in the MTA (Molina et al., 2018). As access to marijuana increases in the United States due to a lifting of legal restrictions, ADHD-related risk of marijuana use and problems should be tracked, particularly given the increasing potency of the drug over time (Compton, Volkow, & Lopez, 2017) and its association with later use of other illicit drugs (Secades-Villa, Garcia-Rodriguez, Chelsea, Wang, & Blanco, 2015).

Other Illicit Drugs

Other illicit drugs include illegal substances such as cocaine, heroin, and crystal methamphetamine. Adolescents are using these illicit drugs less often than in previous years (Johnston et al., 2017), but like marijuana, adolescents with ADHD histories have higher rates of non-marijuana illicit drug use as well (Lee et al., 2011; Molina & Pelham, 2003; Ottosen et al., 2016). Exceptions exist, which could easily be due to sample size limitations given the relative infrequency of street drug use among teens more generally (Barkley, Fischer, Edelbrock, & Smallish, 1990; Grant & Dawson, 1998; Hartsough & Lambert, 1987). When differences are found, youth with ADHD histories start using illegal drugs at younger ages than do their peers (Molina & Pelham, 2003; Molina et al., 2018), and once initiated, drug use progresses to more problematic use and disorder more quickly than for those without ADHD (Molina et al., 2018). Similar to other substances, early onset of illicit drug use is associated with increased risk for eventual drug dependence and disorder (Grant & Dawson, 1998), which raises serious concern about the potential for ensuing addiction and legal problems. Adolescents with ADHD are also more likely to combine drugs: 10.6% of teens with ADHD and 3% without ADHD in the PALS reported using at least two different classes of drugs (Molina et al., 2013; Molina & Pelham, 2003), which is much riskier than taking any one substance in isolation and portends more substance-related future problems (e.g., Moss, Chen, & Yi, 2014).

There is substantial interest in understanding how ADHD may increase risk for illicit stimulants in particular (e.g., cocaine, amphetamines), although few prospective studies examine ADHD risk for use of specific drug classes. Theoretically, adolescents who have taken stimulant medication for the treatment of their ADHD symptoms throughout childhood may become sensitized to its effects and become vulnerable to the addictive properties of illicit stimulants (e.g., Kollins, English, Robinson, Hallyburton, & Chrisman, 2009; Lambert, 2005; Lambert & Hartsough, 1998). Animal studies suggest an ADHD-like biologically based predilection for stimulants (Kantak & Dwoskin, 2016). Across the five studies included in Lee and colleagues' (2011) meta-analysis that examined cocaine use as a function of childhood ADHD diagnosis, those with ADHD were twice as likely to develop a cocaine use disorder by adolescence or adulthood; however, the risk was not specific to stimulant drugs and may simply reflect the general pattern of increased risk for substance use among youth with ADHD. Head-to-head comparisons of preference for stimulants versus nonstimulant drugs are needed, including among individuals well-diagnosed as children and followed longitudinally.

Misuse of Prescription Drugs

Misuse of prescription drugs encapsulates use of medication in greater quantities or in a manner different from that prescribed, or use of medication without a prescription. Due to their psychoactive effects, three classes of prescription drugs are most commonly misused: opioids (e.g., oxycodone, morphine), depressants (e.g., benzodiazepines, barbiturates), and stimulants (e.g., methylphenidate and amphetamine medications). The current epidemic of opioid misuse and associated deaths (Rudd, Aleshire, Zibbel, & Gladden, 2016), as well as increased stimulant-related admissions to emergency departments (Substance Abuse and Mental Health Services Administration [SAMHSA], 2013), have increased concern about misuse of these medications. Prescription stimulants are of particular interest, since they are a first-line treatment for adolescents with ADHD (see Brinkman, Froehlich, & Epstein, Chapter 18, this volume). Given their potential for abuse, there is concern that adolescents with ADHD may be vulnerable to stimulant addiction. Among adolescents generally, the most frequently endorsed forms of amphetamine use in 2016 were misuse of the stimulant medications Adderall (3.9%) and Ritalin (1.1%; Johnston et al., 2017). Most research investigating stimulant misuse, however, has focused on college populations and has found that an ADHD diagnosis, more severe ADHD symptoms, and comorbid ADHD and CD are associated with a higher risk for stimulant misuse (Benson, Flory, Humphreys, & Lee, 2015; Van Eck, Markle, & Flory, 2012). For instance, the results of a meta-analysis suggest that 17% of college students misuse stimulant medication—a risk that is 4.5 times more likely among individuals with an ADHD diagnosis (Benson et al., 2015). This association may reflect a general propensity toward substance use rather than a risk for stimulant misuse specifically (Benson et al., 2015). Importantly, these studies differ from longitudinal follow-up studies of children with ADHD who tend to stop using stimulant medication by adulthood (Barkley, Fischer, Smallish, & Fletcher, 2003); when stimulant medications continue to be used, rates of misuse are low (Wilens, Gignac, Swezey, Monuteaux, & Biederman, 2006)—about 1% (Molina et al., 2018). Thus, there appears to be a demarcation in risk of misuse between individuals who began their treatment as children versus those who initiate treatment in adulthood. The latter may include some adults (particularly college students) who seek medication for cognitive enhancement in the context of a profile of poor academic performance, abuse of other substances, and uncertain ADHD diagnosis (Blevins, Stephens, & Abrantes, 2017; Wilens et al., 2017).

General Substance Use

Some studies aggregate across substance use classes rather than examine substance-specific outcomes. Much like the precocious patterns observed for specific substances, adolescents with childhood ADHD in two large, prospective longitudinal studies tended to try substances at younger ages than adolescents without ADHD (Groenman et al., 2013; Molina et al., 2018). In several other prospective, longitudinal studies, adolescents with ADHD used substances at a higher frequency (Molina et al., 2007a) and were more likely to have a SUD than those without ADHD (Groenman et al., 2013; Tarter et al., 2004). Other studies reveal similar findings for clustered substance use variables (e.g., alcohol/drug abuse: Katusic et al., 2005; any drug use disorder, including marijuana: Mannuzza et al., 1991;

nonalcohol substance use disorder: Mannuzza, Klein, Bessler, Malloy, & LaPadula, 1998), but there are exceptions (Biederman et al., 1997; Hinshaw et al., 2012).

Summary

In summary, adolescents with ADHD use substances across classes at moderately higher levels than their peers without ADHD, especially nicotine. However, rates of prescription stimulant misuse are low. Even more notable, teens with ADHD tend to start using substances *earlier* than their peers, which places them at risk for more rapid progression to high-risk levels of use and worse consequences. In addition to these substances of abuse, limited research to date suggests that adolescents with ADHD consume more caffeine (e.g., coffee, caffeinated soft drinks) than their peers as well; future research should examine whether high rates of caffeine use in adolescence similarly serves as a "gateway" to other stimulant drugs such as nicotine for individuals with ADHD (Van Eck et al., 2012; Walker, Abraham, & Tercyak, 2010).

Moderators and Protective Effects

To be sure, adolescents with ADHD are not doomed to addiction. Several factors may interact with childhood ADHD to buffer against substance use risk. In addition to the role of age, discussed earlier, gender appears to moderate the association between ADHD and substance use. Although they represent a minority of children diagnosed with ADHD, girls across several prospective longitudinal studies—the Berkeley Girls with ADHD Longitudinal Study (Hinshaw et al., 2012), the MTA (Molina, Flory, et al., 2007), and the PALS (Babinski et al., 2011)—did *not* exhibit higher rates of substance use and disorder relative to comparison girls, in contrast to boys. One possible explanation for this pattern may be that girls tend to display lower levels of delinquency and disruptive behavior than do boys, even among those with ADHD (Molina, 2011); indeed, oppositional defiant disorder (ODD) and CD consistently exacerbate the link between ADHD and substance use across substances (Burke et al., 2001; Groenman et al., 2013; Lee et al., 2011; Molina, Pelham, et al., 2007). However, in one prospective longitudinal study in Europe, girls with ADHD were at heightened risk of AUD and SUD by adulthood, although the sample included only 25 girls (Dalsgaard, Mortensen, Frydenberg, & Thomsen, 2014). In a larger registry study of nearly 20,000 individuals in Denmark, females with ADHD also had higher rates of SUD than males with ADHD (Ottosen et al., 2016). Thus, protective effects of gender in adolescence may dissipate by adulthood, but this finding requires replication in more generalizable samples.

Several factors exert protective effects by buffering youth with ADHD from problematic substance use outcomes. One of the strongest is parenting. For instance, successful parental monitoring that results in knowledge of children's whereabouts, friendships, and activities dampens the association between childhood ADHD and adolescent alcohol use (Molina et al., 2012; Walther et al., 2012). Parental warmth is also protective against SUD in the context of ADHD (Tandon, Tillman, Spitznagel, & Luby, 2014), whereas parent–teen conflict increases risk (Sibley et al., 2014). Others have found that parental monitoring *mediates* the link between ADHD and adolescent risk-taking behaviors more broadly, including substance use, dangerous driving, and unprotected sex, suggesting that parental knowledge is more likely to be compromised when teens have ADHD, leading teens to behave more dangerously (Pollak, Poni, Gershy, & Aran, 2018). Developmentally, parental monitoring should be decreasing while teen autonomy increases in adolescence, but it is unclear whether this normative pattern is conducive to healthy outcomes for teens with ADHD. Research addressing this question is needed. Beyond the family environment, although the social impairment common in ADHD predicts a plethora of negative outcomes, social isolation might, paradoxically, serve a protective role for teens with ADHD by limiting their exposure to substance-using peers (Molina et al., 2012).

Pathways from ADHD to Adolescent Substance Use

The psychosocial mechanisms underlying the link between ADHD and adolescent substance use are many and complex (e.g., Flory & Lynam, 2003; Wilens & Biederman, 2006), but we have summarized them by grouping them into two, non-mutually exclusive broad categories: ADHD-related impairment pathways (e.g., conduct problems, delinquency, academic failure) and negative affect, expectancies, and coping pathways (Molina & Pelham, 2014). Here, we discuss several of these pathways.

Perhaps the most robust and well-studied of these pathways is the "deviance proneness" pathway, in which conduct problems, including delinquency, mediate the link between ADHD and substance use (Flory & Lynam, 2003). Across several studies including both community and clinical samples, CD and ODD symptoms fully mediated the positive association between ADHD and substance use outcomes among adolescents (Bussing, Mason, Bell, Porter, & Garvan, 2010; Molina & Pelham, 2003; Sibley et al., 2014). In fact, the results of a meta-analysis suggested that ADHD does not increase risk for illicit substance use independent of CD or ODD, but notably, power was inadequate to detect small effects that may have existed (Serra-Pinheiro et al., 2013). Therefore, some have suggested that behavioral deviance is solely responsible for ADHD-related risk for substance use rather than ADHD per se. Nonetheless, in other studies in which researchers controlled for CD and delinquency, ADHD was an independent predictor of substance use (Elkins, McGue, & Iacono, 2007;

Lambert, 2005; Rhodes et al., 2016; Sibley et al., 2014). As noted earlier, effects of ADHD may be primarily driven by hyperactivity–impulsivity rather than inattention symptoms (Chang et al., 2012; Molina, Smith, & Pelham, 1999; Quinn et al., 2016), which also creates risk of downstream behavior problems, including substance use. Impulsivity may therefore be the core trait of greatest concern—a finding that is supported by both behavioral and functional neurobiological evidence (Adisetiyo & Gray, 2017; Castellanos-Ryan et al., 2014).

Whereas isolation from peers may be protective, exposure to substance-using peers and vulnerabilities to their influence is one of the strongest predictors of adolescent substance use (Chassin & Barrera, 1997)—and it appears to be even *stronger* among adolescents with ADHD histories (Belendiuk, Pedersen, King, Pelham, & Molina, 2016). In one prospective longitudinal study, deviant peer affiliation (tolerance of and perceived peer substance use) *mediated* the association between childhood ADHD symptoms and adolescent substance misuse (Marshal & Molina, 2006). This socially mediated, peer use risk pathway is especially pronounced for adolescents (Marshal & Molina, 2006) and young adults (Van Eck, Markle, Dattilo, & Flory, 2014) with ADHD who have more comorbid CD and ODD symptoms.

Beliefs regarding the anticipated positive and negative effects of substances, such as better sex or fuzzy headedness after drinking alcohol, are known as "expectancies." A large literature exists on the development of these cognitions and their prospective associations with substance use, especially alcohol, as well as their changing nature with substance use experience and exposure (Voogt et al., 2017). Impulsivity is associated with positive expectancies (Hayaki et al., 2011), which may be a function of neurobiological vulnerability or environmental exposures (e.g., a family history of substance dependence) that are known to correlate with impulsivity traits. As such, a steadily growing literature is accumulating on substance expectancies among individuals with ADHD. Some research suggests increased positive expectancies in association with ADHD (Dattilo, Murphy, Van Eck, & Flory, 2013; Elmore, Nikolas, & Canu, 2018), but in other research not conducted with community samples, expectancies do not operate as expected. Two studies conducted in the PALS found lower levels of alcohol (Pedersen, Harty, Pelham, Gnagy, & Molina, 2014) and marijuana (Harty, Pedersen, Gnagy, Pelham, & Molina, 2015) expectancies, as well as weakened associations with substance use. Ultimately, continued research in these two populations, including additional methods such as measures of implicit expectancies (Pedersen et al., 2014), may be needed to determine whether cognitions about substances are driving use and reflecting different subjective experiences, and in what ways age and experience affect these associations.

Beliefs about the effects of marijuana, in particular, may explain heightened rates of marijuana use among adolescents with ADHD. Some young adults with ADHD who use marijuana perceive a beneficial, therapeutic effect of the drug on their ADHD symptoms—a perception that adolescent users may share. For instance, qualitative findings of young adults with ADHD reveal perceptions that marijuana improves negative mood and ADHD symptoms, and these perceptions may be one reason individuals with ADHD are at heightened risk for frequent and problematic cannabis use (Mitchell et al., 2018; Mitchell, Sweitzer, Tunno, Kollins, & McClernon, 2016). Research on this potential motivating perception among adolescents is needed, particularly as adolescents with ADHD are less likely to access medication treatment despite continued impairment over the teen years (e.g., Molina et al., 2013), at the same time that marijuana is becoming increasingly accessible and acceptable (Keyes et al., 2016). Moreover, the neurological and cognitive effects of adolescent marijuana use are not yet fully understood, especially for individuals with ADHD, and should be a priority for research on the outcomes of changing marijuana legislation (Compton et al., 2017). Preliminary evidence suggests that marijuana use in adolescence, especially early use, impairs neurocognitive abilities such as attention, memory, and cognitive control, along with their neural substrates (Ganzer, Broning, Kraft, Sack, & Thomasius, 2016; Gray & Squeglia, 2018), in contrast to the therapeutic effects that some users *perceive*; thus, these impairments may exacerbate the same preexisting deficits in youth with ADHD, though this theory lacks support to date (Kelly et al., 2017).

These pathways all reflect generalized mechanisms of substance use risk; that is, they are theorized to apply equally across substance classes. However, substance-specific pathways may play important roles as well (Chassin, Sher, et al., 2013; Molina & Pelham, 2014). For instance, adolescents with ADHD may experience unique responses to the effects of alcohol (e.g., greater sensitivity to its disinhibiting effects), which in turn may explain ADHD teens' risk for problematic alcohol use in particular (Weafer, Fillmore, & Milich, 2009). Similarly, the potentially symptom-reducing effects of stimulants (Ioannidis, Chamberlain, & Muller, 2014) or perceptions of marijuana's therapeutic effects specific to ADHD (Mitchell et al., 2016, 2018) may contribute to risk for the abuse of those specific substances, respectively.

Finally, clinical lore and public curiosity have heightened interest in the possible mediating role of stimulant medication in ADHD-related substance use risk. Stimulants effectively manage ADHD symptoms and should theoretically reduce substance use outcomes that might result from those symptoms (e.g., impulsively joining in with substance-using peers). Alternatively, it is possible that ADHD medication sensitizes youths' developing brains to its stimulating properties, thereby increasing their vulnerability to addiction, either to stimulants specifically, such as nicotine and cocaine, or to substances more generally (Kantak & Dwoskin, 2016; Kollins et al., 2009; Lambert, 2005; Lambert & Hartsough, 1998). A meta-analysis that pooled the results of 15 studies concluded that stimulant medication taken in childhood to manage ADHD had no effect on a range of substance use outcomes in adolescence/young adulthood (Humphreys, Eng, & Lee, 2013). One study from the MTA replicated these null effects using propensity score methods to adjust for potentially confounding variables that account for treatment selection effects (Molina et al., 2013). On the other hand, some studies have demonstrated positive effects of stimulant medication on *reducing* risk for substance misuse (e.g., Chang et al., 2014; Dalsgaard et al., 2014; Quinn et al., 2017; Wilens, Faraone, Biederman, & Gunawardene, 2003), with large effect sizes for adolescent samples (Schoenfelder, Faraone, & Kollins, 2014). There are, however, many methodological complexities in attempting to merge the results of these studies, particularly given research that suggests onset of medication after, versus prior to, puberty may differentially increase risk for SUD (Kantak & Dwoskin, 2016; Mannuzza et al., 2008). Additionally, the strict definition of substance misuse (hospitalizations or emergency department visits) used in several health registry studies that have found protective effects (Chang et al., 2014; Dalsgaard et al., 2014; Quinn et al., 2017) may contribute to the discrepancy. Given these mixed findings and the complex interrelations among changing medication regimens, ADHD symptoms, and covariates across time, studies are needed that appropriately analyze effects of timing, dosage, and type of ADHD medication.

Additional risk pathways certainly exist and likely operate in combination with one another. For example, a negative affect or negative reinforcement pathway, whereby individuals use substances to relieve unpleasant emotions rather than to actively foster positive ones, may develop later in adulthood (e.g., Koob, 2013; see Molina & Pelham, 2014, for review).

TREATMENT IMPLICATIONS

Substance Use Screening and Prevention

The substantial overlap between ADHD and substance use has important implications for treating adolescents with ADHD. First, practitioners should expand assessments of impairment for teens with ADHD beyond academic, social, familial, and behavioral domains to include substance use. ADHD is often treated in primary care, and brief substance abuse screening tools for use in this setting have been validated for adolescent patients irrespective of ADHD (e.g., for reviews, see Gray & Squeglia, 2018; Levy, Williams, & AAP Committee on Substance Use and Prevention, 2016). Importantly, however, impairment from substance use may sometimes mimic "late-onset" ADHD; thus, practitioners must rigorously diagnose both SUD and ADHD in adolescence by conducting a thorough assessment, including developmental history to track the emergence of ADHD symptoms and the co-occurrence of substance use (Riggs, 1998; Sibley et al., 2017).

Substance use screening should occur *early* (e.g., at the transition into middle school), before risk develops into entrenched substance use patterns (e.g., SUD) that become increasingly difficult to modify over time, because ADHD hastens escalation from initial experimentation to SUD across substance classes (Chassin et al., 2002; Kollins & Adcock, 2014; Molina et al., 2018; Rhodes et al., 2016; Sibley et al., 2014). Given overlap in risk factors for both ADHD-related impairment and substance use, effective treatment for ADHD and its related impairments (e.g., academic failure, delinquency) may in turn reduce risk for substance use.

One potential strategy for mitigating risk for substance use is to target malleable mediators and moderators of the link between ADHD and SUD. For instance, interventions that help caregivers bolster their effective parenting strategies, increase parental monitoring, and foster emotionally supportive relationships with their teens should not only reduce impairment due to ADHD symptoms but also buffer risk for substance abuse (Molina et al., 2012; Pollak, Poni, Gershy, & Aran, 2017; Sibley et al., 2014; Tandon et al., 2014). In fact, several parenting-based prevention programs specifically designed to target adolescent substance use have proven to be efficacious (Allen et al., 2016; Stanger, Scherer, Babbin, Ryan, & Budney, 2017; Winters, Fahnhorst, Botzet, Lee, & Lalone, 2012). Future research should test whether these programs are particularly helpful for teens with ADHD whose substance use risk may only be buffered by especially strong parenting.

Adolescent Substance Use Treatment

Although mental health providers focusing on ADHD as a primary treatment target may feel more comfortable referring patients for separate substance abuse treatment, an integrated multisystemic approach addressing both ADHD and substance use may prove more effective than treatments provided by isolated providers (Riggs, 1998). Despite fears by substance abuse treatment providers that stimulants will be abused, clinical studies of children with ADHD followed longitudinally do not support high rates of stimulant misuse (Molina et al., 2018; Wilens et al., 2006). Nonetheless, a clear ADHD diagnosis must be obtained by a thorough assessment (see DuPaul, Anastopoulos, & Kipperman, Chapter 13, this volume); cautious prescribing and surveillance are warranted; and in high-risk cases, physicians may wish to consider nonstimulant pharmacotherapy to deter abuse (Carpentier & Levin, 2017; Riggs, 1998).

Cognitive-behavioral therapy (CBT) and ecological family-based interventions are the most well-established, efficacious treatments for adolescent substance abuse (for reviews, see Gray & Squeglia, 2017; Hogue, Henderson, Ozechowski, & Robbins, 2014). Combining multiple treatment components is particularly beneficial. For instance, several efficacious intervention programs combine individual or group CBT with parent training, capitalizing on the important role of parents in adolescents' substance use outcomes (e.g., Winters et al., 2012). Others enhance parent- and group-based treatments with contingency management elements, which maximizes beneficial outcomes (e.g., Stanger et al., 2017). These treatments include some of the same components that are efficacious in treating ADHD and target common risk factors (e.g., rule-abiding behaviors, parenting), making them well-suited for the treatment of substance use problems in teens with ADHD (Sibley et al., 2014). However, treatment completion and outcomes are weakened in substance using adolescents with comorbid externalizing disorders (such as ADHD), indicating that these youth may benefit most from more comprehensive, multi-component interventions (Hogue et al., 2014). Brief substance use interventions (i.e., a few sessions) are generally not effective for adolescents (Gray & Squeglia, 2017), but one brief intervention that added a parent component demonstrated positive effects (Winters et al., 2012), again emphasizing the critical role of parents in reducing adolescent substance use.

Given the influence of peers on substance use among youth with ADHD (Belendiuk et al., 2016; Marshal & Molina, 2006), targeting social contexts in prevention efforts and involving peers in treatment programs may be warranted. Such peer-enhanced interventions have shown promise with young adults with SUD (Smith, Davis, Ureche, & Dumas, 2016), as have universal peer-led prevention programs with adolescents (MacArthur, Harrison, Caldwell, Hickman, & Campbell, 2016). There is some support for interactive school-based cannabis prevention programs among young adolescents—particularly more interactive as opposed to didactic programs (Lize et al., 2017). The efficacy of peer intervention programs for teens with ADHD specifically remains to be determined.

More recently, the portable electronic delivery of evidence-based treatments for adolescent substance use, such as text messaging and smartphone applications, has generated positive outcomes (Mason, Ola, Zaharakis, & Zhang, 2015; Gray & Squeglia, 2017). These types of eHealth and mHealth (electronic and mobile health) interventions may be especially engaging and acceptable to adolescents with ADHD, who might benefit from the active, stimulating characteristics of these game-like tools.

Future Directions

After three decades of research, substantial progress has been made in understanding the unique risk for substance abuse that ADHD confers and the various developmental pathways that either exacerbate or limit that susceptibility. With some exceptions, adolescents with ADHD tend to initiate substance use at younger ages, progress more quickly to heavy use, and are at higher risk for developing an SUD than their typically developing peers. Numerous mechanistic pathways have been identified, including delinquency, peer influences, expectancies, and distinct responses to the effects of substances. Protective factors, such as involved parenting and gender, can help offset this risk. However, considerable gaps remain in our knowledge. Examining the consequences of, and reasons for, marijuana use by youth with ADHD is an important avenue of future research, as access to marijuana and acceptability of use continue to increase. Future studies should examine the long-term effects of high-concentration caffeine, such as coffee and energy drinks, for youth with ADHD. In particular, the possible role of caffeine as a gateway to other stimulants of abuse should be explored. Moreover, it is important to measure adolescents' substance use *developmentally* in future research and practice to identify clinically relevant early signs of risk (Molina, Pelham, et al., 2007; Molina, Sibley, Pedersen, & Pelham, 2017; Sibley et al., 2014). Finally, the intersection between substance use and other risk-taking behaviors that are common in ADHD (e.g., driving while intoxicated, unsafe sex) should be investigated.

In addition to the need for research on the prevention and treatment of substance abuse for adolescents with ADHD, we encourage studies of resilience in ADHD. Identifying mutable factors that protect adolescents with ADHD from developing SUDs can help practitioners, parents, and policymakers prevent substance misuse and disorder for youth with ADHD. Additionally, research to date paints an unclear picture of the relation between stimulant treatment and risk for substance use in adolescents with ADHD. Rigorous studies that account for ADHD symptoms, the timing, dosage, and type of ADHD medication, as well as changing covariates over time will be necessary to draw more definitive conclusions about the protective or risk-exacerbating nature of stimulant medications. Finally, developing and promoting effective substance use treatments for teens with ADHD will likely require well-designed studies testing tailored, multipronged interventions that address a range of treatment targets.

References

Adisetiyo, V., & Gray, K. M. (2017). Neuroimaging the neural correlates of increased risk for substance use disorders in ADHD: A systematic review. *American Journal on Addictions, 26,* 99–111.

Allen, M. L., Garcia-Huidobro, D., Porta, C., Curran, D., Patel, R., Miller, J., & Borowsky, I. (2016). Effective parenting interventions to reduce youth substance use: A systematic review. *Pediatrics, 138*(2), e20154425.

American Psychiatric Association. (2013). *Diagnostic and statistical manual of mental disorders* (5th ed.). Arlington, VA: Author.

Arcos-Burgos, M., Vèlez, J. I., Solomon, B. D., & Muenke, M. (2012). A common genetic network underlies substance use disorders and disruptive or externalizing disorders. *Human Genetics, 131,* 917–929.

Babinski, D. E., Pelham, W. E., Jr., Molina, B. S. G., Gnagy, E. M., Waschbusch, D. A., Yu, J., . . . Karch, K. M. (2011). Late adolescent and young adult outcomes of girls diagnosed with ADHD in childhood: An exploratory investigation. *Journal of Attention Disorders, 15*(3), 204–214.

Barkley, R. A., Fischer, M., Edelbrock, C. S., & Smallish, L. (1990). The adolescent outcome of hyperactive children diagnosed by research criteria: I. An 8-year prospective follow-up study. *Journal of the American Academy of Child and Adolescent Psychiatry, 29*(4), 546–557.

Barkley, R. A., Fischer, M., Smallish, L., & Fletcher, K. (2003). Does the treatment of attention-deficit/hyperactivity disorder with stimulants contribute to drug use/abuse?: A 13-year prospective study. *Pediatrics, 111*(1), 97–109.

Barnes, G. M., Hoffman, J. H., Welte, J. W., Farrell, M. P., & Dintcheff, B. A. (2007). Adolescents' time use: Effects on substance use, delinquency and sexual activity. *Journal of Youth and Adolescence, 36,* 697–710.

Beauchaine, T. P., & McNulty, T. (2013). Comorbidities and continuities as ontogenic processes: Toward a developmental spectrum model of externalizing psychopathology. *Development and Psychopathology, 25*(4, Pt. 2), 1505–1528.

Belendiuk, K. A., Pedersen, S. L., King, K. M., Pelham, W. E., & Molina, B. S. G. (2016). Change over time in adolescent and friend alcohol use: Differential associations for youth with and without childhood attention-deficit/hyperactivity disorder (ADHD). *Psychology of Addictive Behaviors, 30*(1), 29–38.

Benson, K., Flory, K., Humphreys, K. L., & Lee, S. S. (2015). Misuse of stimulant medication among college students: A comprehensive review and meta-analysis. *Clinical Child and Family Psychology Review, 18,* 50–76.

Biederman, J., Petty, C. R., Wilens, T., Fraire, M. G., Purcell, C. A., Mick, E., . . . Faraone, S. V. (2008). Familial risk analysis of attention deficit hyperactivity disorder and substance use disorders. *American Journal of Psychiatry, 165*(1), 107–115.

Biederman, J., Wilens, T., Mick, E., Faraone, S. V., Weber, W., Curtis, S., . . . Soriano, J. (1997). Is ADHD a risk factor for psychoactive substance use disorders?: Findings from a four-year prospective follow-up study. *Journal of the American Academy of Child and Adolescent Psychiatry, 36*(1), 21–29.

Blevins, C. E., Stephens, R., & Abrantes, A. M. (2017). Motives for prescription stimulant misuse in a college sample: Characteristics of users, perception of risk, and consequences of use. *Substance Use and Misuse, 52*(5), 555–561.

Burke, J. D., Loeber, R., & Lahey, B. B. (2001). Which aspects of ADHD are associated with tobacco use in early adolescence? *Journal of Child Psychology and Psychiatry, 42*(4), 493–502.

Bussing, R., Mason, D. M., Bell, L., Porter, P., & Garvan, C. (2010). Adolescent outcomes of childhood attention-deficit/hyperactivity disorder in a diverse community sample. *Journal of the American Academy of Child and Adolescent Psychiatry, 49*(6), 595–605.

Carpentier, P., & Levin, F. R. (2017). Pharmacological treatment of ADHD in addicted patients: What does the literature tell us? *Harvard Review of Psychiatry, 25*(2), 50–64.

Castellanos-Ryan, N., Struve, M., Whelan, R., Banaschewski, T., Barker, G. J., Bokde, A. L. W., . . . IMAGEN Consortium. (2014). Neural and cognitive correlates of the common and specific variance across externalizing problems in young adolescence. *American Journal of Psychiatry, 171,* 1310–1319.

Center for Behavioral Health Statistics and Quality. (2016). Key substance use and mental health indicators in the United States: Results from the 2015 National

Survey on Drug Use and Health (HHS Publication No. SMA 16-4984, NSDUH Series H-51). Retrieved from *www.samhsa.gov/data.*

Chang, Z., Lichtenstein, P., Halldner, L., D'Onofrio, B., Serlachius, E., Fazel, S., . . . Larsson, H. (2014). Stimulant ADHD medication and risk for substance abuse. *Journal of Child Psychology and Psychiatry, 55*(8), 878–885.

Chang, Z., Lichtenstein, P., & Larsson, H. (2012). The effects of childhood ADHD symptoms on early-onset substance use: A Swedish twin study. *Journal of Abnormal Child Psychology, 40,* 425–435.

Chassin, L., & Barrera, M. (1997). Substance use escalation and substance use restraint among adolescent children of alcoholics. *Psychology of Addictive Behaviors, 7,* 3–20.

Chassin, L., Colder, C., Hussong, A., & Sher, K. J. (2016). Substance use and substance use disorders. In D. Cicchetti (Ed.), *Developmental psychopathology: Maladaptation and psychopathology* (pp. 833–897). Hoboken, NJ: Wiley.

Chassin, L., Pitts, S. C., & Prost, J. (2002). Binge drinking trajectories from adolescence to emerging adulthood in a high-risk sample: Predictors and substance abuse outcomes. *Journal of Consulting and Clinical Psychology, 70*(1), 67–78.

Chassin, L., Sher, K. J., Hussong, A., & Curran, P. (2013). The developmental psychopathology of alcohol use and alcohol disorders: Research achievements and future directions. *Development and Psychopathology, 25,* 1567–1584.

Compton, W. M., Volkow, N. D., & Lopez, M. F. (2017). Medical marijuana laws and cannabis use: Intersections of health and policy. *JAMA Psychiatry, 74*(6), 559–560.

Dalsgaard, S., Mortensen, P. B., Frydenberg, M., & Thomsen, P. H. (2014). ADHD, stimulant treatment in childhood and subsequent substance abuse in adulthood: A naturalistic long-term follow-up study. *Addictive Behaviors, 39*(1), 325–328.

Dattilo, L., Murphy, K. G., Van Eck, K., & Flory, K. (2013). Do ADHD symptoms moderate the relation between positive alcohol expectancies and alcohol-related outcomes? *ADHD Attention Deficit and Hyperactivity Disorders, 5,* 93–104.

Derefinko, K. J., Charnigo, R. J., Peters, J. R., Adams, Z. W., Milich, R., & Lynam, D. R. (2016). Substance use trajectories from adolescence through the transition to college. *Journal of Studies on Alcohol and Drugs, 77*(6), 924–935.

DeWit, D. J., Adlaf, E. M., Offord, D. R., & Ogborne, A. C. (2000). Age at first alcohol use: A risk factor for the development of alcohol disorders. *American Journal of Psychiatry, 157*(5), 745–750.

Donovan, J. E. (2009). Estimated blood alcohol concentrations for child and adolescent drinking and their implications for screening instruments. *Pediatrics, 123*(6), e975–e981.

Elkins, I. J., McGue, M., & Iacono, W. G. (2007). Prospective effects of attention-deficit/hyperactivity disorder, conduct disorder, and sex on adolescent substance use and abuse. *Archives of General Psychiatry, 64*(10), 1145–1152.

Elmore, A., Nikolas, M., & Canu, W. (2018). Positive alcohol expectancies mediate associations between ADHD behaviors and alcohol-related problems among college students. *Attention Deficit and Hyperactivity Disorders, 10*(1), 65–75.

Ernst, M. (2014). The triadic model perspective for the study of adolescent motivated behavior. *Brain and Cognition, 89,* 104–111.

Flory, K., & Lynam, D. R. (2003). The relation between attention deficit hyperactivity disorder and substance abuse: What role does conduct disorder play? *Clinical Child and Family Psychology Review, 6*(1), 1–16.

Galvan, A. (2013). The teenage brain: Sensitivity to rewards. *Current Directions in Psychological Science, 22*(2), 88–93.

Ganzer, F., Broning, S., Kraft, S., Sack, P., & Thomasius, R. (2016). Weighing the evidence: A systematic review on long-term neurocognitive effects of cannabis use in abstinent adolescents and adults. *Neuropsychological Review, 26,* 186–222.

Gittelman, R., Mannuzza, S., Shenker, R., & Bonagura, N. (1985). Hyperactive boys almost grown up: I. Psychiatric status. *Archives of General Psychiatry, 42*(10), 937–947.

Grant, B. F., & Dawson, D. A. (1998). Age of onset of drug use and its association with DSM-IV drug abuse and dependence: Results from the National Longitudinal Alcohol Epidemiologic Survey. *Journal of Substance Abuse, 10,* 163–173.

Gray, K. M., & Squeglia, L. M. (2018). Research review: What have we learned about adolescent substance use? *Journal of Child Psychology and Psychiatry, 59*(6), 618–627.

Groenman, A. P., Oosterlaan, J., Rommelse, N., Franke, B., Roeyers, H., Oades, R. D., . . . Faraone, S. V. (2013). Substance use disorders in adolescents with attention deficit hyperactivity disorder: A 4-year follow-up study. *Addiction, 108*(8), 1503–1511.

Hartsough, C. S., & Lambert, N. M. (1987). Pattern and progression of drug use among hyperactives and controls: A prospective short-term longitudinal study. *Journal of Child Psychology and Psychiatry, 28*(4), 543–553.

Harty, S. C., Pedersen, S. L., Gnagy, E. M., Pelham, W. E., & Molina, B. S. G. (2015). ADHD and marijuana-use expectancies in young adulthood. *Substance Use and Misuse, 50*(11), 1470–1478.

Hayaki, J., Herman, D. S., Hagerty, C. E., de Dios, M. A., Anderson, B. J., & Stein, M. D. (2011). Expectancies and self-efficacy mediate the effects of impulsivity on marijuana use outcomes: An application of the acquired preparedness model. *Addictive Behaviors, 36,* 389–396.

Hechtman, L., Weiss, G., & Perlman, T. (1984). Hyperactives as young adults: Past and current substance abuse and antisocial behavior. *American Journal of Orthopsychiatry, 54*(3), 415–425.

Hinshaw, S. P., Owens, E. B., Zalecki, C., Huggins, S. P., Montenegro-Nevado, A. J., Schrodek, E., & Swanson, E. N. (2012). Prospective follow-up of girls with attention-deficit/hyperactivity disorder into early adulthood: Continuing impairment includes elevated risk for suicide attempts and self-injury. *Journal of Consulting and Clinical Psychology, 80*(6), 1041–1051.

Hogue, A., Henderson, C. E., Ozechowski, T. J., & Robbins, M. S. (2014). Evidence base on outpatient behavioral treatments for adolescent substance use: Updates and recommendations 2007–2013. *Journal of Clinical Child and Adolescent Psychology, 43*(5), 695–720.

Humphreys, K. L., Eng, T., & Lee, S. S. (2013). Stimulant medication and substance use outcomes: A meta-analysis. *JAMA Psychiatry, 70*(7), 740–749.

Hussong, A., Bauer, D., & Chassin, L. (2008). Telescoped trajectories from alcohol initiation to disorder in children of alcoholic parents. *Journal of Abnormal Psychology, 117*(1), 63–78.

Ioannidis, K., Chamberlain, S. R., & Muller, U. (2014). Ostracising caffeine from the pharmacological arsenal for attention-deficit hyperactivity disorder—Was this a correct decision?: A literature review. *Journal of Psychopharmacology, 28*(9), 830–836.

Johnston, L. D., O'Malley, P. M., Miech, R. A., Bachman, J. G., & Schulenberg, J. E. (2017). *Monitoring the Future national survey results on drug use, 1975–2016: Overview, key findings on adolescent drug use.* Ann Arbor: Institute for Social Research, University of Michigan.

Kantak, K. M., & Dwoskin, L. (2016). Necessity for research directed at stimulant type and treatment-onset age to access the impact of medication on drug abuse vulnerability in teenagers with ADHD. *Pharmacology, Biochemistry and Behaviors, 145,* 24–26.

Katusic, S. K., Barbaresi, W. J., Colligan, R. C., Weaver, A. L., Leibson, C. L., & Jacobson, S. J. (2005). Psychostimulant treatment and risk for substance abuse among young adults with a history of attention-deficit/hyperactivity disorder: A population-based, birth cohort study. *Journal of Child and Adolescent Psychopharmacology, 15*(5), 764–776.

Kelly, C., Castellanos, F. X., Tomaselli, O., Lisdahl, K., Tamm, L., Jernigan, R., . . . MTA Neuroimaging Group. (2017). Distinct effects of childhood ADHD and cannabis use on brain functional architecture in young adults. *NeuroImage: Clinical, 13,* 188–200.

Keyes, K. M., Wall, M., Cerdá, M., Schulenberg, J., O'Malley, P. M., Galea, S., . . . Hasin, D. S. (2016). How does state marijuana policy affect US youth?: Medical marijuana laws, marijuana use and perceived harmfulness: 1991–2014. *Addiction, 111*(12), 2187–2195.

King, S. M., Iacono, W. G., & McGue, M. (2004). Childhood externalizing and internalizing psychopathology in the prediction of early substance use. *Addiction, 99,* 1548–1559.

Kollins, S. H., & Adcock, R. A. (2014). ADHD, altered dopamine neurotransmission, and disrupted reinforcement processes: Implications for smoking and nicotine dependence. *Progress in Neuro-Psychopharmacology and Biological Psychiatry, 52,* 70–78.

Kollins, S. H., English, J., Robinson, R., Hallyburton, M., & Chrisman, A. K. (2009). Reinforcing and subjective effects of methylphenidate in adults with and without attention deficit hyperactivity disorder (ADHD). *Psychopharmacology, 204,* 73–83.

Komro, K. A., Maldonado-Molina, M. M., Tobler, A. L., Bonds, J. R., & Muller, K. E. (2007). Effects of home access and availability of alcohol on young adolescents' alcohol use. *Addiction, 102*(10), 1597–1608.

Koob, G. F. (2013). Addiction is a reward deficit and stress surfeit disorder. *Frontiers in Psychiatry, 4,* 72.

Lambert, N. (2005). The contribution of childhood ADHD, conduct problems, and stimulant treatment to adolescent and adult tobacco and psychoactive substance abuse. *Ethical Human Psychology and Psychiatry,* 7(3), 197–221.

Lambert, N. M., & Hartsough, C. S. (1998). Prospective study of tobacco smoking and substance dependencies among samples of ADHD and non-ADHD participants. *Journal of Learning Disabilities, 31*(6), 533–544.

Lee, S. S., Humphreys, K. L., Flory, K., Liu, R., & Glass, K. (2011). Prospective association of childhood attention-deficit/hyperactivity disorder (ADHD) and substance use and abuse/dependence: A meta-analytic review. *Clinical Psychology Review, 31*(3), 328–341.

Levy, S. J., Williams, J. F., & AAP Committee on Substance Use and Prevention. (2016). Substance use screening, brief intervention, and referral to treatment. *Pediatrics, 138*(1), e20161211.

Lize, S. E., Iachini, A. L., Tang, W., Tucker, J., Seay, K. D., Clone, S., . . . Browne, T. (2017). A meta-analysis of the effectiveness of interactive middle school cannabis prevention programs. *Prevention Science, 18,* 50–60.

MacArthur, G. J., Harrison, S., Caldwell, D. M., Hickman, M., & Campbell, R. (2016). Peer-led interventions to prevent tobacco, alcohol and/or drug use among young people aged 11–21 years: A systematic review and meta-analysis. *Addiction, 111,* 391–407.

Mannuzza, S., Klein, R., Bessler, A., Malloy, P., & LaPadula, M. (1998). Adult psychiatric status of hyperactive boys grown up. *American Journal of Psychiatry, 155*(4), 493–498.

Mannuzza, S., Klein, R., Bonagura, N., Malloy, P., Giampino, T. L., & Addalli, K. A. (1991). Hyperactive boys almost grown up: V. Replication of psychiatric status. *Archives of General Psychiatry, 48*(1), 77–83.

Mannuzza, S., Klein, R., Truong, N. L., Moulton, J. L., Roizen, E. R., Howell, K. H., & Castellanos, F. X. (2008). Age of methylphenidate treatment initiation in children with ADHD and later substance abuse: Prospective follow-up into adulthood. *American Journal of Psychiatry, 165*(5), 604–609.

Marshal, M. P., & Molina, B. S. G. (2006). Antisocial behaviors moderate the deviant peer pathway to substance use in children with ADHD. *Journal of Clinical Child and Adolescent Psychology, 35*(2), 216–226.

Martel, M. M., Nigg, J. T., & von Eye, A. (2009). How do trait dimensions map onto ADHD symptom domains? *Journal of Abnormal Child Psychology, 37,* 337–348.

Martel, M. M., Pierce, L., Nigg, J. T., Jester, J. M., Adams, K., Puttler, L. I., . . . Zucker, R. A. (2009). Temperament pathways to childhood disruptive behavior and adolescent substance abuse: Testing a cascade model. *Journal of Abnormal Child Psychology, 37,* 363–373.

Mason, M., Ola, B., Zaharakis, N., & Zhang, J. (2015). Text messaging interventions for adolescent and young adult substance use: A meta-analysis. *Prevention Science, 16,* 181–188.

Masten, A. S., Faden, V. B., Zucker, R. A., & Spear, L. P. (2008). Underage drinking: A developmental framework. *Pediatrics, 121*(S4), S235–S251.

McCarty, C. A., Ebel, B. E., Garrison, M. M., DiGiuseppe, D. L., Christakis, D. A., & Rivara, F. P. (2004). Continuity of binge and harmful drinking from late adolescence to early adulthood. *Pediatrics, 114*(3), 714–719.

Milberger, S., Biederman, J., Faraone, S. V., Chen, L., & Jones, J. (1997). ADHD is associated with early initiation of cigarette smoking in children and adolescents. *Journal of the American Academy of Child and Adolescent Psychiatry, 36*(1), 37–44.

Mitchell, J. T., Belendiuk, K. A., Howard, A. L., Stehli, A., Lu, B., Swanson, J. M., . . . Molina, B. S. G. (2019). Tobacco smoking progression among young adults diagnosed with ADHD in childhood: A 16-year longitudinal study of children with and without ADHD. *Nicotine and Tobacco Research, 21*(5), 638–647.

Mitchell, J. T., Sweitzer, M., Tunno, A., Hagmann, C., Kollins, S. H., & McClernon, F. J. (2016). "I use weed for my ADHD": A qualitative analysis of online forum discussions on cannabis and ADHD. *PLOS ONE, 11*(5), e0156614.

Mitchell, J. T., Weisner, T. S., Jensen, P. S., Murray, D. W., Molina, B. S. G., Arnold, L. E., . . . Nguyen, J. L. (2018). How substance users with ADHD perceive the relationship between substance use and emotional functioning. *Journal of Attention Disorders, 22*(Suppl. 9), 49S–60S.

Moffitt, T. E., Arseneault, L., Belsky, D., Dickson, N., Hancox, R. J., Harrington, H., . . . Caspi, A. (2011). A gradient of childhood self-control predicts health, wealth, and public safety. *Proceedings of the National Academy of Sciences of the USA, 108*(7), 2693–2698.

Molina, B. S. G. (2011). Delinquency and substance use in attention deficit hyperactivity disorder: Adolescent and young adult outcomes in developmental context. In S. W. Evans & B. Hoza (Eds.), *Treating attention deficit hyperactivity disorder: Assessment and intervention in developmental context* (pp. 19-1–19-52). Kingston, NJ: Civic Research Institute.

Molina, B. S. G., Flory, K., Hinshaw, S. P., Greiner, A. R., Arnold, L. E., Swanson, J. M., . . . Wigal, T. (2007a). Delinquent behavior and emerging substance use in the MTA at 36 months: Prevalence, course, and treatment effects. *Journal of the American Academy of Child and Adolescent Psychiatry, 46*(8), 1027–1039.

Molina, B. S. G., Gnagy, E. M., Joseph, H. M., & Pelham, W. E. (2016, November 27).

Antisocial alcoholism in parents of adolescents and young adults with childhood ADHD. *Journal of Attention Disorders*. [Epub ahead of print]

Molina, B. S. G., Hinshaw, S. P., Arnold, L. E., Swanson, J. M., Pelham, W. E., Hechtman, L., . . . MTA Cooperative Group. (2013). Adolescent substance use in the Multimodal Treatment Study of Attention-Deficit/Hyperactivity Disorder (ADHD) (MTA) as a function of childhood ADHD, random assignment to childhood treatments, and subsequent medication. *Journal of the American Academy of Child and Adolescent Psychiatry, 52*(3), 250–263.

Molina, B. S. G., Howard, A. L., Swanson, J. M., Stehli, A., Mitchell, J. T., Kennedy, T. M., . . . Hoza, B. (2018). ADHD-related substance use in early adulthood is rooted in adolescence: Findings from the MTA longitudinal study. *Journal of Child Psychology and Psychiatry, 59*(6), 692–702.

Molina, B. S. G., Marshal, M. P., Pelham, W. E., Jr., & Wirth, R. J. (2005). Coping skills and parent support mediate the association between childhood attention-deficit/hyperactivity disorder and adolescent cigarette use. *Journal of Pediatric Psychology, 30*(4), 345–357.

Molina, B. S. G., & Pelham, W. E. (2003). Childhood predictors of adolescent substance use in a longitudinal study of children with ADHD. *Journal of Abnormal Psychology, 112*(3), 497–507.

Molina, B. S. G., & Pelham, W. E. (2014). Attention-deficit/hyperactivity disorder and risk of substance use disorder: Developmental considerations, potential pathways, and opportunities for research. *Annual Review of Clinical Psychology, 10*(1), 607–639.

Molina, B. S. G., Pelham, W. E., Cheong, J., Marshal, M. P., Gnagy, E. M., & Curran, P. J. (2012). Childhood attention-deficit/hyperactivity disorder (ADHD) and growth in adolescent alcohol use: The roles of functional impairments, ADHD symptom persistence, and parental knowledge. *Journal of Abnormal Psychology, 121*, 922–935.

Molina, B. S. G., Pelham, W. E., Gnagy, E. M., Thompson, A. L., & Marshal, M. P. (2007). Attention deficit/hyperactivity disorder risk for heavy drinking and alcohol use disorder is age-specific. *Alcoholism: Clinical and Experimental Research, 31*(4), 643–654.

Molina, B. S. G., Sibley, M. H., Pedersen, S. L., & Pelham, W. E., Jr. (2017). The Pittsburgh ADHD Longitudinal Study (PALS). In L. Hechtman (Ed.), *Attention deficit hyperactivity disorder: Adult outcome and its predictors* (pp. 105–156). New York: Oxford University Press.

Molina, B. S. G., Smith, B. H., & Pelham, W. E. (1999). Interactive effects of attention deficit hyperactivity disorder and conduct disorder on early adolescent substance use. *Psychology of Addictive Behaviors, 13*(4), 348–358.

Moss, H. B., Chen, C. M., & Yi, H. (2014). Early adolescent patterns of alcohol, cigarettes, and marijuana polysubstance use and young adult substance use outcomes in a nationally representative sample. *Drug and Alcohol Dependence, 136*, 51–62.

Moss, H. B., Chen, C. M., & Yi, H. (2014). Early adolescent patterns of alcohol, cigarettes, and marijuana polysubstance use and young adult substance use outcomes in a nationally representative sample. *Drug and Alcohol Dependence, 136*, 51–62.

Ottosen, C., Petersen, L., Larsen, J. T., & Dalsgaard, S. (2016). Gender differences in associations between attention-deficit/hyperactivity disorder and substance use disorder. *Journal of the American Academy of Child and Adolescent Psychiatry, 55*(3), 227–234.

Pagano, M. E., Delos-Reyes, C. M., Wasilow, S., Svala, K. M., & Kurtz, S. P. (2016). Smoking cessation and adolescent treatment response with comorbid ADHD. *Journal of Substance Abuse Treatment, 70*, 21–27.

Palmer, R. H. C., Young, S. E., Hopfer, C. J., Corley, R. P., Stallings, M. C., Crowley, T. J., & Hewitt, J. K. (2009). Developmental epidemiology of drug use and abuse in adolescence and young adulthood: Evidence of generalized risk. *Drug and Alcohol Dependence, 102*(1–3), 78–87.

Pedersen, S. L., Harty, S. C., Pelham, W. E., Gnagy, E. M., & Molina, B. S. G. (2014). Differential associations between alcohol expectancies and adolescent alcohol use as a function of childhood ADHD. *Journal of Studies on Alcohol and Drugs, 75,* 145–152.

Pierce, J. P., & Gilpin, E. (1996). How long will today's new adolescent smoker be addicted to cigarettes? *American Journal of Public Health, 86*(2), 253–256.

Pollak, Y., Poni, B., Gershy, N., & Aran, A. (2017). The role of parental monitoring in mediating the link between adolescent ADHD symptoms and risk-taking behavior. *Journal of Attention Disorders.* [Epub ahead of print]

Quinn, P. D., Chang, Z., Hur, K., Gibbons, R. D., Lahey, B. B., Rickert, M. E., . . . D'Onofrio, B. M. (2017). ADHD medication and substance-related problems. *American Journal of Psychiatry, 174*(9), 877–885.

Quinn, P. D., Pettersson, E., Lundström, S., Anckarsäter, H., Långström, N., Gumpert, C. H., . . . D'Onofrio, B. M. (2016). Childhood attention-deficit/hyperactivity disorder symptoms and the development of adolescent alcohol problems: A prospective, population-based study of Swedish twins. *American Journal of Medical Genetics B: Neuropsychiatric Genetics, 171,* 958–970.

Rhodes, J. D., Pelham, W. E., Gnagy, E. M., Shiffman, S., Derefinko, K. J., & Molina, B. S. G. (2016). Cigarette smoking and ADHD: An examination of prognostically relevant smoking behaviors among adolescents and young adults. *Psychology of Addictive Behaviors, 30*(5), 588–600.

Riggs, P. D. (1998). Clinical approach to treatment of ADHD in adolescents with substance use disorders and conduct disorder. *Journal of the American Academy of Child and Adolescent Psychiatry, 37*(3), 331–332.

Rudd, R. A., Aleshire, N., Zibbell, J. E., & Gladden, R. M. (2016). Increases in drug and opioid overdose deaths—United States, 2000–2014. Retrieved from *www.cdc.gov/mmwr/preview/mmwrhtml/mm6450a3.htm.*

Schoenfelder, E. N., Faraone, S. V., & Kollins, S. H. (2014). Stimulant treatment of ADHD and cigarette smoking: A meta-analysis. *Pediatrics, 133*(6), 1070–1080.

Secades-Villa, R., Garcia-Rodriguez, O., Chelsea, J. J., Wang, S., & Blanco, C. (2015). Probability and predictors of the cannabis gateway effect: A national study. *International Journal of Drug Policy, 26*(2), 135–142.

Serra-Pinheiro, M. A., Coutinho, E. S. F., Souza, I. S., Pinna, C., Fortes, D., Araújo, C., . . . Mattso, P. (2013). Is ADHD a risk factor independent of conduct disorder for illicit substance use?: A meta-analysis and meta-regression investigation. *Journal of Attention Disorders, 17*(6), 459–469.

Sibley, M. H., Pelham, W. E., Jr., Molina, B. S. G., Coxe, S., Kipp, H., Gnagy, E. M., . . ., & Lahey, B. B. (2014). The role of early childhood ADHD and subsequent CD in the initiation and escalation of adolescent cigarette, alcohol, and marijuana use. *Journal of Abnormal Psychology, 123*(2), 362–374.

Sibley, M. H., Rohde, L. A., Swanson, J. M., Hechtman, L. T., Molina, B. S. G., Mitchell, J. T., . . . Stehli, A. (2018). Late-onset ADHD reconsidered with comprehensive repeated assessments between ages 10 and 25. *American Journal of Psychiatry, 175*(2), 140–149.

Skoglund, C., Chen, Q., Franck, J., Lichtenstein, P., & Larsson, H. (2015). Attention-deficit/hyperactivity disorder and risk for substance use disorders in relatives. *Biological Psychiatry, 77,* 880–886.

Smith, D. C., Davis, J. P., Ureche, D. J., & Dumas, T. M. (2016). Six month outcomes of a peer-enhanced community reinforcement approach for emerging adults with substance misuse: A preliminary study. *Journal of Substance Abuse Treatment, 61,* 66–73.

Spear, L. P. (2000). The adolescent brain and age-related behavioral manifestations. *Neuroscience and Biobehavioral Reviews, 24,* 417–463.

Stanger, C., Scherer, E. A., Babbin, S. F., Ryan, S. R., & Budney, A. J. (2017). Abstinence based incentives plus parent training for adolescent alcohol and other substance misuse. *Psychology of Addictive Behaviors.* [Epub ahead of print]

Steinberg, L. (2010). A dual systems model of adolescent risk-taking. *Developmental Psychobiology, 52*(3), 216–224.

Substance Abuse and Mental Health Services Administration, Center for Behavioral Health Statistics and Quality. (2013, January 24). *The DAWN Report: Emergency department visits involving attention deficit/hyperactivity disorder stimulant medications.* Rockville, MD: Author.

Tandon, M., Tillman, R., Spitznagel, E., & Luby, J. (2014). Parental warmth and risks of substance use in children with attention-deficit/hyperactivity disorder. *Addiction Research and Theory, 22*(3), 239–250.

Tarter, R. E., Kirisci, L., Habeych, M., Reynolds, M., & Vanyukov, M. (2004). Neurobehavior disinhibition in childhood predisposes boys to substance use disorder by young adulthood: Direct and mediated etiologic pathways. *Drug and Alcohol Dependence, 73,* 121–132.

Tercyak, K. P., Lerman, C., & Audrain, J. (2002). Association of attention-deficit/hyperactivity disorder symptoms with levels of cigarette smoking in a community sample of adolescents. *Journal of the American Academy of Child and Adolescent Psychiatry, 41*(7), 799–805.

Van Eck, K., Markle, R. S., Dattilo, L., & Flory, K. (2014). Do peer perceptions mediate the effects of ADHD symptoms and conduct problems on substance use for college students? *Psychology of Addictive Behaviors, 28*(2), 431–442.

Van Eck, K., Markle, R. S., & Flory, K. (2012). Do conduct problems and sensation seeking moderate the association between ADHD and three types of stimulant use in a college population? *Psychology of Addictive Behaviors, 26*(4), 939–947.

Vitulano, M. L., Fite, P. J., Hopko, D. R., Lochman, J., Wells, K., & Asif, I. (2014). Evaluation of underlying mechanisms in the link between childhood ADHD symptoms and risk for early initiation of substance use. *Psychology of Addictive Behaviors, 28*(3), 816–827.

Voogt, C. M. Beusink, M., Kleinjan, R., Otten, R., Engels, K., Smit, & Kuntsche, E. (2017). Alcohol-related cognitions in children (aged 2–10) and how they are shaped by parental alcohol use: A systematic review. *Drug and Alcohol Dependence, 177,* 277–290.

Walker, L. R., Abraham, A. A., & Tercyak, K. P. (2010). Adolescent caffeine use, ADHD, and cigarette smoking. *Children's Health Care, 39,* 73–90.

Walther, C. A. P., Cheong, J., Molina, B. S. G., Pelham, W. E., Jr., Wymbs, B. T., Belendiuk, K. A., & Pedersen, S. L. (2012). Substance use and delinquency among adolescents with childhood ADHD: The protective role of parenting. *Psychology of Addictive Behaviors, 26*(3), 585–598.

Weafer, J., Fillmore, M. T., & Milich, R. (2009). Increased sensitivity to the disinhibiting effects of alcohol in adults with ADHD. *Experimental and Clinical Psychopharmacology, 17,* 113–121.

Wilens, T. E., & Biederman, J. (2006). Alcohol, drugs, and attention-deficit/hyperactivity disorder: A model for the study of addictions in youth. *Journal of Psychopharmacology, 20*(4), 580–588.

Wilens, T. E., Faraone, S. V., Biederman, J., & Gunawardene, S. (2003). Does stimulant therapy of attention-deficit/hyperactivity disorder beget later substance abuse?: A meta-analytic review of the literature. *Pediatrics, 111*(1), 179–185.

Wilens, T. E., Carrellas, N. W., Martelon, M., Yule, A. M., Fried, R., Anselmo, R., McCabe, S. E. (2017). Neuropsychological functioning in college students who misuse prescription stimulants. *American Journal on Addictions, 26*(4), 379–387.

Wilens, T. E., Gignac, M., Swezey, A., Monuteaux, M. C., & Biederman, J. (2006). Characteristics of adolescents and young adults with ADHD who divert or misuse their prescribed medications. *Journal of the American Academy of Child and Adolescent Psychiatry, 45*(4), 408–414.

Winters, K. C., Fahnhorst, T., Botzet, A., Lee, S., & Lalone, B. (2012). Brief intervention for drug-abusing adolescents in a school setting: Outcomes and mediating factors. *Journal of Substance Abuse Treatment, 42*, 279–288.

Zapolski, T. C. B., Pedersen, S. L., McCarthy, D. M., & Smith, G. T. (2014). Less drinking, yet more problems: Understanding African American drinking and related problems. *Psychological Bulletin, 140*(1), 188–233.

CHAPTER 12

Driving in Adolescents with ADHD and the Road to Intervention

Annie A. Garner

The study of driver behavior, driving outcomes, and traffic-related injury requires collective knowledge drawn from various disciplines, including engineering, human factors, cognitive psychology, epidemiology, among others. When driving behavior and safety are studied in the context of adolescence, knowledge of how brain development (Steinberg, 2007) and the social context of adolescence (Shope & Bingham, 2008) influence risk taking is also critical. The study of adolescent driving in the context of attention-deficit/hyperactivity disorder (ADHD) requires knowledge regarding the etiology and developmental pathways of ADHD, cognitive deficits associated with ADHD, and risk and protective factors associated with other domains of functioning that may likewise contribute to—or buffer against—driving risk in this population.

The developmental psychopathology framework has not been applied to the study of adolescent driving in ADHD, but it could help researchers looking to integrate knowledge and methods from various disciplines. First, a brief review of adolescent driving literature highlights that driving risk, driving problems, and poor driving outcomes are common in adolescence. Consistent with the developmental psychopathology concept that *normal and maladaptive behaviors exist on a continuum,* research comparing adolescents with ADHD to typically developing adolescents is reviewed and demonstrates that adolescents with ADHD are along the more impaired line of the continuum among adolescents with regard to their driving difficulties. The review of *risk and protective factors* is also consistent with the developmental psychopathology framework and sets the stage for discussion of interventions that target risk factors, mechanisms, and moderators of driving problems in adolescents with ADHD.

Driving Risk and Driving Problems in Adolescence

In 2014, an estimated six adolescents, ages 16–19 years, died every day due to a motor vehicle crash, and another 221,313 sustained injuries requiring an emergency room visit (Centers for Disease Control and Prevention [CDC], 2017). In comparison to older drivers, adolescent drivers exhibit more deficits in hazard recognition, maintenance of speed, navigation of intersections, and maintenance of lane position (Senserrick, 2006). In addition, adolescent drivers are more prone to exhibit inattention during driving, including looking away from the road for extended periods of time (Lee, Olsen, & Simons-Morton, 2006). These deficits in driving abilities play a significant role in the occurrence of crashes. One study of 795 serious crashes involving adolescents determined that adolescents were responsible for the error in nearly 80% of the crashes, with errors in recognition and performance being the most common (Curry, Hafetz, Kallan, Winston, & Durbin, 2011). Another study revealed that half of adolescents reported that they misjudged stopping distance needed to keep from rear-ending a driver (Olsen, Shults, & Eaton, 2013). A significant portion of adolescents also engage in risky driving behaviors, with up to 90% of adolescent drivers reporting that they engaged in at least one form of risky driving (Fergusson, Swain-Campbell, & Horwood, 2003). In this study, the most common risky driving behavior reported by adolescents was speeding (83%), followed by tailgating (49%), changing lanes without signaling (48%), and driving without a seat-belt (35%) (Fergusson et al., 2003). It is important to note that this study was conducted before personal smartphones became ubiquitous. In a more recent study, 45% of adolescents reported texting while driving at least once in the past month (Olsen et al., 2013). Similarly, up to half of adolescents in one study were classified as moderate- to high-risk drivers based on 3 years of driving data (Roman, Poulter, Barker, McKenna, & Rowe, 2015). These findings indicate that poor driving outcomes and risky driving behaviors are quite common among adolescents.

Adolescents with ADHD: A Higher Risk Group

Adolescent drivers with ADHD represent a subpopulation within the adolescent driving population that is likely at even greater risk for driving problems. A review of the literature highlights one major obstacle in understanding the nature and scope of driving risk among adolescents with ADHD: a lack of focus on adolescent drivers specifically. The majority of the research examining the impact of ADHD on driving problems includes samples of adults with some inclusion of adolescents, typically ages 18 years and older. In most these studies, the effects of age are controlled for statistically and on rare occasions are examined directly as a moderator. An even smaller literature focuses specifically on drivers with ADHD who are known to be most at risk: newly licensed drivers.

From a developmental psychopathology lens, drawing conclusions about the adolescent driving of individuals with ADHD based on samples that range in age from adolescence to adulthood is clearly problematic. Sroufe (2009) discussed the importance of examining maladaptation within the developmental stage of interest, in this case adolescence, rather than extending what is known about adult maladaptation downward to younger age ranges. Additionally, it is now well known that the prefrontal cortex continues to mature well beyond the adolescent years (Steinberg, 2007). Driving requires the integration of various cognitive functions, including rapid perception and integration of information, as well as rapid decision making and planning, which are largely governed by the still developing prefrontal cortex (Keating, 2007). Moreover, tasks that are repeated frequently, such as driving, can become more automatic and potentially require less executive function with age and experience. Given the differences in brain functioning and driving experience between adolescents and adults, it does not make sense to lump adolescent drivers with ADHD in with adult drivers with ADHD without a careful examination of the effect of age and development on driving outcomes. Yet much of what is known about driving problems among individuals with ADHD is based on adult samples. When possible, in this chapter I review studies that specifically used adolescent samples, but I also include studies that included adolescents (≤ 19 years old) in their samples. I note when age was examined as a moderator or when analyses were conducted separately for different age groups.

Motor Vehicle Crashes

Given its public health relevance, much of the literature on ADHD driving outcomes has emphasized crash involvement as a primary outcome of interest. Estimates of the risk of crash associated with ADHD vary widely across studies. The earliest studies examining driving outcomes involved adolescents and young adults who were recruited from a university medical center specializing in ADHD (Weiss, Hechtman, Perlman, Hopkins, & Wener, 1979; Barkley, Guevremont, Anastopoulos, DuPaul, & Shelton, 1993; Barkley, Murphy, & Kwasnik, 1996). In a particularly influential study (Barkley et al., 1993), parents of 35 individuals with ADHD and 36 individuals without ADHD, who were part of a research study at ages 12–18 years were mailed a packet of questionnaires when children were between ages 16 and 22 (M = 19.1, SD = 1.7). These questionnaires assessed current symptoms of ADHD, oppositional defiant disorder (ODD), conduct disorder (CD), and driving behavior and outcomes. Although individuals with ADHD did not differ between controls in terms of involvement in at least one crash (57.1 and 39.8%, respectively), they were significantly more likely to be involved in multiple crashes (40.0 and 5.6%, respectively) and were more likely to be deemed at fault for these car crashes than were controls (48.6 and 11.1%, respectively). The authors reported the startling statistic that the average frequency of crashes was four times greater in the ADHD group than in the control group. In a second study, Barkley et al. (1996), using a small clinic-based sample (ADHD n = 25 and control n = 23) with a broader age range (17–30 years), replicated the earlier findings and also found that individuals with ADHD had a fourfold increased risk of being the driver in a crash involving physical injuries, suggesting that the types of crashes individuals with ADHD experience are quite serious. Although much credit is due to these early studies for highlighting an area of ADHD impairment not previously considered, the sample sizes were quite small and may have represented a sample that was more severely impaired than might be typically seen in general clinic-based samples.

A recent study included a large sample of adolescent and young adult drivers identified from six New Jersey primary care practices (Curry, Metzger, Pfeiffer, Elliott, Winston, & Power, 2017). The relation between ADHD status and crash involvement in a sample of 2,479 drivers with ADHD and 15,865 drivers without ADHD was assessed. Electronic medical records data indicating ADHD status was linked to individuals' New Jersey driving police-reported crash records. Findings indicated that male and female adolescents and young adults with ADHD were more likely to crash at earlier ages and at greater frequencies than adolescents and young adults without ADHD. Notably, the hazard ratios (1.42 and 1.25 for males and females, respectively) reported in this longitudinal study were more modest than those reported in previous cross-sectional studies (Barkley et al., 1993, 1996). Differences in estimates of risk might be explained by differences in study design. As a longitudinal study, Curry et al. (2017) were able to use statistics (e.g., hazard ratio) that were less subject to bias than statistics used by cross-sectional studies. Similarly, findings from a meta-analysis, which is also designed to integrate findings across studies and reduce bias, were also more modest (Vaa, 2014). Specifically, combining results of 16 studies, with a mix of clinic- and community-based samples, Vaa found that ADHD status does increase risk of crashes but reported a less startling statistic (relative risk = 1.23) than did early studies (e.g., Barkley et al., 1996). Comparison of estimates across these various methodologies highlight the importance of using larger samples, longitudinal studies, and statistical methods designed to reduce bias—approaches that have been favored methods of developmental psychopathologists.

Studies involving other designs, such as population-based case–control studies and longitudinal birth cohort studies, have also found a significant relationship between ADHD diagnosis and crash risk. For example, a Canadian study used universal health care databases to compare rates of disruptive behavior disorders among males between ages 16 and 19 hospitalized for road trauma to those hospitalized for appendicitis (Redelmeir, Chan, & Lu, 2010). Males hospitalized for road trauma exhibited significantly higher rates of disruptive behavior disorder, including ADHD, than individuals hospitalized for appendicitis. Furthermore, having received psychopharmacological treatment for ADHD in the last 5 years was associated with increased risk for road trauma, further supporting the link between ADHD and crash risk (Redelmeier et al., 2010). Similarly, in a longitudinal birth cohort study of 941 children followed from birth to age 21 in New Zealand, researchers examined the association between parent- and teacher-rated symptoms of ADHD (termed *attentional difficulties* in the study) at age 13 and driving outcomes, including crashes involving injury at ages 18 and 21 (Woodward, Fergusson, & Horwood, 2000). After controlling for relevant demographic variables and correcting for multiple comparisons, several previously significant associations were reduced to nonsignificance. ADHD symptoms remained a significant predictor of only 1 of 11 driving outcomes; specifically, ADHD symptom severity at age 13 significantly predicted motor vehicle crashes involving injury 5–8 years later.

In another study using data from several longitudinal, population-based registers in Sweden, Chang, Lichtenstein, D'Onofrio, Sjölander, and Larsson (2014) found that individuals with ADHD experience significantly higher rates of crashes resulting in an emergency hospital visit or death than did those without ADHD, with hazards ratios ranging from 1.45 to 1.47 adjusted for covariates. Of note, given that the age of the sample ranged from ages 18–46, analyses were conducted separately by age groups (young and middle aged) and no significant differences with regard to the risk associated with ADHD and crashes were found across age groups (Chang et al., 2014). However, the authors did not specify how the young and middle-aged groups were defined, making it difficult to determine whether the null finding was influenced by potentially grouping adult drivers with adolescent and young adult drivers.

A final national study (Aduen, Kofler, Cox, Sarver, & Lunsford, 2015) recruited participants ages 16–75 years for a prospective naturalistic study of driver behavior and used baseline self-report data to determine whether participants met diagnostic criteria for ADHD. The relationship between baseline diagnosis and self-reported crash involvement at baseline was examined. Individuals meeting diagnostic criteria for ADHD were at increased risk for multiple collisions (odds ratio = 2.21). Since this sample does not suffer from potential biases in recruitment that might occur when studies recruit specifically based on ADHD status, the findings are especially compelling. However, a notable limitation of this study is that rather than calculating odds ratios separately for age groups, age was only controlled for in analyses.

Although the body of existing studies indicates an association between ADHD and crash risk, additional studies examining this association across development are needed. A focus on *developmental pathways* is sorely needed in this regard. Developmental pathways include trajectories of both adaptive and maladaptive functioning exhibited by individuals across the lifespan (Rutter & Sroufe, 2000). Applied to driving research, an examination of various trajectories of driving outcomes (e.g., crashes, tickets) using latent growth curve modeling, a person-oriented statistical approach commonly used in developmental psychopathology research (Sterba & Bauer, 2010), has recently been used to understand adolescent driving in nonclinical samples of adolescents (Roman et al., 2015; Simmons-Morton, Cheon, Guo, & Albert, 2013). Applying this approach to samples of individuals with ADHD across development could lead to a better understanding of the heterogeneity in driving outcomes experienced by individuals with ADHD. For example, one pathway could represent a group of individuals with ADHD who exhibit a high number of crashes/tickets across development. Another pathway could represent a group of individuals with ADHD who have high numbers of crashes/tickets as newly licensed/early drivers. A third pathway could include individuals with ADHD with a low number of crashes/tickets across development (i.e., individuals with ADHD who are not prone to poor/risky driving). While treatment studies with long-term follow-ups have been used to examine differences in driving outcomes across individuals with and without ADHD (Roy et al., in press; Thompson, Molina, Pelham, & Gnagy, 2007), they have yet to be used to identify driving trajectories experienced by individuals with ADHD across the lifespan.

Other Driving Outcomes

Many of the previously reviewed studies also examined other driving outcomes, including history of traffic violations or citations, general driving behaviors, and engagement in risky driving behaviors. As such, our knowledge of the relationship between ADHD in adolescents and these driving outcomes suffers from many of the same limitations (e.g., studies not focusing on adolescent populations). Still, the evidence suggests that ADHD, generally as well as in adolescence, is linked to negative driving outcomes beyond crash risk.

Analyses of driving violations reported by adolescents and young adults who participated in the Multimodal Treatment of ADHD (MTA) study revealed that ADHD diagnosis predicted greater frequency of driving violations (Hoza et al., 2013). It appears that speeding violations are most commonly experienced by individuals with ADHD (Vaa, 2014). Violations for driving under the influence of a substance are not statistically significant in most studies (Barkley et al., 1993; Lambert, 1995; Barkley et al., 1996), with one exception (Woodward et al., 2000). A study of newly licensed adolescent drivers with ADHD (Narad et al., 2015) highlights that negative driving outcomes, such as fines and points on licenses, start early in the driving histories of individuals with ADHD. Moreover, the consequences reported by newly licensed adolescent drivers with ADHD are more severe (e.g., required to take remedial driving classes and having greater fines) than those reported by their peers, suggesting that the type of infractions adolescents with ADHD engage in are more serious (Narad et al., 2015).

Other studies have assessed problematic driving behaviors of individuals with ADHD using psychometrically valid measures developed by driving researchers. For example, the Manchester Driving Behavior Questionnaire (DBQ; Reason, Manstead, Stradling, Baxter, & Campbell, 1990) was developed to assess three domains of driving problems: violations that reflect deliberate rule-breaking behaviors; errors defined as failures in observation or judgment that pose a hazard for self and others on road; and lapses, defined as absentminded behaviors with consequences mainly for the perpetrator, posing no threat to other road users. Some researchers have used a shorter version of the questionnaire containing two domains: violations and faults (combining lapses and errors) (Rosenbloom & Wultz, 2011). Researchers using this measure in adult samples that include some adolescents (≥ 18 years old) have found that individuals with ADHD report higher total DBQ scores, as well as higher subscale scores (Fried et al., 2006; Groom, van Loon, Chapman, & Hollis, 2015; Reimer et al., 2005; Rosenbloom & Wultz, 2011), though these differences do not always reach statistical significance (Rosenbloom & Wultz, 2011). One study found that males, but not females, with ADHD reported greater levels of faults (e.g., lapses and errors) in driving than controls, and that individuals with ADHD, regardless of sex, did not differ from controls with regard to their violation scores (Rosenbloom & Wultz, 2011). Only one study has compared newly licensed adolescents with and without a childhood history of ADHD on driving problems, and no statistical differences between the two groups were found (Garner et al., 2014). The lack of differences in driving problems across groups could be interpreted in two ways. First, null findings could indicate that all newly licensed drivers experience driving problems, and that differences in driving problems do not emerge until later in adolescence or even adulthood. Alternatively, it may be that current ADHD, rather than childhood ADHD, increases driving problems. Thus, additional studies with narrower age ranges, with individuals currently meeting criteria for ADHD, are needed to better understand the impact of ADHD on problematic driving behaviors in adolescence.

Simulated and Naturalistic Driving

Relying on self- and other-report of driving outcomes leads to concerns about bias and accuracy of this report. Driving simulators offer an opportunity to objectively and safely assess driving problems. Many studies have compared driving performance in driving simulators in adult samples that included some adolescents. Consistent with self-report measures, individuals with ADHD experience more crashes in the driving simulator than do individuals without ADHD (Barkley et al., 1996; Fischer, Barkley, Smallish, & Fletcher, 2007; Oliver, Nigg, Cassavaugh, & Backs, 2012; Reimer, D'Ambrosio, Coughlin, Fried, & Biederman, 2007). Individuals with ADHD also have difficulty maintaining lane positioning or have increased swerving (Fuermaier et al., 2017; Groom et al., 2015). Other indicators of driving performance, including driving speed, steering control, and break reaction time, are at times found to be statistically different across groups (Fischer et al., 2007; Groom et al., 2015; Reimer, Mehler, D'Ambrosio, & Fried, 2010) but not consistently (Barkley, Murphy, DuPaul, & Bush, 2002). The two studies comparing driving simulator performance across adolescents with and without ADHD yielded inconsistent findings (Narad et al., 2013; Stavrinos et al., 2016). Again, the issue of whether adolescents currently meet diagnostic criteria for ADHD and whether this difference across studies explains mixed findings is raised. Although neither study reported significant differences in terms of crashes in the driving simulator across groups (Narad et al., 2013; Stavrinos et al., 2016), the study sample with adolescents currently meeting criteria for ADHD indicated that adolescents with ADHD exhibit greater swerving and difficulty maintaining speed than those without ADHD (Narad et al., 2013). In contrast, the study comparing adolescents with a childhood history of ADHD to controls did not replicate these differences (Stavrinos et al., 2016). Thus, it appears that current, not past, ADHD symptoms confer risk of driving problems.

Naturalistic studies, which use in-car technologies to record continuous driving data over extended periods of time, are an ecologically valid method of studying driving behavior and offer an opportunity to document true rates of crashes and near crashes. These types of studies are rare given the logistical challenges and costs. A recent study of 15.5- to 16-year-old adolescents examined differences in naturalistic driving among adolescents with (n = 10) and without (n = 45) ADHD for 15–24 months across the permit and early licensure (first 6 months) phases of driving (Klauer, Ollendick, Ankem, & Dingus, 2017). Findings indicated that adolescents with ADHD were significantly more likely to be involved in a crash or near-crash and exhibit greater levels of risky driving and driving behaviors characterized as "inexperienced" than their peers (Klauer et al., 2017). Adolescents with ADHD were also significantly more likely than their peers to engage in secondary tasks known to increase crash risk, including cell phone use and interacting with passengers (Klauer et al., 2017). A naturalistic driving study of young adults found similar results and also reported differences in the causes of abrupt stopping (g-force events) across individuals with and without ADHD (Merkel et al., 2016). Specifically, events experienced by young adults with ADHD were due to risky, illegal, hyperactive–impulsive, and distracted behaviors, and tended to occur more frequently in the presence of peers and adverse driving conditions (e.g., rain) in comparison to controls (Merkel et al., 2016). The causes of events experienced by controls were attributable to defensive driving or lapses in attention (Merkel et al., 2016).

Summary

In summary, having an ADHD diagnosis is associated with an increased risk for involvement in multiple motor vehicle crashes, tickets/citations, and impaired driving in both driving simulations and real-world driving. The increased risk for crash involvement appears to be more modest than reported by early studies involving ADHD clinic-referred samples, which may not have been representative of the heterogeneity in impairments experienced by individuals with ADHD. With regard to tickets/citations, individuals with ADHD most consistently receive tickets/citations for speeding. Some studies report that individuals with ADHD also have more tickets/citations for particularly dangerous violations such as driving while intoxicated, but not consistently. Studies examining the relationship between tickets/violations and ADHD status use different methods of assessing history of tickets/violations, and this may account for differences in study findings. Finally, driving simulation studies and naturalistic studies indicate that individuals with ADHD exhibit problems with driving abilities (e.g., increased swerving, problems with steering control), and exhibit riskier driving behaviors and greater distraction while driving than individuals without ADHD. Although many of the reviewed studies included adolescent drivers in their samples, few studies examined age differences in a manner that honed in on the risk of adolescent independent drivers (ages 16–19 years).

Risk and Protective Factors in Adolescent Drivers with ADHD

The developmental psychopathology concept of disorders being *probabilistic, not deterministic* (Rutter & Sroufe, 2000) is relevant to research examining driving outcomes of individuals with ADHD, as these individuals display significant variability with regard to their driving outcomes, behaviors, and abilities (Fuermaier et al., 2017). In fact, experts in ADHD and driving remind the public, parents, and clinicians that drivers with ADHD are not destined to experience poor driving behaviors or outcomes (Aduen, Cox, Fabiano, Garner, & Kofler, 2019). Despite the variability in driving outcomes experienced by individuals with ADHD (Fuermaier et al., 2017), less attention has been given to examining risk and protective factors of driving problems among adolescents with ADHD.

Studies have examined the relationship between ADHD symptom dimensions and driving outcomes/problems to determine whether symptoms of inattention or hyperactivity–impulsivity confer risk for driving problems in ADHD samples. Study findings have been mixed. One study found that symptoms within the ADHD inattentive dimension, but not the hyperactive–impulsive dimension, were uniquely predictive of self-reported driving problems (e.g., errors, violations), as well as official crashes/tickets, in a sample of newly licensed adolescent drivers (Garner et al., 2014). However, other studies have reported that hyperactivity–impulsivity is predictive of self-report of driving problems (Groom et al., 2015; Thompson et al., 2007). A possible explanation for these study differences might be that studies using samples recruited from clinics (Groom et al., 2015; Thompson et al., 2007) might have been characterized by a restricted range of symptoms of inattention in adolescents, as these symptoms are known to persist at higher rates in this stage of development in comparison to symptoms of hyperactivity–impulsivity, which generally decrease (Holbrook et al., 2016; see Willcutt, Chapter 3, this volume) but likely have a greater variability. Additional research is needed given the inconclusiveness of the current literature on ADHD symptom dimensions and risk for driving problems.

Evidence suggests that comorbidity increases risk of driving problems for individuals with ADHD. For example, Vaa (2014) conducted a separate set of analyses in his meta-analysis of ADHD crash risk to estimate crash risk in samples with ADHD only and in ADHD samples with ODD and CD comorbidity. Relative risk was greater in samples with ODD and CD comorbidity (1.86) than in ADHD-only samples (1.35); however, both relative risks were significant, suggesting that ADHD alone is associated with increased risk for crash involvement, but that ODD and CD comorbidity confers additional risk for crashes in ADHD samples. It is possible that other psychiatric conditions commonly comorbid with ADHD might also increase risk for poor driving outcomes among adolescents with ADHD. In fact, one study found that depression alone increased risk of injury due to crash by a factor of 2.25 (Aduen et al., 2015). Thus, it is possible that adolescents with ADHD and depression could be especially at risk. One might posit that anxiety could be a protective, similar to the literature finding that comorbid anxiety lowers risk of aggression/delinquency among youth with ADHD (Falk, Lee, & Chorpita, 2017; Murray, Booth, Eisner, Obsuth, & Ribeaud, 2018; see Becker & Fogleman, Chapter 9, this volume). While this research has yet to be conducted with ADHD samples and driving specifically, one can look at research with non-ADHD samples to make predictions. For example, in a simulator study, Stephens and Groeger (2009) found that adult drivers with high levels of trait anxiety drove more carefully in the simulator (e.g., fewer speed violations, greater control of their steering wheel) than did adults with low levels of trait anxiety. However, a downward extension of these findings to adolescent drivers would be an error that developmental psychopathologists have cautioned against (Cicchetti & Rogosch, 2002). In nonclinical adolescent samples, anxiety symptoms and disorders have been linked to *increased* risk of driving problems, including greater levels of risky driving (Oltedal & Rundmo, 2006) and committing errors more frequently (Shahar, 2009). Moreover, in a study of 390 novice drivers, Scott-Parker, Watson, King, and Hyde (2013) found that anxiety, but not depression, uniquely predicted greater levels of risky driving. While an empirical question, research with adolescents without ADHD suggests that comorbid ADHD and anxiety would be associated with poorer driving outcomes. Finally, autism spectrum disorder (ASD) has also recently been identified as a comorbidity that increases risk of driving problems among individuals with ADHD (Classen, Monahan, & Wang, 2013). Examination of the impact of comorbidities on risk for driving problems in adolescents with ADHD is an area in need of additional research; particularly needed are studies that examine multiple comorbidities and consider both independent and interactive effects.

Researchers are beginning to look beyond the individual to consider relational factors that increase risk of driving problems among adolescents with ADHD. Specifically, parenting behaviors in childhood, including low monitoring/supervision and increased parental stress, predict risky driving (e.g., driving illegally, traffic violations) in adolescence and young adulthood in ADHD samples (Johnson, Jakubovski, Reed, & Bloch, 2017). In this study, empirically derived prognostic subgroups were identified, and adolescents who were considered to be at low risk for risky driving behaviors had a stronger parent–child relationship and parents who reported low levels of parent stress. Affiliation with deviant peers is another relational factor associated with crashes, citations, and illegal driving in adolescents with ADHD (Cardoos, Loya, & Hinshaw, 2013).

Contextual factors related to the driving environment have also been examined as potential protective/risk factors for drivers with ADHD. For example, in an experimental study, manual transmission was found to improve simulated driving performance relative to automatic transmission in a sample of adult licensed drivers with ADHD (Cox, Punja, et al., 2006). Another study found that low-demand monotonous drives, such as highway driving, were associated with poorer simulated driving performance than shorter drives characterized by frequent stopping and going (Reimer et al., 2010). Finally, a study of adolescent drivers with and without ADHD highlighted that whereas texting and driving negatively impact all adolescents' driving, this activity was particularly risky for adolescents with ADHD given that their baseline driving was already impaired (Narad et al., 2013). These studies highlight that changing the driving environment by reducing distractions, making driving a more engaging experience (e.g., manual transmission use), and choosing routes based on length and level of monotony could be another method of reducing risk for drivers with ADHD. However, all of these studies were conducted in controlled laboratory environments, so whether findings may be replicated in real-world conditions is a key area for future research.

Assessment of mediators and moderators of the relationship between ADHD and driving outcomes is an emerging area of study. For example, Kingery et al. (2015) examined the role of *visual inattention*, defined as eye glances lasting longer than 2 seconds (Klauer, Dingus, Neale, Sudweeks, & Ramsey 2006), as a mediator of driving simulator performance among adolescents with ADHD. Kingery et al. (2015) reported that extended eye glances mediated the relationship between ADHD status and poor driving in the simulator. Another study involving a sample of adolescents and young adults with a childhood history of ADHD found that current hyperactive–impulsive, not inattentive, symptoms mediated the relationship between having childhood ADHD and crashes/tickets (Thompson et al., 2007). Hoza et al. (2013) identified childhood positive self-perceptual bias as a mediator of the relationship between childhood ADHD and greater illegal driving frequency, traffic violations, and license suspensions in adolescence and young adulthood. In a final study, deviant peer affiliation mediated the relationship between greater inattention and crashes and citations (Cardoos et al., 2013). Moderation analyses in this study suggested that greater hyperactivity–impulsivity symptoms were predictive of crashes, but only for girls who do not affiliate with deviant peers. Studies of mediation and moderation offer clues into potential targets for intervention, including reduction of extended eye glances during driving and increased parental involvement and parental stress. Increased parental involvement could also have the added benefit of limiting adolescents' affiliation with deviant peers, who appear to be an important risk factor for poor driving outcomes in adolescents with ADHD.

The Road to Intervention

Delaying Licensure

Given the negative driving outcomes associated with ADHD, it may be tempting to encourage adolescents with ADHD to delay obtaining their license as a method to prevent these outcomes. The principle of *development as hierarchical* denotes that at each stage of development, individuals are tasked with stage-salient issues that build on previous stage-salient tasks and set the stage for the next developmental period's stage-salient tasks (Sroufe, 2009). Driving is one stage-salient task of adolescence and/or emerging adulthood that, if not resolved, could impact subsequent development. In the United States, driving has historically been one method of establishing autonomy from parents, and in many parts of the country, driving affords more opportunities for vocation and leisure (Keating, 2007). These are all important tasks for adolescents and emerging adults that set the stage for healthy development.

Whether intentional or not, it appears that adolescents with ADHD do in fact put off obtaining their license (Thompson et al., 2007; Curry et al., 2017). For example, in the Pittsburgh ADHD Longitudinal Study (PALS), the mean age for obtaining a license was 20.51 in the ADHD sample versus 17.52 for controls (Thompson et al., 2007). It is worth noting that adolescents in general appear to be postponing obtaining their license for a variety of reasons, including not having a car, the high cost of gas, the cost of driver's education, which is required by most Graduated Driver's License (GDL) laws, and "not getting around to it" (Teft, Williams, & Grabowski, 2013). Adolescents with ADHD face challenges related to obtaining their license that are unique (e.g., difficulty passing the written exam) (Almberg et al., 2015). Potential challenges to obtaining licensure for adolescents with ADHD that have not been examined in the literature but seem probable include difficulty keeping up with paperwork necessary to obtain a license (e.g., tracking hours spent in supervised driving) and parents not allowing them to pursue a license due to poor school performance.

Some researchers have called for increasing the driving age for all adolescent drivers (Steinberg, 2007). This recommendation is based on the dual systems framework of adolescence in which socioemotional networks that promote engagement in rewarding behaviors, including risk taking, peak earlier in development than cognitive control networks that regulate the aforementioned networks (Steinberg, 2007). However, individuals with ADHD exhibit a lag in brain development, particularly in the prefrontal cortex, which is part of the cognitive control network, compared to their peers (Shaw et al., 2007). Thus, increasing the driving age may not have the same effect for all adolescents, especially adolescents with ADHD, who may take longer to develop mature cognitive control networks. Even if this approach were to work, it would target only risky driving behaviors, not other types of driving problems experienced by adults with ADHD, such as impairments in driving performance (Fuermaier et al., 2017). As such, at this point, increasing the driving age for all adolescents may not be as effective in reducing risky driving as would be hoped.

It is also important to note that delaying licensure does not necessarily keep adolescents with ADHD from driving (Thompson et al., 2007), nor does it protect them from experiencing negative driving outcomes (Curry et al., 2017). In fact, adolescents and young adults with ADHD report driving without a license more frequently than do individuals without ADHD (Barkley et al., 1993; Hoza et al., 2013; Nada-Raja et al., 1997; Woodward et al., 2000; Fischer et al., 2007; Thompson et al., 2007). Practitioners and parents are encouraged to consider that driving is a skill that requires deliberate, guided practice with scaffolding and an emphasis on learning from errors in increasingly complex and risky situations to develop expertise (Keating, 2007). State GDL laws are in place for adolescents (under the age of 18) to allow practice under conditions known to reduce risk (e.g., restricting driving to daytime hours, limiting peers in the vehicle). Thus, an individual with ADHD who delays licensure until adulthood misses out on the opportunity to gain experience driving under safer conditions. The decision of when to allow adolescents with ADHD to obtain their license is a sensitive matter with serious implications for safety. As I discuss below, practitioners are encouraged to provide psychoeducation regarding the driving risks associated with ADHD and to work with parents (and adolescents) to weigh the pros and cons of the available choices.

Learning to Drive

GDL requirements often involve multiple steps that include studying for the written exam and tracking hours spent in practice driving with an adult. These steps can feel overwhelming and might deter an adolescent with ADHD who lacks motivation or who exhibits deficits in planning abilities. Moreover, given the high-risk nature of driving, one might hypothesize that to practice driving with a parent could be a recipe for conflict. Thus, it would not be surprising if adolescents with ADHD and their parents avoid or postpone practice driving. To my knowledge, there is a lack of empirically based recommendations for tackling the potential challenges faced during the learning-to-drive period for adolescents with ADHD. However, the following recommendations are offered for clinicians who are working with adolescents with ADHD and their parents as they break down tasks into manageable goals. With regard to obtaining a permit/license, the following recommendations are offered: (1) Direct the family to your state's Department of Motor Vehicles, so that families can find reliable and accurate information about the steps for licensure, as well as GDL restrictions, once they obtain their permit/license; (2) help break down the task of obtaining one's permit and driver's license by conducting a *task analysis* (breaking down a complicated task into its concrete, manageable components); and (3) make a plan for each step of the requirements, including filling out paperwork, studying for exams, and practicing driving with an adult. Each step should have SMART (specific, measurable, achievable, relevant, and time-bound) goals tied to them. If the adolescent is lacking in motivation, help him or her identify ways to reward themselves for reaching each goal.

As previously mentioned, teaching typically developing adolescents to drive involves scaffolding and guided practice. Adolescents with ADHD might require additional scaffolding and direct, objective feedback in real time. The Children's Hospital of Philadelphia has great resources to scaffold learning and set learning goals for each driving lesson (*https://injury.research.chop.edu/sites/default/files/documents/tdp_chop_2.5.18_3.pdf*).

Behavioral Contracts

Behavioral contracts are a commonly used tool in interventions targeting adolescents with ADHD, as they clearly outline both behavioral expectations and consequences for not meeting said expectations (e.g., Sibley et al., 2016). Such contracts could be useful in the context of driving as well. In fact, using behavioral contracts to set up expectations about driving is consistent with recommendations made by experts with regard to promoting driving safety in typically developing adolescents (Keating, 2007). Aside from sample contracts that are readily available online, this recommendation is typically given to families without much guidance on how to develop contracts. As clinicians work with adolescents with ADHD and their parents, they are encouraged to adapt behavioral contracts for typically developing adolescent drivers in a manner that directly targets the unique needs of adolescents with ADHD. Specifically, a contract that establishes the expectation that adolescents with ADHD will not be allowed to obtain their license until they have taken their ADHD medication as prescribed can be set up (e.g., adolescent takes medication as prescribed for at least 5 of 7 days per week for 2 months before being allowed to get a driver's permit). For adolescents with substance use history, parents might consider setting a contract that establishes that their adolescent with ADHD must agree to monthly drug tests before and after they obtain their license. Similarly, adolescent must agree to video monitoring in the car.

Medication

A systematic review of 15 randomized clinical trials, totaling 338 subjects (ADHD = 283; healthy controls = 34; ADHD participants not taking medication = 21), reviewed studies examining the effects of stimulants and nonstimulants on driving among individuals with ADHD (Gobbo & Louzã, 2014). Of these studies, five were conducted with exclusively adolescent samples (Cox, Humphrey, Merkel, Penberthy, & Kovatchev, 2004; Cox, Merkel, Penberthy, Kovatchev, & Hankin, 2004; Cox, Merkel, Moore, et al., 2006; Cox et al., 2008; Mikami et al., 2009), one was conducted with adolescents and young adults (Cox, Davis, Mikami, Singh, & Merkel,

2012), and two comprised adult samples that included adolescents (Biederman et al., 2012a, 2012b). The remainder of the studies included in the Gobbo and Louzã (2014) review comprised adults.

Studies of adolescent-only samples indicate that driving is improved under conditions of treatment with methylphenidate (MPH) extended release (OROS) relative to no medication (Cox, Humphrey, et al., 2004; Cox, Merkel, et al., 2006), and that OROS is more effective than immediate release (IR), particularly in the evening hours (Cox, Humphrey, et al., 2004; Cox, Merkel, et al., 2006). Drivers with ADHD also exhibit better driving performance when taking OROS compared to extended release mixed amphetamine salts (Cox, Merkel, et al., 2006). Moreover, extended release mixed amphetamine salts improved performance in the morning but worsened performance by the evening when compared to placebo (Cox, Merkel, et al., 2006). Studies that did not comprise exclusively adolescent samples, but included some adolescents, have found that lisdexamfetamine dimesylate (LDX; Vyvanse) and MPH transdermal system (MTS) also improve self-report of driving behaviors (Biederman et al., 2012a), driving simulation performance (Biederman et al., 2012b), and real-world driving performance (Cox et al., 2012). The review concludes that treatment with stimulants improves driving performance, and that these improvements appear to be stronger in studies involving adolescent and young adult samples in comparison to adult samples (Gobbo & Louzã, 2014).

Multifaceted Intervention

The Supporting a Teen's Effective Entry to the Roadway (STEER) program is a multifaceted, behavioral parenting training intervention that focuses on reducing risk for crashes, violations, and risky driving behavior in adolescent drivers with ADHD (Fabiano et al., 2011). This 8-week program includes skills training for parents and adolescents in communication and negotiation in order to promote safe independent driving. Driving simulation provides additional practice in a safe environment and is a method of providing objective feedback regarding driving skills to adolescents with ADHD, who may underestimate their difficulties in other domains (Owens, Goldfine, Evangelista, Hoza, & Kaiser, 2007). Parents are coached during the simulation drive to use positive behavioral strategies (e.g., specific praise) to reinforce safe driving practices. In-car technology is used to monitor adolescents' driving in the real world. Data obtained from in-car technology are reviewed throughout the intervention with parents and adolescents in order to increase parental monitoring of driving behaviors. Behavioral contracts targeting driving safety behaviors are created by adolescents and their parents with the coaching of therapists. Given the high level of conflict between many parents and adolescents with ADHD (Edwards, Barkley, Laneri, Fletcher, & Metevia, 2001), the need for an intervention such as STEER that provides communication and negotiation training is likely to be key for successful development of such contracts.

Results from a recently published randomized controlled trial indicate that relative to a driver education/practice intervention, adolescents in the STEER intervention engaged in fewer self-reported risky driving behaviors 6 months and 12 months postintervention, with a moderate effect at both time points (*d*'s = 0.40), though the decrease at 12 months did not reach statistical significance (*p* = .07) (Fabiano et al., 2016). These effects held regardless of whether participants were taking stimulant medication. Naturalistic driving behaviors and incidents (e.g., crashes, tickets) were measured using an in-car event recording device that was installed for 4-week periods of observation following each assessment visit (6-month and 12-month). No significant effects of STEER were observed for naturalistic driving behaviors or for incidents (e.g., crashes, tickets) (Fabiano et al., 2016), though the power to detect differences in the two intervention groups might have been negatively impacted by the study's reliance on relatively short observation periods. Events such as tickets and crashes occur at low base rates, necessitating longer periods of observation in order to capture enough events to make comparisons across intervention groups. As a point of reference, the other ADHD naturalistic driving studies have consisted of 3-month (Merkel et al., 2016) and up to 24-month observation periods (Klauer, Ollendick, Ankem, & Dingus, 2017). Given the positive effect of STEER on self-reported risky driving, the results of STEER are promising and worth exploring with longer naturalistic driving observation periods.

Intervention Targeting Visual Attention during Driving

The enhanced FOcused Concentration and Attention Learning (FOCAL+) intervention is an adaptation of an intervention developed for typically developing adolescents (FOCAL) that has been shown to improve visual attention to the roadway in randomized controlled studies (Fisher et al., 2010; Pradhan et al., 2011). In FOCAL, typically developing adolescents are trained to reduce extended eye glances away from the roadway using a computerized training program. Extended eye glances are targeted because they are a primary cause of crashes in the general population (Klauer et al., 2006) and because driving requires periodic glances away from the roadway to engage in driving-related tasks (e.g., checking mirrors). Given that extended eye glances have been shown to mediate the relationship between ADHD risk and poor driving performance in simulated driving (Kingery et al., 2015), the FOCAL intervention addresses an identified mechanism in ADHD-related driving deficits.

Consistent with the developmental psychopathology framework, the FOCAL intervention was modified to address the unique needs of adolescents with ADHD by an interdisciplinary team. The FOCAL intervention was modified in collaboration with researchers in clinical psychology to enhance effectiveness and generalizability with an ADHD population. Because adolescents with ADHD often exhibit difficulties generalizing skills gained in interventions (Abikoff, 2009), driving simulation with immediate feedback about glance behaviors is used when targeting extended eye glances, in addition to the computerized training in FOCAL. Since driving simulator and in-car technology are utilized in the intervention, collaboration with engineers knowledgeable in this methodology has been essential. A randomized clinical trial of the FOCAL+ intervention in adolescents with ADHD is currently under way. Thus, while targeting visual attention (and extended eye glances specifically) appears to be a promising, theoretically driven approach, it remains to have empirical support for its use.

Summary

Adolescent drivers are the highest risk group of drivers, and adolescent drivers with ADHD are at an even higher risk than their peers. Adolescents with ADHD experience higher rates of crashes and citations, and exhibit greater deficits in driving than their peers. The majority of research on the impact of ADHD on driving has yet to focus on those with the highest risk, adolescents with ADHD. Furthermore, the literature on mediators and moderators of this increased risk is in its infancy, as is the literature on interventions targeting driving outcomes of adolescents with ADHD. In keeping with the developmental psychopathology framework, researchers are encouraged to collaborate across fields to more effectively tackle this public health concern.

References

Abikoff, H. (2009). ADHD psychosocial treatments: Generalization reconsidered. *Journal of Attention Disorders, 13*(3), 207–210.

Aduen, P. A., Cox, D. J., Fabiano, G. A., Garner, A. A., & Kofler, M. (2019). Expert recommendations for improving driving safety for teens and adult drivers with ADHD. *ADHD Report, 27*(4), 8–14.

Aduen, P. A., Kofler, M. J., Cox, D. J., Sarver, D. E., & Lunsford, E. (2015). Motor vehicle driving in high incidence psychiatric disability: Comparison of drivers with ADHD, depression, and no known psychopathology. *Journal of Psychiatric Research, 64*, 59–66.

Almberg, M., Selander, H., Falkmer, M., Vaz, S., Ciccarelli, M., & Falkmer, T. (2015). Experiences of facilitators or barriers in driving education from learner and novice drivers with ADHD or ASD and their driving instructors. *Developmental Neurorehabilitation, 20*(2), 59–67.

Barkley, R. A., Guevremont, D. C., Anastopoulos, A. D., DuPaul, G. J., & Shelton, T.

L. (1993). Driving-related risks and outcomes of attention deficit hyperactivity disorder in adolescents and young adults: A 3- to 5-year follow-up survey. *Pediatrics, 92*(2), 212–218.

Barkley, R. A., Murphy, K. R., DuPaul, G., & Bush, T. (2002). Driving in young adults with attention deficit hyperactivity disorder: Knowledge, performance, adverse outcomes, and the role of executive functioning. *Journal of the International Neuropsychological Society, 8*(5), 655–672.

Barkley, R. A., Murphy, K. R., & Kwasnik, D. (1996). Motor vehicle driving competencies and risks in teens and young adults with attention deficit hyperactivity disorder. *Pediatrics, 98*(6), 1089–1095.

Biederman, J., Fried, R., Hammerness, P., Surman, C., Mehler, B., Petty, C. R., . . . Reimer, B. (2012a). The effects of lisdexamfetamine dimesylate on the driving performance of young adults with ADHD: A randomized, double-blind, placebo-controlled study using a validated driving simulator paradigm. *Journal of Psychiatric Research, 46,* 484–491.

Biederman, J., Fried, R., Hammerness, P., Surman, C., Mehler, B., Petty, C. R., . . . Reimer, B. (2012b). The effects of lisdexamfetamine dimesylate on driving behaviors in young adults with ADHD assessed with the Manchester driving behavior questionnaire. *Journal of Adolescent Health, 51*(6), 601–607.

Cardoos, S. L., Loya, F., & Hinshaw, S. P. (2013). Adolescent girls' ADHD symptoms and young adult driving: The role of perceived deviant peer affiliation. *Journal of Clinical Child and Adolescent Psychology, 42*(2), 232–242.

Centers for Disease Control and Prevention. (2017). Teen drivers: Get the facts. Retrieved from *www.cdc.gov/motorvehiclesafety/teen_drivers/teendrivers_factsheet.html.*

Chang, P. D., Lichtenstein, P., D'Onofrio, B. M., Sjölander, A., & Larsson, H. (2014). Serious transport accidents in adults with attention-deficit/hyperactivity disorder and the effect of medication: A population-based study. *JAMA Psychiatry, 71*(3), 319–325.

Cicchetti, D., & Rogosch, F. A. (2002). A developmental psychopathology perspective on adolescence. *Journal of Consulting and Clinical Psychology, 70*(1), 6–20.

Classen, S., Monahan, M., & Wang, Y. (2013). Driving characteristics of teens with attention deficit hyperactivity and autism spectrum disorder. *American Journal of Occupational Therapy, 67*(6), 664–673.

Cox, D. J., Davis, M., Mikami, A. Y., Singh, H., & Merkel, R. L. (2012). Long-acting methylphenidate reduces collision rates of young adult ADHD drivers. *Journal of Clinical Psychopharmacology, 32,* 225–230.

Cox, D. J., Humphrey, J. W., Merkel, L., Penberthy, J. K., & Kovatchev, B. (2004). Controlled-release methylphenidate improves attention during on-road driving by adolescents with attention-deficit/hyperactivity disorder. *Journal of the American Board of Family Medicine, 17*(4), 235–239.

Cox, D. J., Merkel, R. L., Moore, M., Thorndike, F., Muller, C., & Kovatchev, G. (2006). Relative benefits of stimulant therapy with OROS methylphenidate vs mixed amphetamine salts extended release in improving the driving performance of adolescent drivers with ADHD. *Pediatrics, 118,* e704–e710.

Cox, D. J., Merkel, R. L., Penberthy, J. K., Kovatchev, B., & Hankin, C. S. (2004). Impact of methylphenidate delivery profiles on driving performance of adolescents with attention-deficit/hyperactivity disorder: A pilot study. *Journal of the American Academy of Child and Adolescent Psychiatry, 43*(3), 269–275.

Cox, D. J., Moore, M., Burket, R., Merkel, R. L., Mikami, A. Y., & Kovatchev, B. (2008). Rebound effects with long acting amphetamine or methylphenidate stimulant medication preparations among adolescent male drivers. *Journal of Child and Adolescent Psychopharmacology, 18,* 1–10.

Cox, D. J., Punja, M., Powers, K., Merkel, R. L., Burket, R., Moore, M., . . . Kovatchev, B. (2006). Manual transmission enhances attention and driving performance of ADHD adolescent males. *Journal of Attention Disorders, 10*(2), 212–216.

Curry, A. E., Hafetz, J., Kallan, M. J., Winston, F. K., & Durbin, D. R. (2011). Prevalence of teen driver errors leading to serious motor vehicle crashes. *Accident Analysis and Prevention, 43,* 1285–1290.

Curry, A. E., Metzger, K. B., Pfeiffer, M. R., Elliott, M. R., Winston, F. K., & Power, T. J. (2017). Motor vehicle crash risk among adolescents and young adults with attention-deficit/hyperactivity disorder. *JAMA Pediatrics, 171*(8), 756–763.

Edwards, G., Barkley, R. A., Laneri, M., Fletcher, K., & Metevia L. (2001). Parent–adolescent conflict in teenagers with ADHD and ODD. *Journal of Abnormal Child Psychology, 29,* 557–572.

Fabiano, G. A., Hulme, K., Linke, S., Nelson-Tuttle, C., Pariseau, M., Gangloff, B., . . . Buck, M. (2011). The Supporting a Teen's Effective Entry to the Roadway (STEER) program: Feasibility and preliminary support for a psychosocial intervention for teenage drivers with ADHD. *Cognitive and Behavioral Practice, 18,* 267–280.

Fabiano, G. A., Schatz, N. K., Morris, K. L., Vujnovic, R. K., Hulme, K. F., Riordan, J., . . . Wylie, A. (2016). Efficacy of a family-focused intervention for young drivers with attention-deficit hyperactivity disorder. *Journal of Consulting and Clinical Psychology, 84*(12), 1078–1093.

Falk, A. E., Lee, S. S., & Chorpita, B. F. (2017). Differential association of youth attention-deficit/hyperactivity disorder and anxiety with delinquency and aggression. *Journal of Clinical Child and Adolescent Psychology, 46*(5), 653–660.

Fergusson, D., Swain-Campbell, N., & Horwood, J. (2003). Risky driving behavior in young people: Prevalance, personal characteristics and traffic accidents. *Australian and New Zealand Journal of Public Health, 27*(3), 337–342.

Fischer, M., Barkley, R. A., Smallish, L., & Fletcher, K. (2007). Hyperactive children as young adults: Driving abilities, safe driving behavior, and adverse driving outcomes. *Accident Analysis and Prevention, 39,* 94–105.

Fisher, D. L., Thomas, F. D., Pradhan, A. K., Pollatsek, A., Blomber, R. D., & Reagan, I. (2010). Development and evaluation of a PC-based attention maintenance training program (Research Report N. DOT HS 811 252). Retrieved from *https://trid.trb.org/view.aspx?id=915936.*

Fried, R., Petty, C., Surman, C. B., Reimer, B., Aleardi, M., Martin, J. M., . . . Biederman, J. (2006). Characterizing impaired driving in adults with attention-deficit/hyperactivity disorder: A controlled study. *Journal of Clinical Psychiatry, 67,* 567–574.

Fuermaier, A. B. M., Tucha, L., Evans, B. L., Koerts, J., de Waard, D., Brookhuis, K., . . . Tucha, O. (2017). Driving and attention deficit hyperactivity disorder. *Journal of Neural Transmission, 124*(1), 55–67.

Garner, A. A., Gentry, A., Welburn, S. C., Fine, P. R., Franklin, C. A., & Stavrinos, D. (2014). Symptom dimensions of disruptive behavior disorders in adolescent drivers. *Journal of Attention Disorders, 18*(6), 496–503.

Gobbo, M. A., & Louzã, M. R. (2014). Influence of stimulant and non-stimulant drug treatment on driving performance in patients with attention deficit hyperactivity disorder: A systematic review. *European Neuropsychopharmacology, 24,* 1425–1443.

Groom, M. J., van Loon, E., Daley, D., Chapman, P., & Hollis, C. (2015). Driving behavior in adults with attention deficit/hyperactivity disorder. *BMC Psychiatry, 15,* 175.

Holbrooke, J. R., Cuffe, S. P., Cai, B., Vasser, S. N., Forthofer, M. S., Bottai, M., . . .

McKeown, R. E. (2016). Persistence of parent-reported ADHD symptoms from childhood through adolescence in a community sample. *Journal of Attention Disorders, 20*(1), 11–20.

Hoza, B., McQuade, J. D., Murray-Close, D., Shoulberg, E., Molina, B. S. G., Arnold, L. E., . . . Hechtman, L. (2013). Does childhood positive self-perception bias mediate adolescent risky behavior in youth from the MTA study? *Journal of Consulting and Clinical Psychology, 81*(5), 846–858.

Johnson, J. A., Jakubovski, E., Reed, M. O., & Bloch, M. H. (2017). Predictors of long-term risky driving behavior in the multimodal treatment study of children with attention-deficit/hyperactivity disorder. *Journal of Child and Adolescent Psychopharmacology, 27*(8), 747–754.

Keating, D. P. (2007). Understanding adolescent development: Implications for driving safety. *Journal of Safety Research, 38,* 147–157.

Kingery, K. M., Narad, M., Garner, A. A., Antonini, T. N., Tamm, L., & Epstein, J. N. (2015). Extended visual glances away from the roadway are associated with ADHD- and texting-related driving performance deficits in adolescents. *Journal of Abnormal Child Psychology, 43*(6), 1175–1186.

Klauer, C., Ollendick, T., Ankem, G., & Dingus, T. (2017). Improving driving safety for teenagers with attention deficit and hyperactivity disorder (ADHD) (Research Report No. 17-UM-053). Retrieved from *https://vtechworks.lib.vt.edu/bitstream/handle/10919/79137/adhd%20stsce%20report_final.pdf?sequence=1&isallowed=y.*

Klauer, S. G., Dingus, T. A., Neale, V. L., Sudweeks, J. D., & Ramsey, D. J. (2006). The impact of driver inattention on near-crash/crash risk: An analysis using the 100-car naturalistic driving study data (Research Report No. DOT HS 810 594). Retrieved from *https://vtechworks.lib.vt.edu/handle/10919/55090.*

Lambert, N. M. (1995). Analysis of driving histories of ADHD subjects (Research Report DOT HS No. 808 417). Retrieved from *https://rosap.ntl.bts.gov/view/dot/1556.*

Lee, S. E., Olsen, E. C. B., & Simons-Morton, B. (2006). Eyeglance behavior of novice teen and experienced adult drivers. *Transportation Research Record, 1980,* 57–64.

Merkel, R. L., Nichols, J. Q., Fellers, J. C., Hidalgo, P., Martinez, L. A., Putziger, I., . . . Cox, D. J. (2016). Comparison of on-road driving between young adults with and without ADHD. *Journal of Attention Disorders, 20*(3), 260–269.

Mikami, A. Y., Cox, D. J., Davis, M. T., Wilson, H. K., Merkel, R. L., & Burket, R. (2009). Sex differences in effectiveness of extended-release stimulant medication among adolescents with attention-deficit/hyperactivity disorder. *Journal of Clinical Psychology in Medical Settings, 16,* 233–242.

Murray, A. L., Booth, T., Eisner, M., Obsuth, I., & Ribeaud, D. (2018, May 22). Quantifying the strength of general factors in psychopathology: A comparison of CFA with maximum likelihood estimation, BSEM, and ESEM/EFA bifactor approaches. *Journal of Personality Assessment.* [Epub ahead of print]

Nada-Raja, S., Langley, J. D., McGee, R., Williams, S. M., Begg, D. J., & Reeder, A. I. (1997). Inattentive and hyperactive behaviors and driving offenses in adolescence. *Journal of the American Academy of Child and Adolescent Psychiatry, 36*(4), 515–522.

Narad, M. E., Garner, A. A., Antonini, T. N., Kingery, K. M., Tamm, L., Calhoun, H. R., & Epstein, J. N. (2015). Negative consequences of poor driving outcomes reported by adolescents with and without attention deficit hyperactivity disorder. *Journal of Attention Disorders, 22*(12), 1109–1112.

Narad, M. E., Garner, A. A., Brassell, A. A., Saxby, D., Antonini, T. N., O'Brien, K.

M., . . . Epstein, J. N. (2013). Impact of distraction on the driving performance of adolescents with and without attention-deficit/hyperactivity disorder. *JAMA Pediatrics, 167*(10), 933–938.

Oliver, M. L., Nigg, J. T., Cassavaugh, N. D., & Backs, R. W. (2012). Behavioral and cardiovascular responses to frustration during simulated driving tasks in young adults with and without attention disorder symptoms. *Journal of Attention Disorders, 16*(6), 478–490.

Olsen, E. O., Shults, R. A., & Eaton, D. K. (2013). Texting while driving and other risky motor vehicle behaviors among US high school students. *Pediatrics, 131*(6), e1708–e1715.

Oltedal, S., & Rundmo, T. (2006). The effects of personality and gender on risky driving behavior and accident involvement. *Safety Science, 44*(7), 621–628.

Owens, J. S., Goldfine, M. E., Evangelista, N. M., Hoza, B., & Kaiser, N. M. (2007). A critical review of self-perceptions and the positive illusory bias in children with ADHD. *Clinical Child and Family Psychology Review, 10*(4), 335–351.

Pradhan, A. K., Divekar, G., Masserang, K., Romoser, M., Zafian, T., Blomberg, R. D., . . . Fisher, D. L. (2011). The effects of focused attention training on the duration of novice drivers' glances inside the vehicle. *Ergonomics, 54*(10), 917–931.

Reason, J., Manstead, A., Stradling, S., Baxter, J., & Campbell, K. (1990). Errors and violations on the roads: A real distinction? *Ergonomics, 33*(10–11), 1315–1332.

Redelmeier, D. A., Chan, W. K., & Lu, H. (2010). Road trauma in teenage male youth with disruptive behavior disorders: A population based analysis. *PLOS Medicine, 7*(11), e1000369.

Reimer, B., D'Ambrosio, L. A., Coughlin, J. F., Fried, R., & Biederman, J. (2007). Task-induced fatigue and collisions in adult drivers with attention deficit hyperactivity disorder. *Traffic Injury Prevention, 8*(3), 290–299.

Reimer, B., D'Ambrosio, L. A., Gilbert, J., Coughlin, J. F., Biederman, J., Surman, C., . . . Aleardi, M. (2005). Behavior differences in drivers with attention deficit hyperactivity disorder: The driving behavior questionnaire. *Accident Analysis and Prevention, 37*(6), 996–1004.

Reimer, B., Mehler, B., D'Ambrosio, L. A., & Fried, R. (2010). The impact of distractions on young adult drivers with attention deficit hyperactivity disorder (ADHD). *Accident Analysis and Prevention, 42*(3), 842–851.

Roman, G. D., Poulter, D., Barker, E., McKenna, F. P., & Rowe, R. (2015). Novice drivers' individual trajectories of driver behavior over the first three years of driving. *Accident Analysis and Prevention, 82,* 61–69.

Rosenbloom, T., & Wultz, B. (2011). Thirty-day self-reported risky driving behaviors of ADHD and non-ADHD drivers. *Accident Analysis and Prevention, 43,* 128–133.

Roy, A., Garner, A. A., Epstein, J. N., Hoza, B., Nichols, J. Q., Molina, B. S. Q., . . . Hechtman, L. (in press). Effects of childhood and adult persistent attention-deficit/hyperactivity disorder or risk of motor vehicle crashes. Results from the Multimodal Treatment Study of ADHD. *Journal of the American Academy of Child and Adolescent Psychiatry.*

Rutter, M., & Sroufe, A. (2000). Developmental psychopathology: Concepts and challenges. *Development and Psychopathology, 12,* 265–296.

Scott-Parker, B., Watson, B., King, M. J., & Hyde, M. K. (2013). A further exploration of sensation seeking propensity, reward sensitivity, depression, anxiety, and the risky behavior of young novice drivers in a structural equation model. *Accident Analysis and Prevention, 50,* 465–471.

Senserrick, T. M. (2006). Reducing young driver road trauma: Guidance and optimism for the future. *Injury Prevention, 12,* i56–i60.

Shahar, A. (2009). Self-reported driving behaviors as a function of trait anxiety. *Accident Analysis and Prevention, 41*(2), 241–245.

Shaw, P., Eckstrand, K., Sharp, W., Lumenthal, J., Lerch, J. P., Greenstein, D., . . . Rapoport, J. L. (2007). Attention-deficit/hyperactivity disorder is characterized by a delay in cortical maturation. *Proceedings of the National Academy of Sciences of the USA, 104*(49), 19649–19654.

Shope, J. T., & Bingham, R. (2008). Teen driving: Motor-vehicle crashes and factors that contribute. *American Journal of Preventative Medicine, 35*(Suppl. 3), S261–S271.

Sibley, M. H., Graziano, P. A., Kuriyan, A. B., Coxe, S., Pelham, W. E., Rodriguez, L., . . . Ward, A. (2016). Parent–teen behavior therapy + motivational interviewing for adolescents with ADHD. *Journal of Consulting and Clinical Psychology, 84*(8), 699–712.

Simmons-Morton, B. G., Cheon, K., Guo, F., & Albert, P. (2013). Trajectories of kinematic risky driving among novice teenagers. *Accident Analysis and Prevention, 51,* 27–32.

Sroufe, L. A. (2009). The concept of developmental psychopathology. *Child Development Perspectives, 3*(3), 178–183.

Stavrinos, D., Garner, A. A., Franklin, C. A., Johnson, H. D., Welburn, S. C., Griffin, R., . . . Fine, P. R. (2016). Distracted driving in teens with and without attention-deficit/hyperactivity disorder. *Journal of Pediatric Nursing, 30*(5), e183–e191.

Steinberg, L. (2007). Risk taking in adolescence: New perspectives from brain and behavioral science. *Current Directions in Psychological Science, 16*(2), 55–59.

Sterba, S. K., & Bauer, D. J. (2010). Matching method with theory in person-oriented developmental psychopathology research. *Development and Psychopathology, 22,* 239–254.

Stephens, A. N., & Groeger, J. A. (2009). Situational specificity of trait influences on drivers' evaluations and driving behavior. *Transportation Research Part F: Traffic Psychology and Behaviour, 12*(1), 29–39.

Teft, B. C., Williams, A. F., & Grabowski, J. G. (2013). Timing of driver's license acquisition and reasons for delay among young people in the United States, 2012. Retrieved from *www.aaafoundation.org/sites/default/files/teen%20licensing%20survey%20final_0.pdf.*

Thompson, A. L., Molina, B. S. G., Pelham, W., & Gnagy, E. M. (2007). Risky driving in adolescents and young adults with childhood ADHD. *Journal of Pediatric Psychology, 32*(7), 745–759.

Vaa, T. (2014). ADHD and relative risk of accidents in road traffic: A meta-analysis. *Accident Analysis and Prevention, 62,* 415–425.

Weiss, G., Hechtman, L., Perlman, T., Hopkins, J., & Wener, A. (1979). Hyperactives as young adults: A controlled prospective ten-year follow-up of 75 children. *Archives of General Psychiatry, 36*(6), 675–681.

Woodward, L., Fergusson, D., & Horwood, L. J. (2000). Driving outcomes of young people with attentional difficulties in adolescence. *Journal of the American Academy of Child and Adolescent Psychiatry, 39*(5), 627–634.

PART II

ASSESSING AND TREATING ADOLESCENTS WITH ADHD

CHAPTER 13

Assessing and Diagnosing ADHD in Adolescence

George J. DuPaul
Arthur D. Anastopoulos
Kristen Kipperman

Comprehensive assessment of attention-deficit/hyperactivity disorder (ADHD) involves systematic collection of data from multiple sources using a variety of methods. The aim of assessment is not only to inform diagnostic decisions but also to support the development, implementation, and evaluation of effective intervention strategies. Many assessment methods and measures have been developed for evaluation of symptoms of ADHD and related disorders, and, to a lesser extent, the measurement of symptom-related impairments and functional outcomes. In general, most ADHD assessment measures have been designed in the context of assessing symptomatic behaviors in elementary school-age children, presumably because this is the developmental period when most referrals for ADHD evaluation are generated (i.e., consonant with school entry; Barkley, 2015). Given the growing, ample evidence that ADHD continues throughout the lifespan (Sibley, Mitchell, & Becker, 2016; see Willcutt, Chapter 3, this volume), measures to assess symptoms of this disorder and related impairment in adolescence and adulthood have emerged.

Our purpose in this chapter is to provide an overview of the process, methods, and measures used to assess and diagnose ADHD in adolescents. We first describe the process, methods, and measures used to assess ADHD in the context of the *Diagnostic and Statistical Manual of Mental Disorders* (DSM-5; American Psychiatric Association, 2013) diagnostic system. Given the importance of establishing functional impairment in association with symptomatic behaviors, we discuss measures to assess adolescent performance in several key areas, including academic, social, emotional, family, sleep, and executive functioning. We also describe measures to assess areas of emerging importance for adolescents, including alcohol abuse, substance use, sexually risky behavior, and driving performance. Because ADHD rarely occurs in isolation, it also is important to comprehensively assess for symptoms of possible comorbid disorders, including disruptive behavior, anxiety, and mood disorders. Next, we discuss challenges associated with assessing and diagnosing ADHD during a time of rapid development transition from childhood to emerging adulthood. One of these challenges may involve adolescents malingering or "faking" ADHD symptoms in order to obtain desirable accommodations and/or stimulant medication. We conclude the chapter with several generic/composite case examples ranging from early adolescence to emerging adulthood.

Assessment Process in the Context of DSM-5

Assessment of ADHD at any age involves gathering data using multiple measures, with input from multiple respondents (Barkley, 2015). The primary objective is to determine whether the reasons for an adolescent's referral for clinical services are due to ADHD and/or related disorders. Clinicians conduct diagnostic interviews with the teen and his or her parents, administer behavior rating scales with parents and teachers, and gather archival data whenever possible (e.g., school and medical records) in the context of a comprehensive psychological evaluation (Anastopoulos & Shelton, 2001; Barkley, 2015). Assessment data are interpreted using DSM-5 (American Psychiatric Association, 2013) criteria in order to reach a diagnostic decision. Data are also used to identify and prioritize functioning areas in need of intervention. Treatment targets typically go beyond symptomatic behaviors and focus on academic, social, and/or occupational functioning. In addition, assessment and treatment may be directed at ameliorating executive functioning deficits, sleep disturbances, and risky behaviors (e.g., alcohol and substance use, sexual activity, driving performance) that often are associated with ADHD symptoms in adolescence. Finally, assessment of ADHD does not end with diagnosis; rather, it continues in an iterative manner to monitor treatment effects and to inform possible changes to intervention strategies over time.

DSM-5 outlines current diagnostic criteria for ADHD. Although there were not many major changes in symptomatology from the DSM-IV-TR (American Psychiatric Association, 2000), minor changes reflect a more developmental approach to understanding ADHD. Unlike previous DSM editions, DSM-5 defines ADHD as a neurodevelopmental disorder, emphasizes the persistence of ADHD across the lifespan, and acknowledges that the manifestation of symptoms and impairment varies throughout development. Additionally, symptom definitions were expanded to include developmentally appropriate illustrations of ADHD across the lifespan (e.g., internal restlessness rather than overt hyperactivity for adolescents). ADHD "subtypes" were changed to "presentations" to demonstrate the fluidity of symptom presentation over time. Last, age of onset was changed from 7 years of age to 12 years to reflect evidence regarding the typical development of the disorder (Barkley, 2015).

As described in greater detail in DSM-5, there are five major criteria that must be met to diagnose ADHD in individuals at any age. The first of these, Criterion A, stipulates that there be evidence of a "persistent pattern of inattention and/or hyperactivity–impulsivity that interferes with functioning or development," characterized by the presence of a high frequency of inattention and/or hyperactive symptoms (i.e., six or more, if below age 17, and five or more, if 17 or older) that persist for at least 6 months and are inconsistent with developmental level. Criterion B requires that several of these inattentive or hyperactive–impulsive symptoms emerge before age 12 years. Criterion C addresses the pervasiveness of ADHD, requiring that several inattentive or hyperactive–impulsive symptoms be evident in two or more settings. There must also be clear evidence that these symptoms interfere with, or reduce the quality of, daily functioning (Criterion D). Finally, it is also necessary to consider whether the symptoms and their interference with functioning might better be explained by another mental disorder (Criterion E). All of these criteria must be met to establish an ADHD diagnosis.

Although it is commonly the case that these criteria are addressed in the order in which DSM-5 presents them, such an approach lends itself to an overemphasis on counting symptoms (Criterion A), often at the expense of appropriate attention to Criteria B–E. Adhering to this ordering of the criteria also runs counter to the realities of clinical practice in which impairment in school, home, and social functioning, more so than the symptoms themselves, are what prompts parents and teachers to request professional consultation and evaluation. For these and many other reasons, a reordering of the DSM-IV Criteria A–E was previously put forth as a more clinically logical way to assess ADHD (Anastopoulos & Shelton, 2001); Table 13.1 outlines steps for suggested diagnostic process.

The starting point for this reordering is Criterion D, especially based on evidence that impairment should be given greater weight than symptom counts in making ADHD diagnostic decisions in adolescents (Sibley, Pelham, Molina, Gnagy, Waschbusch, et al., 2012). Fundamentally, this is a two-part criterion that examines whether there is (1) any evidence of

TABLE 13.1. Steps to Assessment Process for ADHD in Adolescents

1. *Assess functional impairment*
   - Academic functioning
     Archival records: report cards, school evaluations, attendance records
     WJ-IV (Schrank, Mather, & McGrew, 2014)
     AAPC (Sibley, Altszuler, Morrow, & Merrill, 2014)
     LASSI-2 (Weinstein, Palmer, & Shulte, 2002)
   - Social functioning
     Interview: peer relationships, involvement in extracurricular activities
     SSIS-RS (Gresham & Elliott, 2008)
     CADRI (Wolfe et al., 2001)
   - Executive functioning
     Conners Continuous Performance Test (Conners, 2000)
     BRIEF-2 (Gioia, Isquith, Guy, & Kenworthy, 2015)
   - Emotion regulation
     DERS (Gratz & Romer, 2004)
   - Family relationships
     Interview: family medical, psychiatric, and substance use history
     IFR (Hudson, 1997)
   - Sleep functioning
     Interview: bedtime routines, sleep environment, behavior, time to fall asleep
     ASWS (LeBourgeois et al., 2005)
   - Substance use and risk taking
     SASSI-3 (Miller & Lazowski, 1999)
     HSBQ (Flory et al., 2006)
     DBQ (Donovan, 1993)

2. *Determine pervasiveness*

   Evidence that symptoms are present in two or more settings (home, school, peers, work)

3. *Evaluate ADHD symptoms (frequency, severity, duration, age of onset)*

   Diagnostic interview (self-report, parent report)
   - K-SADS-PL DSM-5 (Kaufman et al., 2016)
   - P-ChIPS (Weller, Weller, Fristad, Rooney, & Schechter, 2000)

   Narrowband rating scales (multiple informants)
   - Conners Rating Scale (Conners, 2008)
   - ADHD-RS-5 (DuPaul, Power, Anastopoulos, & Reid, 2016)

   Observation
   - BOSS (Shapiro, 2011)

4. *Evaluate whether symptoms are better explained by alternative cause*

   Diagnostic interview (self-report, parent report; see above)

   Broad-band rating scales to assess behaviors related to various mental health disorders
   - BASC-3 (Kamphaus & Reynolds, 2015)
   - CBCL (Achenbach & Rescorla, 2001)

   Administer narrow-band rating scales to follow up on broad-band scales
   - Beck Youth Inventories of Emotional and Social Impairment (Beck, Beck, & Jolly, 2001)
   - RADS (Reynolds, 2002)

interference with, or reduction in the quality of, daily functioning and (2) reason to believe that some symptoms of inattention and/or hyperactivity–impulsivity are directly causing or contributing to (1). Assuming this is to be the case, it then becomes necessary to determine whether these symptoms are of sufficient clinical significance to rise to the level of ADHD. First to be considered among the remaining criteria is Criterion C. This is primarily because, in the process of evaluating Criterion D, information often becomes available that allows for an assessment of the setting contexts in which symptoms are occurring, thereby addressing the pervasiveness requirement of Criterion C. With Criteria D and C met, the next checkpoint in the diagnostic analysis is Criterion A, addressing three questions:

1. Is the frequency of inattention and/or hyperactive–impulsive symptoms above threshold (e.g., five or six or more symptoms from either list depending on the age of the adolescent)?
2. Are the frequency and severity of these symptoms atypical or developmentally deviant, well beyond what would be expected of others of the same age and gender?
3. Have these symptoms been present for the past 6 months or longer?

If the answer to all three questions is "yes," one begins examining Criterion B, which addresses yet another temporal characteristic of ADHD, requiring that symptoms of inattention and/or hyperactivity–impulsivity first emerged prior to 12 years of age. When met, Criteria D, C, A, and B together represent DSM-5's inclusionary criteria for ADHD. Before concluding that ADHD is present, however, one final hurdle must be cleared. More specifically, it remains necessary to consider the possibility that this clinical picture might better be accounted for by another mental disorder. Assuming that such exclusionary conditions can be ruled out, one can then conclude that ADHD is likely the best explanation for the reported patterns of symptoms and functional impairment.

Assessing ADHD Symptoms

The primary methods used to assess the presence, frequency, and severity of ADHD symptoms are independent diagnostic interviews with the parent and adolescent, along with behavior rating scales completed by parents and teachers. Self-report ratings should be obtained from older adolescents (i.e., age 16 and older) and young adults, although informant reports should carry greater weight given the tendency for individuals with ADHD to underreport their symptoms (Sibley, Pelham, Molina, Gnagy, Waxmonsky, et al., 2012). Structured and semistructured diagnostic interviews can be used to identify symptoms and related impairment. Although not all have been updated to conform to DSM-5 criteria, interviews include the Diagnostic Interview Schedule for Children (DISC-IV; Shaffer, Fisher, Lucas, Dulcan, & Schwab-Stone, 2000), Kiddie Schizophrenia and Affective Disorders Schedule—Present and Lifetime DSM-5 version (K-SADS-PL DSM-5; Kaufman et al., 2016), and Parent Version—Children's Interview for Psychiatric Symptoms (P-ChIPS; Weller, Weller, Fristad, Rooney, & Schechter, 2000). Parents and adolescents are interviewed separately regarding the presence of symptoms of ADHD and other externalizing and internalizing disorders (e.g., conduct disorder, major depressive episode). Structured and semistructured interviews provide a standardized format for questions, along with branching logic based on individual responses (e.g., interviewer is prompted to ask questions about symptom-related impairment if individual endorses a symptom as "present"). Semistructured diagnostic interviews (e.g., Barkley, 2015) are an alternative in situations when interview time is limited and/or the clinician desires more flexibility in questioning format. In general, structured and semistructured diagnostic interviews have good psychometric properties, including adequate interclinician agreement. Parent retrospective report of ADHD symptoms and impairment should be corroborated whenever possible by review of school archival records such as report cards, teacher comments, and school evaluations (Sibley, Pelham, Molina, Gnagy, Waschbusch, et al., 2012). If possible, retrospective ADHD symptom ratings can be collected from one or two teachers who previously taught the teen referred for evaluation.

Parents and teachers should complete both broad-band and narrow-band rating scales to identify the frequency of behaviors symptomatic of ADHD and other disorders over a specific time period (typically 1–6 months). Broad-band scales such as the Behavior Assessment System for Children—Third Edition (BASC-3; Kamphaus & Reynolds, 2015) and Child Behavior Checklist (CBCL; Achenbach & Rescorla, 2001) typically include 100 or more items to assess respondent perceptions of behaviors related to a variety of disorders. Clinicians can use broad-band scales not only to gauge the presence and frequency of ADHD symptoms but also to assess whether symptoms of other disorders may better account for inattention and/or hyperactivity–impulsivity, as well as to identify possible comorbid disorders. Narrow-band scales such as the Conners Rating Scales (Conners, 2008) and ADHD Rating Scale–5 (ADHD-RS-5; DuPaul, Power, Anastopoulos, & Reid, 2016) are briefer and more focused on ADHD symptoms. These typically provide more specific information about DSM-5 symptoms of ADHD, including whether symptoms are associated with functional impairment. Broad-band and narrow-band rating scales are particularly helpful in determining whether the symptom frequency of ADHD and other disorders is developmentally inappropriate given the availability of age- and gender-based norms.

The fact that most adolescents have several teachers presents a significant challenge for assessing ADHD symptoms in the school context (Evans, Allen, Moore, & Strauss, 2005). In contrast to elementary schoolteachers, who work with the same children throughout most, if not all, of the school day, secondary schoolteachers typically work with students for only 45–60 minutes per day, thus limiting opportunities to observe ADHD symptoms and associated impairments. Obtaining rating scales from multiple teachers in a reasonable time frame may also be challenging. For these reasons, clinicians should attempt to get behavior ratings from two to four core subject-area teachers (e.g., English, mathematics, science, and social studies), as these academic areas are most critical to school success and may be more likely to elicit ADHD-related difficulties given the importance of sustained attention, organization, and self-regulated behavior. If all else fails, clinicians should obtain ratings from a core academic teacher, preferably from a subject area in which the adolescent is struggling (Sibley, Pelham, Molina, Gnagy, Waschbusch, et al., 2012).

Assessing Functional Impairment

Assessing an individual's ADHD-related symptoms is imperative; however, it is also important to understand how these symptoms interfere with daily life. Assessing functional impairment allows for a more comprehensive understanding of how ADHD impacts an individual's ability to function socially, academically, and occupationally. In fact, assessment of impairment should be emphasized relative to symptom assessment when evaluating adolescents (Sibley, Pelham, Molina, Nagy, Waschbusch, et al., 2012) and young adults (Sibley, Pelham, Molina, Nagy, Waxmonsky, et al., 2012). Furthermore, by understanding the areas of functioning in which an individual is demonstrating impairment, the provider is better able to plan effective treatment.

Assessing Academic Functioning

Adolescents with ADHD typically experience academic impairment, as they are more likely to have lower grade point averages (GPAs), and lower standardized test scores and school grades when compared to peers without ADHD (Kuriyan, Pelham, Molina, Waschbusch, Gnagy, & Sibley, 2013). Furthermore, they demonstrate difficulty with task completion, studying, homework completion, and note taking (Evans et al., 2001; see Evans, Van der Oord, & Rogers, Chapter 8, this volume). When assessing academic functioning, it is important to collect information regarding current school performance. This includes class grades, overall GPA, standardized test scores, attendance records, and current academic accommodations. School archival records can be supplemented with norm-referenced, individual achievement tests such as the Woodcock–Johnson IV (WJ-IV; Schrank, Mather, & McGrew, 2014) and Wechsler Individual Achievement Test—Third Edition (WIAT-III; Wechsler, 2009). Both academic achievement tests can be used across a wide age span to assess a range of achievement domains, including reading comprehension, reading and math fluency, spelling, problem solving, and numerical operations.

Additionally, rating scales can be used to assess other potential areas of academic difficulty, including homework performance and classroom behavior. Parents and teachers can complete the Adolescent Academic Problems Checklist (AAPC; Sibley, Altszuler, Morrow, & Merrill, 2014) to assess behaviors associated with general academic performance (e.g., making careless errors on work, failing to take notes in class). The Classroom Performance Survey (CPS; Brady, Evans, Berlin, Bunford, & Kern, 2012) can be used to obtain teacher perceptions of students' classroom behaviors (e.g., "arrives to class on time") and areas of strength and weakness. To assess possible homework difficulties, parents can complete the Homework Problems Checklist (HPC; Anesko, Schoiock, Ramirez, & Levine, 1987), which includes items regarding homework completion and homework management behaviors. Another option for obtaining parent and teacher report of homework difficulties is the Homework Performance Questionnaire (HPQ; Power, Dombrowski, Watkins, Mautone, & Eagle, 2007). The parent form consists of three factors: student task engagement and efficiency, student competence, and teacher support. The teacher form consists of two factors: student responsibility and student competence. All of these measures have established reliability and validity for specific use in assessment of adolescents with ADHD.

Older adolescents and young adults attending college can complete the Learning and Study Strategies Inventory–2 (LASSI-2; Weinstein, Palmer, & Shulte, 2002). This self-report scale assesses 10 different areas of learning: anxiety and worry about school performance, attitude and interest, concentration, information processing, motivation, preparation, ability to select main ideas, use of support techniques and materials, time management, and test strategies. Not surprisingly, college students with ADHD obtain significantly lower scores on the LASSI-2 relative to their peers without ADHD (Gormley et al., 2018). This measure also can be used to identify areas of specific need for educational accommodations and support services.

Assessing Social Functioning

Social functioning is another area where adolescents with ADHD often demonstrate impairment (see McQuade, Chapter 7, this volume). For example, individuals with ADHD have difficulty understanding cause-and-effect or reciprocity of social relationships, when compared to peers without ADHD, which has been linked to social impairment in adolescence (Lorch, Milich, Astrin, & Berthiaume, 2006; Sibley, Evans, & Zerpell, 2010).

Social history can be gathered through interview. The clinician can ask about current peer relationships and involvement in extracurricular activities (i.e., sports teams, employment, clubs or social organizations). General information regarding friendships or committed relationships can also be gathered through an interview format. In addition, parents, teachers, and teens can complete the Social Skills Improvement System—Rating Scale (SSIS-RS; Gresham & Elliott, 2008) to obtain information about the frequency and perceived importance of various social skills (e.g., self-control, responding appropriately to conflict and nonconflict situations). The Conflict in Adolescent Dating Relationships Inventory (CADRI; Wolfe, Scott, Reitzel-Jaffe, Wekerle, Grasley, & Straatman, 2001) is a self-report scale that measures abusive behavior between adolescent dating partners. The scale addresses five factors: sexual abuse, threatening behavior, verbal or emotional abuse, relational abuse, and physical abuse. This scale is appropriate for use in middle and late adolescence, with different versions for males and females. Furthermore, the scale requires the individual to answer introductory dating questions, including whether the individual has begun dating and in how many relationships he or she has participated. Although not recommended for use on a routine basis, the CADRI may provide helpful information if concerns around dating behavior are warranted.

Assessing Executive Functioning

Typically, adolescents with ADHD also exhibit executive skills dysfunction, which is not surprising given that inattention symptoms directly impact core executive functioning areas such as organization and planning. Thus, individuals with ADHD often experience difficulty in self-regulation, decision making, and engaging in goal-directed behavior (Biederman et al., 2004; Miller, Ho, & Hinshaw, 2012; in this volume, see Doidge, Saoud, & Toplak, Chapter 4, and Sibley, Chapter 14). Executive functioning deficits interfere with learning due to difficulties with assignment tracking, planning of academic activities (e.g., homework, long-term projects), and organization of school materials (see Weyandt & Gudmundsdottir, 2015).

Although clinic-based tests of executive function are available (e.g., Conners Continuous Performance Test; Conners, 2000), behavior ratings offer cost and time efficiency. For example, parents, teachers, and adolescents can complete the Behavior Rating Inventory of Executive Function, Second Edition (BRIEF-2; Gioia, Isquith, Guy, & Kenworthy, 2015; Roth, Isquith, & Gioia, 2005). The BRIEF-2 parent and teacher reports comprise nine clinical scales including Inhibit, Self-Monitor, Shift, Emotional Control, Initiate, Working Memory, Plan/Organize, Task-Monitor, and

Organization. The self-report consists of seven clinical scales, including Inhibit, Self-Monitor, Shift, Emotional Control, Task Completion, Working Memory, and Plan/Organize. The BRIEF—Adult version comprises nine clinical scales: Inhibit, Self-Monitor, Plan/Organize, Shift, Initiate, Task Monitor, Emotional Control, Working Memory, and Organization of Materials. For both child and adult scales, composite scores are derived for emotion regulation, behavioral regulation, and cognitive regulation, in addition to an overall global executive functioning. Another option for young adolescents in middle school, the Children's Organizational Skills Scale (COSS; Abikoff & Gallagher, 2009) can be used to assess parent, teacher, and teen perceptions of task planning, organized actions, and memory and materials management. The latter often are important targets for intervention in middle and high school (see Sibley, Chapter 14, and Sprich & Burbridge, Chapter 16, this volume).

Assessing Emotion Regulation

Emotion regulation also is important to assess in adolescents suspected of having ADHD (see Bunford, Chapter 5, this volume). Research indicates that emotion dysregulation can mediate the relationship between ADHD and the development of internalizing disorders, such as depression (Seymour et al., 2012). Self-report ratings can be obtained using the Difficulties in Emotion Regulation Scale (DERS; Gratz & Roemer, 2004) and/or the Emotion Regulation Index for Children and Adolescents (ERICA; MacDermott, Gullone, Alle, King, & Tonge, 2010). The DERS includes six subscales: Nonacceptance of Emotional Responses, Difficulties Engaging in Goal-Directed Behavior, Impulse Control Difficulties, Lack of Emotional Awareness, Limited Access to Emotion Regulation Strategies, And Lack of Emotional Clarity. The briefer ERICA comprises three subscales: Emotional Control, Emotional Self-Awareness, and Situation Responsiveness. These measures can be used to identify possible emotion regulation difficulties that could be targeted for intervention.

Assessing Family Relationships

Family relationships often are strained for adolescents with ADHD (see Wiener, Chapter 6, this volume). Families of adolescents with ADHD are exposed to higher levels of stress that impact various relationships within the home and increase familial conflict (Theule, Wiener, Rogers, & Marton, 2011). High levels of stress can compromise parenting behaviors such that increased use of ineffective parenting strategies can further deleteriously affect family functioning and relationships (Johnston & Mash, 2001).

It is important to collect information regarding the current family structure and living situation, as well as family medical, psychiatric, and substance use history. This information can help contextualize how family experiences may affect adolescent functioning. In addition, several rating scales are available to assess family conflict and parenting stress. Parents and teens can complete the Index of Family Relations (IFR; Hudson, 1997) to measure the perceived magnitude of difficulty in relationships amongst family members. Parents can complete the Stress Index for Parents of Adolescents (SIPA; Sheras, Abidin, & Konold, 1998) to evaluate parenting stress across three domains, including Adolescent (i.e., stress as a function of adolescent characteristics), Parent (i.e., effect of parenting on other life roles), and Adolescent–Parent Relationship (i.e., quality of parent–teen relationship). Again, these measures can provide data regarding family interaction impairment resulting from teen ADHD symptoms, as well as valuable information regarding family functioning areas to target in treatment.

Assessing Sleep Functioning

Adolescents with ADHD are more likely to have difficulties with sleep hygiene and functioning than their non-ADHD peers (Cortese, Faraone, Konofal, & Lecendreux, 2009; see Mulraney, Sciberras, & Becker, Chapter 10, this volume). Additionally, sleep problems can be predictive of comorbid internalizing and externalizing symptoms, suggesting that sleep difficulties contribute to the developmental trajectory of psychopathology over time (Becker, Langberg, & Evans, 2015). Thus, it is important to assess sleep functioning of adolescents being evaluated for ADHD.

Interviews, sleep diaries, and rating scales can be used to assess sleep functioning (in some clinical settings, actigraphy may also be available). Interviews should focus on the quantity and quality of sleep an individual receives. This information can be obtained by asking questions regarding bedtime routines, sleep environment, behavior at bedtime, and the amount of time it takes the individual to fall asleep (Laracy, Ridgard, & DuPaul, 2015). Sample questions include "What happens in the 30–60 minutes before you get into bed?"; "Describe your sleep environment"; "Do you wake independently, or do you need assistance?"; "Do you nap?"; and "Does anything bother you when trying to fall asleep?" These questions can be adapted depending on the adolescent's age and whether parent information also is being collected. Sleep diaries often are used to track an individual's sleep and include information regarding bedtime, whether the individual awakes in the night, how long it takes to return to sleep, and wake-up time.

Several self-report rating scales can be used to assess sleep functioning and daytime sleepiness. The Adolescent Sleep Hygiene Scale (ASHS; LeBourgeois, Gianotti, Cortesi, Wolfson, & Harsh, 2005) includes a combination of qualitative and quantitative items assessing behaviors related to bedtime across nine subscales: Physiological, Cognitive, Emotional, Sleep Environment, Daytime Sleep, Substances, Sleep Stability, Bedtime Routine, and Bed Sharing. The Adolescent Sleep–Wake Scale (ASWS; LeBourgeois et al., 2005) measures several factors associated with sleep quality, including Going to Bed, Falling Asleep, Maintaining Sleep, Reinitiating Sleep, and Returning to Sleep. The Epworth Sleepiness Scale (ESS; Johns, 1998) is a brief, self-report measure that is used to evaluate daytime sleepiness in children, adolescents, and adults. Respondents rate their likelihood of dozing off during specific activities (e.g., "sitting and reading"; "as a passenger in a car for an hour without a break"; "sitting, inactive in a public place"). Another brief measure of daytime sleepiness is the Pediatric Daytime Sleepiness Scale (PDSS; Drake et al., 2003). Sample items include "How often do you fall asleep or get drowsy during class periods?" and "How often do you have trouble getting out of bed in the morning?" All of these rating scales have adequate reliability and validity for use with adolescents.

Assessing Substance Use and Risk-Taking Behavior

Another potential area of concern for adolescents with ADHD is risk-taking behavior, such as substance use, sexual activity, and reckless driving behaviors (Flory, Molina, Pelham, Gnagy, & Smith, 2006; Lee, Humphreys, Flory, Liu, & Glass, 2011; Thompson, Molina, Pelham, & Gnagy, 2007; see Kennedy, McKone, & Molina, Chapter 11, and Garner, Chapter 12, this volume). Self-report rating scales can be used to assess the degree to which an adolescent or young adult engages in these various risky behaviors.

The Substance Abuse Subtle Screening Inventory–3 (SASSI-3; Miller & Lazowski, 1999) includes both adolescent and adult versions and is designed to identify individuals with a high probability of having a substance use disorder, including abuse and dependence. Sample items include: "taken drugs to improve your thinking and feeling", "gotten into trouble at school, at home, on the job, or with police because of your drug use", and "many of my friends drink or get high repeatedly." The SASSI-3 provides insight into family and social risk factors, level of defensive responding, and consequences of substance misuse (Laux, Piazza, Saylers, & Roseman, 2012). The World Health Organization—Alcohol, Smoking and Substance Involvement Screening Test (WHO-ASSIST; WHO ASSIST Working Group, 2002) is a brief scale to measure substance and alcohol use. Each question is focused on the use and consequences of use of a variety of substances, including tobacco products, alcoholic beverages, cannabis, and other drugs.

The Health and Sexual Behavior Questionnaire (HSBQ; Flory et al., 2006) asks individuals about their sexual history including: sexual activity, frequency of sexual behaviors, how often they have engaged in casual sex, use of birth control, and presence of sexually transmitted diseases. This measure has been used extensively in research with adolescents (Flory et al., 2006; Hoza et al., 2013). The Sexual Risk Survey (SRS; Turchik & Garske, 2009) specifically examines the frequency of sexual risk behaviors of adolescents and young adults. Respondents are asked to respond with the number of times they have engaged in a particular sexual activity (e.g., unexpected and unanticipated sexual experience, use of alcohol or drugs before or during sex) over the past 6 months. Administration of this measure includes a glossary of terms and a calendar of the last 6 months to help participants remember their experiences.

Multiple measurement methods, including self-report rating scales, can be used to assess driving-related skills and the degree to which adolescents and young adults engage in risky driving behavior (for review, see Fabiano & Schatz, 2015). The Driving Behavior Questionnaire (DBQ; Donovan, 1993) asks respondents to report the frequency with which they engage in behaviors that represent driving errors, attention lapses, and traffic law violations. The DBQ has been used in studies examining driving deficits associated with ADHD (e.g., Reimer et al., 2005). The Driving Performance Rating Scale (DPRS; Barkley, Guevremont, Anastopoulos, DuPaul, & Shelton, 1993) assesses a similar set of driving behaviors and was developed specifically for use with adolescents and adults with ADHD. The DPRS can be used as either a self-report or a collateral report measure. The Jerome Driving Questionnaire (JDQ; Jerome, Segal, & Habinski, 2006) was also specifically developed for the assessment of driving behaviors in individuals with ADHD. Respondents report on driving history and answer items regarding driving behaviors under a variety of conditions (e.g., city or highway) using a visual analogue scale.

Assessing Comorbid Symptoms and Disorders in Adolescence

It is of critical clinical importance for researchers and practitioners alike to be keenly aware that ADHD is frequently accompanied by co-occurring, or comorbid, psychiatric and learning conditions (see Becker & Fogleman, Chapter 9, this volume). For example, up to 44% of children and adolescents with ADHD drawn from a large community sample exhibited at least one comorbid condition, and as many as 43% of this same sample displayed two or more comorbid disorders (Willcutt et al., 2012). Even higher comorbidity rates occur in clinic-referred samples, with 60–80% of children and adolescents with ADHD having one additional diagnosis and as many as 50% displaying two or more comorbid conditions (Pliszka, 2014). Disruptive behavior disorders, such as oppositional defiant disorder (ODD) and conduct disorder (CD), are especially common comorbid conditions in youth with ADHD. Although occurring less frequently, mood and anxiety disorders, learning disabilities, and other psychiatric and developmental conditions have been found to co-occur with ADHD at rates higher than that in the general child population (Angold, Costello, & Erkanli, 1999; Nigg & Barkley, 2014). High rates of comorbidity (55%) have also been found among emerging adults with ADHD in their first year of college, primarily involving various depression and anxiety disorders (Anastopoulos et al., 2018).

Although it is well established that ADHD often is accompanied by other psychiatric and learning disorders that occur throughout the lifespan, the exact manner in which comorbid conditions arise across development is not well understood. The extent to which comorbid conditions contribute to functional impairment, above and beyond that accounted for by ADHD, also is unclear. Until such issues are clarified in future research, it remains critically important for researchers and clinicians to bear in mind that adolescents with ADHD are at substantially increased risk for displaying comorbid conditions. Such a possibility necessitates the inclusion of developmentally appropriate assessment procedures for identifying comorbid disorders during the initial evaluation. Therein lies the challenge. What assessment procedures are "appropriate" for this segment of the population with ADHD?

Given the types of comorbidity that research has identified within the population with ADHD, initial assessments, at a minimum, should include measures that address not only ODD and CD but also various mood and anxiety disorders. Regarding the latter, routine clinical attention should focus on psychiatric conditions that have the highest probability of being present within an adolescent population with ADHD, including persistent depressive disorder (PDD), major depressive disorder (MDD), generalized anxiety disorder (GAD), and social anxiety disorder (SAD). Initial assessments should also screen for the possibility that less frequently occurring conditions, such as substance use, obsessive–compulsive, and bipolar disorders, may be present.

How might information about these potential comorbid conditions be gathered? Consistent with the approach recommended for assessing ADHD symptoms and impairment, a multimethod assessment strategy should be used, encompassing clinical interviews; standardized rating scales that allow for normative comparisons; and reviews of past school, mental health, and medical records. Such information should be gathered from multiple informants who provide not only overlapping but unique perspectives on the functioning of the adolescent in the multiple contexts in which the adolescent functions (i.e., in school, at home, and with friends). Ideally, this would include input from both parents, from at least two teachers in two of the adolescent's core classes (e.g., math, English, science, or social studies), and from the adolescent him- or herself. The older the adolescent, the more important it is to solicit self-report, especially as it relates to depression, anxiety, and other internalizing disorders. That said, in our experience, self-reporting adolescents are not always keenly aware of the details surrounding their own internalizing problems related to onset, duration, impact on functioning, and treatment history. For this reason, it remains important to include parents in the assessment process, regardless of how old the adolescent may be.

Yet another critically important factor to take into consideration is how best to determine whether reported co-occurring symptoms are clinically significant and worthy of being formally diagnosed as a comorbid disorder. At a minimum, there needs to be evidence that what the adolescent is displaying is developmentally deviant, that is, outside the boundaries of what might be considered normal or typical adolescent life experiences. Thus, it is not just that the adolescent is feeling very sad, for example; it must be a level of sadness that goes beyond what many typically developing adolescents experience. Having extensive knowledge of typical adolescent development is immensely helpful in making this determination. Even more helpful, primarily because they are more objective, are comparisons of the adolescent's clinical presentation with that of individuals of the same age and gender. Such comparative information is readily available from standardized rating scales and questionnaires for which normative data, grouped by age, gender, and informant, are available (e.g., Beck Youth Inventories of Emotional and Social Impairment: Beck, Beck, & Jolly, 2001; Reynolds Adolescent Depression Scale: Reynolds, 2002).

In addition to considering the issue of developmental deviance, it also is necessary to address the degree to which comorbid features are impacting daily academic, social, and/or vocational functioning. In particular, the degree to which an adolescent's daily functioning is impaired must be clinically significant, exceeding that which would be expected for most adolescents. Thus, for an adolescent who is experiencing anxiety and earning a grade of B+ in an advanced placement course, it would be a difficult to label this type of performance as "impaired" functioning.

Issues with Assessment in Adolescence

It is critically important to be mindful of the many dramatic changes that take place during typical adolescent development, as they provide a background against which developmental deviance (i.e., clinical significance of ADHD symptoms and associated impairment) can be judged. A particularly salient developmental challenge facing adolescents is their emerging need for greater independence (Arnett, 1999). This push for independence can put adolescents on a collision course with parents, teachers, and other authority figures who set rules and have expectations for behavior. Another developmental challenge is related to the transitions into middle school, then high school that result in greater demands for self-regulation in terms of remembering what to bring from one class to another, getting to and from classes in a timely fashion, avoiding the temptation to talk to classmates in the hallways, and so forth. In the classroom, there is an increased emphasis on working independently. Completion of homework takes on increased importance as well, with most assignments requiring systematic planning, organization, and sustained effort over long periods of time. These developmental challenges become a major focus of relationships with family. Choice of friends, decisions about curfews, driving privileges, what to wear, and whether to complete chores are some of the many issues that have great potential for bringing adolescents into conflict with parents. A related developmental change that takes place during adolescence is the important influence of friends, even more important than that of family (Fuligni & Eccles, 1993). Relationships with same-sex and opposite-sex peers, are both important, as the adolescent sorts out what sexuality will mean for him or her. Additional opportunities for independence and freedom arise in terms of facing the temptations of alcohol and drugs, acquiring a driver's license, and taking on part-time jobs. Finally, adolescence also brings with it many physical changes, including major disruptions in hormonal functioning, which can lead to new emotional experiences, or at the very least, intensify previously learned emotional reactions.

Emerging from the preceding discussion is an important theme emphasizing adolescence as a developmental period in which demands for self-regulation increase over time across multiple contexts. Awareness of this theme can provide clinically relevant guidance to those conducting evaluations to determine the presence or absence of adolescent ADHD. This includes, for example, insight into the various behavioral, academic, family, social, and emotional contexts in which adolescents with ADHD are at increased risk for displaying not only ADHD symptoms but also impairments in daily functioning related to these symptoms. Equally important to keep in mind, however, is that these developmental challenges are by no means specific to adolescents with ADHD. Many typically developing adolescents experience similar challenges (Ausubel, 2002). Thus, to establish an ADHD diagnosis, it is incumbent on evaluators to gather compelling evidence attesting to the fact that such difficulties are in excess of what typically developing adolescents display.

When approaching assessment of ADHD through a developmental lens, it also is imperative to account for several different stages within adolescence. Generally, adolescence spans from ages 11–21 years and is further broken down into three stages: early adolescence (11–14), middle adolescence (14–17), and late adolescence/emerging adulthood (17–21) (Barrett, 1996). To effectively assess ADHD symptoms and associated functional impairment, it is critical to use measures and methods that accurately reflect an individual's current stage within adolescence, and it also is important to consider diagnostic thresholds (Sibley, Pelham, Molina, Gnagy, Waschbusch, et al., 2012). When diagnosing children with ADHD, multimethod and multi-informant methods are the recommended guidelines for comprehensive assessment (American Academy of Pediatrics, 2011). Although similar recommendations are relevant for comprehensive assessment in adolescents, it is important to consider unique characteristics within each stage of adolescence. In early and middle stages of adolescence, youth are likely still enrolled in secondary education and living with their parents. Therefore, it is important to collect data from the individual, the parents of the individual, and the teacher(s) of the individual (Barkley, 2015). In contrast, in the later stage of adolescence, it is probable that the teen has moved away from home and is either attending postsecondary education or has joined the workforce. Therefore, information may be gathered from other respondents, such as roommates, significant others, and/or employers (Sibley, Pelham, Molina, Gnagy, Waxmonsky, et al., 2012).

There are several methods of data collection used when conducting a comprehensive assessment, including diagnostic interviews, surveys regarding symptomatology and associated impairment, cognitive ability tests, achievement tests, and permanent records review. Similarly, multiple informants are asked to respond about the individual being assessed to evaluate impairment in multiple settings (American Academy of Pediatrics, 2011; Pelham, Fabiano, & Massetti, 2005). With younger adolescents, it is relatively simple to collect data from multiple sources, as minors require consent from a legal guardian to undergo an evaluation process. However, individuals in late adolescence/emerging adulthood can likely legally consent, themselves, and it is more difficult to obtain data from multiple sources. For late adolescence, research indicates that retrospective rating scales of childhood ADHD can be effective in providing accurate diagnosis when these are completed by both individuals being assessed and their parents (Dvorsky, Langberg, Molitor, & Bourchtein, 2016). Furthermore, collecting data from multiple sources can help to prevent malingering (Dvorsky et al., 2016; Green & Rabiner, 2012).

Malingering refers to feigning or exaggerating symptoms of ADHD to obtain services and accommodations associated with diagnosis such as academic services and access to prescription medication (Booksh, Pella, Singh, & Gouvier, 2010; Green & Rabiner, 2012; see Brinkman, Froehlich, & Epstein, Chapter 18, this volume). Research indicates that malingering increases in late adolescence, typically with college students. Often, students believe receiving these services, especially access to stimulant medication, will enhance their academic performance (Rabiner et al., 2009). The possibility of malingering raises concerns regarding the misuse of stimulant medication and potential ethical implications of using medication to improve academics (Advokat, Lane, & Luo, 2011). Furthermore, it calls to question the assessment methods being utilized to provide a diagnosis of ADHD. Research conducted by Booksh and colleagues (2010) demonstrates that undergraduate students were able to successfully feign ADHD symptoms on a retrospective report of childhood ADHD. This illustrates the importance of collecting information from multiple sources and of using multiple methods beyond self-report. By collecting objective data (e.g., permanent product review) and data from other reporters, there is greater protection from malingering (Booksh et al., 2010; Dvorsky et al., 2016).

Case Examples

James

James was a 14-year-old, non-Hispanic white male attending ninth grade in a large suburban high school serving a predominantly middle- to upper-class population. He was referred by his parents for services due to chronic difficulties getting along with parents and authority figures, problems completing and returning homework, and feeling bad about himself (i.e., low self-esteem). School records indicated that despite above-average intellectual abilities (IQ = 122), he consistently earned average to below-average grades in school and obtained WJ-IV scores in the average to low-average range for reading and math achievement. Maternal interview on the P-ChIPS indicated significant symptoms and associated impairment for ADHD combined presentation, ODD, and SAD. Brief telephone interviews with James's English and math teachers indicated that he was frequently off-task in class, had problems completing assigned work in a timely fashion, and often verbally disrupted class activities. Clinically significant scores (i.e., 93rd percentile or above) on the BASC-3 were found for parent and teacher ratings of externalizing problems, as well as parent ratings of internalizing problems. ADHD-RS-5 ratings from James's mother and two of his four core academic teachers indicated significant frequency of inattention and hyperactivity–impulsivity symptoms along with symptom-related impairment in relationships with adults and peers, as well as homework performance. On the P-ChIPS diagnostic interview, James reported significant symptoms and distress related to SAD, along with a few inattentive symptoms of ADHD; however, self-reported symptoms did not meet DSM-5 criteria for ADHD or ODD. Self-report ratings were elevated on the Beck Youth Inventory Anxiety scale. Neither James nor his mother reported alcohol or substance use difficulties on the SASSI. Based on this assessment, James was diagnosed with ADHD combined presentation, ODD, and SAD with treatment recommendations including behavioral parent training to address ODD and homework performance difficulties, teacher behavioral consultation to address classroom disruption, and cognitive-behavioral therapy to help James to cope with anxiety symptoms. He was also referred to a developmental and behavioral pediatrician for possible medication to ameliorate ADHD symptoms.

Florence

Florence was a 17-year-old Latina student attending 11th grade in a large urban high school serving a predominantly lower working-class population. Her parents referred her for an evaluation due to teacher report of chronic academic underachievement and frequent daydreaming in class. She also was reported to be somewhat socially withdrawn, with only a few friends. Although her parents primarily spoke Spanish at home, Florence was fluent in both English and Spanish. A school psychoeducational evaluation conducted when Florence was in middle school indicated that she had average intellectual abilities, along with low-average range math and reading skills. She was not found to have a learning disability and, as a result, did not receive any school services. The P-ChIPS interview with her mother revealed clinically significant inattentive symptoms that were associated with primarily academic impairment. Alternatively, she was not reported to exhibit significant problems with hyperactivity–impulsivity, oppositional behavior, or rule breaking and conduct disturbance. A telephone interview with three of Florence's teachers indicated similar reports of frequent inattentiveness in class, problems getting assignments completed in a timely fashion, and often seeming to be lost in her own thoughts. Parent and teacher ratings on the BASC-3 were elevated only for the Attention Problems subscale and did not indicate clinically significant internalizing or externalizing difficulties. On the ChIPS, Florence reported minor difficulties with concentration and attention that she attributed to her boredom with school activities. She did not report significant internalizing symptoms on the Beck Youth Inventory Anxiety scale or the Reynolds Adolescent Depression Scale. Neither Florence nor her mother reported significant alcohol or substance use difficulties. In fact, she rarely left home and only occasionally associated with peers. Based on this assessment, Florence was diagnosed with ADHD predominantly inattentive presentation, with daydreaming and social withdrawal suggesting that co-occurring sluggish cognitive tempo (SCT) symptoms might also be present (Becker et al., 2016; see Becker & Fogleman, Chapter 9, this volume). Treatment recommendations included joint sessions with Florence and her parents to develop and implement a behavioral contract designed to increase her motivation to complete assigned schoolwork and homework, teacher consultation to develop parallel motivational strategies in the classroom to increase Florence's task-related attention, and meetings with her school counselor to identify her interests and plan for the transition from high school to possible postsecondary education. A plan was also developed with Florence's family to identify out-of-home activities that might be of interest to her as a way to build stronger connections to her peers.

Allen

Allen was a 19-year-old non-Hispanic white male first-year student at a moderate-size, private 4-year university. Due to struggles in keeping up with course assignments and managing his time, Allen has been receiving failing grades in most classes. He sought support services and educational accommodations through the college's students with disabilities office. In order to obtain those services, he first needed to complete a diagnostic evaluation to establish eligibility as well as identify other potential interventions. Allen and his mother independently completed ADHD rating scales regarding both current (i.e., past 6 months) and retrospective (childhood) symptoms. He reported six out of nine inattentive symptoms both currently and in childhood, while his mother reported six inattentive symptoms in childhood only. Allen also reported six out of nine hyperactive–impulsive symptoms in childhood but only one symptom currently, while his mother reported five hyperactive–impulsive symptoms in childhood but only one currently. Current symptom reports were confirmed through a semistructured diagnostic interview with Allen; specifically, he reported seven inattentive symptoms to have been present since childhood and only two hyperactive–impulsive symptoms. Notably, he reported having been diagnosed with a learning disability in reading in elementary school and thus received special education services through middle school. Allen denied any symptomatic behaviors associated with ODD or CD, and self-report ratings on the Beck Anxiety Inventory (Beck & Steer, 1993) and Beck Depression Inventory–II (Beck, Steer, & Brown, 1996) were not in the clinical range. Scores were in the clinical range across all LASSI-2 subscales, indicating significant difficulties with all aspects of studying and academic preparation. Although he reported occasional alcohol and cannabis use, self-report ratings on the SRS and WHO-ASSIST did not indicate any elevated risk with respect to sexual behavior and use of alcohol and illicit substances. Given the history, chronicity, and cross-respondent reports, as well as impairment related to inattentive symptoms, Allen was diagnosed with ADHD, predominantly inattentive presentation and was thus deemed eligible for academic support services (e.g., study skills support, time management coaching) and educational accommodations (e.g., provided with lecture notes).

CONCLUSIONS

Given the plethora of difficulties typically experienced by adolescents with ADHD across home, school, and community settings, it is critically important that diagnostic evaluations involve multiple methods, measures, and respondents. Furthermore, the diagnostic process should emphasize assessing possible impairment across a variety of functioning areas, in addition to symptomatic behaviors. The primary objective is to determine whether the reasons for an adolescent's referral for clinical services are due to ADHD and/or related disorders. In addition, assessment should be directed toward identifying and prioritizing areas of functioning (e.g., academic, social, occupational) that require intervention. Furthermore, assessment and treatment may be directed at ameliorating executive functioning deficits, sleep disturbances, and risky behaviors (e.g., alcohol and substance use, sexual activity, driving performance) that often are associated with ADHD symptoms in adolescence. Thus, clinicians can not only reach reliable and valid diagnostic decisions but also develop and implement potentially effective interventions that can be evaluated by periodically assessing ADHD symptoms and symptom-related impairment over time.

REFERENCES

Abikoff, H., & Gallagher, R. (2009). *Children's Organizational Skills Scales: Technical manual.* North Tonawanda, NY: Multi-Health Systems.

Achenbach, T. M., & Rescorla, L. A. (2001). *Manual for the ASEBA school-age forms and profiles.* Burlington: University of Vermont, Department of Psychiatry.

Advokat, C., Lane, S. M., & Luo, C. (2011). College students with and without ADHD: Comparison of self-report of medication usage, study habits, and academic achievement. *Journal of Attention Disorders, 15,* 656–666.

American Academy of Pediatrics. (2011). ADHD: Clinical practice guideline for the diagnosis, evaluation, and treatment of attention-deficity/hyperactivity disorder in children and adolescents. *Pediatrics, 128,* 1–16.

American Psychiatric Association. (2000). *Diagnostic and statistical manual of mental disorders* (4th ed., text rev.). Washington, DC: Author.

American Psychiatric Association. (2013). *Diagnostic and statistical manual of mental disorders* (5th ed.). Arlington, VA: Author.

Anastopoulos, A. D., DuPaul, G. J., Weyandt, L. L., Morrissey-Kane, E., Sommer, J. L., Rhoads, L. H., . . . Gudmundsdottir, B. G. (2018). Rates and patterns of comorbidity among first-year college students with ADHD. *Journal of Clinical Child and Adolescent Psychology, 47,* 236–247.

Anastopoulos, A. D., & Shelton, T. L. (2001). *Assessing attention-deficit/hyperactivity disorder.* New York: Kluwer Academic/Plenum Press.

Anesko, K. M., Schoiock, G., Ramirez, R., & Levine, F. M. (1987). The Homework Problem Checklist: Assessing children's homework difficulties. *Behavioral Assessment, 9,* 179–185.

Angold, A., Costello, E. J., & Erkanli, A. (1999). Comorbidity. *Journal of Child Psychology and Psychiatry, 40,* 57–87.

Arnett, J. J. (1999). Adolescent storm and stress, reconsidered. *American Psychologist, 54,* 317– 326.

Ausubel, D. P. (2002). *Theory and problems of adolescent development* (3rd ed.). Bloomington, IN: iUniverse.

Barkley, R. A. (2015). Psychological assessment of children with ADHD. In R. A. Barkley (Ed.), *Attention-deficit hyperactivity disorder: A handbook for diagnosis and treatment* (3rd ed., pp. 455–474). New York: Guilford Press.

Barkley, R. A., Guevremont, D. C., Anastopoulos, A. D., DuPaul, G. J., & Shelton, T. L. (1993). Driving-related risks and outcomes of attention-deficit hyperactivity disorder in adolescents and young adults: A 3- to 5-year follow-up survey. *Pediatrics, 92,* 212–218.

Barkley, R. A., Murphy, K. R., & Fischer, M. (2008). *ADHD in adults: What the science says.* New York: Guilford Press.

Barrett, D. E. (1996). The three stages of adolescence. *High School Journal, 79,* 333–339.

Beck, A., & Steer, T. (1993). *Beck Anxiety Inventory.* San Antonio, TX: Psychological Corporation.

Beck, A., Steer, T., & Brown, G. K. (1996). *Beck Depression Inventory–II.* San Antonio, TX: Psychological Corporation.

Beck, J. S., Beck, A., & Jolly, J. (2001). *Manual for the Beck Youth Inventories of Emotional and Social Impairment.* San Antonio, TX: Psychological Corporation.

Becker, S. P., Langberg, J. M., & Evans, S. W. (2015). Sleep problems predict comorbid externalizing behaviors and depression in young adolescents with attention-deficit/hyperactivity disorder. *European Child Adolescent Psychiatry, 24,* 897–907.

Becker, S. P., Leopold, D. R., Burns, G. L., Jarrett, M. A., Langberg, J. M., Marshall, S. A., . . . Willcutt, E. G. (2016). The internal, external, and diagnostic validity of sluggish cognitive tempo: A meta-analysis and critical review. *Journal of the American Academy of Child and Adolescent Psychiatry, 55,* 163–178.

Biederman, J., Monuteaux, M. C., Doyle, A. E., Seidman, L. J., Wilens, T. E., Ferrero, F., . . . Faraone, S. V. (2004). Impact of executive function deficits and attention-deficit/hyperactivity disorder (ADHD) on academic outcomes in children. *Journal of Consulting and Clinical Psychology, 72,* 757–766.

Booksh, R. L., Pella, R. D., Singh, A. N., & Gouvier, W. D. (2010). Ability of college students to simulate ADHD on objective measures of attention. *Journal of Attention Disorders, 13,* 325–338.

Brady, C. E., Evans, S. W., Berlin, K. S., Bunford, N., & Kern, L. (2012). Evaluating school impairment with adolescents using the Classroom Performance Survey. *School Psychology Review, 41,* 429–446.

Conners, C. K. (2000). *Conners Continuous Performance Test.* North Tonawanda NY: Multi-Health Systems.

Conners, C. K. (2008). *Conners 3rd edition.* Toronto, ON, Canada: Multi-Health Systems.

Cortese, S., Faraone, S. V., Konofal, E., & Lecendreux, M. (2009). Sleep in children with attention-deficit/hyperactivity disorder: Meta-analysis of subjective and objective studies. *Journal of the American Academy of Child and Adolescent Psychiatry, 48,* 894–908.

Donovan, J. E. (1993). Young adult drinking–driving: Behavioral and psychosocial correlates. *Journal of Studies on Alcohol, 54,* 600–613.

Drake, C., Nickel, C., Burduvali, E., Roth, T., Jefferson, C., & Badia, P. (2003). The Pediatric Daytime Sleepiness Scale (PDSS): Sleep habits and school outcomes in middle-school children. *Sleep, 26,* 455–458.

DuPaul, G. J., Power, T. J., Anastopoulos, A. D., & Reid, R. (2016). *ADHD Rating Scale–5 for children and adolescents: Checklists, norms, and clinical interpretation.* New York: Guilford Press.

Dvorsky, M. R., Langberg, J. M., Molitor, S. J., & Bourchtein, E. (2016). Clinical utility and predictive validity of parent and college student symptom ratings in predicting an ADHD diagnosis. *Journal of Clinical Psychology, 72,* 401–418.

Evans, S. W., Allen, J., Moore, S., & Strauss, V. (2005). Measuring symptoms and functioning of youth with ADHD in middle schools. *Journal of Abnormal Child Psychology, 33,* 695–706.

Evans, S. W., Pelham, W. E., Smith, B. H., Bukstein, O., Gnagy, E. M., Greiner, A. R., . . . Baron-Myak, C. (2001). Dose–response effects of methylphenidate on ecologically valid measures of academic performance and classroom behavior in adolescents with ADHD. *Experimental and Clinical Psychopharmacology, 9,* 163–175.

Fabiano, G. A., & Schatz, N. K. (2015). Driving risk interventions for teens with ADHD. In R. A. Barkley (Ed.), *Attention-deficit hyperactivity disorder: A handbook for diagnosis and treatment* (4th ed., pp. 705–727). New York: Guilford Press.

Flory, K., Molina, S. G., Pelham, W. E., Gnagy, E., & Smith, B. (2006). Childhood ADHD predicts risky sexual behavior in young adulthood. *Journal of Clinical Child and Adolescent Psychology, 35,* 571–577.

Fuligni, A. J., & Eccles, J. S. (1993). Perceived parent–child relationships and early adolescents' orientation toward peers. *Developmental Psychology, 29*(4), 622–632.

Gioia, G. A., Isquith, P. K., Guy, S. C., & Kenworthy, L. (2015). *Behavior Rating Inventory of Executive Function* (2nd ed.). Lutz, FL: Psychological Assessment Resources.

Gormley, M. J., Pinho, T., Pollack, B., Puzino, K., Franklin, M., Busch, C., . . . Anastopoulos, A. D. (2018). Impact of study skills and parent education on first-year GPA among college students with and without ADHD: A moderated mediation model. *Journal of Attention Disorders, 22*(4), 334–348.

Gratz, K. L., & Roemer, L. (2004). Multidimensional assessment of emotion regulation and dysregulation: Development, factor structure, and initial validation of the difficulties in emotion regulation scale. *Journal of Psychopathology and Behavioral Assessment, 26,* 41–54.

Green, A. L., & Rabiner, D. L. (2012). What do we really know about ADHD in college students? *Neurotherapeutics, 9,* 559–568.

Gresham, F. M., & Elliott, S. N. (2008). *Social Skills Improvement System.* Minneapolis, MN: Pearson Assessments.

Hoza, B., McQuade, J. D., Murray-Close, D., Shoulberg, E., Molina, B. S. G, Arnold, L. E., . . . Hechtman, L. (2013). Does childhood positive self-perceptual bias mediate adolescent risky behavior in youth from the MTA study? *Journal of Consulting Clinical Psychology, 81,* 846–858.

Hudson, W. W. (1997). Index of family relations. In J. Fischer & K. J. Corcoran (Eds.), *Measures for clinical practice and research: A sourcebook* (pp. 351–352). New York: Oxford University Press.

Jerome, L., Segal, A., & Habinski, L. (2006). What we know about ADHD and driving risk: A literature review, meta-analysis and critique. *Journal of the Canadian Academy of Child and Adolescent Psychiatry, 15,* 105–125.

Johns, M. W. (1998). Rethinking the assessment of sleepiness. *Sleep Medical Review, 2,* 3–15.

Johnston, C., & Mash, E. J. (2001). Families of children with attention-deficit/hyperactivity disorder: Review and recommendations for future research. *Clinical Child and Family Psychology Review, 4,* 183–207.

Kamphaus, R. W., & Reynolds, C. R. (2015). *Behavior Assessment System for Children—Third Edition (BASC-3).* Bloomington, IN: Psychological Corporation.

Kaufman, J., Birmaher, B., Axelson, D., Perepletchikova, F., Brent, D., & Ryan, N. (2016). *Kiddie SADS—Present and Lifetime DSM-5 November 2016 version.* New Haven, CT: Advanced Center for Intervention and Services Research for Early Onset Mood and Anxiety Disorders, Western Psychiatric Institute and Clinic, Child and Adolescent Research and Education Program, Yale University.

Kuriyan, A. B., Pelham, W. E., Jr., Molina, B. S., Waschbusch, D. A., Gnagy, E. M., Sibley, M. H., . . . Kent, K. M. (2013). Young adult educational and vocational outcomes of children diagnosed with ADHD. *Journal of Abnormal Child Psychology, 41*(1), 27–41.

Laracy, S. D., Ridgard, T. J., & DuPaul, G. J. (2015, June). Sleep and school functioning: Guidelines for assessment and intervention. *NASP Communique, 43*(8), 1, 18–21.

Laux, J. M., Piazza, N. J., Salyers, K., & Roseman, C. P. (2012). The Substance Abuse Subtle Screening Inventory–3 and stages of change: A screening validity study. *Journal of Addictions and Offender Counseling, 33,* 82–92.

LeBourgeois, M. K., Giannotti, F., Cortesi, F., Wolfson, A. R., & Harsh, J. (2005). The relationship between reported sleep quantity and sleep hygiene in Italian and American adolescents. *Pediatrics, 115,* 257–265.

Lee, S. S., Humphreys, K. L., Flory, K., Liu, R., & Glass, K. (2011). Prospective association of childhood attention-deficit/hyperactivity disorder and substance use and abuse/dependence: A meta-analytic review. *Clinical Psychology Review, 31,* 328–341.

Lorch, E. P., Milich, R., Astrin, C. C., & Berthiaume, K. S. (2006). Cognitive engagement and story comprehension in typically developing children and children with ADHD from preschool through elementary school. *Developmental Psychology, 42,* 1206–1219.

MacDermott, S. T., Gullone, E., Allen, J. S., King, N. J., & Tonge, B. (2010). The Emotion Regulation Index for Children and Adolescents (ERICA): A psychometric investigation. *Journal of Psychopathology and Behavioral Assessment, 32,* 301–314.

Miller, F. G., & Lazowski, L. E. (1999). *The Substance Abuse Subtle Screening Inventory 3 (SASSI-3) manual.* Springville, IN: SASSI Institute.

Miller, M., Ho, J., & Hinshaw, S. P. (2012). Executive functions in girls with ADHD followed prospectively into young adulthood. *Neuropsychology, 26,* 278–287.

Nigg, J. T., & Barkley, R. A. (2014). Attention deficit hyperactivity disorder. In E. Mash & R. A. Barkley (Eds.), *Child psychopathology* (pp. 75–144). New York: Guilford Press.

Pelham, W. E., Fabiaon, G. A., & Massetti, G. M. (2005). Evidence-based assessment of attention deficit hyperactivity disorder in children and adolescents. *Journal of Clinical Child and Adolescent Psychology, 34,* 449–476.

Pliszka, S. R. (2015). Comorbid psychiatric disorders in children. In R. A. Barkley (Ed.), *Attention-deficit hyperactivity disorder: A handbook for diagnosis and treatment* (4th ed., pp. 140–168). New York: Guilford Press.

Power, T. J., Dombrowski, S. C., Watkins, M. W., Mautone, J. A., & Eagle, J. W. (2007). Assessing children's homework performance: Development of multi-dimensional, multi-informant rating scales. *Journal of School Psychology, 45,* 333–348.

Rabiner, D. L., Anastopoulos, A. D., Costello, E. J., Hoyle, R. H., McCabe, S. E., & Swartzwelder, H. S. (2009). Motives and perceived consequences of nonmedical ADHD medication use by college students. *Journal of Attention Disorders, 13,* 259–270.

Reimer, B., D'Ambrosio, L. A., Gilbert, J., Coughlin, J. F., Biederman, J., Surman, C., . . . Aleardi, M. (2005). Behavior differences in drivers with attention deficit hyperactivity disorder: The Driving Behavior Questionnaire. *Accident Analysis and Prevention, 37,* 996–1004.

Reynolds, W. M. (2002). *Reynolds Adolescent Depression Scale—Second Edition: Professional manual.* Odessa FL: Psychological Assessment Resources.

Roth, R. M., Isquith, P. K., & Gioia, G. A. (2005). *Behavior Rating Inventory of Executive Function—Adult Version (BRIEF-A).* Lutz, FL: Psychological Assessment Resources.

Schrank, F. A., Mather, N., & McGrew, K. S. (2014). *Woodcock–Johnson IV Tests of Achievement.* Rolling Meadows, IL: Riverside.

Seymour, K. E., Chronis-Tuscano, A., Halldorsdottir, T., Stupica, B., Owens, K., & Sacks, T. (2012). Emotion regulation mediates the relationship between ADHD and depressive symptoms in youth. *Journal of Abnormal Child Psychology, 40,* 595–606.

Shaffer, D., Fisher, P., Lucas, C., Dulcan, M., & Schwab-Stone, M. (2000). NIMH Diagnostic Interview Schedule for Children Version IV (NIMH DISC-IV): Description, differences from previous versions, and reliability of some common diagnoses. *Journal of the American Academy of Child and Adolescent Psychiatry, 39,* 28–38.

Shapiro, E. S. (2011). *Academic skills problems, fourth edition workbook.* New York: Guilford Press.

Sheras, P. L., Abidin, R. R., Konold, T. R. (1998). *Stress Index for Parents of Adolescents: Professional manual.* Lutz, FL: Psychological Assessment Resources.

Sibley, M. H., Altszuler, A. R., Morrow, A. S., & Merrill, B. M. (2014). Mapping the academic problem behaviors of adolescents with ADHD. *School Psychology Quarterly, 29,* 422–437.

Sibley, M. H., Evans, S. W., & Zerpell, Z. N. (2010). Social cognition and interpersonal impairment in young adolescents with ADHD. *Journal of Psychopathology and Behavioral Assessment, 32,* 193–202.

Sibley, M. H., Mitchell, J. T., & Becker, S. P. (2016). Method of adult diagnosis influences estimated persistence of childhood ADHD: A systematic review of longitudinal studies. *Lancet Psychiatry, 3,* 1157–1165.

Sibley, M. H., Pelham, W. E., Molina, B. S. G., Gnagy, E. M., Waschbusch, D. A., Garefino, A. C., . . . Karch, K. M. (2012). Diagnosing ADHD in adolescence. *Journal of Consulting and Clinical Psychology, 80,* 139–150.

Sibley, M. H., Pelham, W. E., Molina, B. S. G., Gnagy, E. M., Waxmonsky, J. G., Waschbusch, D. A., . . . Kuriyan, A. B. (2012). When diagnosing ADHD in young adults emphasize informant reports, DSM items, and impairment. *Journal of Consulting and Clinical Psychology, 80,* 1052–1061.

Theule, J., Weiner, J., Rogers, M. A., & Marton, I. (2011). Predicting parenting stress in families of children with ADHD: Parent and contextual factors. *Journal of Child and Family Studies, 20,* 640–647.

Thompson, A. L., Molina, B. S. G., Pelham, W., & Gnagy, E. M. (2007). Risky driving in adolescents and young adults with childhood ADHD. *Journal of Pediatric Psychology, 32,* 745–759.

Turchik, J. A., & Garske, J. P. (2009). Measurement of sexual risk taking among college student. *Archives of Sexual Behavior, 38*(6), 936–948.

Wechsler, D. (2009). *Wechsler Individual Achievement Test—III.* San Antonio, TX: Psychological Corporation.

Weinstein, C. E., Palmer, D. P., & Schulte, A. C. (2002). *Learning and Study Strategies Inventory* (LASSI). Clearwater, FL: H & H Publishing.

Weller, E. B., Weller, R. A., Fristad, M. A., Rooney, M. T., & Schecter, J. (2000). Children's Interview for Psychiatric Syndromes (ChIPS). *Journal of the American Academy of Child and Adolescent Psychiatry, 39,* 76–84.

Weyandt, L. L., & Gudmundsdottir, B. G. (2015). Developmental and neuropsychological deficits in children with ADHD. In R. A. Barkley (Ed.), *Attention-deficit hyperactivity disorder: A handbook for diagnosis and treatment* (4th ed., pp. 116–139). New York: Guilford Press.

WHO ASSIST Working Group. (2002). The Alcohol, Smoking and Substance Involvement Screening Test (ASSIST): Development, reliability and feasibility. *Addiction, 97,* 1183–1184.

Willcutt, E. G., Nigg, J. T., Pennington, B. F., Solanto, M. V., Rohde, L. A., Tannock, R., . . . Lahey, B. B. (2012). Validity of DSM–IV attention deficit/hyperactivity disorder symptom dimensions and subtypes. *Journal of Abnormal Psychology, 121,* 991–1010.

Wolfe, D. A., Scott, K., Reitzel-Jaffe, D., Wekerle, C., Grasley, C., & Straatman, A. L. (2001). Development and validation of the Conflict in Adolescent Dating Relationships Inventory. *Psychological Assessment, 13,* 277–293.

CHAPTER 14

Motivational and Executive Functioning Considerations When Treating Adolescents with ADHD

Margaret H. Sibley

When adolescents with attention-deficit/hyperactivity disorder (ADHD) arrive for clinical treatment, perhaps the most common presenting issue stated by parents and teachers is a lack of motivation in schoolwork, daily responsibilities, and socialization. Other common concerns are problems with disorganization, forgetfulness, and time management. As discussed by Doidge, Saoud, and Toplak (Chapter 4, this volume) findings from neuroimaging and basic cognition studies match the intuitions of parents, teachers, and adolescents during clinical assessment. ADHD is empirically linked to key deficits in executive functioning (EF) and rewards processing, which are associated with structural and functional abnormalities in the prefrontal cortex (PFC) and striatal dopamine circuitry. Impairment relative to household responsibilities (Wiener, Chapter 6, this volume), peers (McQuade, Chapter 7, this volume), and schoolwork (Evans, Van der Oord, & Rogers, Chapter 8, this volume) often stems from these motivational and EF deficits. There is also increasing evidence that the effects of these difficulties extend to additional domains such as risky behavior (Kennedy, McKone, & Molina, Chapter 11, this volume) and driving (Garner, Chapter 12, this volume).

EF and Motivation Deficits in Adolescents with ADHD: An Inextricable Interplay

Below is a review of five ways in which EF and motivational deficits produce behavioral impairments in adolescents with ADHD. I discuss how each domain links to the neurocognitive literature and influences daily life during the adolescent developmental period. These psychological impairments stem from brain-based and cognitive deficits that interact with environmental and developmental contextual factors. As depicted in Figure 14.1, multiple levels of interactions contribute to the complex presentations of adolescents with ADHD.

Organization, Time Management, and Planning Problems

During adolescence, EF deficits that are characteristic of ADHD (see Doidge et al., Chapter 4, this volume) often manifest as organization and time management problems (Barkley, Edwards, Laneri, Fletcher, & Metevia, 2001a). Middle school and high school students need greater self-management than elementary school students and are required to keep track of their own schedule and school materials, turn in assignments with minimal prompts, remember page numbers and worksheets that are given across the day by multiple teachers, and plan for long-term projects (Eccles, 2004). Parental expectations increase during the teen years to include independent completion of daily chores without reminders and self-management of homework. Social interactions become more complicated. Adolescence is a time of normative adjustment problems as teens struggle to master this new environmental context (Eccles, 2004). As a result of these mounting environmental demands, it is not surprising that organization, time management, and planning (OTP) deficits are the most consistently identified mechanisms of school failure among adolescents with ADHD (Langberg, Dvorsky, & Evans, 2013; Sibley, Altszuler, Morrow, & Merrill, 2014). For example, Sibley, Altszuler, Morrow, et al. (2014) reported that teachers rated time management problems and difficulties keeping track of homework deadlines as the most common behavioral impairments of adolescents with ADHD. Langberg et al. (2011) reported that management of school materials predicts homework problems in middle school students with ADHD, while Langberg et al. (2013) reported that organization and planning problems in middle school predict reductions in grade point average (GPA) beyond the contribution of ADHD symptoms. OTP deficits persist in college students with ADHD and are associated with college performance (Kern, Rasmussen, Byrd, & Wittschen, 1999; Meaux, Green, & Broussard, 2009; Schwanz, Palm, & Brallier, 2007), mediating the relationship between ADHD and GPA in college students (Dvorsky &

Brain Level

Impairment in regions and pathways involved in executive functioning and rewards processing such as prefrontal cortex and frontal–striatal dopamine circuits.

Cognitive Level

Impairment in basic cognitive processes such as rewards sensitivity, working memory, and inhibitory control.

Environmental Level

Childhood learning history characterized by negative environmental feedback and effort failing to yield success. Potential imbalance between environmental demands and availability of resources to support cognitive deficits.

Developmental Level

Hypersensitivity to social and emotional rewards. Increased expectations for self-reliance at school and home. Developmental mismatch between cognitive maturity and complexity of academic and social demands.

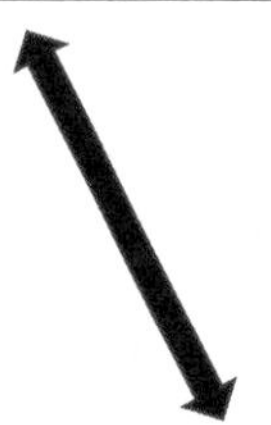

Psychological Level

Low intrinsic and extrinsic motivation. Impairment in goal-directed behavior, willpower, grit, and delay of gratification. Poor self-efficacy and locus of control. Impairment pursuing long-term goals or rewards.

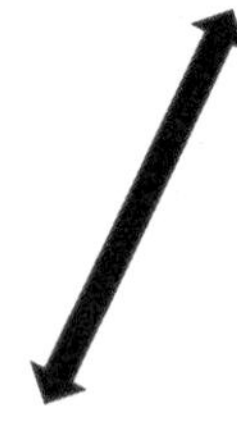

Behavioral Level

Low effort on academic and household tasks. Decreased social approach. Organization, time management, and planning problems at home and school.

FIGURE 14.1. Complex causal pathways between ADHD neurocognitive deficits and their consequences for adolescent behavior.

Langberg, 2014). When already struggling adolescents with ADHD experience added developmental maladjustment, serious long-term consequences may ensue (e.g., course failure, deviant behavior, and school disengagement; Kuriyan et al., 2013; Molina et al., 2012).

Goal-Directed Behavior

Aside from OTP problems (Langberg et al., 2013), EF deficits also may lead to problems with *goal-directed behavior,* or using top-down executive functions to implement actions in support of one's goals and suppress counterproductive motivational states (Kim, 2013). Whereas *motivation* encompasses one's decision to engage in an activity or pursue an outcome, goal-directed behavior involves the ability to persist at this pursuit (Kuhl, 1987). Goal-directed behavior involves excising cognitive (e.g., persisting in the face of boredom) and emotional (e.g., persisting in the face of frustration) control, as well as higher order planning to implement environmental control (e.g., avoiding environments that might lead to distractions). At the heart of conceptual models of ADHD (Barkley, 1997; Nigg, 2001) are EF-related and self-control deficits that are reflected by poor performance on tasks that measure cognitive (Desman, Petermann, & Hampel, 2008; Willcutt, Doyle, Nigg, Faraone, & Pennington, 2005) and emotional control (Musser et al., 2011; Sobanski et al., 2010), as well as poor higher order planning when self-selecting work-completion strategies (Alvarado, Puente, Jiménez, & Arrebillaga, 2011). ADHD-related deficits in goal-directed behavior may be particularly pernicious in adolescence, because rewards circuitry matures earlier than does the PFC (Casey, Jones, & Hare, 2008). Typically developing adolescents are challenged to use immature EFs (i.e., inhibitory control and planning) to exert self-control in the face of socially and emotionally salient stimuli (e.g., smartphones, peer interactions, substances). Thus, ADHD and the adolescent brain are a double threat to goal-directed behavior.

Intrinsic Motivation

Intrinsic motivation is the level of enjoyment experienced while completing a task (Oudeyer, Kaplan, & Hafner, 2007). Plamondon and Martinussen (2015) reported that ADHD symptoms are negatively correlated with intrinsic motivation and engagement in learning. Morsink et al. (2017) reported that, compared to adolescents without ADHD, those with the diagnosis reported reduced intrinsic motivation for learning and were more likely to perceive slow or long-lasting academic tasks as boring or aversive. Intrinsic motivation is significantly related to task performance—the more an adolescent enjoys a task, the more likely he or she is to engage in it for natural rewards (i.e., acquiring new information, the subjective feeling of accomplishment; Gottfried, 1985; Vallerand et al., 1993).

The rewards processing deficits of adolescents with ADHD (see Doidge et al., Chapter 4, this volume) may have a direct impact on intrinsic motivation. As a result of these deficits, natural rewards embedded in school and household tasks may be less salient to adolescents with ADHD. Teens with ADHD may experience lower intrinsic motivation to complete work, because they experience reduced sensitivity to endogenous rewards associated with learning or other daily activities (e.g., household responsibilities, extracurricular programs, social events). Rewards sensitivity deficits are also theorized to reduce learning from the natural consequences of one's behavior. For example, on the occasion that a teen with ADHD enjoys an academic task, he or she still may not properly store the task as positively rewarding (Sonuga-Barke, 2003). The learning history of an adolescent with ADHD may also influence intrinsic motivation. Years of cross-situational impairments may create learned associations between daily responsibilities (i.e., schoolwork, chores, social interactions) and aversive intrinsic consequences (i.e., feelings of incompetent, boredom). Learned associations between academic work and subjective feelings of enjoyment are the basis of stable intrinsic motivation for learning (Oudeyer et al., 2007).

Extrinsic Motivation

Extrinsic motivation is the value that an individual places on an outcome. Whereas the rewards associated with intrinsic motivation are *endogenous*, or fused with the activity itself, the rewards associated with extrinsic motivation are *exogenous*, or separate from the activity (Kruglanski, Stein, & Riter, 1977). Intrinsic motivation appears to decline at the transition to adolescence (Anderman & Midgley, 1997) as schoolwork and daily responsibilities grow more challenging and less enjoyable. As a result, there is an important role for extrinsic motivation (e.g., desire to achieve a high grade, desire to please adults) in adolescent success (Anderman, Maehr, & Midgley, 1999). Extrinsic motivation may be *self-initiated* (i.e., performing a task to get high school grades) or *other-initiated* (i.e., performing a task to obtain a reward that has been offered by an adult). Self-directed extrinsic motivation may be particularly protective for adolescents with ADHD. Gut, Heckmann, Meyer, Schmid, and Grob (2012) found that the relationship between the desire to achieve in school and academic performance was stronger in students with ADHD than in typically developing students. Similarly, Merkt and Gawrilow (2016) reported that young adults with ADHD who were enrolled in a 4-year university had higher extrinsic academic motivation than peers without the disorder. These finding may indicate that individuals with ADHD experience lower levels of intrinsic motivation; therefore, to compensate, the value adolescents with ADHD place on their performance (extrinsic motivation) must be especially high to ensure success.

As with intrinsic motivation, adolescents with ADHD may find lower reward value in the extrinsic outcomes associated with success (i.e., social or tangible rewards from adults, making the honor roll, being known as a good student) due to rewards sensitivity deficits. Once again, their impaired response to rewards also may leave them with a less salient learning history: Students with ADHD may show lower extrinsic motivation to repeat a positive behavior if they have a weaker internal representation of its exogenous benefits. Furthermore, deficits may lead to learned associations between daily responsibilities and a range of aversive extrinsic consequences (i.e., adult reprimands, academic probation, taunting by peers).

Self-Efficacy

Individuals with ADHD have reduced self-esteem compared to peers (Newark, Elsässer, & Stieglitz, 2016; Philipsen et al., 2007; Ramsay & Rostain, 2008). This is not surprising, as youth with ADHD typically receive high levels of negative environmental feedback from parents (Johnston & Mash, 2001), teachers (Nelson & Roberts, 2000), and peers (Hoza, 2007). As a result of reduced self-esteem, individuals with ADHD may have lower *self-efficacy,* or the belief that they are capable of achieving desired outcomes (Newark et al., 2016). In a recent study, in a sample of 285 young adolescents with ADHD who self-reported expectancies about their ability to successfully complete homework (i.e., homework self-efficacy), Langberg et al. (2017) positively predicted teacher-rated homework completion. Students with ADHD may not attempt to pursue an outcome if they do not believe they will be successful (Zimmerman, 2000). Thus, the life experiences associated with ADHD may influence teens' beliefs about the self. In turn, these beliefs may undercut adolescent motivation.

A Complex Clinical Presentation

Most frequently, adolescents with ADHD present with both EF deficits and motivation problems. When parents or teachers state that an adolescent with ADHD experiences a problem with *motivation,* they often choose this word to describe perceived difficulties with task effort. As I discussed earlier, reduced effort may be a consequence of a number of combined EF and motivation-related cognitive deficits. The impairing nature of these deficits in adolescence represents an agglomeration of factors related to development stage, environmental fit, cognitive functions, and learning history (see Figure 14.1). Because OTP problems and reduced effort arise from so many sources, it is not just teens with rewards sensitivity deficits (i.e., those with ADHD combined presentation) who struggle to initiate tasks and sustain effort. Furthermore, for the reasons I described earlier, the unique developmental context of adolescence may elevate both OTP problems and goal-directedness–motivation difficulties as central features of ADHD during this life stage.

TREATMENT APPROACHES

Because EF and motivational deficits can influence teen functioning in diverse and interrelated ways, most psychosocial treatment approaches for adolescent ADHD are multimodal. Despite shared impairments, the lives and difficulties of teens with ADHD are heterogeneous and dynamic. To promote a personalized approach to treatment (Gray, 2013), below are descriptions of intervention components that have been integrated in empirically supported treatments for adolescents with ADHD. Following these descriptions is a discussion of how these components may be blended in treatment to address the intertwined deficits that aggregate to produce impairments, as well as key issues when devising a treatment approach.

Improving Environmental Fit

The demands of the adolescent environment may exacerbate symptoms of ADHD (Turgay, Lasser, Goodman, & Asherson, 2012). At the same time, a teen's natural strengths and interests may mitigate the effects of his or her deficits. For example, encouraging adolescents with ADHD to pursue high-interest educational tracks and extracurricular activities maximizes intrinsic motivation to learn and extrinsic motivation to achieve desired outcomes in these activities. When adolescents with ADHD are given opportunities to develop their strengths, they may increase their global self-efficacy and experience successes that lead to opportunities that capitalize on strengths, while diminishing the influence of deficits. They may also internalize the link between high effort and success. Devoting time in treatment to identifying strengths, discussing how to cultivate them, and finding best-fit environments may improve the adolescent's functioning long term.

OTP Skills Instruction

Interventions that target OTP problems in teens with ADHD typically involve remedial training and daily repetition of strategies that compensate for EF deficits. The aim of this skills-based approach is to increase compensatory abilities to offset the effects of EF deficits. These strategies include systematically recording daily homework, maintaining a bookbag organization system, applying time management strategies, using active studying techniques, using lists to complete daily responsibilities, and taking notes in class (Evans, Axelrod, & Langberg, 2004; Langberg, Epstein, Becker, Girio-Herrera, & Vaughn, 2012).

Teaching Cognitive and Self-Regulation Skills

Due to burgeoning metacognitive abilities (Blakemore & Choudhury, 2006), adolescence marks the first time that cognitive-behavioral techniques may be developmentally appropriate in the treatment of ADHD (see Sprich & Burbridge, Chapter 16, this volume). These strategies can be particularly useful in the treatment of deficits in goal-directed behavior and include identifying and replacing cognitions that promote procrastination (Antshel, Faraone, & Gordon, 2014), introducing problem-solving strategies that promote metacognition and strategy selection (Barkley, Edwards, Laneri, Fletcher, & Metevia, 2001b), and diffusing emotional reactivity by teaching self-control strategies and communication skills (i.e., reflective listening, "I" statements; Barkley et al., 2001b). Teaching these compensatory skills may allow teens to exercise greater self-control in the face of tempting distractions, thereby increasing the diligence with which they pursue their goals. These strategies may also prevent EF-related emotional difficulties (Bunford, Chapter 5, this volume) and metacognitive deficits from undermining sustained effort on daily tasks.

Goal Setting and Implementation Intentions

Low extrinsic motivation may arise when the adolescent is unaware of the full range of positive outcomes associated with a task. One way to increase extrinsic motivation for daily tasks is to allow an adolescent to select personal goals and to plan the steps needed to achieve the goal (i.e., implementation intentions; Gollwitzer & Brandstätter, 1997). Goals provide an important link between tasks and outcome. In addition, working memory and other EF deficits may lead to difficulties recalling salient reasons to persist on aversive tasks in the moment. Interventions for adolescents with ADHD that utilize implementation intentions (Gawrilow, Morgenroth, Schultz, Oettingen, & Gollwitzer, 2013) may circumvent deficits in goal-directed behavior by creating if–then decision rules (e.g., "If my friends text me during homework, then I will say I cannot talk until after I finish") that are mentally available for adolescents to implement in situations that test their self-control.

Motivational Interviewing

Motivational interviewing (MI; Miller & Rollnick, 2013) uses social psychology principles as conversational strategies that enhance patients' motivation to achieve outcomes that they value and want to prioritize. Like goal setting, MI has been used to increase the teen's perceived value of academic and behavioral success. However, in addition to identifying a desired outcome, MI includes mental contrasting (Oettingen et al., 2009) that juxtaposes a desired future with a present reality. MI also includes exploration of personal values and priorities to enhance awareness of one's identity and desired future—which supports the adolescent developmental goal of identity development (Steinberg & Morris, 2001). MI targets teen openness to trying new strategies and increasing effort on daily responsibilities—even when these tasks may feel aversive. MI emphases on autonomy support, respectful collaboration as equals, and affirming a client's worth contribute to a treatment atmosphere that reduces skepticism and oppositional attitudes in adolescents. MI targets self-efficacy by increasing an adolescent's awareness of his or her successes and affirming efforts during treatment. MI is designed to increase self-initiated extrinsic motivation. However, for adolescents with ADHD, increasing self-motivation may be insufficient to create long-term behavioral change. Additional intervention may be necessary to help the adolescent follow through on steps required to meet his or her goals.

Adult-Implemented Monitoring and Contingency Management

First-generation interventions to address the motivation problems of adolescents with ADHD targeted extrinsic motivation through adult-delivered contingency management (see Smith, Waschbusch, Willoughby, & Evans, 2000, for review). When adolescents lack intrinsic and extrinsic self-motivation to complete required daily tasks, adult-implemented contingency management creates new, adult-initiated, sources of extrinsic motivation. These interventions utilize classic behavioral principles that set clear expectations for task performance and titrate the immediacy and strength of environmental rewards associated with meeting these expectations (e.g., access to electronics and privileges at home) until the teen reliably demonstrates the appropriate behavior (Kazdin, 2001). By enhancing rewards for aversive tasks, contingency management can create consequences that are impossible to ignore, overriding EF deficits in working memory and inhibitory control that can impede sustained mental effort (see Figure 14.1). These treatments are upward extensions of childhood behavioral treatments for ADHD (Fabiano et al., 2009). Adolescent adaptations of adult-implemented contingency management include converting naturally rewarding aspects of the adolescent's environment (i.e., social time with friends, electronics and social media use, use of the car) to privileges that are contingent on meeting expectations. To uphold adolescent autonomy, use of behavioral contracts (these emphasize equality between the adult and teen and a need for mutual compromise; Forgatch

& Patterson, 1989) replaces point charts and Daily Report Cards used in childhood (Fabiano et al., 2009).

Blended Approaches

Given the complexity of EF and motivation deficits, nearly all empirically supported treatments for adolescents with ADHD take a blended approach—integrating multiple previously discussed components. For example, one of the first empirically supported treatments for adolescent ADHD, the Challenging Horizons afterschool program (Evans et al., 2016), includes OTP skills instruction, problem-solving skills, social goal setting, and contingency management (i.e., providing snacks to students who demonstrate good organization skills, enhanced social reinforcement by staff members, allowing students with completed assignments to participate in recreational activities). Another, more recent program (Plan My Life; Boyer, Geurts, Prins, & Van der Oord, 2015) includes OTP skill instruction, cognitive-behavioral skills, goal setting, and motivational interviewing. Both of these treatments engage multiple approaches to simultaneously target a range of EF and motivation deficits in adolescents with ADHD. Doing so maximizes efficacy and may be necessary to create detectable changes in functioning. Early single-modality approaches were substantially less efficacious than these modern blended approaches (for reviews, see Smith et al., 2000; Sibley, Kuriyan, Evans, Waxmonsky, & Smith, 2014). One disadvantage of these blended approaches is an inability to disentangle active intervention ingredients when conducting treatment outcome research—just like the deficits, components are interwoven rather than distinct. Also, given the heterogeneity of youth with ADHD and their daily contexts, there is no optimal approach to sequencing and combining these treatments—youth are treated in a personalized manner when treatment planning (Kazdin, 2016).

Selecting an Engagement-Based Implementation Strategy

In addition to selecting treatment components that align with an adolescent's presenting difficulties, an implementation strategy must be selected. Implementation strategies are key to maximizing engagement in treatment. Existing treatments for adolescents with ADHD that utilize the components I reviewed earlier include afterschool programming (Evans, Schultz, DeMars, & Davis, 2011), pull-out meetings with a school counselor (Langberg et al., 2012), intensive summer programs (Sibley et al., 2011), school consultation interventions (Evans, Serpell, Schultz, & Pastor, 2007), parent training programs (Barkley et al., 2001b), parent–teen therapy sessions (Sibley, Graziano, et al., 2016), individual therapy sessions with the teen (Antshel et al., 2014; Boyer et al., 2015; Sprich, Saften, Finkelstein, Remmert, & Hammerness, 2016), and simultaneously held parent and teen therapy groups (Sibley, Altszuler, Ross, et al., 2014). Though these formats have advantages, each may invite a number of population-specific barriers that may threaten engagement and implementation. Thus, implementation strategies must also be customized to the adolescent's context and give attention to engagement barriers.

Balancing Adolescent Autonomy with Adult Involvement

Autonomy development is a critical goal for adolescents as they prepare for adult life (Steinberg & Morris, 2001). By young adulthood, individuals with ADHD lag behind peers in independence from parents and autonomous functioning (Altszuler et al., 2016). As a part of autonomy development, adolescent norms stipulate self-management and formation of personal values (Ryan & Deci, 2000). One dilemma when treating adolescents with ADHD is whether to rely on adult-initiated, rather than self-initiated, sources of motivation. There are concerns that using manipulated external rewards to motivate behavior can undermine adolescent self-determination and intrinsic motivation (Deci, Koestner, & Ryan, 1999). On the other hand, the long-term goal of contingency management is to create self-motivation in the adolescent by newly exposing the teen to natural intrinsic and extrinsic rewards associated with increased effort. For example, a student who does not value grades or enjoy learning may be incentivized by a parent to complete a school project with the promise of a social outing. Once the project is complete, it is hoped that the adolescent will encode and store additional benefits of performing the task (e.g., intellectual fulfillment, pride, praise from teachers, reduced hovering from parents) that in turn increase his or her likelihood of repeating the behavior without an adult-imposed consequence. Without the adult-administered reward, it is possible that the student might never initiate the project in the first place. Unfortunately, there has been no research examining the long-term effects of contingency management on self-motivation in adolescents with ADHD. Thus, the extent to which there is a transfer of motivation from adult to self-initiated sources remains unknown.

If an adolescent is unable to cultivate sufficient self-directed motivation (i.e., through environmental modification, goal setting, skills building, implementation intentions, or motivational interviewing) to overcome impairments in task completion, generating adult-initiated motivation through adult monitoring and contingency management may be advantageous. It is important to recognize that a monitoring and contingency management approach is contrasted with an adult-assistance approach. In the former, adolescents are expected to self-correct their behavior (e.g., using new organization strategies, contacting teachers for themselves to learn of forgotten assignments, completing homework independently) and accept negative consequences of failing to meet expectations (e.g., privilege removal, sitting out on activities in a group treatment program). In the latter, an adult might correct the problem for the adolescent (e.g., reorganizing a student's materials for him or her, personally contacting teachers to learn of homework assignments that the student failed to record or remember) or remind and assist the teen with tasks until they are completed. The former preserves the important adolescent goal of autonomy development; the latter fails to transfer responsibility onto the student and may create dependence on the adult.

Whether an adult monitoring and contingency management approach is advisable elicits a number of dilemmas. Resolution of these dilemmas requires prioritization of conflicting values, which can only be determined by the adolescent and the adults in his or her unique cultural and familial context. With respect to using adult-implemented rewards and consequences to enhance motivation and goal-directed behavior, families must weigh the relative importance of adolescent self-determination and autonomy development against desires to see an immediate change in teen behavior. This predicament is particularly complicated for adolescents with ADHD. For example, academic failure in secondary school begets a cascade of negative outcomes for youth with ADHD that may include school disengagement, risk behaviors, substance use, and dropout (Barkley, Fischer, Smallish, & Fletcher, 2002; Kent et al., 2011; Molina et al., 2012). Utilization of contingency management is an effective strategy to create immediate behavioral change—potentially offsetting negative developmental trajectories that begin with school failure (Molina et al., 2012). Though this strategy may come at a cost of student autonomy development, evaded risk trajectories may outweigh this cost for some families. In another dilemma, there is evidence that adults' use of contingency management to set limits on adolescents with ADHD may lead to conflict between the teen and the adult (Barkley et al., 2001b; Edwards, Barkley, Laneri, Fletcher, & Metevia, 2001). Chronic conflict in families of youth with ADHD catalyzes negative adult outcomes (Barkley, Anastopoulos, Guevremont, & Fletcher, 1991; Sibley, Pelham, et al., 2014). Thus, self-directed motivation strategies, which may be slower to change behavior, may be preferable to families who want to avoid conflict at all costs—even if it means reduced or slower behavioral change in treatment. It is also important to consider that different families and cultural contexts place varying degrees of importance on adolescent autonomy, rule following and deference to authority, and academic success. Because these decisions are personal, treatment planning for an adolescent with ADHD cannot be unilaterally conducted by the clinician—it must involve collaboration from the adolescent and the adults in his or her life.

When contingency management is implemented with adolescents, several techniques may preserve autonomy and promote teen consent. Adults may consider using contingency management as a last resort when self-motivation is insufficient and stakes are sufficiently high to justify costs to self-determination (Deci et al., 1999). Contingency management may be more amenable to teens when posed as a strategy for self-motivation (e.g., "To stay motivated, I am making a decision to remove my distracting phone until after homework by giving it to my mom") rather than imposed limits (e.g., "My mom is taking away my phone after school"). Offering an explanation for why a task is necessary (e.g., "Completing homework daily helps you retain information") and acknowledging when tasks may be boring, difficult, or uninteresting also may increase teen consent to contingency management. Finally, adults can allow as much choice as possible in *how* a task is completed as long as the teen meets expectations. In fact, adults may actively expand opportunities for choice (e.g., allowing the teen to decide when and where homework is done, reducing parental involvement in the steps to task completion).

Overcoming Resource and Environmental Barriers

Some of the blended treatment packages developed for adolescents with ADHD, including summer and after school programs (i.e., Challenging Horizon's program; Evans et al., 2016; summer treatment program for adolescents with ADHD; Sibley et al., 2011) are intensive and require large quantities of staff time, space, and supplies to implement. These treatments provide a holistic and immersive treatment experience in high-resource environments that can support these models. One advantage of these models is that program staff members, rather than natural adult stakeholders (i.e., parents and teachers) can be engaged to conduct monitoring and contingency management. This may reduce arguments noted in treatments that seek to engage parents as purveyors of contingency management (Barkley et al., 2001b)—as might hiring an organization coach to provide daily monitoring and contingency management. When family, school, or community resources permit these approaches, they maximize treatment comprehensiveness. At the same time, these models have been criticized as not being realistic in most communities. There are also concerns that these approaches are not sustainable after treatment is discontinued, because they fail to engage natural stakeholders in the teen's environment. However, these concerns have not been examined empirically.

Less intensive treatments involve weekly meetings between the adolescent and a mental health professional. These can be resource-efficient alternatives in contexts that cannot sustain intensive programming. When school districts can devote 30 minutes to an hour of weekly staff time to a student with ADHD, pull-out organization skills programs such as Homework, Organization, and Planning Skills (HOPS; Langberg et al., 2012) can be a fitting implementation package. When families have access to mental health care through insurance or public funding, clinical therapists can deliver any of the noted intervention components in individual, family, or group formats (Antshel et al., 2014; Boyer et al., 2015; Sibley, Altszuler, Ross, et al., 2014; Sibley, Olson, Morley, Campez, & Pelham, 2016; Sprich et al., 2016). Treatment delivery becomes challenging when adolescents attend schools with low resources, do not possess insurance that covers mental health services, and cannot qualify for community grant funding. It is important to remember that our ability to treat ADHD in adolescence, regardless of approach, fully relies on available resources.

Overcoming Interfering Stakeholder Beliefs and Behaviors

Adult stakeholders in the treatment of adolescent EF and motivational deficits typically include parent figures and teachers. These adults are naturally present in the adolescent's daily environment and their expectations define adolescent success. Though involvement of parents and teachers can enhance the success of treatments for adolescent EF and motivational deficits, a number of stakeholder beliefs and behaviors can interfere with a teen's success in treatment.

Middle and high school teachers typically teach over 100 students and spend less than an hour a day in the presence of each student. As a result, they often state that they have much less available time, attention, and resources to offer individual students than do elementary teachers (Benner & Graham, 2009; Eccles, 2004). Unlike in earlier grades, secondary school teachers typically identify as teachers of "content" (e.g., Algebra, Chemistry). Embedded in this school culture is the view that interventionists, and not academic teachers, are expected to provide support services to struggling students (National Center on Response Intervention, 2013). Additionally, secondary teachers typically expect students to be self-reliant, citing that teens are sufficiently mature to complete academic tasks without adult support. Secondary teachers are known to refuse participation in interventions due to philosophical reasons (DuPaul & Weyandt, 2006), which may be exacerbated by teacher burnout (Hakanen, Baker, & Schaufeli, 2006). Successful efforts to overcome these barriers have included involving teachers who have a special relationship with the student (e.g., an athletic coach), setting expectations that the adolescent must approach the teacher to prompt his or her involvement (e.g., the teen asks the teacher to sign a planner, rather than the teacher being expected to approach the teen), and emphasizing teacher voice and expertise in designing school-based intervention components (Sibley, Olson, et al., 2016).

As previously mentioned, parenting an adolescent requires a precarious autonomy support balance: Too much parental involvement can stifle teen independence, while too little may prevent the teen from being held accountable for his or her actions (Baumrind, 2005). Through latent class analysis, our team (Sibley, Campez, et al., 2016) demonstrated that a subset of parents of adolescents with ADHD (20.4%) appeared to achieve this balance (termed *parent–teen collaboration*) characterized by pairing consistent but noninvasive monitoring with collaborative planning and as-needed use of contingency management strategies to promote independent task completion. However, the majority of parents displayed one of three maladaptive styles: (1) *parental control* (18.7%), characterized by pervasive overmonitoring, directing, and assisting with school activities; (2) *homework assistance* (20.4%), in which the parent provides invasive assistance with homework, such as completing assignments for the adolescent; and (3) *uninvolved* (40.5%), characterized by minimal to no monitoring, assistance, or involvement in academics. All three maladaptive patterns were associated with higher levels of parent and youth psychopathology than the more balanced parent–teen collaboration style; therefore, treatment for adolescents with ADHD may be impeded if parents display maladaptive parenting profiles—regardless of teen efforts in treatment.

Another key barrier when engaging parents in the treatment of EF and motivational deficits is parental confidence in the intervention. Based on past attempts to treat teens' chronic difficulties, parents of adolescents with ADHD may believe that organization or behavioral strategies work only for a short while (if at all). This belief is grounded in the reality that no long-term effects have been found for behavioral intervention delivered in childhood (Molina et al., 2009). Therefore, parents may believe that strategies introduced by therapists are not realistic long-term solutions. Parents also may have low confidence in the teen's abilities to change and in their own abilities to successfully influence their teen's behavior. After witnessing a decade of ADHD-related impairments, parents may believe that the teen is incapable of independently managing his or her life, and that parental attempts at influencing teen behavior are bound to be fruitless.

In addition, ADHD possesses a genetic component (see Willcutt, Chapter 3, this volume) and, as such, parents of teens with ADHD may struggle with their own EF deficits (Nigg, Blaskey, Stawicki, & Sachek, 2004) and may forget to reinforce daily skills at home or struggle to provide the adolescent with a consistent home routine. Even without parental ADHD, contingency management for adolescents with ADHD can be complicated and challenging to refine due to dilemmas that include (1) difficulties restricting electronics access when electronics are required for homework completion or communicating with parents, (2) the reality that adolescents are often left unattended after school, leaving parents unavailable to monitor teen skills practice and contingency management in person, and (3) ADHD-related deficits in reward sensitivity that limit the range of reinforcers that are incentivizing to the adolescent (see Doidge et al.,

Chapter 4, this volume). Parents may struggle to troubleshoot contingency management when things do not go according to plan, become impatient with gradual (instead of rapid) behavioral change, or believe that treatment is ineffective at the first sign of a setback. As previously noted, parents may believe that asking teens to complete treatment activities could become a source of additional arguments (Weisz & Hawley, 2002)—a fear that our research has substantiated in the short-term (Garcia, Medina, & Sibley, in press). Therefore, parents of teens with an oppositional attitude may fail to monitor and reinforce practice of new skills to avoid negative reactions from teens. Any of these factors may impact parent efforts, leading to premature treatment disengagement. Strategies to overcome these parent-related barriers are discussed below in the context of an example intervention.

A Blended, Engagement-Oriented Intervention: Supporting Teens' Autonomy Daily

In consideration of the information discussed in this chapter, my team and I undertook the task of developing a blended, engagement-oriented intervention for the EF and motivation deficits of adolescents with ADHD. Our model was empirically informed by extant research on adolescents with ADHD and evolved to address the unique engagement barriers that appeared in our societal and community context. Undoubtedly, there are alternative methods of combining empirically supported components using novel engagement strategies that match the unique demands of other cultures and communities. Description of our treatment—Supporting Teens' Autonomy Daily (STAND; Sibley, 2016)—might serve as a starting point for professionals constructing their own intervention approaches for adolescents with ADHD.

STAND was designed as a weekly, time-limited (typically 10–12 one-hour sessions) parent–teen therapy that targets EF and motivational deficits in adolescents. In our context, we selected a clinic-based model due to insufficient intervention delivery resources in our surrounding schools paired with widespread community access to mental health services through Medicaid, private, and state health insurance programs. We opted for a blended modular treatment approach, so that therapists could collaborate with family members to tailor treatment plans to the unique deficits of each teen in his or her distinct environmental context. Understanding that EF and motivational deficits in teens with ADHD may stem from different sources and require different treatments, STAND includes optional modules in all of the intervention components reviewed at the beginning of this chapter. MI is implemented throughout both to directly treat motivation and EF deficits and to increase parent and teen engagement in treatment. Knowing that many adolescents require contingency management to change their behavior, and understanding that interfering parental behaviors can undermine treatment, we chose to engage a parent as a stakeholder with specific efforts to address parent-related barriers. We felt that a parent should be involved, because parents are available, invested, and create continuity—interacting with the teen for more than just a single school year. Working directly with parents and teens together also allows for remediation of parent–teen relationship problems, maladaptive parenting practices, and homework problems (key predictors of outcome for adolescents with ADHD; Langberg et al., 2011; Molina et al., 2012).

STAND occurs in three phases with a few sessions devoted to each—engagement, skills, and planning. In the *engagement phase,* parents and teens explore their personal goals, values, and priorities, while parents share their current parenting tendencies and philosophy. A strengths-based approach is used that identifies environments in which the teen feels most successful and helps the teen and parent identify and recognize unique teen strengths that may be harnessed to overcome the effects of deficits. MI is implemented heavily throughout this phase, including mental contrasting designed to increase a perceived discrepancy between parent and teen current behaviors and their goals and values. Importantly, the parent discusses personal goals for him- or herself as a parent (e.g., becoming more consistent with rules, yelling less, finding more time to spend with the teen), rather than setting goals for teen improvement. The therapist is trained to listen to the parent and the teen's stories to learn about their unique familial and cultural context and to honor their worldview during therapy. At the end of the engagement phase, parent and teen review a menu that contains a list of OTP, cognitive, and behavioral skills that could be learned and practiced in the context of STAND (e.g., bookbag organization, using a daily planner, active study skills, problem solving). The therapist collaborates with the family members as equals in selecting two or three skills that seem most relevant to the teen's difficulties.

The *skills phase* begins with an introduction of the basics of parent–teen conflict management and behavioral contracting to parents and teens. Equipping all families with these skills facilitates corrective efforts when sessions become emotionally escalated and provide parents and teens with initial tools for setting rules at home and rewarding teen successes. Each week, the parent and teen are asked to devise a home practice activity that will serve as a trial-and-error approach to integrating new skills into the home and school routine—frequently with a behavioral contract to increase adolescent motivation to practice new strategies.

In the *planning phase,* parents and teens reflect on progress and lessons learned during weekly home activities to collaboratively set expectations for the teen's daily routine and determine consequences (as needed) for independently practicing new skills and demonstrating self-initiated behaviors (e.g., writing all homework in a planner, waking up independently).

The planning modules also include content on engaging the school in treatment and conclude with MI conversations designed to heighten parent and teen awareness of the link between changes made during treatments and positive improvements in the parent and teen's quality of life.

For parents, one intended outcome of STAND is movement toward the parent–teen collaboration style detected in our latent class analysis (Sibley, Campez, et al., 2016). As part of therapy individualization, therapists and parents discuss the parent's current parenting at the outset of treatment, how these tendencies developed, and what maintains them. The therapist asks the parent to forecast the long-term effects of his or her current parenting practices. The parent considers whether changing aspects of parenting would better support his or her parenting goals and values. Throughout treatment, progress is linked to these parenting goals, which increases parental commitment to a modified and more balanced parenting approach. For overinvolved parents, this may include reducing reminders and assistance despite fears that the teen's grades may drop with reduced parental support. For uninvolved parents, this may include increasing oversight or more consistently enforcing consequences, despite skepticism that efforts will not pay off.

An important component of STAND is that during these activities, the therapist is trained to use deliberate strategies (often through MI) that reduce known barriers and enhance engagement. With respect to parent confidence, STAND therapists are trained to draw parental awareness to small positive changes that the teen makes during treatment, increase parent openness to trying an intervention for a single week, affirm even small parental efforts, and help the parent link new parenting strategies to teen behavioral changes. With respect to sustained parent implementation of new strategies, therapists use therapeutic reflections that reframe parental expectations about progress, helping parents accept a best-case scenario instead of settling only for an ideal. Therapists reframe setbacks as helpful learning moments rather than failures. Parental organization and problem-solving difficulties are addressed by guiding parents through imaginal implementation of weekly contingency management plans and setting implementation intentions (Gollwitzer, 1999) for anticipated challenging scenarios (e.g., "If the teen does not complete homework by dinner, then I will not help him and will take away his phone").

Like all of the treatment packages cited in this chapter, STAND leads to clinically meaningful changes in teen (and parent) behaviors in controlled clinical trials (see reviews by Chan, Fogler, & Hammerness, 2016; Sibley, Kuriyan, et al., 2014). This includes teen OTP skills, ADHD severity, homework behavior, GPA, and the parent–teen relationship. It also includes reduced parent stress level and use of parent–teen contracts at home (Sibley et al., 2013; Sibley, Graziano, et al., 2016). Most effects are noted up to 6 months after treatment ceases.

FUTURE DIRECTIONS

The field knows very little about the long-term impact of psychosocial treatments for ADHD delivered in adolescence. There have been no long-term outcome studies of treatments for adolescent ADHD. There are also unanswered questions about what aspects of motivation and EF change during treatment—future treatment studies should measure a broader range of cognitive and motivational constructs to deepen this understanding. Additional research on ADHD in adolescence should link findings on neurocognition and basic cognitive processes to psychological and behavioral aspects of teen motivation and behavior. Additional work is also needed to identify additional strategies to improve engagement in a broader range of contexts.

REFERENCES

Altszuler, A., Page, T., Gnagy, E., Coxe, S., Arrieta, A., Molina, B., & Pelham, W. E., Jr. (2016). Financial dependence of young adults with childhood ADHD. *Journal of Abnormal Child Psychology, 44,* 1217–1229.

Alvarado, J. M., Puente, A., Jiménez, V., & Arrebillaga, L. (2011). Evaluating reading and metacognitive deficits in children and adolescents with attention deficit hyperactivity disorder. *Spanish Journal of Psychology, 14*(1), 62–73.

Anderman, E., Maehr, M., & Midgley, C. (1999). Declining motivation after the transition to middle school: Schools can make a difference. *Journal of Research and Development in Education, 32*(3), 131–147.

Anderman, E. M., & Midgley, C. (1997). Changes in achievement goal orientations, perceived academic competence, and grades across the transition to middle-level schools. *Contemporary Educational Psychology, 22*(3), 269–298.

Antshel, K. M., Faraone, S. V., & Gordon, M. (2014). Cognitive behavioral treatment outcomes in adolescent ADHD. *Focus, 18*(6), 483–495.

Barkley, R. A. (1997). Behavioral inhibition, sustained attention, and executive functions: Constructing a unifying theory of ADHD. *Psychological Bulletin, 121,* 65–94.

Barkley, R. A., Anastopoulos, A., Guevremont, D., & Fletcher, K. (1991). Adolescents with ADHD: Patterns of behavioral adjustment, academic functioning, and treatment utilization. *Journal of the American Academy of Child and Adolescent Psychiatry, 30,* 752–761.

Barkley, R. A., Edwards, G., Laneri, M., Fletcher, K., & Metevia, L. (2001a). Executive functioning, temporal discounting, and sense of time in adolescents with attention deficit hyperactivity disorder (ADHD) and oppositional defiant disorder (ODD). *Journal of Abnormal Child Psychology, 29,* 541–556.

Barkley, R. A., Edwards, G., Laneri, M., Fletcher, K., & Metevia, L. (2001b). The efficacy of problem-solving communication training alone, behavior management training alone, and their combination for parent–adolescent conflict in teenagers with ADHD and ODD. *Journal of Consulting and Clinical Psychology, 69,* 926–941.

Barkley, R. A., Fischer, M., Smallish, L., & Fletcher, K. (2002). The persistence of attention-deficit/ hyperactivity disorder into young adulthood as a function of reporting source and definition of disorder. *Journal of Abnormal Psychology, 111,* 279–289.

Baumrind, D. (2005). Patterns of parental authority and adolescent autonomy. *New Directions for Child and Adolescent Development, 2005,* 61–69.

Benner, A. D., & Graham, S. (2009). The transition to high school as a developmental process among multiethnic urban youth. *Child Development, 80,* 356–376.

Blakemore, S., & Choudhury, S. (2006). Development of the adolescent brain: Implications for executive function and social cognition. *Journal of Child Psychology and Psychiatry, 47,* 296–312.

Boyer, B. E., Geurts, H. M., Prins, P. J., & Van der Oord, S. (2015). Two novel CBTs for adolescents with ADHD: The value of planning skills. *European Child and Adolescent Psychiatry, 24,* 1075–1090.

Casey, B. J., Jones, R. M., & Hare, T. A. (2008). The adolescent brain. *Annals of the New York Academy of Sciences, 1124,* 111–126.

Chan, E., Fogler, J. M., & Hammerness, P. G. (2016). Treatment of attention-deficit/hyperactivity disorder in adolescents: A systematic review. *Journal of the American Medical Association, 315,* 1997–2008.

Corno, L. (1993). The best-laid plans: Modern conceptions of volition and educational research. *Educational Researcher, 22,* 14–22.

Deci, E. L., Koestner, R., & Ryan, R. M. (1999). The undermining effect is a reality after all—Extrinsic rewards, task interest, and self-determination: Reply to Eisenberger, Pierce, and Cameron (1999) and Lepper, Henderlong, and Gingras (1999). *Psychological Bulletin, 125*(6), 692–700.

Desman, C., Petermann, F., & Hampel, P. (2008). Deficit in response inhibition in children with attention deficit/hyperactivity disorder (ADHD): Impact of motivation? *Child Neuropsychology, 14,* 483–503.

DuPaul, G. J., & Weyandt, L. L. (2006). School-based interventions for children and adolescents with attention-deficit/hyperactivity disorder: Enhancing academic and behavioral outcomes. *Education and Treatment of Children, 29,* 341–358.

Dvorsky, M. R., & Langberg, J. M. (2014, November 17). Predicting impairment in college students with ADHD: The role of executive functions. *Journal of Attention Disorders.* [Epub ahead of print]

Eccles, J. S., & Roeser, R. W. (2009). Schools, academic motivation, and stage–environment fit. In R. M. Lerner & L. Steinberg (Eds.), *Handbook of adolescent psychology: Individual bases of adolescent development* (pp. 404–434). Hoboken, NJ: Wiley.

Edwards, G., Barkley, R. A., Laneri, M., Fletcher, K., & Metevia, L. (2001). Parent–adolescent conflict in teenagers with ADHD and ODD. *Journal of Abnormal Child Psychology, 29*(6), 557–572.

Evans, S., Axelrod, J., & Langberg, J. M. (2004). Efficacy of a school-based treatment program for middle school youth with ADHD: Pilot data. *Behavior Modification, 28,* 528–547.

Evans, S. W., Langberg, J. M., Schultz, B. K., Vaughn, A., Altaye, M., Marshall, S. A., & Zoromski, A. K. (2016). Evaluation of a school-based treatment program for young adolescents with ADHD. *Journal of Consulting and Clinical Psychology, 84*(1), 15–30.

Evans, S. W., Schultz, B. K., DeMars, C. E., & Davis, H. (2011). Effectiveness of the Challenging Horizons after-school program for young adolescents with ADHD. *Behavior Therapy, 42,* 462–474.

Evans, S. W., Serpell, Z. N., Schultz, B. K., & Pastor, D. A. (2007). Cumulative benefits of secondary school-based treatment of students with attention deficit hyperactivity disorder. *School Psychology Review, 36,* 256–273.

Fabiano, G. A., Pelham, W. E., Coles, E. K., Gnagy, E. M., Chronis-Tuscano, A., & O'Connor, B. C. (2009). A meta-analysis of behavioral treatments for attention-deficit/hyperactivity disorder. *Clinical Psychology Review, 29*(2), 129–140.

Forgatch, M. S., & Patterson, G. R. (1989). *Parents and adolescents living together: Part 2. Family problem solving.* Eugene, OR: Castalia.

Garcia, A., Medina, D., & Sibley, M. H. (in press). Conflict between parents and adolescents with ADHD: Situational triggers and the role of comorbidity. *Journal of Child and Family Studies.*

Gawrilow, C., Morgenroth, K., Schultz, R., Oettingen, G., & Gollwitzer, P. M. (2013). Mental contrasting with implementation intentions enhances self-regulation of goal pursuit in schoolchildren at risk for ADHD. *Motivation and Emotion, 37*(1), 134–145.

Gollwitzer, P. M. (1999). Implementation intentions: Strong effects of simple plans. *American Psychologist, 54,* 493–503.

Gollwitzer, P. M., & Brandstätter, V. (1997). Implementation intentions and effective goal pursuit. *Journal of Personality and Social Psychology, 73,* 186–199.

Gottfried, A. E. (1985). Academic intrinsic motivation in elementary and junior high school students. *Journal of Educational Psychology, 77,* 631–645.

Gray, J. A. (2013). The shift to personalised and population medicine. *Lancet, 382,* 200–201.

Gut, J., Heckmann, C., Meyer, C., Schmid, M., & Grob, A. (2012). Language skills, mathematical thinking, and achievement motivation in children with ADHD, disruptive behavior disorders, and normal controls. *Learning and Individual Differences, 22,* 375–379.

Hakanen, J. J., Bakker, A. B., & Schaufeli, W. B. (2006). Burnout and work engagement among teachers. *Journal of School Psychology, 43,* 495–513.

Hoza, B. (2007). Peer functioning in children with ADHD. *Journal of Pediatric Psychology, 32,* 655–663.

Johnston, C., & Mash, E. J. (2001). Families of children with attention-deficit/hyperactivity disorder: Review and recommendations for future research. *Clinical Child and Family Psychology Review, 4,* 183–207.

Kazdin, A. E. (2001). *Behavior modification in applied settings* (6th ed.). Belmont, CA: Wadsworth.

Kazdin, A. E. (2016). Evidence-based psychosocial treatment: Advances, surprises, and needed shifts in foci. *Cognitive and Behavioral Practice, 23,* 426–430.

Kent, K. M., Pelham, W. E., Molina, B. S. G., Sibley, M. H., Waschbusch, D. A., Yu, J., . . . Karch, K. M. (2011). The academic experience of male high school students with ADHD. *Journal of Abnormal Child Psychology, 39,* 451–462.

Kern, R. M., Rasmussen, P. R., Byrd, S. L., & Wittschen, L. K. (1999). Lifestyle, personality, and attention deficit hyperactivity disorder in young adults. *Individual Psychology, 55,* 186–199.

Kim, S. I. (2013). Neuroscientific model of motivational process. *Frontiers in Psychology, 4,* 98.

Kruglanski, A. W., Stein, C., & Riter, A. (1977). Contingencies of exogenous reward and task performance: On the "minimax" strategy in instrumental behavior. *Journal of Applied Social Psychology, 7,* 141–148.

Kuhl, J. (1987). Action control: The maintenance of motivational states. In F. Halisch & J. Kuhl (Eds.), *Motivation, intention, and volition* (pp. 279–291). Berlin: Springer.

Kuriyan, A. B., Pelham, W. E., Molina, B. S. G., Daniel, W. A., Gnagy, E. M., Sibley, M. H., . . . Kent, K. M. (2013). Young adult educational and vocational outcomes of children diagnosed with ADHD. *Journal of Abnormal Child Psychology, 41,* 27–41.

Langberg, J. M., Dvorsky, M. R., & Evans, S. W. (2013). What specific facets of executive function are associated with academic functioning in youth with attention-deficit/hyperactivity disorder? *Journal of Abnormal Child Psychology, 41,* 1145–1159.

Langberg, J. M., Epstein, J. N., Becker, S. P., Girio-Herrera, E., & Vaughn, A. J. (2012). Evaluation of the Homework, Organization, and Planning Skills (HOPS) intervention for middle school students with attention deficit hyperactivity disorder as implemented by school mental health providers. *School Psychology Review, 41,* 342–364.

Langberg, J. M., Epstein, J. N., Girio-Herrera, E., Becker, S. P., Vaughn, A., & Altaye, M. (2011). Materials organization, planning, and homework completion in middle-school students with ADHD: Impact on academic performance. *School Mental Health, 3,* 93–101.

Langberg, J. M., Smith, Z. R., Dvorsky, M. R., Molitor, S. J., Bourchtein, E., Eddy, L. D., . . . Oddo, L. E. (2018). Factor structure and predictive validity of a homework motivation measure for use with middle school students with attention-deficit/hyperactivity disorder. *School Psychology Quarterly, 33*(3), 390–398.

Meaux, J. B., Green, A., & Broussard, L. (2009). ADHD in the college student: A block in the road. *Journal of Psychiatric and Mental Health Nursing, 16*(3), 248–256.

Merkt, J., & Gawrilow, C. (2016). Health, dietary habits, and achievement motivation in college students with self-reported ADHD diagnosis. *Journal of Attention Disorders, 20,* 727–740.

Miller, W. R., & Rollnick, S. (2013). *Motivational interviewing: Helping people change.* New York: Guilford Press.

Molina, B., Hinshaw, S., Swanson, J., Arnold, L., Vitiello, B., Jensen, P., et al. (2009). The MTA at 8 years: Prospective follow-up of children treated for combined-type ADHD in a multisite study. *Journal of the American Academy of Child and Adolescent Psychiatry, 48,* 484–500.

Molina, B. S., Pelham, W. E., Jr., Cheong, J., Marshal, M. P., Gnagy, E. M., & Curran, P. J. (2012). Childhood attention-deficit/hyperactivity disorder (ADHD) and growth in adolescent alcohol use: The roles of functional impairments, ADHD symptom persistence, and parental knowledge. *Journal of Abnormal Psychology, 121,* 922–935.

Morsink, S., Sonuga-Barke, E., Mies, G., Glorie, N., Lemiere, J., Van der Oord, S., & Danckaerts, M. (2017). What motivates individuals with ADHD?: A qualitative analysis from the adolescent's point of view. *European Child and Adolescent Psychiatry, 26*(8), 923–932.

Musser, E. D., Backs, R., Schmitt, C., Ablow, J. C., Measelle, J. R., & Nigg, J. T. (2011). Emotion regulation via the autonomic nervous system in children with attention deficit/hyperactivity disorder (ADHD). *Journal of Abnormal Child Psychology, 39,* 841–852.

National Center on Response to Intervention. (2013). Multi-level prevention system. Retrieved August 2013, from *www.rti4success.org.*

Nelson, J. R., & Roberts, M. L. (2000). Ongoing reciprocal teacher–student interactions involving disruptive behaviors in general education classrooms. *Journal of Emotional and Behavioral Disorders, 8,* 27–37.

Newark, P. E., Elsässer, M., & Stieglitz, R. D. (2016). Self-esteem, self-efficacy, and resources in adults with ADHD. *Journal of Attention Disorders, 20,* 279–290.

Nigg, J. T. (2001). Is ADHD a disinhibitory disorder? *Psychological Bulletin, 127,* 571–598.

Nigg, J. T., Blaskey, L., Stawicki, J., & Sachek, J. (2004). Evaluating the endophenotype model of ADHD neuropsychological deficit: Results for parents and siblings of children with ADHD combined and inattentive subtypes. *Journal of Abnormal Psychology, 113,* 614–625.

Oettingen, G., Mayer, D., Timur Sevincer, A., Stephens, E. J., Pak, H. J., & Hagenah, M. (2009). Mental contrasting and goal commitment: The mediating role of energization. *Personality and Social Psychology Bulletin, 35,* 608–622.

Oudeyer, P. Y., Kaplan, F., & Hafner, V. V. (2007). Intrinsic motivation systems for autonomous mental development. *IEEE Transactions on Evolutionary Computation, 11,* 265–286.

Philipsen, A., Richter, H., Peters, J., Alm, B., Sobanski, E., Colla, M., . . . Hesslinger, B. (2007). Structured group psychotherapy in adults with attention deficit hyperactivity disorder: Results of an open multicentre study. *Journal of Nervous and Mental Disease, 195,* 1013–1019.

Plamondon, A., & Martinussen, R. (2015, June 5). Inattention symptoms are associated with academic achievement mostly through variance shared with intrinsic motivation and behavioral engagement. *Journal of Attention Disorders.* [Epub ahead of print]

Ramsay, J. R., & Rostain, A. L. (2008). Adult ADHD research: Current status and future directions. *Journal of Attention Disorders, 11*(6), 624–627.

Ryan, R. M., & Deci, E. L. (2000). Self-determination theory and the facilitation of intrinsic motivation, social development, and well-being. *American Psychologist, 55*(1), 68–78.

Schwanz, K. A., Palm, L. J., & Brallier, S. A. (2007). Attention problems and hyperactivity as predictors of college grade point average. *Journal of Attention Disorders, 11*(3), 368–373.

Sibley, M. H. (2016). *Parent–teen therapy for executive function deficits and ADHD: Building skills and motivation.* New York: Guilford Press.

Sibley, M. H., Altszuler, A., Morrow, A., & Merrill, B. (2014). Mapping the academic problem behaviors of adolescents with ADHD. *School Psychology Quarterly, 29,* 422–437.

Sibley, M. H., Altszuler, A. R., Ross, J. M., Sanchez, F., Pelham, W. E., & Gnagy, E. M. (2014). A group-based parent–teen collaborative intervention for high school students with ADHD. *Cognitive and Behavioral Practice, 21,* 32–42.

Sibley, M. H., Campez, M., Perez, A., Morrow, A., Merrill, B., Altszuler, A., . . . Yequez, C. E. (2016). Parent management of organization, time management, and planning deficits among adolescents with ADHD. *Journal of Psychopathology and Behavioral Assessment, 38,* 216–228.

Sibley, M. H., Graziano, P. A., Kuriyan, A. B., Coxe, S., Pelham, W. E., Rodriguez, L. M., . . . Ward, A. (2016). Parent–teen behavior therapy + motivational interviewing for adolescents with ADHD. *Journal of Consulting and Clinical Psychology, 84,* 699–712.

Sibley, M. H., Kuriyan, A. B., Evans, S. W., Waxmonsky, J. G., & Smith, B. H. (2014). Pharmacological and psychosocial treatments for ADHD in adolescents: An updated systematic review of the literature. *Clinical Psychology Review, 34,* 218–232.

Sibley, M. H., Olson, S., Morley, C., Campez, M., & Pelham, W. E. (2016). A school consultation intervention for adolescents with ADHD: Barriers and implementation strategies. *Child and Adolescent Mental Health, 21,* 183–191.

Sibley, M. H., Pelham, W. E., Derefinko, K. D., Kuriyan, A. B., Sanchez, F., & Graziano, P. A. (2013). A pilot trial of Supporting Teens' Academic Needs Daily (STAND): A parent–adolescent collaborative intervention for ADHD. *Journal of Psychopathology and Behavioral Assessment, 35,* 436–449.

Sibley, M. H., Pelham, W. E., Evans, S. W., Gnagy, E. M., Ross, J. M., & Greiner, A. R. (2011). Evaluation of a summer treatment program for adolescents with attention deficit/hyperactivity disorder. *Cognitive and Behavioral Practice, 18,* 530–544.

Sibley, M. H., Pelham, W. E., Molina, B. S. G., Coxe, S., Kipp, H., . . . Lahey, B. B. (2014). The role of early childhood ADHD and subsequent CD in the initiation and escalation of adolescent cigarette, alcohol, and marijuana use. *Journal of Abnormal Psychology, 123,* 362–374.

Smith, B. H., Waschbusch, D. A., Willoughby, M. T., & Evans, S. (2000). The efficacy, safety, and practicality of treatments for adolescents with attention-deficit/hyperactivity disorder (ADHD). *Clinical Child and Family Psychology Review, 3*(4), 243–267.

Sobanski, E., Banaschewski, T., Asherson, P., Buitelaar, J., Chen, W., Franke, B., . . . Stringaris, A. (2010). Emotional lability in children and adolescents with attention deficit/hyperactivity disorder (ADHD): Clinical correlates and familial prevalence. *Journal of Child Psychology and Psychiatry, 51*(8), 915–923.

Sonuga-Barke, E. J. (2003). The dual pathway model of AD/HD: An elaboration of neuro-developmental characteristics. *Neuroscience and Biobehavioral Reviews, 27,* 593–604.

Sprich, S. E., Safren, S. A., Finkelstein, D., Remmert, J. E., & Hammerness, P. (2016). A randomized controlled trial of cognitive behavioral therapy for ADHD in medication-treated adolescents. *Journal of Child Psychology and Psychiatry, 57,* 1218–1226.

Steinberg, L., & Morris, A. (2001). Adolescent development. *Annual Review of Psychology, 52,* 83–110.

Turgay, A., Lasser, R., Goodman, D., & Asherson, P. (2012). Lifespan persistence of ADHD: The life transition model and its application. *Journal of Clinical Psychiatry 73,* 192–201.

Vallerand, R. J., Pelletier, L. G., Blais, M. R., Brière, N. M., Senecal, C., & Vallieres, E. F. (1993). On the assessment of intrinsic, extrinsic, and amotivation in education: Evidence on the concurrent and construct validity of the Academic Motivation Scale. *Educational and Psychological Measurement, 53,* 159–172.

Weisz, J. R., & Hawley, K. M. (2002). Developmental factors in the treatment on adolescents. *Journal of Consulting and Clinical Psychology, 70,* 21–43.

Willcutt, E. G., Doyle, A. E., Nigg, J. T., Faraone, S. V., & Pennington, B. F. (2005). Validity of the executive function theory of attention-deficit/hyperactivity disorder: A meta-analytic review. *Biological Psychiatry, 57,* 1336–1346.

Zimmerman, B. J. (2000). Self-efficacy: An essential motive to learn. *Contemporary Educational Psychology, 25,* 82–91.**Conflict between parents and adolescents with ADHD: Situational triggers and the role of comorbidity**

CHAPTER 15

Addressing Homework Problems in Adolescents with ADHD

Joshua M. Langberg
Zoe R. Smith
Cathrin D. Green

Homework problems are ubiquitous among adolescents diagnosed with attention-deficit/hyperactivity disorder (ADHD). Although there is certainly heterogeneity in the impairments adolescents with ADHD exhibit, clinically speaking, it is difficult to envision an adolescent meeting full *Diagnostic and Statistical Manual of Mental Disorders* (DSM-5; American Psychiatric Association, 2013) criteria for ADHD who does *not* experience at least some homework difficulties. Indeed, the inattentive symptoms used to define ADHD, which remain prominent in adolescence (see Willcutt, Chapter 3, this volume), include many behaviors necessary to successfully manage and complete homework. Table 15.1 lists the nine inattentive symptoms used to diagnose ADHD, along with corresponding examples for how they relate to homework problems. It is clear that if an adolescent truly has developmentally inappropriate difficulties with these inattentive symptoms, then it is largely by definition that he or she will also have problems organizing and managing school materials, planning ahead for the completion of homework and tests, implementing and monitoring study plans, and staying focused for extended periods of time to complete work. Homework problems can wax and wane across development, vary as a function of child characteristics (e.g., intelligence), and increase or decrease in severity depending on context (e.g., parent support; Cooper, Lindsay, & Nye, 2000; Rogers, Wiener, Marton, & Tannock, 2009). However, if an adolescent presents for an ADHD evaluation and reports no history of homework problems, at a minimum, alternate conceptualizations should be strongly considered.

Among adolescents with ADHD, homework problems are not only common but they are also associated with a host of negative outcomes. Students with ADHD turn in between 12 to 20% fewer homework assignments in comparison to their peers each academic semester (Kent et al., 2011; Langberg et al., 2016). Multiple longitudinal studies have documented that homework problems predict academic outcomes such as grade point average (GPA), above and beyond a number of other factors. For example, in a sample of 579 children diagnosed with ADHD, Langberg et al. (2011) found that parent-rated homework problems in elementary

TABLE 15.1. Inattentive Symptoms Used to Diagnose ADHD and Homework/Organization-Related Examples from DSM-5

ADHD inattention item	Homework/organization-related examples from DSM-5
1. Fails to give close attention/makes careless mistakes	Overlooks or misses details, work is inaccurate
2. Difficulty sustaining attention	Difficulty remaining focused during lectures or lengthy readings
3. Does not seem to listen when spoken to directly	Mind seems elsewhere
4. Does not follow through on instructions and fails to finish schoolwork	Starts schoolwork but quickly loses focus
5. Difficulty organizing	Disorganized work, poor time management, fails to meet deadlines
6. Avoids, dislikes, or is reluctant to engage in tasks requiring sustained mental effort	Avoids, dislikes, or is reluctant to engage in schoolwork or homework, preparing reports, reading textbook chapters
7. Loses things	Loses school materials, pencils/books/paperwork
8. Easily distracted	Distracting extraneous stimuli, including unrelated thoughts
9. Forgetful	Forgetful in daily activities or remembering assignments

Note. See American Psychiatric Association (2013, p. 59).

school predicted GPA in high school above and beyond ADHD symptom severity, intelligence, and service utilization. Similarly, in a sample of 104 middle school students with ADHD, Langberg et al. (2016) found that homework completion rate predicted GPA 18 months later, controlling for intelligence, reading and math achievement, income, and race. As such, it is clear that homework problems are prevalent in adolescents with ADHD, persistent across time, and associated with significant negative outcomes such as school failure. Accordingly, this chapter is designed to provide the reader with an understanding of (1) the nature of homework problems in adolescents with ADHD and how they manifest across development, (2) strategies for the assessment of homework problems, and (3) the behavioral principles associated with evidence-based intervention for homework problems.

The Multifaceted Nature of Homework: The Homework Completion Cycle

Clinicians who work with families of adolescents with ADHD have no doubt heard parents express frustration and exasperation about their child's homework completion. Parents often say something similar to "I don't get it—when I was their age I completed my homework because that is what I was told to do" or "He is lazy—if he wanted to do his homework, he would." At the root of these statements are beliefs that homework completion is a simple process, and that the skills needed to complete homework are innate rather than learned. Unfortunately, neither of these assumptions is true, as multiple rather advanced skills are needed to successfully complete homework. With the goal of visually displaying the complexity of the homework completion process and the skills involved, we introduce the homework completion cycle shown in Figure 15.1 (Langberg et al., 2016). In this chapter, this figure highlights the multifaceted nature of homework problems and how treatment must vary based on the specific behavior(s) that need improvement. It is important to acknowledge that given the complexity of the homework completion process, many adolescents struggle with aspects of homework completion, not only adolescents with ADHD (Bryan, Burstein, & Bryan, 2001; Toney, Kelley, & Lanclos, 2003). In many ways, difficulty adjusting to homework load and expectations for independence is normative across the transitions from elementary to middle school and again from middle to high school. As such, many of the strategies discussed in this chapter could be applied to all adolescents, not just to adolescents with ADHD. We start in this chapter by considering how the behaviors that comprise the homework completion cycle vary across development, and how student characteristics interact to facilitate or hinder these processes.

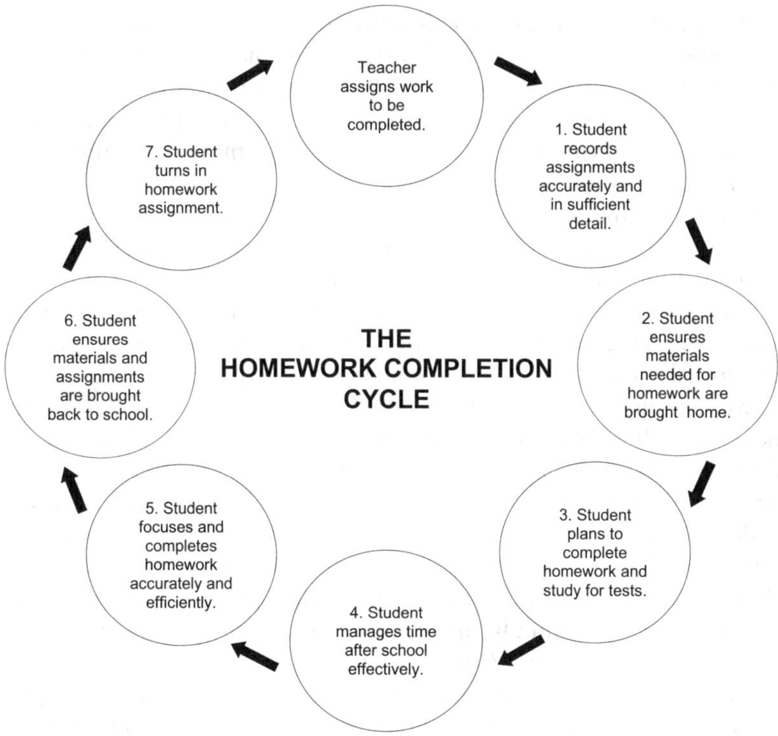

FIGURE 15.1. Visual depiction of the steps necessary to complete homework.

Homework Problems across Development

Homework Recording

The first step in the homework completion cycle is for the student to accurately record homework assignments and in sufficient detail. Essentially, this step highlights the fact that irrespective of ability with focus and organization, if an adolescent does not know what was assigned, he or she will have difficulty completing the necessary tasks. How problematic this first step is can vary considerably based on development and context. Indeed, homework recording is an excellent example of the usefulness of taking a developmental psychopathology approach when studying ADHD, because development and context determine expectations and, therefore, whether the behavior is "abnormal" or problematic. To illustrate, let's consider a clinical example. If a second-grade student with ADHD presents for treatment, is highly unlikely that accurate homework recording is a major concern for the child's parents, because (1) developmentally, second graders are not expected to independently record homework, and (2) if they are, teachers typically provide considerable support through shaping and prompting. It is often not until early adolescence (e.g., sixth grade) that schools and teachers determine that it is developmentally appropriate for students to be recording assignments on their own without teacher support. Accordingly, this is when problems with homework recording typically emerge for students with ADHD.

It is important to acknowledge that a categorical distinction between problem and no problem is a false dichotomy, because homework recording expectations can vary across development and teachers. For example, for a fourth-grade student, writing "complete math homework" may be developmentally appropriate, because the teacher has ensured that the math worksheet is in the child's homework folder and there are completion instructions written on the worksheet. However, for a sixth-grade student, recording "complete math homework" may be problematic if the student and parent do not know what specific page or problems are to be completed. Furthermore, in sixth grade, some teachers may consistently provide detailed information about assigned homework online or at the beginning of the week, whereas others do not view that as their responsibility. In that case, homework recording might easily be a problem in one class but not another. Accordingly, and as discussed in more detail in the section "Assessment of Homework Problems," a critical part of helping adolescents with ADHD succeed with homework recording is helping the family fully understand and clearly define developmentally appropriate expectations.

Organization of Materials

Circles two and six in the homework completion cycle (see Figure 15.1) relate to the student's ability to manage and organize materials. This is differentiated from organization and management of time (circles 3 and 4), which we discuss in the next section. Students typically rely on three or fewer items to manage all of their school materials: binder, bookbag, and locker. Unfortunately, just because students have these three items does not mean they use them well and are organized, just as having a car does not mean that you are a good driver. For materials organization, the devil is in the details in terms of how students *use* bookbags, binders, and lockers to file, transfer, and store materials. Some students carry multiple binders, one for each class, while others carry a single, large binder. Similarly, some students have a single folder in which they put all homework assignments, whereas others have a separate folder for homework for each class. Some students keep all their materials in their bookbag all the time; others store materials in lockers or at home. The main issue is that, usually, a specific system for organizing materials has never been suggested to the student. It was assumed that if the student was provided with a bookbag, binder, and locker, the rest would naturally fall into place. For some adolescents, this is sufficient, as they (or their parents) figure out a specific system that works. However, that is typically an unrealistic assumption for an adolescent with ADHD.

Here again, development and context play an important role. Ask yourself, when during development is it appropriate to expect that a student will manage his or her bookbag, binder, and locker materials independently and effectively, without guidance and support? Unfortunately, if we asked multiple school personnel and teachers this question, we would get many different responses, even across teachers within a particular grade level at the same school. Establishing developmentally appropriate expectations for materials organization is further complicated by the fact that the age/grade at which you would expect these skills to be used independently would likely be later for an adolescent with ADHD in comparison to his or her peers; that is, if we acknowledge and accept that a deficit in organization abilities exists, it then follows logically that the developmentally appropriate expectation for that individual will also have to shift. This is perhaps the clinician's greatest challenge in providing intervention for homework problems with adolescents with ADHD. Because schools and teachers often do not agree on what is developmentally appropriate for materials organization, it can be difficult to get all parties to agree on developmentally appropriate supports and goals. Regardless, and as discussed further in the assessment and treatment sections below, the essential first step in treatment is to define and establish a specific system of organization and expectations for maintenance of that system. Transferring materials and papers to and from school daily is not a simple task, and significant progress can often be made by establishing a system rather than assuming that the student knows what to do.

Time Management and Planning

Circles 3 and 4 in the homework completion cycle (see Figure 15.1) pertain to time management and planning. These are often the skills that parents desperately want their adolescents to learn prior to attending college. Developmentally, they are also the skills that are the last to develop (Boyer, Geurts, Prins, & Van der Oord, 2014; Van der Meer, Jansen, & Torenbeek, 2010). Time management and planning skills develop during the middle and high school years and are never really mastered—they are continually being refined. Consider how you manage your time and task lists effectively and efficiently at work. Does your system always work? Have you always used the same processes, or have you changed your process based on the demands of your job and your responsibilities? In answering these questions, many people acknowledge that effective time management is challenging and, in fact, is something adults often struggle with on a daily basis (even in the absence of ADHD). Despite this, as with materials organization, assumptions exist that by the time students reach middle or high school, they should know how to plan ahead and manage their time. For some reason, we believe this to be true, even though we do not believe that students automatically learn calculus or a foreign language by middle or high school. As with homework recording and materials organization, clinicians can provide an important service to adolescents with ADHD and their families simply by defining time-management skills, teaching students to apply those skills, and establishing clear and realistic expectations.

Adolescents with ADHD often procrastinate and rush to complete tasks at the last minute (Boyer et al., 2014). This occurs both long term (e.g., not studying for a test on Friday until Thursday night) and daily (e.g., not starting homework until bedtime). The homework completion cycle conceptualizes planning as separate from time management. Planning refers to thinking ahead and mapping out a series of smaller steps or behaviors needed to accomplish a long-term goal. For example, for a test on Friday, you can decide that you are going to make flash cards on Tuesday, study half on Tuesday, half on Wednesday, and review on Thursday. In contrast, the homework completion cycle defines time management as *implementation* of the plan. This is an important distinction. A student could develop a clear and detailed plan, then be unable to implement that plan. Perhaps the student has many other competing responsibilities (e.g., extracurricular activities) that impact his or her ability to put the plan into action. Alternatively, the student may have difficulty with perception of time or with forgetfulness, and the day slips by before flash cards have been made. In other words, it is important to teach adolescents not only how to plan but also how to successfully enact that plan when faced with competing responsibilities. As we discuss in the subsequent section, understanding this difference becomes important when assessing homework problems and determining where to intervene.

Focus and Behavior during Homework Completion

Consider for a moment that we have now outlined multiple different behaviors that can be problematic for adolescents with ADHD in completing homework and, as of yet, have not even mentioned the core behaviors many people think of when they think of ADHD: hyperactivity, impulsivity, and difficulties with concentration. Even when students with ADHD record homework, bring it home, and plan ahead to complete work, parents are still faced with the daunting task of having them sit for an extended period of time to complete the work. Let us again take a developmental perspective and start by asking a question. How long should a third-grade student be able to sit and focus on homework? How would your answer change if we told you that student had ADHD? How would the answer change if we had asked about a seventh-grade student? When assessing homework problems, parents of adolescents with ADHD often make statements such as "The teacher says homework should take 30 minutes but it takes us 2 hours" or "I want him to go to bed earlier but even with me sitting with him, we don't finish homework until 9:00 P.M." Here again, whether a behavior is problematic is largely determined by the developmental expectations that are in place. A child with ADHD predominantly inattentive presentation might exhibit minimal impairment in the home setting in early elementary school because expectations that the child focus for extended periods are minimal. That same child may exhibit severe impairment in the home setting during middle school because now the expectation is that students complete 1–2 hours of homework each night. As with the other behaviors in the homework completion cycle, assessment of the problem requires assessment of the expectations and whether they are developmentally appropriate and reasonable for an adolescent with ADHD.

Expanding the Cycle: The Role of Motivation

When we initially published the homework completion cycle it was entirely skills focused (Langberg et al., 2016); that is, each circle represents a skill or ability that a clinician can assess and consider whether there are clear expectations in place, and whether the adolescent has been taught that particular skill. However, as we continue to work with adolescents with ADHD, it has become clear that sometimes skills are present but motivation to implement the skills is lacking and hinders therapeutic progress (see also Doidge et al., Chapter 4, and Sibley, Chapter 14, this volume). There is compelling evidence that students' motivation plays a significant role in their academic success (e.g., Wang & Eccles, 2013). It is also clear that the association between motivation and academics is bidirectional, and that academic failure decreases motivation to engage in school and homework related tasks (e.g., Green et al., 2012). Unfortunately, many adolescents with ADHD experience repeated failures with homework-related tasks, and as a result, start to believe that they cannot be successful ("Why try?"). Indeed, in our own work, we have shown that it is not just homework completion that predicts future academic success; academic success (GPA) also predicts future homework completion (Langberg et al., 2016). Furthermore, we recently found that adolescents' self-reported homework motivation predicted the percentage of homework assignments they turned in, above and beyond ADHD symptoms and achievement scores (Langberg, Smith, et al., 2018). As such, it is important to acknowledge that teaching students homework completion skills is only part of the equation. Ensuring that they are motivated to consistently implement the skills is often equally, if not more, challenging.

Assessment of Homework Problems

As with most psychological constructs, the assessment of homework problems can be approached from both *idiographic* (individual) and *nomothetic* (broad, relative to others) perspectives. Psychology as a research field tends to rely on nomothetic approaches, such as the collection of rating scales from parents and teachers that provide us with normative data based on a large sample of respondents who have completed the measure. This is useful for helping us understand whether a behavior is in the "normal" or "abnormal" range. However, from a practical/clinical perspective, idiographic assessment of homework problems is often sufficient and is typically more consistent with families' treatment goals. For example, parents are more likely to be interested in working to improve their adolescent's percentage of assignments turned in than they are in moving the adolescent into the "normal range" on a measure. That said, both approaches clearly have utility, and examples of each are reviewed below.

Idiographic Assessment and Monitoring of Homework Problems

The main benefit of taking an idiographic approach is the ease with which the teacher, parent, or clinician can measure intervention progress on any aspect of the homework completion cycle. In contrast, no single rating scale adequately assesses all of the behaviors that are required for successful homework completion. As we described earlier in this chapter, the first step in treating any homework problem is to specifically define the behavior. For example, for homework recording (circle 1, Figure 15.1), the definition may be "Homework is recorded in the school planner in sufficient detail, so that the parent can determine what needs to be completed without asking for clarification." Once the definition is established, assessment and treatment monitoring logically follow. For an adolescent in middle school, assessment could involve evaluation of the number of core classes (e.g., math, English) in which this criterion was met out of the total number of core classes on a daily basis (e.g., two out of four). Similarly, if we wanted to assess organization and planning, definitions would first need to be established. Checklists that provide specific measurable organization and planning criteria have been established and are readily available (e.g., Langberg, 2011). However, parents, teachers, and clinicians can certainly come up with their own definitions and criteria for assessing materials organization. For example, a parent might define organization as "There are no loose papers or trash in the bookbag" or "All homework to be completed is filed in a specific homework folder." These behaviors can easily be assessed (i.e., yes–no) on a daily basis to obtain baseline data. Similarly, a parent or teacher might assess planning skills by establishing definitions such as

"The students accurately recorded upcoming tests in his planner (e.g., test Friday in math)" or "The student recorded times to study for tests in her planner (e.g., study 30 minutes for math on Thursday)." The planner could then be reviewed on a daily or weekly basis to evaluate how the student is engaging in planning behaviors.

These are idiographic approaches, because they provide no information on the adolescent's use of these behaviors relative to others. As such, while an idiographic approach is ideal for assessing and tracking homework problems, it is the clinician's role to ensure that the established treatment goals are reasonable and developmentally appropriate. It is common for parents to establish goals that are unrealistic, either because they lack understanding of the deficits inherent to ADHD or, more generally, lack knowledge about developmentally appropriate homework expectations. For example, setting a goal that a fifth-grade student with ADHD will record homework assignments in a planner for all classes or always have homework in the homework folder (i.e., 100% of the time) is unrealistic and sets the adolescent (and parent) up for failure. Another benefit of idiographic measurement is that it tends to be sensitive to change and progress with treatment and, as such, is useful for graphing to show parents progress. In contrast, nomothetic measures often rely on parent perception and may change more slowly or not at all over time. Graphing idiographic progress during treatment is an excellent way to recognize and celebrate progress and to further motivate the adolescent. An example is provided in Figure 15.2, graphing specifically defined binder, bookbag, and locker organization criteria. In this graph, we simply divided the number of criteria met by the number of criteria on the checklist to establish a percentage.

Nomothetic Assessment and Monitoring of Homework Problems

Given the prevalence of homework and organizational skills problems in adolescents with ADHD, multiple nomothetic measures have been developed that specifically assess these concerns. In this section we discuss a few of the most commonly used measures and how they might map onto the homework completion cycle.

The Homework Problems Checklist (HPC; Anesko, Schoiock, Ramirez, & Levine, 1987) is a parent-completed rating scale that contains two factors. The first factor largely assesses circle 5 (see Figure 15.1) of the homework completion cycle: the adolescent's focus, concentration, and behavior during homework completion. The second factor primarily assesses the adolescent's ability to manage homework materials (circles 2 and 6 of the homework completion cycle). This measure is relatively short (20 items) and has undergone multiple psychometric validation studies in youth with ADHD specifically (Langberg et al., 2010; Power, Werba,

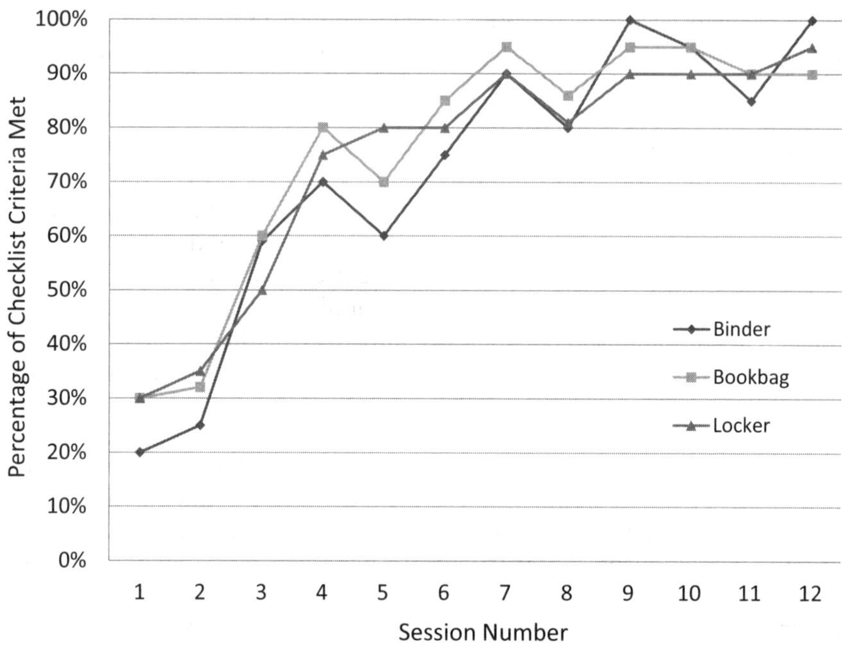

FIGURE 15.2. Example of graphing intervention progress with materials organization.

Watkins, Angelucci, & Eiraldi, 2006). The Homework Performance Questionnaire (HPQ) is an option that contains both parent and teacher versions (23 and 17 items contribute to the factors, respectively) and has also undergone multiple psychometric validation studies (Mautone, Marshall, Costigan, Clarke, & Power, 2012; Power, Dombrowski, Watkins, Mautone, & Eagle, 2007). The teacher version has two factors that assess student self-regulation of homework behaviors and student competence with homework, and the parent version includes the same two factors, along with a third factor assessing teacher support for homework (Power et al., 2015). Multiple items on the Student Self-Regulation factor assess aspects of the homework completion cycle (e.g., "Child wastes time on homework," "Child brings materials home," and "Child returns materials to class"). Unfortunately, neither the HPC nor the HPQ have factors that specifically assess the organization, planning, and time-management behaviors on the homework completion cycle.

The Children's Organizational Skills System (COSS; Abikoff & Gallagher, 2009) is designed to assess organization and planning skills, and provides normative data. The COSS is a 58-item questionnaire that includes three factors: task planning, memory and materials management, and organized actions. However, it is important to note that the items are not specific to homework problems as organization and planning are assessed broadly (e.g., organization of room). Nevertheless, many of the items do assess homework-related behaviors (particularly circles 1, 2, and 3 of the homework completion cycle; see Figure 15.1), and the COSS has been used in multiple studies of adolescents with ADHD and shown to be sensitive to treatment effects (Langberg, Dvorsky et al., 2018). The COSS has parent, youth, and teacher versions available, allowing the assessment of organization and planning skills from multiple perspectives. Limitations include cost and the fact that the proposed three-factor structure may not be valid as applied to adolescents with ADHD (Molitor et al., 2017). Finally, the Adolescent Academic Problems Checklist (AAPC; Sibley, Altzuler, Morrow, & Merrill, 2014) is a relatively recently developed measure with parent, student, and teacher versions that assesses academic impairment broadly as related to ADHD. The overall measure contains 24 items, many of which are specific to aspects of homework and organizational skills (particularly circles 1, 2, and 3; see Figure 15.1). The AAPC contains two factors, representing an academic skills index and a disruptive behavior index. Items pertaining to organization and management of homework load onto the academic skills index and include "Leaves longer-term projects until the last minute," "Fails to record homework in daily planner/agenda," and "Has poorly organized folders and binders." The AAPC has also been used in multiple ADHD treatment studies and has been found to be sensitive to intervention (Sibley et al., 2016). Of the measures reviewed in this section, the AAPC Academic Index contains the most items that clearly map onto the homework completion cycle and is recommended for monitoring treatment progress.

The Importance of Comprehensive, Multimethod Assessment

Overall, a combination of idiographic, nomothetic, and objective measures would be considered the most comprehensive assessment strategy. Objective indicators include metrics such as the percentage of homework assignments turned in or GPA. These are often very meaningful indicators to parents and teachers, but they can be slow to respond to intervention efforts. For example, if an adolescent struggles with multiple behaviors on the homework completion cycle, improving one (e.g., homework recording) may not lead to an increase in assignments turned in until additional behaviors are addressed. For clinicians who are providing homework interventions on a broad scale (e.g., school- or classroomwide), it is important to collect ratings such as the AAPC to facilitate a direct comparison across students. It can also be useful to collect ratings with normative data as a way of helping parents develop and maintain realistic expectations for treatment. For example, if parents see that teacher ratings on the COSS are consistently in the normal range, it may help them understand that their expectations are high and potentially unrealistic. As we stated earlier, however, idiographic assessments should always be included when providing intervention for adolescents with ADHD. Idiographic assessment is the most sensitive to change, and specifically defining and monitoring individual behaviors over time is an essential aspect of all evidence-based behavioral interventions (Wolpert et al., 2012).

Treatment of Homework Problems

We divide our discussion of the treatment of homework problems into two sections. In the first section, we briefly review research on homework interventions for adolescents with ADHD. The interventions are described and evidence supporting intervention efficacy is summarized. In the second section, we discuss the cognitive and behavioral principles on which these interventions are all based. In essence, all homework problem interventions for adolescents with ADHD rely on the same core principles. These principles can be applied by parents, teachers, and clinicians, regardless of whether a specific intervention is used. As such, these principles are reviewed, along with some examples of how they might be applied to improve homework problems.

Summary of Research on Homework Interventions for Adolescents with ADHD

There are multiple interventions that improve the homework and organizational skills of elementary school students with ADHD. Research on these interventions has demonstrated impressive effects on multiple aspects of the homework completion cycle. However, given the significant developmental and contextual differences between elementary school, middle school, and high school in terms of homework expectations and demands, these interventions are not reviewed in this section. Information on interventions for grades K–5 can be found elsewhere (see Abikoff et al., 2013; Pfiffner et al., 2007, 2014; Pfiffner, Villodas, Kaiser, Rooney, & McBurnett, 2013; Power et al., 2012). The three adolescent-focused interventions reviewed in this section target similar aspects of the homework completion cycle but vary in how services are delivered. Multiple randomized trials support the efficacy of the Challenging Horizons Program—After School (CHP-AS) model for improving organizational skills as measured with the COSS and homework problems as measured with the HPC (Evans et al., 2011; Evans, Schultz, DeMars, & Davis, 2016). The CHP-AS is typically delivered as a yearlong afterschool program that meets 2 or 3 days per week for 2 hours after school. All studies of the CHP-AS have focused on middle school students with ADHD who are taught to accurately record homework assignments, organize and manage school materials in a binder, bookbag, and locker; and to plan ahead to study for tests (the CHP-AS also includes a social skills component not reviewed here; see McQuade, Chapter 7, this volume). The Homework, Organization, and Planning Skills (HOPS) intervention targets similar homework skills in middle school students (all aspects of the homework cycle except for circle 5; see Figure 15.1), but is delivered by school counselors or school psychologists during the school day. Students are taught a specific system for managing their school planners and materials in their binders/bookbags, and a school mental health provider completes weekly checklists to evaluate progress and apply contingencies. The HOPS intervention consists of 16 meetings, each 20 minutes in length, and is completed is less than one school semester. The HOPS intervention has only been studied as an individual, 1:1 model, but group- and classroom-based models are described in the manual and have been used in classrooms and schools. Similar to the CHP-AS, the HOPS intervention is associated with large improvements on the HPC and COSS (Breaux et al., 2019; Langberg, Epstein, Becker, Girio-Herrera, & Vaughn, 2012; Langberg, Dvorsky, et al., 2018).

In contrast to CHP and HOPS, which are delivered directly to the adolescent with minimal parent involvement (e.g., two parent meetings in HOPS), the Supporting Teens' Autonomy Daily (STAND) intervention, a clinic-based intervention delivered to parents and adolescents, has been evaluated in individual small-group models and with middle and high school-age adolescents (Sibley et al., 2013, 2014, 2016; see also Sibley, Chapter 14, this volume). The STAND intervention is typically delivered through 8–10 90-minute group sessions. There are typically multiple facilitators/clinicians, as the parents and adolescents meet separately before coming together as a group at the end of each session. Unlike CHP and HOPS, STAND emphasizes parent–adolescent communication in improving homework and organizational problems, and participants practice communicating and problem solving around academic tasks and goals. The STAND intervention is also associated with significant improvements in homework problems and organizational skills (Sibley et al., 2016). One of the limitations of STAND is that it requires two clinicians to implement, as there are separate parent and adolescent activities. However, similar parent–adolescent groups targeting academic skills and parent–adolescent communication in adolescents with ADHD have been evaluated and can be implemented by one clinician (Ciesielski, Tamm, Vaughn, Cyran, & Epstein, 2019). This intervention model was also found to lead to significant improvements in homework and organizational skills. As such, the CHP-AS, HOPS, and STAND interventions all have compelling evidence supporting efficacy for improving the homework problems of adolescents with ADHD. Choices regarding which intervention to use would largely be based on the service delivery model that best fits the setting and available resources.

Core Strategies Used to Improve Homework Problems

All of the interventions described in the previous section largely rely on behavioral therapeutic techniques to teach and reinforce the use of homework, organization, and planning skills. Generally speaking, behavioral therapeutic techniques include specifically defining a behavior, consistently monitoring the behavior, establishing realistic and developmentally appropriate immediate and long-term goals, and applying salient and meaningful contingencies for the adolescent meeting those goals (Fabiano, 2016). Most of the interventions described previously also include specific strategies to facilitate generalization and maintenance of the skills across time. Some of the interventions (e.g., STAND) also incorporate cognitive strategies, such as motivational interviewing, to increase the likelihood that the adolescent applies the skills being taught.

As described earlier in this chapter, Step 1 in any behavioral intervention is to specifically define the target behavior. Having a clear behavioral definition on which all parties agree is the key foundation of homework interventions, as the steps that follow will not work without a definition in place. A specifically defined behavior (e.g., homework recording or organization of the locker) is required before Step 2, monitoring the behavior, can proceed. Often, intervention manuals will suggest monitoring a behavior for a short period of time before goals are set (called *establishing a baseline*). This is not always necessary, but is useful to ensure that the initial goals are realistic and achievable. Step 3 is to set a specific target or goal for the adolescent to aim for during the next week. Here again, the definition is key, because if the goal is vague, there will be confusion and conflict between the adolescent, parent(s), and teachers surrounding goal attainment. This is unfortunately the step during which many homework interventions for adolescents with ADHD fail, because the initial goal is too high. The main objective of setting an initial goal (e.g., three out of seven binder organization criteria met or homework recorded accurately for at least two of four classes) is to establish the adolescent's buy-in and to increase motivation. Most adolescents, and sometimes their parents, approach behavioral systems with skepticism, distrust, and low motivation, and the only way to combat that is to show them that they can be successful. The importance of this cannot be overstated, because when an adolescent tries but fails to reach the initial homework completion target, the chances of future progress are close to zero. This is one of the key developmental differences in working with children compared to adolescents. Children often approach goals and rewards systems with enthusiasm, whereas adolescents typically do not. However, it can be very difficult for parents and teachers to set low, easy-to-achieve goals initially. Understandably, they want to see progress quickly, and they may not want to reinforce the adolescent for meeting a low threshold (e.g., "They can do better, that is not sufficient"). This is why psychoeducation about adolescents with ADHD and developmentally appropriate expectations is incorporated into most evidence-based homework interventions. Psychoeducation is designed to explain the purpose and importance of setting realistic goals to establish motivation and buy-in when working with adolescents with ADHD.

Step 4 is to consistently monitor the behavior to determine whether the homework completion target was met. Unfortunately, this is often easier said than done, as monitoring takes time and effort on the part of a parent or teacher. However, if there is not consistency in monitoring, there is not going to be consistency in the adolescent enacting the desired behavior. Furthermore, monitoring is typically only effective when done frequently. Frequent monitoring facilitates the adolescent having multiple opportunities to succeed. For example, a parent could check the planner each day after school to evaluate whether the adolescent recorded at least two of four homework assignments accurately. Although this takes time and effort, it allows adolescents repeated opportunities for success and, importantly, when they fail, it gives them an opportunity to quickly turn around and to succeed the next day. For example, if the parent chooses to monitor the planner for homework recording once per week and to set a weekly goal (e.g., 12 out of 20 assignments recorded accurately), if the adolescent struggles early in the week with homework recording, there is no motivation for him or her to excel in the second half of the week (i.e., the goal is already out of reach). As such, monitoring plans need to be as frequent as possible, while also ensuring that they are feasible for the parent or teacher to implement consistently—a difficult balance.

Step 5 involves attaching contingencies to the established behavioral targets. Using the previous example, what happens if the adolescent records two of four assignments accurately in the planner, and what happens if he or she does not? With adolescents, the use of contingences and rewards is much more complex in comparison to working with younger children, largely because motivation is typically lower to begin with and fewer salient external motivators are available (e.g., a sticker won't cut it). It is also important to recognize that material rewards are often not necessary. Many adolescents, particularly those with ADHD, have very few positive interpersonal relationships and feel criticized by adults on a daily basis (see Wiener, Chapter 6, and McQuade, Chapter 7, this volume). Sometimes, simply establishing clear and achievable expectations surrounding homework and organization is sufficient to motivate the adolescent. Similarly, positive attention or a strong therapeutic alliance may motivate the adolescent to work to achieve homework-related goals. Overall, making the intervention experience a positive one is of paramount importance when working with adolescents with ADHD.

The ultimate goal for most parents and teachers is for the adolescent to be internally motivated to use effective homework and organization strategies. They often ask questions such as "Will I have to be monitoring and providing rewards forever?" An important part of psychoeducation is helping parents and teachers understand that internal motivation comes from experiencing success. This is why it is essential that short-term, easily achievable goals for homework and organization are initially established. The goal can and should be increased (made more difficult) over time, but unless adolescents with ADHD experience success initially, they will not be motivated to achieve more ambitious goals. Once adolescents experience a series of successes, only then will they begin to truly believe that future success is likely. This is when internal motivation can begin to take over and less frequent monitoring/rewarding may be possible.

One way to increase parent buy-in and motivation to monitor and provide rewards for the adolescent is to frame the purpose of the homework intervention as seeking to increase the adolescent's autonomy. Ask the parent to consider how many times per day or week he or she currently prompts and reminds (or nags) the adolescent to complete homework-related tasks (e.g., to start homework, to put homework back in the folder, to stay on-task during homework completion). Typically, these types of prompts and reminders occur frequently and are exhausting for the parent and quite negative for the adolescent ("They treat me like a baby"). Suggest to the parent or teacher that the goal of the intervention is to decrease how often he or she has to prompt and remind, and to increase the percentage of time the adolescent engages in these behaviors on his or her own. By telling the adolescent exactly what to do and completing the checklists to determine whether homework goals were met, the parents are actually putting more responsibility back on the adolescent. For example, the adolescent now writes down homework on his or her own rather than waiting for parents to ask what he or she has to complete. Similarly, the adolescent organizes his or her bookbag on Sunday before the school week starts rather than having his or her parents nag about the mess each day after school. Indeed, when working with adolescents, the promise that you as the clinician will work to reduce parental "nagging" is a powerful motivator that can facilitate the therapeutic alliance.

Unfortunately, because it is important to ensure that the adolescent has success early with the intervention, and it is critical that the target behavior is monitored frequently, typically only two circles on the homework completion cycle can be addressed simultaneously. If goals are established for more than two behaviors, the likelihood that the adolescent will meet all of the necessary criteria and succeed decreases as the adolescent feels overwhelmed by what he or she is being asked to do. Furthermore, targeting more than two behaviors in the homework cycle simultaneously significantly increases the risk that one or both behaviors will not be monitored consistently for feasibility reasons. Inconsistent monitoring causes the adolescent to believe that the parent–teacher implementing the system is not invested or is not holding up his or her end of the bargain. The adolescent also receives less frequent positive feedback, and it may be unclear whether goals were met. In either scenario, the system will not be successful. For these reasons, targeting only one or two circles on the homework cycle initially is recommended, and providing psychoeducation around the rationale for this strategy is important.

CONCLUSION

In summary, given the prevalence and complexity of homework problems in adolescents with ADHD and how important homework completion is to parents and teachers, clinicians who work with adolescents need to have a solid understanding of evidence-based homework assessment and treatment practices. The homework completion cycle can be printed and used with families in session as a tool to facilitate conversations about developmentally appropriate expectations and to determine where to start with intervention.

REFERENCES

Abikoff, H., & Gallagher, R. (2009). *Children's organizational skills scales: Technical manual.* North Tonawanda, NY: Multi-Health Systems.

Abikoff, H. B., Gallagher, R., Wells, K. C., Murray, D. W., Huang, L., Lu, F., & Petkova, E. (2013). Remediating organizational functioning in children with ADHD: Immediate and long-term effects from a randomized controlled trial. *Journal of Consulting and Clinical Psychology, 81,* 113–128.

American Psychiatric Association. (2013). *Diagnostic and statistical manual of mental disorders* (5th ed.). Arlington, VA: Author.

Anesko, K. M., Schoiock, G., Ramirez, R., & Levine, F. M. (1987). The Homework Problems Checklist: Assessing children's homework difficulties. *Behavioral Assessment, 9,* 179–185.

Boyer, B. E., Geurts, H. M., Prins, P. J., & Van der Oord, S. (2014). Two novel CBTs for adolescents with ADHD: The value of planning skills. *European Child and Adolescent Psychiatry, 24,* 1075–1090.

Breaux, R. P., Langberg, J. M., Bourchtein, E., Eadeh, H. M., Molitor, S. J., & Smith, Z. R. (2019). Brief homework intervention for adolescents with ADHD: Trajectories and predictors of response. *School Psychology Quarterly, 34*(2), 201–211.

Bryan, T., Burstein, K., & Bryan, J. (2001). Students with learning disabilities: Homework problems and promising practices. *Educational Psychologist, 36*(3), 167–180.

Ciesielski, H. A., Tamm, L., Vaughn, A. J., Cyran, J. E., & Epstein, J. N. (2019). Academic skills groups for middle school children with ADHD in the outpatient mental health setting: An open trial. *Journal of Attention Disorders, 23*(4), 409–417.

Cooper, H., Lindsay, J. J., & Nye, B. (2000). Homework in the home: How student, family, and parenting-style differences relate to the homework process. *Contemporary Educational Psychology, 25,* 464–487.

Evans, S. W., Langberg, J. M., Schultz, B. K., Vaughn, A., Altaye, M., Marshall, S. A., & Zoromski, A. K. (2016). Evaluation of a school-based treatment program for young adolescents with ADHD. *Journal of Consulting and Clinical Psychology, 84*(1), 15–30.

Evans, S. W., Schultz, B. K., DeMars, C. E., & Davis, H. (2011). Effectiveness of the challenging horizons after-school program for young adolescents with ADHD. *Behavior Therapy, 42*, 462–474.

Fabiano, G. A. (2016). *Interventions for disruptive behavior disorders: Reducing problems and building skills*. New York: Guilford Press.

Green, J., Liem, G. A. D., Martin, A. J., Colmar, S., Marsh, H. W., & McInerney, D. (2012). Academic motivation, self-concept, engagement, and performance in high school: Key processes from a longitudinal perspective. *Journal of Adolescence, 35*(5), 1111–1122.

Kent, K. M., Pelham, W. E., Jr., Molina, B. S., Sibley, M. H., Waschbusch, D. A., Yu, J., . . . Karch, K. M. (2011). The academic experience of male high school students with ADHD. *Journal of Abnormal Child Psychology, 39*, 451–462.

Langberg, J. M. (2011). *Homework, Organization and Planning Skills (HOPS) interventions: A treatment manual*. Bethesda, MD: National Association of School Psychologists Publications.

Langberg, J. M., Arnold, L. E., Flowers, A. M., Altaye, M., Epstein, J. N., & Molina, B. S. G. (2010). Assessing homework problems in children with ADHD: Validation of a parent-report measure and evaluation of homework performance patterns. *School Mental Health, 2*, 3–12.

Langberg, J. M., Dvorsky, M. R., Molitor, S. J., Bourchtein, E., Eddy, L. D., Smith, Z. R., . . . Eadeh, H. M. (2018). Overcoming the research-to-practice gap: A randomized trial with two brief homework and organization interventions for students with ADHD as implemented by school mental health providers. *Journal of Consulting and Clinical Psychology, 86*(1), 39–55.

Langberg, J. M., Dvorsky, M. R., Molitor, S. J., Bourchtein, E., Eddy, L. D., Smith, Z., . . . Evans, S. W. (2016). Longitudinal evaluation of the importance of homework completion for the academic performance of middle school students with ADHD. *Journal of School Psychology, 55*, 27–38.

Langberg, J. M., Epstein, J. N., Becker, S. P., Girio-Herrera, E., & Vaughn, A. J. (2012). Evaluation of the Homework, Organization, and Planning Skills (HOPS) intervention for middle school students with ADHD as implemented by school mental health providers. *School Psychology Review, 41*, 342–364.

Langberg, J. M., Molina, B. S. G., Arnold, L. E., Epstein, J. N., Altaye, M., Hinshaw, S. P., . . . Hechtman, L. (2011). Patterns and predictors of adolescent academic achievement and performance in a sample of children with attention-deficit/hyperactivity disorder (ADHD). *Journal of Clinical Child and Adolescent Psychology, 40*, 519–531.

Langberg, J. M., Smith, Z. R., Dvorsky, M. R., Molitor, S. J., Bourchtein, E., Eddy, L. D., . . . Oddo, L. E. (2018). Factor structure and predictive validity of a homework motivation measure for use with middle school students with attention-deficit/hyperactivity disorder. *School Psychology Quarterly, 33*(3), 390–398.

Mautone, J. A., Marshall, S. A., Costigan, T. E., Clarke, A. T., & Power, T. J. (2012). Multidimensional assessment of homework: An analysis of students with ADHD. *Journal of Attention Disorders, 16*, 600–609.

Molitor, S. J., Langberg, J. M., Evans, S. W., Dvorsky, M. R., Bourchtein, E., Eddy, L. D., . . . Oddo, L. E. (2017). Evaluating the factor validity of the Children's Organizational Skills Scale in Youth with ADHD. *School Mental Health, 9*(2), 143–156.

Pfiffner, L. J., Hinshaw, S. P., Owens, E., Zalecki, C., Kaiser, N. M., Villodas, M., & McBurnett, K. (2014). A two-site randomized clinical trial of integrated psychosocial treatment for ADHD-inattentive type. *Journal of Consulting and Clinical Psychology, 82*(6), 1115.

Pfiffner, L. J., Mikami, A., Huang-Pollock, C., Easterlin, B., Zalecki, C., & McBurnett, K. (2007). A randomized, controlled trial of integrated home-school behavioral treatment for ADHD, predominantly inattentive type. *Journal of the American Academy of Child and Adolescent Psychiatry, 46,* 1041–1050.

Pfiffner, L. J., Villodas, M., Kaiser, N., Rooney, M., & McBurnett, K. (2013). Educational outcomes of a collaborative school–home behavioral intervention for ADHD. *School Psychology Quarterly, 28,* 25–36.

Power, T. J., Dombrowski, S. C., Watkins, M. W., Mautone, J. A., & Eagle, J. W. (2007). Assessing children's homework performance: Development of multi-dimensional, multi-informant rating scales. *Journal of School Psychology, 45,* 333–348.

Power, T. J., Mautone, J. A., Soffer, S. L., Clarke, A. T., Marshall, S. A., Sharman, J., . . . Jawad, A. F. (2012). A family–school intervention for children with ADHD: Results of a randomized clinical trial. *Journal of Consulting and Clinical Psychology, 80,* 611–623.

Power, T. J., Watkins, M. W., Mautone, J. A., Walcott, C. M., Coutts, M. J., & Shreidan, S. M. (2015). Examining the validity of the Homework Performance Questionnaire: Multi-informant assessment in elementary and middle school. *School Psychology Quarterly, 30,* 260–275.

Power, T. J., Werba, B. E., Watkins, M. W., Angelucci, J. G., & Eiraldi, R. B. (2006). Patterns of parent-reported homework problems among ADHD-referred and nonreferred children. *School Psychology Quarterly, 21,* 13–33.

Rogers, M. A., Wiener, J., Marton, I., & Tannock, R. (2009). Parental involvement in children's learning: Comparing parents of children with and without attention-deficit/hyperactivity disorder (ADHD). *Journal of School Psychology, 47,* 167–185.

Sibley, M. H., Altszuler, A. R., Morrow, A. S., & Merrill, B. M. (2014). Mapping the academic problem behaviors of adolescents with ADHD. *School Psychology Quarterly, 29,* 422–437.

Sibley, M. H., Graziano, P. A., Kuriyan, A. B., Coxe, S., Pelham, W. E., Rodriguez, L., . . . Ward, A. (2016). Parent–teen behavior therapy + motivational interviewing for adolescents with ADHD. *Journal of Consulting and Clinical Psychology, 84,* 699–712.

Sibley, M. H., Pelham, W., Derefinko, K., Kuriyan, A., Sanchez, F., & Graziano, P. (2013). A pilot trial of Supporting Teens Academic Needs Daily (STAND): A parent–adolescent collaborative intervention for ADHD. *Journal of Psychopathology and Behavior Assessment, 35,* 436–449.

Toney, L. P., Kelley, M. L., & Lanclos, N. F. (2003). Self-and parental monitoring of homework in adolescents: Comparative effects on parents' perceptions of homework behavior problems. *Child and Family Behavior Therapy, 25*(1), 35–51.

Van der Meer, J., Jansen, E., & Torenbeek, M. (2010). "It's almost a mindset that teachers need to change": First-year students' need to be inducted into time management. *Studies in Higher Education, 35*(7), 777–791.

Wang, M., & Eccles, J. S. (2013). School context, achievement motivation, and academic engagement: A longitudinal study of school engagement using a multidimensional perspective. *Learning and Instruction, 28,* 12–23.

Wolpert, M., Ford, T., Trustam, E., Law, D., Deighton, J., Flannery, H., & Rew, J. B. (2012). Patient-reported outcomes in Child and Adolescent Mental Health Services (CAMHS): Use of idiographic and standardized measures. *Journal of Mental Health, 21,* 165–173.

CHAPTER 16

Cognitive-Behavioral Therapy for Adolescents with ADHD

Susan E. Sprich
Jennifer A. Burbridge

The prevalence rate of attention-deficit/hyperactivity disorder (ADHD) in adolescence is estimated to be between 5 and 10% (Centers for Disease Control and Prevention, 2010; Fergusson, Horwood, & Lynskey, 1993; Murphy & Barkley, 1996; Verhulst, van der Ende, Ferdinand, & Kasius, 1997). ADHD is a psychiatric disorder characterized by impairment in attention, hyperactivity, and impulsivity (American Psychiatric Association, 2013). Previous research suggested that ADHD is a disorder seen only in childhood, because as children mature, they often gain symptom remission (Hill & Schoener, 1996). However, more recent research suggests that 50–80% of individuals diagnosed with ADHD as children continue to be symptomatic in adolescence and adulthood (Barkley, Fischer, Smallish, & Fletcher, 2006; Biederman, Petty, Evans, Small, & Farone, 2010; Sibley, Mitchell, & Becker, 2016). While ADHD persists into teenage and adult years, psychosocial treatments have been understudied in teens and adults relative to younger children (Chronis, Jones, & Raggi, 2006; Cuffe et al., 2001).

In this chapter, we discuss cognitive-behavioral therapy (CBT) for adolescents with ADHD. We briefly review psychosocial treatments for adults and adolescents before discussing our CBT intervention for adolescents with ADHD. We then describe our intervention in detail before presenting two case studies illustrating its use.

Review of Psychosocial Treatments for ADHD in Adults

It was once thought that ADHD symptoms are found only in children and that ADHD symptoms disappear when children grow up (Wolraich et al., 2005). We now know that this is not true. ADHD symptoms can be significantly impairing to adults, affecting work performance, relationships, and comorbid symptoms such as anxiety and depression (Barkley, Murphy, & Fischer, 2008; Skirrow et al., 2014).

Steele, Jensen, and Quinn (2006) reported that while stimulant medications remain the first-line treatment for adults with ADHD, not everyone responds positively to medication treatments or reaches the 30% reduction in symptoms needed to be considered a responder in most medication studies. Thus, there is a strong need for psychosocial treatments for adults with ADHD. Our group at Massachusetts General Hospital completed two successful trials of CBT for adults with ADHD who were taking medications but still had residual ADHD symptoms (Safren, Otto, et al., 2005; Safren et al., 2010). Similarly, in a randomized controlled trial, Emilsson et al. (2011) found that CBT not only reduced ADHD symptoms in adults but also resulted in functional improvements and fewer comorbid symptoms. While individual and group CBT have been shown to be effective treatments for adult ADHD (Safren et al., 2010; Solanto et al., 2010), new approaches and forms of delivery of CBT are being tested (see Canu & Wymbs, 2015). For example, Pettersson, Soderstrom, Edlund-Soderstrom, and Nilsson (2017) found promising treatment effects with an Internet-based self-help CBT program (iCBT).

In a recent meta-analysis of CBT for adult ADHD, Knouse, Teller, and Brooks (2017) found that CBT treatments in 32 studies showed medium-to-large effect sizes when comparing pre- and posttreatment symptoms. Furthermore, they found that CBT effect sizes were comparable whether patients were taking medications or not. Finally, they observed a pattern of results indicating that CBT may have greater effects on inattentive symptoms than on hyperactivity–impulsivity symptoms. Thus, given the effectiveness of psychosocial treatments for adult ADHD, extending adult protocols for use in adolescence is a fast-growing area of psychological research.

The Need for Psychosocial Treatments for Adolescents with ADHD

There has been far more research with children with ADHD than with adolescents or adults with ADHD. The literature that does exist consists primarily of studies of children with ADHD who were followed as they entered adolescence. Previous research looked at psychosocial interventions that focused primarily on parent training and school support, and was derived from childhood psychosocial treatment protocols (see Evans, Owens, & Bunford, 2014, for a review). Increasingly, and as indicated elsewhere in this volume by Sibley (Chapter 14) and Davis and Mitchell (Chapter 17), researchers are emphasizing the need for additional studies on psychosocial treatments for adolescents with ADHD (Chronis et al., 2006; Evans et al., 2014).

Developmental and Theoretical Rationale for CBT in Adolescents with ADHD

There are several reasons why it is so important to study the effectiveness of psychosocial treatments in adolescents with ADHD. First, adolescence is a time marked by increasingly less adult supervision and emerging independence. Thus, allowing adolescents to take ownership and have increased responsibility for their own goals and treatment can be vital to setting up a strong foundation of skills and is in line with this stage of development. By first learning and applying these skills in middle and high school, adolescents can practice skills and learn to overcome obstacles when there are still opportunities for teacher and parent supervision. Cuffe et al. (2001) found that more than 80% of their sample of seventh, eighth, and ninth graders continued to experience ADHD symptoms and functional impairment as they entered their late teens/early 20s. In our own work with adults with ADHD (Safren et al., 2010), many of our study participants reported to us that they wished they had been taught these strategies when they were younger, because they might have made different decisions regarding education, career choices, and relationships.

Second, there are short- and long-term risks of having ADHD. Specifically, having ADHD in adolescence increases the risk of poor grades, negative school experiences, suspensions, needing to repeat grades, dropping out of school (see Evans, Van der Oord, & Rogers, Chapter 8, this volume), and experiencing increased stress in relationships with teachers, parents (see Wiener, Chapter 6, this volume), and even friends (see McQuade, Chapter 7, this volume; Barkley, Anastopoulos, Guevremont, & Fletcher, 1991; Barkley, Fischer, Edelbrock, & Smallish, 1991; Fischer, Barkley, Edelbrock, & Smallish, 1990). Adolescents with untreated or undertreated ADHD are also at higher risk for tobacco, alcohol, and substance use (see Kennedy, McKone, & Molina, Chapter 11, this volume) and are more likely to engage in behaviors such as antisocial activities (see Becker & Fogleman, Chapter 9, this volume) and riskier sexual behaviors (see McQuade, Chapter 7, this volume; Barkley, Fischer, Smallish, & Fletcher, 2004, 2006; Tercyak, Peshkin, Walker, & Stein, 2002). In a meta-analysis and review of the long-term risks associated with childhood diagnosed ADHD, Mohr-Jensen and Steinhausen (2016) found a substantial increase in the risk of later antisocial activities. They also found that ADHD is associated with increased arrests, convictions, and incarcerations, and with an earlier age of onset of antisocial activities and risk of multiple offenses. McCabe, Dickinson, West, and Wilens (2016) conducted a multicohort national study of adolescent ADHD and substance use. They found that there were higher rates of substance use behaviors when stimulant medications were initiated at later ages of adolescence, suggesting that closer monitoring of this subgroup of adolescents would be beneficial.

Third, because ADHD is a neurobiological disorder, medications may allow for a sufficient reduction in symptoms, so that adolescents can optimally learn and implement these strategies in their daily lives. Stimulant medications have been widely used as an effective treatment for decades in children, adolescents, and adults. However, despite medication treatment, most adolescents continue to have residual symptoms; thus, there is an important need to add psychosocial evidence-based strategies to provide comprehensive treatment of ADHD in adolescence (Chronis et al., 2006; Wilens et al., 2006). Medications cannot replace the skills and strategies that must be acquired in order to cope successfully with the complexities of twenty-first century school, work and family life. Specifically, Murphy (2005) identified a number of effective skills-based interventions: using electronic organizer devices to emphasize daily school planning and task lists; cognitive strategies to break down overwhelming tasks into smaller, more manageable tasks; visual reminders; and employing more adaptive "coaching" techniques to keep teens on task. He concluded that adolescents with ADHD manage their symptoms most effectively when given treatment that includes stimulant medication and skills-based cognitive and behavioral strategies.

A fourth reason to pursue psychosocial treatments for ADHD in adolescents is that for some individuals, the medication side effects (e.g., weight loss and sleep problems) may outweigh the benefits of medication (see Lerner & Wigal, 2008, for a review). There may also be a problem with medication adherence if adolescents do not have a system for remembering to take their medication (see Brinkman, Froehlich, & Epstein, Chapter 18, this volume).

In a review, Evans et al. (2014) divided psychosocial treatments into two types: "behavioral treatments," in which consequences/rewards are provided by others (e.g., parents and teachers) and "training interventions," in which skills are taught directly to the adolescents themselves. They suggest that training interventions may be the preferred mode of treatment for adolescents for three reasons: (1) Adolescents frequently have many different teachers, so it can be difficult to create consistent contingencies; (2) parents monitor adolescents less closely as there are increased opportunities for independence (afterschool activities, greater time spent with peers, driving, etc.); and (3) it is sometimes difficult for others to come up with relevant and impactful rewards for adolescents.

In examining behavioral treatments, Barkley, Edwards, Laneri, et al. (2001) compared problem-solving communication training (PSCT) alone with PSCT plus behavior management training in a sample of 97 families who had a teenager with ADHD and oppositional defiant disorder (ODD). Their results indicated improvement in parent–teen conflicts for both conditions. Evans, Schultz, Demars, and Davis (2011) conducted a study of their Challenging Horizons Program (CHP), an after-school program for young adolescents with ADHD. They found that students in the CHP showed greater improvement on measures of ADHD symptoms and impairment than did the students in the community care condition. The CHP program has demonstrated efficacy across several randomized trials (see Langberg et al., 2016). Most recently, Langberg et al. examined potential predictors of a positive response to CHP and found that strong working alliance and lower levels of parenting stress and lower parent–adolescent conflict predicted a strong treatment response.

There has also been promising research on CBT-specific training interventions for adolescents with ADHD. Antshel, Faraone, and Gordon (2014) modified our CBT for adult ADHD protocol (Safren, Sprich, Perlman, & Otto, 2005; Safren, Perlman, Sprich, & Otto, 2005) for adolescents and found improvement at posttreatment in the following areas: adolescent self-report of self-esteem, and parent and teacher ratings of inattentive symptoms. Antshel and Olszewski (2014) observed that many prior studies of ADHD in adolescence rely more on behavioral principles than on cognitive ones. They suggest that cognitive interventions be paired with reinforcement principles in order to be an effective treatment. Given that adolescence is a time of increasing independence from and conflict with parents, interventions that use this tendency toward independence as an opportunity to do more adolescent cognitive individual interventions might be more successful. Furthermore, pairing cognitive interventions with reinforcement principles further increases the likelihood that the interventions will be practiced and learned. They also suggest that parent involvement in the session with adolescents who have comorbid ODD may be less effective than parent involvement with adolescents who have ADHD in addition to a comorbid internalizing disorder, such as depression. Again, the authors reason that given the developmental task of adolescence of separating and individuating from parents, those adolescents with ODD, who have a propensity to act out conflicts and difficult emotions, might be better off with less parental involvement, while those adolescents with depression, who might be more likely to internalize conflicts with parents, might be more successful having parents involved while the therapist assists them in discussing conflicts and challenging aspects of ADHD.

More recently, in a randomized controlled trial of group CBT for adolescents with ADHD, Vidal et al. (2015) found a reduction in both ADHD symptoms and functional impairment for the CBT group relative to the waitlist control group. This study suggests that group CBT may be comparable to individual CBT for the reduction in ADHD symptoms and impairment in adolescents with ADHD.

We (Sprich, Safren, Finkelstein, Remmert, & Hammerness, 2016) modified our adult CBT treatment protocol for use with adolescents. Our approach is primarily a training intervention, in that we mainly work to teach skills to the adolescents themselves. We did incorporate a behavioral component, however, in that we included some work with parents on managing contingencies around adolescent skills use. In our treatment program, we started with a neurobiological model of ADHD symptoms, which hypothesizes that symptoms of inattention, hyperactivity, and impulsivity are maintained or exacerbated by a lack of effective coping strategies (Safren, Sprich, Chulvick, & Otto, 2004).

Our results show that for adolescents with ADHD, CBT is an effective psychosocial treatment. Our study was one of the first to show that CBT based on an adult protocol and primarily having individual sessions with the adolescents themselves can be effective. Study participants included 46 adolescents ages 14–18 with a primary diagnosis of ADHD who were stabilized on medication for ADHD. Participants completed 10 individual CBT sessions (with parents coming in for the last 10 minutes of each session), and two sessions that included both the adolescents and their parents. We also offered two optional sessions with parents only. Our results indicate improvements on three outcome measures: independent evaluator (IE)-rated parent assessment of symptoms, IE-rated adolescent assessment of symptoms, and IE-rated overall stress and impairment of adolescent symptoms.

Description of CBT for Adolescents with ADHD

The treatment consists of twelve 45- to 50-minute sessions of individual therapy. The intervention was informed by our CBT intervention work with adults and adolescents with ADHD over the past 14 years as detailed in our published therapist guide and client workbook (Safren, Perlman, et al., 2005; Safren, Sprich, Perlman & Otto, 2017a; Safren, Sprich, Perlman, & Otto, 2005, 2017b). The manualized treatment includes skills drawn from traditional cognitive-behavioral approaches and approaches used to foster behavioral change in substance abuse, and additionally interventions that target health behavior change where motivations may vary (e.g., Fisher, Fisher, Williams, & Malloy, 1994; Safren, Otto, & Worth, 1999).

The adult treatment includes twelve 45- to 50-minute sessions that are divided into three core modules (organization/planning, distractibility, and cognitive restructuring), two optional modules (procrastination and involvement of a spouse/partner), and a one-session relapse prevention module. We retained the structure and content of the adult protocol, but we adapted it for adolescents based on the clinical experience of the team and a review of the literature.

Specifically, for adolescent clients, we opted to include parents in several full treatment sessions and at the end of each session. We hypothesized that it would be important to involve parents, so that they could be aware and supportive of the skills the adolescents were learning. Parents and adolescents with ADHD often have difficulties with communication (Robin, 1998). Involving the parents gives the clinician an opportunity to provide guidance to both parents and adolescents around these issues.

We try to have the first parent–child session early in the treatment (Session 2 or Session 3, if possible) and the second parent session toward the end of treatment (Session 7, Session 8, or Session 9). We realize that flexibility in scheduling is required for the sessions involving the parents, due to family logistical constraints. We also invite parents into each session for several minutes, so that the adolescent can review the skills that were covered in session and let the parents know the CBT homework he or she will be working on for the next session. This allows the parents insight into the therapy goals and provides an opportunity for the therapist to ensure that the adolescent understands the session's skills and homework, and to provide corrective feedback, if needed.

Based on the clinical experience of the team, we felt that adolescents might be less receptive to the cognitive restructuring strategies we used in the adult protocol (e.g., traditional cognitive restructuring involving detailed self-monitoring of negative automatic thoughts, thinking errors, and the development of rational responses), so we reduced the number of sessions devoted to adaptive thinking from three to two, and we switched from a formal "thought record" to emphasizing a coaching metaphor (Otto, 2000). Finally, we felt that adolescents might be more interested/engaged in using technology (smartphones, laptops) to keep track of their tasks and meetings/appointments, so we changed the language in the protocol to reflect these options.

Each intervention session builds on previous material. The beginning of each session also contains a review of all previous material and a review of homework, with additional review and problem-solving regarding any material that was not completed or helpful. Similarly, we review adherence to medication treatment, and assist with reducing barriers to consistent medication use.

Prior to initiating treatment, it is important to assess whether the adolescent is a good fit for CBT. The therapist should ascertain whether the adolescent is bothered by his or her ADHD symptoms and is willing to be an active participant in therapy. ADHD symptoms can be assessed using the Adult ADHD Self-Report Scale (ASRS), a checklist based on the 18 DSM-IV-TR symptoms (the symptoms for ADHD did not change in the DSM-5). This scale was developed in conjunction with the World Health Organization (Adler et al., 2006) and can be accessed at *med.nyu.edu/psych/sites/default/files/psych_adhd_checklist_0.pdf*. We recommend that parents and adolescents fill out the scale independently. To obtain information on functional impairment, the Weiss Functional Impairment Rating Scale Self-Report (WFIRS-S; Weiss, 2000) can be used. Since psychosocial treatment of ADHD focuses on organization and planning, rather than on hyperactivity, it is important to assess whether the adolescent with ADHD has difficulties in these areas. If the adolescent is not on medication for ADHD, it might be useful to suggest a medication evaluation prior to starting CBT. In our study evaluating this treatment (Sprich et al., 2016), we required that adolescents be stabilized on ADHD medications prior to initiating treatment, though this approach may not always be feasible in clinical practice. We have not formally evaluated this treatment in adolescents who were not on medications for ADHD.

Psychoeducation and Organization/Planning (Four Sessions)

The first module of treatment is tailored to introduce adolescents to a CBT model of treatment, to promote credibility of the approach and motivation, and to provide psychoeducation about ADHD, as well as training in organization and planning. This process involves helping the adolescent set up an organizational system for keeping track of appointments, assignments, and tests, as well as a task list. This may involve using a paper system or a smartphone to set up a system that is effective for each adolescent. We note that many of these strategies may be familiar to adolescents (e.g., utilizing a task list); however, the fact that individuals are accountable to the therapist and will return for 12 therapy sessions increases the chances that they will engage in the behaviors long enough to have them become personal habits.

As adolescents move through middle school, high school, and into college, the expectations for independence from parents and teachers increase. Thus, younger adolescents (e.g., those in middle school) generally receive more help from others in developing their task lists and setting goals and priorities. The therapist may work more closely with parents and/or school personnel to help the younger adolescent develop a workable system. As adolescents near the end of high school, and certainly when they enter college, it is important that they learn to become more independent in keeping track of their own tasks and independently setting priorities. It is crucial that adolescents understand the differences between high school and college in terms of how homework is assigned (by giving a syllabus at the beginning of the semester in college vs. on a daily or weekly basis in high school). The individual preferences and limitations of each adolescent need to be taken into consideration when choosing a system. For example, some adolescents prefer to use a paper planner, because it is inherently less distracting than an electronic system. In other cases, schools prohibit the use of electronics in class, so even if the adolescent would prefer an electronic system to schedule appointments or track assignments, this is not feasible. Generally, as adolescents move from high school to college, the use of electronic systems becomes more acceptable and often is even encouraged.

Once adolescent and therapist have agreed on a system for keeping track of tasks and appointments, the adolescent is instructed to use the system and to bring the paper or electronic system to each session. This enables the therapist to see exactly what the adolescent is working on and to observe any difficulties the youth might be having. For example, if the adolescent has large projects listed that keep getting carried over from one daily task list to the next, the therapist would instruct him or her to break this down into more manageable chunks that might have a better chance of being completed in a single day (e.g., "Make outline for English paper" instead of "Write English paper"). If the therapist observes that the adolescent does not seem to have a clear plan for completing the task (e.g., the adolescent has not chosen a topic for the English paper, which is why he or she has not been able to start it), the therapist would instruct him or her in problem solving to find a solution.

The initial module focuses on organizing both tasks and environments, both home and school. If the adolescent does not have an organized room, backpack, and school locker, it is difficult for him or her to be successful. We start with this module so that the skills taught in this module can be reinforced throughout the rest of the treatment, and so that parents can be enlisted to help generalize the skills outside of the treatment sessions.

Distractibility (Two Sessions)

The distractibility module builds on the skills used in the first module on organizing and planning. Commonly, adolescents with ADHD find that they do not complete important tasks such as homework and chores because they get distracted by other, less important or more appealing tasks or activities. In this module, the therapist works with the adolescent to set a realistic goal for the amount of time they want to focus on a task such as homework. The adolescent is then taught to set an alarm for that amount of time and to use a technique that involves writing down the distraction, so that the adolescent can deal with it once the alarm goes off. Similar procedures are commonly used in anxiety management and worry control procedures (see Craske & Barlow, 2006).

In this module, adolescents are also taught to set alarms on smartphones, watches, or other devices to go off at regular intervals. Whenever the alarm sounds, adolescents are instructed to ask themselves whether they have been distracted from the task at hand, and, if so, to return to that task. Last, this module teaches techniques for reducing external environmental distractions (e.g., social media, Internet, phone) and finding designated spots for important items (e.g., backpack, phone, keys) to reduce time spent looking for those items when leaving the house.

As in the previous module, younger adolescents may require more assistance from parents or other adults in implementing these strategies. A middle school student is less likely to independently set alarms and set up systems than a high school or college student. In cases where the younger adolescent is not motivated to use skills independently, the therapist can work with the parents to develop a contingency management system to reward the adolescent for use of skills until the skills have become habitual. As older adolescents start to see the value of using these skills (getting homework completed earlier, not having to take extra time looking for car keys in the morning), they tend to become more willing to use the skills.

Cognitive Restructuring/Adaptive Thinking (Two Sessions)

In the third module of treatment, adolescents are taught adaptive thinking skills. Although this module is based on the work of Aaron Beck and colleagues (for a full description of this approach, see Beck, 2011), for this treatment, we use a coaching metaphor to describe the cognitive restructuring approach (Otto, 2000) rather than trying to teach adolescents the traditional method of completing thought records. In our clinical experience, adolescents are often noncompliant with completing thought records and therefore do not achieve the maximum benefit from cognitive restructuring. Accordingly, adolescents are instructed to observe and modify their own internal "coaching style" and learn the best ways to coach or encourage themselves when they notice that they are coaching themselves in a negative or unhelpful fashion. Although we typically think of a need to change "negative thoughts," individuals with ADHD can, at times, engage in overly optimistic thinking that may be equally problematic (Knouse & Mitchell, 2015). For example, if an adolescent who has a project due in a week starts to think about needing to work on the project and becomes distressed, then has the thought, "I don't need to work on it today, because I have all afternoon free on Sunday and I can most certainly finish the whole project on Sunday," he or she might feel relieved and decide not to start working on the project. However, when Sunday comes around, the adolescent might realize that he or she needs to go to a cousin's birthday party for a couple of hours, doesn't have all the needed supplies, and that the project requires more than a single afternoon. If the adolescent can learn to recognize these "red flag" thoughts, he or she will be in a stronger position to modify the thoughts. The idea is that adolescents will understand that simply because their internal "coach" is saying something to them, it is not necessarily true and they can learn to coach themselves in a more accurate and/or helpful fashion. The goal is for them to generalize this skill to many situations (e.g., homework or other school-related situations, social situations, family situations).

The cognitive restructuring skills also build on previous modules—particularly organizing and planning. If unhelpful self-statements get in the way of completing tasks, these skills are used in conjunction with the problem solving and related material to help participants with task completion. As with the earlier modules, parental involvement is likely to be greater with the younger adolescents. Parents may need to prompt the younger adolescents when they hear them verbalizing negative or unhelpful self-statements and ask them whether they can change the statement to a more helpful or accurate coaching style.

Procrastination

This one-session module focuses on procrastination, using skills from previous modules. For the adolescent population, targets include tasks such as homework, college applications (if appropriate), and organizing "stuff" (e.g., backpack, locker, bedroom). The skills include adaptive thinking to challenge perfectionistic thoughts, breaking down large tasks into smaller steps, and learning to set realistic goals for completing tasks. Generally, this session is a review of previous skills, but with the focus on procrastination.

Parent Involvement

The parents participate fully in two sessions of the treatment, along with the adolescent. The first parent session takes place early on in treatment, and the second session takes place toward the end of treatment. The scheduling of the parent sessions is flexible due to the complex logistics of family and parental schedules. Parents are also brought in at the end of the other sessions to briefly discuss the content of the sessions, as well as home practice assignments. In instances when the therapist observes a lot of parent–adolescent conflict, the parents may be invited in for one or more session without the adolescent present. Parents can, understandably, feel frustrated when dealing with adolescents with ADHD. But at times, this can lead them to react in unhelpful and invalidating ways, so it may be helpful for the therapist to provide education and coaching about the best ways to handle problematic situations. The parent-only and parent–adolescent sessions consist of psychoeducation about ADHD, as well as the content of the treatment. Although one emphasis of the treatment is to help adolescents transition to self-regulation and prepare for future independence, the parent sessions are used to extend the treatment outside of the sessions during the active treatment phase and after completion of the formal treatment. Specifically, parents learn the organizational system that the adolescent is using, and can help support their teen with this. As with the other modules, parents are generally more involved with younger adolescents in terms of supporting their use of organizational systems. With older adolescents, parents' attempts to force them into using a specific organizational system may be counterproductive and simply anger the adolescent, and possibly even make the adolescent less likely to use that system.

Parents are also provided with suggestions regarding how to interact with their child's school and how to advocate for their child with ADHD. Many adolescents with ADHD have 504 plans (legal documents in which the school describes how it will meet the needs of a specific student) or an individualized education program (IEP; a plan developed by a team consisting of parents and school personnel that outlines goals for the school year, as well as any special supports that are needed to help achieve these goals). Examples of supports or accommodations that might be included in these plans are giving the student duplicate sets of books for home and school, giving parents frequent progress reports from teachers, e-mailing assignments to parents or placing them on a website, or giving the adolescent extended time on assignments or tests. There is currently some controversy around the provision of accommodations to adolescents with ADHD, with some experts raising concerns that services provided to teens with ADHD through the schools are often not those supported by research (Spiel, Evans, & Langberg, 2014).

Relapse Prevention

We end the treatment with a discussion of relapse prevention. In this session, the adolescent is asked to review each of the skills covered and rate the usefulness of each skill. The adolescent is then given a "troubleshooting form" that matches potential difficulties that may arise with skills that can be implemented to target those difficulties. Finally, adolescents are asked to think about how they will continue to apply the techniques they have learned and schedule a 2-week self-check-in to assess ongoing use of skills. Parents are informed about this, and parents of younger adolescents are asked to facilitate the scheduling of the self-check-in session. It is a common practice in CBT that individuals are invited to schedule "booster sessions" to review skills and to assist with generalization to new situations. For example, if an adolescent completes a course of treatment while in high school but then is transitioning to college, he or she might come in for one or more booster sessions to discuss how he or she is going to adapt the skills to the college environment. This is encouraged and viewed as a normal part of treatment rather than as any type of treatment failure.

Case Examples

Please note that these case examples are composites based on various clients we have treated in our research studies and clinic. Any identifying information has been changed to protect privacy.

Jack

Jack was a 14-year-old boy who presented to the clinic with ADHD combined subtype/presentation. He lived in the suburbs with his parents and two younger brothers. Jack was on stimulant medication to treat his ADHD. He and his parents reported that the medication was helpful in managing his ADHD symptoms while he was taking it, although they noticed a decrease in productivity when the medication was wearing off. Jack reported that he had trouble with procrastination and with time management. He said that he often wanted to do other things (e.g., sports or going out with friends after school) and would put off doing his homework until later in the evening, when it was more challenging. He said that he often didn't finish his homework in the evening; sometimes he got up early to finish it and other times he did not complete it at all. Jack's mother noted that this was a frequent source of conflict in the family—she said that she felt she was always "nagging" Jack to do his homework and it still didn't seem to be very effective.

Initially, treatment with Jack and his parents focused on developing his organizational system. Jack opted to use a paper planner, because he was not allowed to use electronics in school. He was instructed to write down his assignments for every class, then to review and prioritize his tasks when he got home. The therapist worked with Jack to help him learn how to break down large tasks such as science projects and English papers into smaller chunks. At first, Jack had a lot of difficulty with this, and he did not bring his planner to sessions or he brought the planner without the assignments written in. However, after repeated discussions in the sessions, Jack was able to begin using his planner consistently.

In the parent sessions, Jack and his parents talked about how they could have a family meeting every week to go over the weekly schedule, and how Jack's parents could remind him to use his organizational skills without "nagging." They opted to use a shared electronic calendar for family and individual activities. They agreed on a contingency management system whereby Jack would get a privilege of his choice (trip to the mall or a sporting event with friends, going out to dinner at a favorite restaurant) on the weekend if he used skills during the week. Jack and his parents had a brief review meeting at the end of each day so that Jack could let his parents know which skills he had used that day. If he had used skills, he would get a point, and he could trade points toward the weekend privileges. As part of the therapy, Jack organized his personal spaces (desk, bedroom, closet) and identified specific places for important objects. He reported that he felt calmer knowing that he could find the things he needed and that he was getting more sleep since he wasn't staying up as late. Jack's parents reported that things were less contentious at home and that the whole family was benefiting from the reduced frequency of bickering about Jack's homework assignments.

Kate

Kate was an 18-year-old girl who presented to the clinic with ADHD inattentive subtype/presentation. She lived with her parents in the city. She had an older brother, who lived in an apartment on his own. Her mother accompanied her to the first session, but generally Kate took public transportation to the sessions and came alone. She had comorbid diagnoses of generalized anxiety disorder and major depression. She was on stimulant medication for ADHD, along with antidepressant medication to address her anxiety and depression. However, she reported that she often forgot to take her medication. Kate was a senior in high school and planned on attending college out of state. Kate said that she wanted to work on becoming more independent of her parents and better able to manage her own schedule. Kate noted that she was aware that college would present challenges, and she was worried about how she would be able to handle the transition to a less structured environment.

The focus of the early stages of treatment was on helping Kate develop systems for managing her appointments and tasks. Kate opted to use apps on her phone to keep track of her schedule and tasks, with the rationale that she always had her phone with her and thus would never be without access to her systems. The therapist worked with Kate on breaking down large tasks into smaller steps and scheduling out long-term tasks. They talked about the differences between high school and college in terms of how assignments are given (e.g., "Read three books before the midterm" in college vs. "Read Chapters 1–3 tonight" in high school) and how Kate might manage the longer time frame for college assignments.

While Kate seemed engaged in the treatment during sessions, she often did not practice skills outside of session. When questioned, she reported that, at times, she became anxious about doing her assignments perfectly, and this led to procrastination. She noted that, at other times, she felt down and did not have the energy she needed to complete the home practice of skills. The therapist used motivational interviewing strategies (see Sibley, Chapter 14, this volume) to help Kate increase her motivation to take her medications regularly, and incorporated behavioral activation strategies into Kate's schedule (e.g., helped Kate identify pleasurable activities, as well as activities that would give her a sense of mastery, and put them onto her schedule) to help reduce her depressive symptoms. The therapist moved the cognitive strategies earlier in the treatment and talked with Kate about how she could use adaptive thinking when she was feeling urges to avoid or withdraw. They also talked about how to apply adaptive thinking to the topic of perfectionism.

Kate had indicated that she did not wish her parents to be very involved in treatment. However, there were some instances when it seemed that the lack of communication with her parents was causing difficulties. For example, a source of friction in the family was that frequently Kate did not communicate her plans to her parents, so they were unsure whether she remembered appointments, whether she would be home for dinner, or whether she had a school event scheduled that her parents needed to attend. The therapist and Kate invited her parents to a session so that they could problem-solve about how they could develop a shared calendar, so that Kate's parents could see her appointments/plans and communicate more effectively.

Kate and her parents reported that having better organizational and communication systems, along with Kate taking her medications more regularly, improved not only Kate's ADHD symptoms but also her symptoms of anxiety and depression. She noted that she felt better prepared to start college following treatment.

This example illustrates several factors that can complicate treatment of adolescents with ADHD, specifically the presence of comorbid conditions, medication and homework noncompliance, and problematic communication patterns within the family. Another factor that might complicate treatment in teens with ADHD is the presence of substance use disorders.

Future Directions

Although the existing studies of CBT for ADHD are promising, more research is clearly needed on this topic. For example, studies with larger sample sizes, randomized trials that compare CBT to a time-matched comparison treatment, and studies with adolescents who are not on ADHD medications would be useful. Furthermore, the impact of psychosocial treatment for ADHD on functional impairment should be examined in more detail, and medication compliance should be formally assessed. Given the high rates of comorbidity with ADHD and other psychiatric disorders (see Becker & Fogleman, Chapter 9, this volume), the impact of comorbidity on treatment should be studied. Finally, it would be useful to study the use of school supports in tandem with CBT interventions to further improve the outcomes of adolescents with ADHD.

REFERENCES

Adler, L. A., Spencer, T., Faraone, S. V., Kessler, R. C., Howes, M. J., Biederman, J., & Secnik, K. (2006). Validity of a pilot Adult ADHD Self-Report Scale (ASRS) to rate adult ADHD symptoms. *Annals of Clinical Psychiatry, 18*(3), 145–148.

American Psychiatric Association. (2013). *Diagnostic and statistical manual of mental disorders* (5th ed.). Arlington, VA: Author.

Antshel, K. M., Faraone, S. V., & Gordon, M. (2014). Cognitive behavioral treatment outcomes in adolescent ADHD. *Journal of Attention Disorders, 18*(6), 483–495.

Antshel, K. M., & Olszewski, A. K. (2014). Cognitive behavioral therapy for adolescents with ADHD. *Child and Adolescent Psychiatric Clinics of North America, 23,* 825–842.

Barkley, R. A., Anastopoulos, A. D., Guevremont, D. C., & Fletcher, K. E. (1991). Adolescents with ADHD: Patterns of behavioral adjustment, academic functioning, and treatment utilization. *Journal of the American Academy of Child and Adolescent Psychiatry, 30*(5), 752–761.

Barkley, R. A., Edwards, G., Laneri, M., Fletcher, K., & Metevia, L. (2001). The efficacy of problem-solving communication training alone, behavior management training alone, and their combination for parent–adolescent conflict in teenagers with ADHD and ODD. *Journal of Consulting and Clinical Psychology, 69*(6), 926–941.

Barkley, R. A., Fischer, M., Edelbrock, C., & Smallish, L. (1991). The adolescent outcome of hyperactive children diagnosed by research criteria: III. Mother–child interactions, family conflicts and maternal psychopathology. *Journal of Child Psychology and Psychiatry and Allied Disciplines, 32*(2), 233–255.

Barkley, R. A., Fischer, M., Smallish, L., & Fletcher, K. (2004). Young adult follow-up of hyperactive children: Antisocial activities and drug use. *Journal of Child Psychology and Psychiatry, 45,* 195–211.

Barkley, R. A., Fischer, M., Smallish, L., & Fletcher, K. (2006). Young adult outcome of hyperactive children: Adaptive functioning in major life activities. *Journal of the American Academy of Child and Adolescent Psychiatry, 45*(2), 192–202.

Barkley, R. A., Murphy, K. R., & Fischer, M. (2008). *ADHD in adults: What the science says.* New York: Guilford Press.

Beck, J. S. (2011). *Cognitive behavior therapy: Basics and beyond* (2nd ed.). New York: Guilford Press.

Biederman, J., Petty, C. R., Evans, M., Small, J., & Farone, S. V. (2010). How persistent is ADHD?: A controlled 10-year follow-up study of boys with ADHD. *Psychiatry Research, 177,* 299–304.

Canu, W. H., & Wymbs, B. T. (2015). Novel approaches to cognitive-behavioral therapy for adult ADHD. *Cognitive and Behavioral Practice, 22,* 111–115.

Centers for Disease Control and Prevention. (2010). Increasing prevalence of parent-reported attention-deficit/hyperactivity disorder among children—United States, 2003 and 2007. *Morbidity and Mortality Weekly Report, 59*(44), 1439–1443.

Chronis, A. M., Jones, H. A., & Raggi, V. L. (2006). Evidence-based psychosocial treatments for children and adolescents with attention-deficit/hyperactivity disorder. *Clinical Psychology Review, 26*(4), 486–502.

Craske, M. H., & Barlow, D. H. (2006). *Mastery of your anxiety and worry, client workbook* (2nd ed.). New York: Oxford University Press.

Cuffe, S. P., McKeown, R. E., Jackson, K. L., Addy, C. L., Abramson, R., & Garrison, C. Z. (2001). Prevalence of attention-deficit/hyperactivity disorder in a community sample of older adolescents. *Journal of the American Academy of Child and Adolescent Psychiatry, 40,* 1037–1044.

Emilsson, B., Gudjonsson, G., Sigurdsson, J. F., Baldursson, G., Einarsson, E., Ofafsdottir, H., & Young, S. (2011). Cognitive behaviour therapy in medication-treated adults with ADHD and persistent symptoms: A randomized controlled trial. *BMC Psychiatry, 11,* 116.

Evans, S. W., Owens, J. S., & Bunford, N. (2014). Evidence-based psychosocial treatments for children and adolescents with attention-deficit/hyperactivity disorder. *Journal of Clinical Child and Adolescent Psychology, 43,* 527–551.

Evans, S. W., Schultz, B. K., Demars, C. E., & Davis, H. (2011). Effectiveness of the Challenging Horizons After-School Program for young adolescents with ADHD. *Behavior Therapy, 42*(3), 462–474.

Fergusson, D. M., Horwood, L. J., & Lynskey, M. T. (1993). Prevalence and comorbidity of DSM-III-R diagnoses in a birth cohort of 15 year olds. *Journal of the American Academy of Child and Adolescent Psychiatry, 32*(6), 1127–1134.

Fischer, M., Barkley, R. A., Edelbrock, C. S., & Smallish, L. (1990). The adolescent outcome of hyperactive children diagnosed by research criteria: II. Academic, attentional, and neuropsychological status. *Journal of Consulting and Clinical Psychology, 58,* 580–588.

Fisher, J. D., Fisher, W. A., Williams, S. S., & Malloy, T. E. (1994). Empirical tests of an information–motivation–behavioral skills model of AIDS-preventive behavior with gay men and heterosexual university students. *Health Psychology, 13*(3), 238–250.

Hill, J. C., & Schoener, E. P. (1996). Age-dependent decline of attention deficit hyperactivity disorder. *American Journal of Psychiatry, 153*(9), 1143–1146.

Knouse, L. E., & Mitchell, J. T. (2015). Incautiously optimistic: Positively valenced cognitive avoidance in adults with ADHD. *Cognitive and Behavioral Practice, 22*(2), 192–202.

Knouse, L. E., Teller, J., & Brooks, M. A. (2017). Meta-analysis of cognitive-behavioral treatments for adult ADHD. *Journal of Consulting and Clinical Psychology, 85*(7), 737–750.

Langberg, J. M., Evans, S. W., Schultz, B. K., Becker, S. P., Altaye, M., & Girio-Herrera, E. (2016). Trajectories and predictors of response to the Challenging Horizons Program for adolescents with ADHD. *Behavior Therapy, 47,* 339–354.

Lerner, M., & Wigal, T. (2008). Long-term safety of stimulant medications used to treat children with ADHD. *Journal of Psychosocial Nursing and Mental Health Services, 46*(8), 38–48.

McCabe, S. E., Dickinson, K., West, B. T., & Wilens, T. E. (2016). Age of onset, duration, and type of medication therapy for attention-deficit/hyperactivity disorder and substance use during adolescence: A multi-cohort national study. *Journal of the American Academy of Child and Adolescent Psychiatry, 55*(6), 479–486.

Mohr-Jensen, C., & Steinhausen, H. (2016). A meta-analysis and systematic review of the risks associated with childhood attention-deficit hyperactivity disorder on long-term outcome of arrests, convictions, and incarcerations. *Clinical Psychology Review, 48,* 32–42.

Murphy, K. (2005). Psychosocial treatments for ADHD in teens and adults: A practice-friendly review. *Journal of Clinical Psychology/In Session, 61,* 607–619.

Murphy, K., & Barkley, R. A. (1996). Attention deficit hyperactivity disorder adults: Comorbidities and adaptive impairments. *Comprehensive Psychiatry, 37*(6), 393–401.

Otto, M. W. (2000). Stories and metaphors in cognitive-behavioral therapy. *Cognitive and Behavioral Practice, 7,* 172–177.

Pettersson, R., Soderstrom, S., Edlund-Soderstrom, K., & Nilsson, K. W. (2017). Internet-based cognitive behavioral therapy for adults with ADHD in outpatient psychiatric care: A randomized trial. *Journal of Attention Disorders, 21*(6), 508–521.

Robin, A. L. (1998). Training families with ADHD adolescents. In R. A. Barkley (Ed.), *Attention deficit hyperactive disorder: A handbook for diagnosis and treatment* (2nd ed., pp. 413–457). New York: Guilford Press.

Safren, S. A., Otto, M. W., Sprich, S. E., Winett, C. L., Wilens, T. E., & Biederman, J. (2005). Cognitive-behavioral therapy for ADHD in medication-treated adults with continued symptoms. *Behaviour Research and Therapy, 43*(7), 831–842.

Safren, S. A., Otto, M. W., & Worth, J. L. (1999). Life-Steps: Applying cognitive-behavioral therapy to patient adherence in HIV medication treatment. *Cognitive Behavioral Practice, 6*, 332–341.

Safren, S. A., Perlman, C. A., Sprich, S. E., & Otto, M. W. (2005). *Mastering your adult ADHD: A cognitive behavioral treatment program, therapist guide.* New York: Oxford University Press.

Safren, S. A., Sprich, S., Chulvick, S., & Otto, M. W. (2004). Psychosocial treatments for adults with attention-deficit/hyperactivity disorder. *Psychiatric Clinics of North America, 27*(2), 349–360.

Safren, S. A., Sprich, S., Mimiaga, M. J., Surman, C., Knouse, L., Groves, M., & Otto, M. W. (2010). Cognitive behavioral therapy vs relaxation with educational support for medication-treated adults with ADHD and persistent symptoms: A randomized controlled trial. *Journal of the American Medical Association, 304*(8), 875–880.

Safren, S. A., Sprich, S. E., Perlman, C. A., & Otto, M. W. (2005). *Mastering your adult ADHD: A cognitive-behavioral treatment program, client workbook.* New York: Oxford University Press.

Safren, S. A., Sprich, S. E., Perlman, C. A., & Otto, M. W. (2017a). *Mastering your adult ADHD: A cognitive behavioral treatment program, therapist guide* (2nd ed.). New York: Oxford University Press.

Safren, S. A., Sprich, S. E., Perlman, C. A., & Otto, M. W. (2017b). *Mastering your adult ADHD: A cognitive behavioral treatment program, client workbook* (2nd ed.). New York: Oxford University Press.

Sibley, M. H., Mitchell, J. T., & Becker, S. P. (2016). Method of adult diagnosis influences estimated persistence of childhood ADHD: A systematic review of longitudinal studies. *Lancet Psychiatry, 3*, 1157–1165.

Skirrow, C., Ebner-Priemer, U., Reinhard, I., Malliaris, Y., Kuntsi, J., & Asherson, P. (2014). Everyday emotional experience of adults with ADHD: Evidence for reactive and endogenous lability. *Psychological Medicine, 44*, 3571–3583.

Solanto, M. V., Marks, D. J., Wasserstein, J., Mitchell, K., Abikoff, H., Alvir, J. M., & Kofmann, M. D. (2010). Efficacy of metacognitive therapy (MCT) for adult ADHD. *American Journal of Psychiatry, 167*, 958–968.

Spiel, C. F., Evans, S. W., & Langberg, J. M. (2014). Evaluating the content of individualized education programs and 504 plans of young adolescents with attention deficit/hyperactivity disorder. *School Psychology Quarterly, 29*(4), 452–468.

Sprich, S. E., Safren, S. A., Finkelstein, D., Remmert, J. E., & Hammerness, P. (2016). A randomized controlled trial of cognitive behavioral therapy for ADHD in medication-treated adolescents. *Journal of Child Psychology and Psychiatry, 57*(11), 1218–1226.

Steele, M., Jensen, P. S., & Quinn, D. M. P. (2006). Remission versus response as the goal of therapy in ADHD: A new standard for the field? *Clinical Therapeutics, 28*, 1892–1908.

Tercyak, K. P., Peshkin, B. N., Walker, L. R., & Stein, M. A. (2002). Cigarette smoking among youth with attention-deficit/hyperactivity disorder: Clinical phenomenology, comorbidity, and genetics. *Journal of Clinical Psychology in Medical Settings, 9*, 35–50.

Verhulst, F. C., van der Ende, J., Ferdinand, R. F., & Kasius, M. C. (1997). The prevalence of DSM-III-R diagnoses in a national sample of Dutch adolescents. *Archives of General Psychiatry, 54*(4), 329–336.

Vidal, R., Castells, J., Richarte, V., Palomar, G., Garcia, M., Nicolau, R., . . . Ramos-Quiroga, J. A. (2015). Group therapy for adolescents with attention-deficit/hyperactivity disorder: A randomized controlled trial. *Journal of the American Academy of Child and Adolescent Psychiatry, 54*(4), 275–282.

Weiss, M. D. (2000). Weiss Functional Impairment Rating Scale Self-Report (WFIRS-S) (Measurement Instrument). Retrieved from *http://naceonline.com/adultadhd-toolkit/assessmenttools/wfirs.pdf.*

Wilens, T. E., Biederman, J., Prince, J., Spencer, T., Schleifer, D., Harding, M., . . . Hatch, M. (1996). A double blind, placebo controlled study of desipramine for adult attention deficit hyperactivity disorder. *American Journal of Psychiatry, 153,* 1147–1153.

Wilens, T. E., McBurnett, K., Bukstein, O., McGough, J., Greenhill, L., Lerner, M., . . . Lynch, J. M. (2006). Multisite controlled study of OROS methylphenidate in the treatment of adolescents with attention-deficit/hyperactivity disorder. *Archives of Pediatrics and Adolescent Medicine, 160*(1), 82–90.

Wolraich, M. L., Wibbelsman, C. J., Brown, T. E., Evans, S. W., Gotlieb, E. M., Knight, J. R., . . . Wilens, T. (2005). Attention-deficit/hyperactivity disorder among adolescents: A review of the diagnosis, treatment, and clinical implications. *Pediatrics, 115*(6), 1734–1746.

CHAPTER 17

Mindfulness Meditation Training for Adolescents with ADHD

Naomi Ornstein Davis
John T. Mitchell

Attention-deficit/hyperactivity disorder (ADHD) is a developmental condition involving deficits in the regulation of attention, activity level, and impulses, and is defined, in part, by its childhood onset. Although previously thought of as "outgrown" during adolescence, ADHD typically persists into adolescence (and even adulthood) for the majority of cases (Barkley, Murphy, & Fischer, 2008). In one longitudinal cohort, ADHD persisted at a clinical level into adolescence for up to 70% of cases (Sibley et al., 2012). Symptom-driven impairment actually appears to increase during this developmental stage (Howard et al., 2016), and symptom persistence through adolescence is a strong predictor of a range of negative outcomes (Hechtman et al., 2016). Indeed, the manifestations of ADHD and its impairments become more distinct during adolescence. Impairments in the academic, personal, and social domains evolve in the context of increased expectations for independence, and new impairments may emerge as adolescents are expected to function in new ways (e.g., driving, finances, romantic relationships) (Graziano et al., 2015; Howard et al., 2016; VanderDrift, Antshel, & Olszewski, 2017).

Pharmacotherapy is a well-established treatment for individuals of all ages with ADHD, but medications do not always normalize functioning (Nolan & Gadow, 1997). Furthermore, a review of adolescent treatment suggests that behavioral therapy may be more effective than medication at reducing ADHD impairments for adolescents, despite recommendations from prominent practice organizations that prioritize medication (Sibley, Kuriyan, Evans, Waxmonsky, & Smith, 2014). As described by Brinkman, Froehlilch, and Epstein (Chapter 18, this volume), many adolescents discontinue medication due to a variety of motivations, including intentional and unintentional reasons (Emilsson, Gustafsson, & Marteinsdottir, 2017; Hodgkins, Sasane, Christensen, Harley, & Liu, 2011; Marcus & Durkin, 2011). At the same time, parents often seek to minimize and/or supplement use of medications with alternative or complementary approaches (Pellow, Solomon, & Barnard, 2011). Despite a clear need for this population, nonmedication treatments are not as well established as medication for adolescents with ADHD (Antshel & Olszewski, 2014). Overall, adolescence and the subsequent transition to adulthood appear to be a particularly vulnerable stage of development, and one for which novel ADHD treatments are needed (Buitelaar, 2017).

Mindfulness meditation training is a nonmedication intervention that is gaining increasing scientific attention in clinical and nonclinical populations, as evidenced by the special issues devoted to the topic (e.g., Baer, 2016; Black, 2014; Davidson & Kaszniak, 2015; DeSole, 2011; Renshaw & Cook, 2016; Tang & Posner, 2013), and is receiving growing clinical interest for ADHD. Our goal in this chapter is to describe the current state of research on mindfulness training for adolescents with ADHD. We define mindfulness-based interventions (MBIs), describe the rationale for applying mindfulness to ADHD, review the types of mindfulness training that have been developed for this population, describe treatment outcomes from clinical trials, and identify needed future directions for this research.

Overview of MBIs

MBIs are considered relatively recent additions to the field of behavior therapy (i.e., part of the "third wave"), though they are derived from the long-standing Eastern tradition of Vipassana meditation (Hayes, Follette, & Linehan, 2004; Hayes, Luoma, Bond, Masuda, & Lillis, 2006). MBIs teach mindfulness via formal and informal meditation practices. Although the field has yet to define the construct of mindfulness in a way that fully addresses the complex, multifaceted Buddhist phenomenology from which it is derived (Grossman, 2008, 2011; Kang & Whittingham, 2010), some widely adopted definitions capture aspects of this construct. One widely used definition is that mindfulness involves adopting nonjudgmental attention to one's experience(s) in the present moment (Kabat-Zinn, 1990). Others have defined it as a psychological process that comprises two components: orienting one's attention purposefully to the present moment, and approaching one's experience in the present moment with curiosity, openness, and acceptance (Bishop et al., 2004). Another commonly cited definition conceptualizes mindfulness as a trait or set of skills, such as being nonreactive, observing with awareness, acting with awareness, describing with awareness, and adopting a nonjudgmental approach towards one's experience (Baer et al., 2008). Each of these different definitions includes elements that are particularly relevant to ADHD, namely, an emphasis on present-moment regulation of attention.

Early in their development in Western psychological practices, MBIs such as mindfulness-based stress reduction (MBSR; Kabat-Zinn, 1990) and mindfulness-based cognitive therapy (Segal, Williams, & Teasdale, 2002) were developed for adults. For example, the first clinical application of mindfulness was for the treatment of chronic pain in adults via MBSR (Kabat-Zinn, 1982; Kabat-Zinn, Lipworth, & Burney, 1985). Since that time, mindfulness has been adopted for treatment of adults with various mental health conditions, such as anxiety disorders, mood disorders, and substance use disorders (Bowen et al., 2014; Goldin & Gross, 2010; Kuyken et al., 2016). Systematic reviews and meta-analyses indicate that these mindfulness-based treatments are effective for a variety of mental health treatment targets in adults (Bohlmeijer, Prenger, Taal, & Cuijpers, 2010; Chiesa & Serretti, 2011, 2014; Fjorback, Arendt, Ornbol, Fink, & Walach, 2011), which is likely due in part to the proposed impact of MBIs on transdiagnostic processes across different forms of psychopathology (Greeson, Garland, & Black, 2014).

Extending MBIs to Adolescents

Despite wide dissemination of MBIs for adults, notably fewer studies have examined the use of mindfulness training among adolescents (Burke, 2010; Kallapiran, Koo, Kirubakaran, & Hancock, 2016). However, MBIs are likely to confer similar benefits for adolescents as for adults. For instance, Tan and Martin (2016) suggested that trait mindfulness likely has positive benefits on adolescent mental health based on findings that trait mindfulness is associated with greater well-being, including positive emotion and psychological flexibility, in adolescents just as in adults (Tan & Martin, 2016). Furthermore, as observed in the adult literature, mindfulness training for adolescents may also influence clinically relevant transdiagnostic processes such as impulsivity, rumination, and emotion regulation (Deplus, Billieux, Scharff, & Philippot, 2016). Similarly, Perry-Parrish, Copeland-Linder, Webb, Shields, and Sibinga (2016) posited that training adolescents in the use of mindfulness strategies leads to improvements in overall psychological functioning, which leads to enhanced coping processes and subsequently yields improvements in cognitive function (i.e., attention, impulse control, and cognitive flexibility).

Among the adult-focused MBIs that have been extended downward for youth, multiple studies suggest they are acceptable to a wide range of adolescents (Ahola Kohut, Stinson, Davies-Chalmers, Ruskin, & van Wyk, 2017; Zoogman, Goldberg, Hoyt, & Miller, 2015). Intervention results are promising, but many studies have been underpowered to adequately examine efficacy (Ahola Kohut et al., 2017). In a meta-analysis on mindfulness meditation interventions for youth, larger effects were observed for psychological symptoms compared to other types of outcomes (e.g., blood pressure), and more benefit was noted for clinical samples as compared to nonclinical samples (Zoogman et al., 2015). Other reviews have focused on implementation of MBIs in the educational setting and have demonstrated feasibility and acceptability when treatments are delivered in schools (Felver, Celis-de Hoyos, Tezanos, & Singh, 2016). Like other broad reviews, methodological issues precluded clear assessment of efficacy, but some patterns can be observed. For example, in studies that included secondary students and used both intervention and control groups, results indicated reduced depression and anxiety symptoms, improved emotion regulation, improved mindfulness, decreased hostility, and decreased blood pressure (Felver et al., 2016).

MBIs for Adolescent Psychopathology

MBIs have also been used with adolescents with a range of psychiatric symptoms. Bögels, Hoogstad, van Dun, de Schutter, and Restifo (2008) piloted an intervention with adolescents ($N = 14$) with externalizing disorders including ADHD, autism spectrum disorder (ASD), oppositional defiant disorder (ODD), or conduct disorder. Bögels's MYmind intervention, which is described in further detail below, involves parallel youth and parent sessions that instruct and provide practice in a set of mindfulness skills. Results indicated substantial improvement on measures of attention, awareness, and impulsivity following the intervention, and positive outcomes were maintained at an 8-week follow-up assessment. A more recent study examined MYmind in a sample of 23 adolescents with ASD (de Bruin, Blom, Smit, van Steensel, & Bögels, 2015). Although ASD core symptoms did not change following the intervention, parents reported improved social behaviors, and adolescents reported improved quality of life following the intervention. Using a different MBI with another psychiatric sample, Ames, Richardson, Payne, Smith, and Leigh (2014) examined the impact of mindfulness on adolescents ($N = 11$) who were experiencing residual symptoms of depression or low mood following psychological treatment. Qualitative findings suggest that treatment was acceptable to these adolescents, and quantitative analyses suggest reduction in depression, and modest improvements in worry and quality of life. Although limited by the lack of a control group, findings across these studies demonstrate feasibility, acceptability, and preliminary support for efficacy in clinical adolescent samples.

Cautions and Considerations for Mindfulness Research

Despite widespread enthusiasm for integrating mindfulness meditation into clinical practice, a number of cautions are also warranted. To date, the methodology used in mindfulness intervention trials has some limitations, and future research should consider refining definitions of mindfulness, developing appropriate measures of mindfulness constructs, and using more rigorous study designs (Van Dam et al., 2018). In addition, as some have observed, many of the current practices that are designated as "mindfulness" differ from the original meditation practices from which they were derived. Based on research to date, it is not clear whether these adaptations may undermine the effectiveness of the practice (Farb, 2014). Finally, given the application of mindfulness to children and adolescents, including youth with ADHD, it is important to note the continued need for an improved developmental orientation. As noted by Greenberg and Harris (2012), factors such as normative shorter attention span, need for movement, and metacognitive strategy capacity among children and adolescents are likely to impact the ability of young people to engage with mindfulness interventions.

Rationale for Applying MBIs to ADHD

Attentional Functioning

Multiple general reviews on the topic of MBIs have identified ADHD as a particularly appropriate psychiatric disorder to target given the purported impact of MBIs on attentional functioning and, more broadly, cognitive control (Chiesa, Calati, & Serretti, 2011; Hölzel et al., 2011; Keng, Smoski, & Robins, 2011). As reviewed in Mitchell, Zylowska, and Kollins (2015), even some of the formal meditation practices demonstrate potential application and relevance to attention regulation in ADHD. For example, mindfulness meditation practices involve focusing attention on a particular object (e.g., one's own breath) and returning to this object after becoming distracted, which is proposed to improve attentional control abilities (Keng et al., 2011). Indeed, this practice requires top-down regulation of attention and conflict detection, which can be thought of as a regulatory approach to attention that improves executive processes (Chiesa et al., 2011). Since poor attentional functioning is a core symptom cluster of ADHD (see Willcutt, Chapter 3, this volume; American Psychiatric Association, 2013) and executive functioning deficits are common in ADHD (see Doidge, Saoud, & Toplak, Chapter 4, this volume; Barkley, 1997; Boonstra, Oosterlaan, Sergeant, & Buitelaar, 2005; Hervey, Epstein, & Curry, 2004; Poletti, 2009), any treatment that strengthens these processes seems appropriate for adolescents with ADHD.

The proposal that MBIs improve attentional functioning and, more broadly, cognitive control is consistent with findings in clinical and nonclinical child and adolescent samples (Mak, Whittingham, Cunningham, & Boyd, 2018). Combining mindfulness training with traditional cognitive-behavioral therapy (CBT) mitigates attention deficits (i.e., decline on a computerized attention task) that can result from prolonged high stress among incarcerated adolescents (Leonard et al., 2013). Using a more traditional mindfulness model, Quach, Mano, and Alexander (2016) demonstrated that a school-based mindfulness training program among 12- to 15-year-olds yielded improvements in working memory via a computerized task in comparison to an active treatment comparison group and a waitlist control group. Similar findings have been shown in female adolescents with elevated ADHD symptoms, who received a mindfulness intervention, with better planning and inhibition on laboratory tasks of executive functioning compared to a waitlist control group (Kiani, Hadianfard, & Mitchell, 2017). Overall, findings are consistent with a recent meta-analysis by Mak et al. (2018), who concluded that MBIs are a promising approach to targeting attentional processes and executive functioning in adolescents.

Emotion Dysregulation

Emotion regulation is an additional process that implicates ADHD as an appropriate psychiatric disorder to target using MBIs (Mitchell et al., 2015). Emotion regulation difficulties, though not a core diagnostic criteria for ADHD, are often present across the lifespan and contribute to significant impairment for children and adolescents (see Bunford, Chapter 5, this volume; Barkley, 2010; Shaw, Stringaris, Nigg, & Leibenluft, 2014; van Stralen, 2016). According to one model for ADHD, poor response inhibition results in greater difficulty resisting impulsive urges to act out on emotions and leads to emotional impulsivity (Barkley, 2010). This model is consistent with others described in the mindfulness literature, which argue that improving executive functioning will have a downstream beneficial effect on emotion regulation (Teper, Segal, & Inzlicht, 2013). MBIs are proposed to improve emotion regulation, because they teach individuals to observe emotional states as temporary and passing phenomenon that can be responded to in a nonreactive or compassionate manner (Chambers, Gullone, & Allen, 2009; Gratz & Tull, 2010; Guendelman, Medeiros, & Rampes, 2017). In nonclinical adolescent samples, researchers have suggested that mindfulness training may promote emotion regulation and reduce stress (Black, 2014; Zenner, Herrnleben-Kurz, & Walach, 2014). Galla (2016) conducted 5 day-long intensive meditation retreats with adolescents and found improvements in mindfulness, along with self-compassion and several aspects of emotion regulation, immediately following the retreat. Many of these improvements were maintained at follow-up 3 months later (Galla, 2016). Metz and colleagues (2013) conducted a school-based mindfulness intervention and demonstrated improved emotion regulation via a six-session program. In a study of female adolescents with elevations in ADHD symptoms, self-reported emotion dysregulation improved following participation in an MBI in comparison to a waitlist control condition (Kiani et al., 2017).

Intervention Studies Using MBIs for ADHD

Across mindfulness studies for ADHD, mindfulness has been implemented as either a component of a broader treatment or as a stand-alone intervention. Examples of the former include a mixed mindfulness meditation, CBT, and martial arts intervention (Haydicky, Wiener, Badali, Milligan, & Ducharme, 2012), a mixed yoga, meditation, and behavioral play therapy (Mehta et al., 2011, 2012), or acceptance and commitment therapy (Murrell, Steinberg, Connally, Hulsey, & Hogan, 2015). With regard to stand-alone MBI programs, some child and adolescent studies have yielded promising outcomes based on very small samples (e.g., ranging from four to six participants) (Carboni, Roach, & Fredrick, 2013; Singh et al., 2016). Other MBIs for ADHD have not intervened directly with children or adolescents but have instead provided the intervention for parents (Anderson & Guthery, 2015) or parents and teachers of students with ADHD (Miller & Brooker, 2017).

This burgeoning literature on MBIs for ADHD has been described in past reviews (Baijal & Gupta, 2008; Black, Milam, & Sussman, 2009; Cassone, 2015; Evans et al., 2018; Krisanaprakornkit, Ngamjarus, Witoonchart, & Piyavhatkul, 2010; Mitchell et al., 2015; Modesto-Lowe, Farahmand, Chaplin, & Sarro, 2015; Mukerji Househam & Solanto, 2016; Searight, Robertson, Smith, Perkins, & Searight, 2012). One relatively recent meta-analysis indicated medium effect sizes of MBIs for ADHD samples, indicating that MBIs are a promising intervention for this population (Cairncross & Miller, 2016). To date, however, prior reviews have been limited by a number of factors, such as a lack of unique focus on clinically diagnosed ADHD, inclusion of heterogeneous interventions that include but are not limited to mindfulness practices, and a predominant focus on adults with ADHD.

MBI Treatment Studies for Adolescents with ADHD

For the current summary, we provide an updated review of the treatment outcome literature on MBIs for ADHD—specifically for adolescents (defined herein as ages 10–19 years). Five clinical trials have examined the effects of an MBI in clinical samples with ADHD. Given the small body of literature, mixed-age samples (i.e., adolescents plus adults or adolescents plus children) were included. Table 17.1 summarizes these treatment outcome studies.

TABLE 17.1. Treatment Outcomes Studies of MBIs That Included Adolescents with ADHD

Study	Sample size	Mean age (range)	Male/female	ADHD subtype[a]	Intervention	Caregiver mindfulness training	Assessments	Outcome measures[b]	Findings[c]
Zylowska et al. (2008)	8	15.6 (range: 15–17)	3/5	3 IA 5 C 0 HI	MAPs	No	Pretreatment Posttreatment	CDI, RCMAS	n/a[d]
Haydicky et al. (2015)	18	15.5 (range: 13–18)	13/5	5 IA 12 C 1 HI	MYmind	Yes	Control baseline[e] Pretreatment Posttreatment 6-week f/u	C3, RCADS, SIPA, FAD, IC, AAQ, IM-P	*Conduct disorder symptoms* (post: parent [C3]) *Peer relations* (post: parent [C3]) *Depression, anxiety, and internalizing symptoms* (6-week: self [RCADS]) *Parental stress outcomes* (2 of 12 at posttreatment: SIPA, 3 of 12 at 6-week f/u) *Mindful parenting* (post: IM-P) *Parent acceptance* (post: AAQ)
Van de Weijer-Bergsma et al. (2012)	10	13.4 (range: 11–15)	5/5	4 IA 5 C 1 HI	MYmind	Yes	Pretreatment Posttreatment 8-week f/u 16-week f/u	YSR/CBCL/TRF, BRIEF, MAAS, PSI, PS, FFS, SHS, AmNT	*Attention problems* (8-week: self [YSR], paternal [CBCL]) *Externalizing problems* (post and 8-week: paternal [CBCL]) *Executive functioning* (8-week: paternal [BRIEF]) *Parenting stress* (post and 8-week: paternal [PSI]) *Parental overreactivity* (post: maternal and paternal [PS]) *Visual sustained attention reaction speed* (post)

TABLE 17.1. *(continued)*

									Auditory sustained attention false-alarm responses (post) *Auditory sustained attention number of misses* (8-week)
Van der Oord et al. (2012)	22	9.55 (range: 8–12)	16/6	7 IA 12 C 3 HI	MYmind	Yes	Control baseline[e] Pretreatment Posttreatment 8-week f/u	DBDRS, PSI, PS	**ADHD symptoms** (post, 8-week: parent [DBDRS]) *Parental stress* (8-week: parent [PSI]) *Parental overreactivity* (8-week: parent [PS])
Zhang et al. (2017)	11	9.5 (range: 8–12)	8/3	Not reported	MYmind	Yes	Pretreatment Posttreatment	CPT, TEA-Ch, ECBI, BRIEF, PSI, PS, IM-P	*Attention* (CPT omission, TEA-Ch time per target, TEA-Ch attention score, TEA-Ch map mission) *Disruptive behavior* (parent [ECBI])

Note. AAQ, Acceptance and Action Questionnaire; AmNT, Amsterdam Neuropsychological Tasks (Baseline Speed, Sustained Attention Dots, Sustained Attention Auditory); BRIEF, Behavior Rating Inventory of Executive Function; CBCL, Child Behavior Checklist; CDI, Child Depression Inventory; C3, Conners 3 Parent Rating Scale and Conners 3 Adolescent Self-Report; CPT 3, Conners' Continuous Performance Test 3rd Edition; DBDRS, Disruptive Behavior Disorder Rating Scale; ECBI, Eyberg Child Behavior Inventory; FAD, Family Assessment Device; FFS, Flinders Fatigue Scale; f/u, follow-up; IC, Issues Checklist; IM-P, Interpersonal Mindfulness in Parenting Scale; MAAS, Mindfulness Attention and Awareness Scale; PS, Parenting Scale; PSI, Parenting Stress Index; RCADS, Revised Child Anxiety and Depression Scale—Youth and Parent Report; RCMAS, Revised Children's Manifest Anxiety Scale; SIPA, Stress Index for Parents of Adolescents; TEA-Ch, Test of Everyday Attention for Children; TRF, Teacher Report Form; SHS = Subjective Happiness Scale; YSR = Youth Self-Report.

[a]IA, inattentive; C, combined; HI, hyperactive–impulsive.

[b]Child/adolescent-focused outcomes are listed (not parent outcomes).

[c]Only statistically significant effects are listed.

[d]Inferential statistical analyses were not conducted for these adolescent-specific reported findings—all other treatment outcome findings were reported in the combined adult and adolescent sample.

[e]Control baseline indicates a waitlist-control baseline assessment for the treatment group.

Zylowska and colleagues (2008) conducted the first clinical trial of an MBI for ADHD using a mixed sample of adolescents and adults with ADHD. The Mindful Awareness Practices (MAPS) program included an 8-week group intervention consisting of 2.5-hour weekly sessions accompanied by daily at-home practice. While informed by existing models for mindfulness training (Kabat-Zinn, 1990), MAPS was adapted for individuals with ADHD in specific ways (Zylowska et al., 2008). Adaptations included the addition of psychoeducation about ADHD, reducing the length of certain activities, use of visual aids, emphasis on mindful awareness in daily living, and use of a loving-kindness meditation to address the low self-esteem that can accompany ADHD. This study utilized a within-subjects design and examined outcomes at pretreatment and posttreatment. Regarding feasibility and acceptability among the adolescent sample (n = 8), 87% attended at least six sessions and reported high treatment satisfaction (M = 9.35, SD = 1.04) on a scale of 1 (*least satisfied*) to 10 (*most satisfied*). While self-reported ADHD symptoms and laboratory tasks of cognitive functioning improved at posttreatment, these effects were reported only for the full sample (N = 32) and were not presented separately for the adolescents. However, in a regression model examining the impact of age (among other variables) on a measure of attentional set shifting and inhibition, younger age was associated with greater improvement. The only symptom outcome measures reported separately for the adolescent sample were self-reported depression and anxiety. Although scores were reduced on both measures, these changes were described qualitatively as minor and were not analyzed statistically given the small sample size.

The four remaining MBI studies for adolescents with ADHD all implemented the MYmind intervention. MYmind is an 8-week group intervention that comprises 1.5-hour sessions for child or adolescent participants, along with a parallel mindful parent training group (for details, see Bögels et al., 2008; Bögels, Lehtonen, & Restifo, 2010; van der Oord, Bögels, & Peijnenburg, 2012). Both youth and parent participants learn formal mindfulness meditation techniques. In the youth training group, formal mindfulness meditation techniques are taught and connected to goals of reducing distractibility, impulsive responding, and hyperactivity. These techniques are also taught in the context of struggles that adolescents with ADHD typically experience (e.g., homework, parent–teen interactions), for example, practicing the "breathing space" exercise during conflict situations with parents. For parent groups, caregivers are taught formal mindfulness meditation techniques as a foundation to improve parent–child interactions, such as changing how parents approach an interaction and helping parents accept the difficulties their child is experiencing. These approaches are contrasted with automatic negative reactions parents may typically have to their child's behavior. Parents also learn about specific issues involved with parenting a child with ADHD and a common paradoxical dilemma for many parents—while adolescents typically desire autonomy, adolescents with ADHD tend to underperform when given more autonomy. Parents are taught how to balance close monitoring and support with granting greater independence to their child with ADHD (see also Sibley, Chapter 14, this volume).

Haydicky, Schecter, Wiener, and Ducharme (2015) examined MYmind in a sample of 18 adolescents (ages 13–18 years) with ADHD and 17 caregivers. Assessments were completed at four time points: 4 weeks prior to pretreatment, pretreatment, posttreatment, and 6-week follow-up. A within-group waitlist condition was also included to consider the effects of time. Session attendance was good both for adolescents ($M = 6.78$, $SD = 1.11$) and caregivers ($M = 6.94$, $SD = 0.9$). Analyses examined time effects across 4 weeks prior to pretreatment, pretreatment, posttreatment, and 6-week follow-up, and pairwise comparisons were conducted on any outcomes that were significant or approaching significance. Results indicated that parent report of conduct disorder and peer relations were significantly improved at posttreatment with medium or large effect sizes, and that self-reported depression, anxiety, and internalizing symptoms improved at 6-week follow-up with medium to large effect sizes. Regarding inattention, parent report demonstrated trend-level improvement from pre- to posttreatment ($p = .07$) with a medium effect size.

With regard to parenting characteristics, significant time effects were observed across four weeks prior to pre-treatment, pre-treatment, post-treatment, and 6-week follow-up on subscales of a parenting stress measure. At the 6-week follow-up, significant improvement was observed in the area of total parenting stress, the total parent domain, and a specific subscale that assesses life restrictions (all medium to large effect sizes). Significant time effects were observed for mindfulness and parenting mindfulness variables, with significant changes in mindful parenting at post-treatment with a large effect size and parental acceptance at 16-week follow-up with a medium effect size.

van de Weijer-Bergsma, Formsma, de Bruin, and Bögels (2012) examined the impact of MYmind in a sample of 10 child/adolescent participants (mean age 13.4 years) and 11 caregivers. This study utilized a within-subjects design that involved assessments at pretreatment, posttreatment, 8-week follow-up, and 16-week follow-up. Feasibility and acceptability were not reported, but symptom ratings were obtained from multiple sources, including self-report (all assessment points), parent report (pretreatment, posttreatment, 8-week follow-up), and teacher report (pretreatment and posttreatment). Results indicated mixed outcomes depending on the rater and the time point. For example, ratings of attention improved and approached significance, with a medium effect size, by paternal report at posttreatment and at 8-week follow-up, and by self-report, with large effect sizes at 8-week follow-up. Similarly, paternal report showed significant improvement in externalizing symptoms at posttreatment and 8-week follow-up, with small effect sizes, and self-report of externalizing symptoms approached significance, with a medium effect size at 8-week follow-up and a large effect size at 16-week follow-up. Notably, neither teacher report nor maternal report showed improvements in ratings of attention or externalizing symptoms. With regard to parental characteristics, parenting stress improved per paternal report but not maternal report at posttreatment and 8-week follow-up, with large effect sizes. However, parental overreactivity improved per both maternal and paternal ratings, with large effect sizes at posttreatment but not at the 8-week follow-up.

Additional outcomes examined aspects of neuropsychological functioning. Executive functioning approached significance at posttreatment and was significant at 8-week follow-up, with large effect sizes for paternal ratings, whereas teacher ratings approached significance at posttreatment, with a medium effect size. On objective neuropsychological tasks, visual sustained attention improved, with a large effect size for speed of responses at posttreatment, although this did not extend to 8- and 16-week follow-ups. In addition, performance on indices of auditory attention improved, with a medium effect size at posttreatment. These effects were large at both follow-ups, but were only approaching statistical significance. Another index of auditory attention indicated improvement at 8-week follow-up, with a large effect.

van der Oord and colleagues (2012) implemented MYmind using a within-group, quasi-experimental waitlist-control design with 22 participants (ages 8–12 years) and 21 caregivers. This design involved a pretreatment assessment at least 6 weeks prior to the treatment for 11 families; the full sample completed pretreatment, posttreatment, and 8-week follow-up assessments. Fourteen percent of the sample (n = 3) did not complete the treatment. Among the participating families that completed the treatment and were assessed at any point posttreatment (n = 1 elected not to participate in assessments after completing treatment), overall session attendance was 94%. Paired t-tests indicated that no significant changes emerged between waitlist and pretreatment except for teacher report of ODD symptoms, which increased with a small effect size. From pretreatment to posttreatment, there was a significant reduction in parent ratings of inattention (large effect size) and hyperactivity–impulsivity (medium effect size), and this reduction was maintained at the 8-week follow-up. Teacher ratings indicated improvement in inattention that approached significance, with a small effect size at posttreatment, though this finding was not maintained at the 8-week follow-up. There were no treatment effects for ODD symptoms based on parent or teacher ratings.

Zhang and colleagues (2017) conducted a within-subjects pre- and posttreatment trial with 11 youth (ages 8–12 years) and their caregivers. In terms of feasibility and acceptability, 91% of families attended at least six sessions with high treatment satisfaction ratings (i.e., on a 10-point Likert scale, mean ratings were 7.2 [*SD* = 2.1] and 8.0 [*SD* = 1.2] for children and parents, respectively). Statistical analyses included correction for multiple comparisons and indicated that attentional performance on a continuous performance test (omission errors) improved with large effect sizes and reached clinical remission (i.e., posttreatment *T*-score below 60). Scores on another laboratory task of attentional functioning improved with large effect sizes. Parent report of disruptive behavior improved with a small effect size, although intensity and problem scores did not fall below cut-off scores. However, improvements were not found in a number of other domains, including parent report of executive functioning, parenting stress, parenting style, or mindful parenting skills.

Summary of Adolescent MBI Intervention Findings

In summary, across five trials of a mindfulness intervention for adolescents with ADHD, MBIs appear both feasible and acceptable. For example, attendance of at least six out of eight sessions ranged from 87 to 94% (van der Oord et al., 2012; Zhang et al., 2017; Zylowska et al., 2008). In addition, treatment satisfaction averages (10-point Likert scale, with higher scores indicating higher satisfaction) ranged from 7.2 (Zhang et al., 2017) to 9.35 (Zylowska et al., 2008). The majority of these studies administered the same intervention, MYmind, which involved parents in addition to the child or adolescent diagnosed with ADHD (Haydicky et al., 2015; van de Weijer-Bergsma et al., 2012; van der Oord et al., 2012; Zhang et al., 2017)—the other study involved adolescents only, without parent involvement (Zylowska et al., 2008). Regarding ADHD symptom outcome analyses, three reported improvements in attentional functioning on at least one measure (van de Weijer-Bergsma et al., 2012; van der Oord et al., 2012; Zhang et al., 2017). Among the remaining two studies, one trial yielded improvement in inattentive symptoms that approached significance (Haydicky et al., 2015) and the other study reported improvement in ADHD symptoms, but findings were presented for the combined sample of adolescents and adults (Zylowska et al., 2008). Although some of these trials utilized a waitlist-control condition within groups to address the effects of time to overcome some limitations of within-group designs (i.e., assessments 4–6 weeks pretreatment and immediately pretreatment) (Haydicky et al., 2015; van der Oord et al., 2012), no adolescent ADHD studies to date have compared individuals receiving mindfulness to a comparison condition.

Discussion

Despite accumulating evidence that indicates MBIs may be beneficial for individuals with ADHD, only five trials examined the effects of mindfulness interventions with clinical samples of adolescents with ADHD. Importantly, only two of these studies included adolescent-only samples rather than samples of adolescents mixed with children or with adults. Based on these existing studies, and consistent with the literature on MBIs with other groups of adolescents, MBIs appear both feasible and acceptable for this population. However, preliminary findings on ADHD outcomes are mixed.

Overall, this small but promising literature on mindfulness interventions for adolescent ADHD is limited by a number of study design issues. Sample sizes have been small, with the largest sample of 22 participants (van der Oord et al., 2012), which limits generalization of results. In addition, at the time of this review, all studies utilized a within-subjects design, with no randomized controlled studies comparing an MBI to a comparison condition. Although several trials addressed limitations of within-group designs by using a waitlist-control condition, (Haydicky et al., 2015; van der Oord et al., 2012), future studies will benefit from more rigorous study design by including a treatment comparison group. This limitation is currently being addressed in a multicenter, randomized controlled trial (RCT) that will compare the effects of mindfulness training to the effects of medication treatment with methylphenidate (Meppelink, de Bruin, & Bögels, 2016). Using the MYmind protocol, youth with ADHD (ages 9–18) will be randomized to either mindfulness or medication, and outcomes will include ADHD symptoms (primary outcome), co-occurring psychopathology (secondary outcomes), and mechanisms of change (e.g., mindfulness, emotion regulation, parenting). This study will fill an important gap in the literature, but additional RCTs with adolescent samples will also be important, to examine the impact of mindfulness as an alternative to other behavioral therapies and as an adjunctive treatment (e.g., with behavioral therapy or with medication management) (Cassone, 2015).

Among the studies that have explored MBIs with adolescents, including both clinical and nonclinical samples, few trials have specified ways to downward-extend interventions to meet the needs of the adolescent population (Tan, 2016). Treatment modifications are likely necessary given developmental differences between adults and adolescents with regard to normative attention, cognitive skills, and need for movement and physical activity (Tan, 2016). Importantly, four of the five clinical trials for adolescent ADHD used the MYmind program, which was designed specifically for youth while drawing on MBSR developed for adults. Further study of the distinct components of MYmind (e.g., parent-only, youth-only, and combined treatments) may be important to further understand the active ingredients of mindfulness treatment and to identify any needed developmental modification.

Understanding the symptom targets of any intervention is critical for treatment outcomes research, and determining these targets is similarly important when considering use of MBIs in this adolescent population. Treatment goals may vary widely, from determining whether MBIs can be as effective as stimulant medication for reducing ADHD symptoms to determining whether MBIs can sufficiently reduce parenting stress and other functional domains (but may not necessarily reduce symptoms) (Becker, Chorpita, & Daleiden, 2011). These different goals will impact the measurement tools used and reporting sources employed in a given study (e.g., self-, parent, or teacher report, or laboratory task performance). Similarly, if increased adolescent mindfulness is a treatment goal, then measurement must include more reliable and valid tools that address challenges such as respondent developmental level and ways to integrate self-report with other reporters (Goodman, Madni, & Semple, 2017; Pallozzi, Wertheim, Paxton, & Ong, 2017). In addition to employing multiple informants to assess outcomes, other novel methods, such as ecological momentary assessment, may provide valuable information that cannot otherwise be measured (Davidson & Kaszniak, 2015). Indeed, some of these methods have been adopted in the adult ADHD treatment literature (Mitchell et al., 2017).

Finally, although the adult literature includes a robust discussion of mechanisms of action for MBIs, less work has examined these mechanisms for adolescents. In adults, individuals who are experienced meditators show reduced activation in the brain's default mode network, which is a network of several brain structures that are dysfunctional in the context of ADHD. Furthermore, meditation is associated with stronger connectivity in brain regions that are implicated in cognitive control and self-monitoring (Brewer et al., 2011). Based on a review of the literature, Bachmann, Lam, and Philipsen (2016) concluded that mindfulness meditation may lead to reductions in adult ADHD symptoms and may cause neuroplastic changes in brain regions affected by ADHD. To date, none of this research has been conducted with adolescents, but downward extensions of this literature will be very important to understand potential brain changes at this earlier stage in development. Importantly, findings from the adult literature suggest neuroplastic changes in brain regions that support emotion regulation (Tang, Holzel, & Posner, 2015). These findings are consistent with those of Kiani and colleagues (2017), in which adolescents with elevated ADHD symptoms showed improvement in emotion regulation and executive functioning following mindfulness intervention, though brain imaging was not conducted in that study.

In summary, although current research suggests a high degree of feasibility and acceptability of mindfulness treatments for adolescents with ADHD, a number of considerations need to be addressed before these interventions can be widely disseminated and efficacy is demonstrated. Nonetheless, adolescents with ADHD are a unique group for whom novel treatments are needed as a complement or alternative to existing treatments. Current treatment studies indicate that MBIs for adolescents with ADHD are feasible and acceptable. Findings support preliminary efficacy, but methodological issues need to be addressed, including treatment randomization to an MBI or a comparison condition, larger samples for greater statistical power, consideration of primary outcome variables, and measurement of these primary outcome variables. Future studies that address these issues are needed to inform empirically supported treatment options for adolescents with ADHD and their families. Such research is crucial to improving the lives of adolescents with ADHD as they navigate this critical developmental period.

References

Ahola Kohut, S., Stinson, J., Davies-Chalmers, C., Ruskin, D., & van Wyk, M. (2017). Mindfulness-based interventions in clinical samples of adolescents with chronic illness: A systematic review. *Journal of Alternative and Complementary Medicine, 23*(8), 581–589.

American Psychiatric Association. (2013). *Diagnostic and statistcal manual of mental disorders* (5th ed.). Arlington, VA: Author.

Ames, C. S., Richardson, J., Payne, S., Smith, P., & Leigh, E. (2014). Innovations in practice: Mindfulness-based cognitive therapy for depression in adolescents. *Child and Adolescent Mental Health, 19*(1), 74–78.

Anderson, S. B., & Guthery, A. M. (2015). Mindfulness-based psychoeducation for parents of children with attention-deficit/hyperactivity disorder: An applied clinical project. *Journal of Child and Adolescent Psychiatric Nursing, 28*(1), 43–49.

Antshel, K. M., & Olszewski, A. K. (2014). Cognitive behavioral therapy for adolescents with ADHD. *Child and Adolescent Psychiatric Clinics of North America, 23*(4), 825–842.

Bachmann, K., Lam, A. P., & Philipsen, A. (2016). Mindfulness-based cognitive therapy and the adult ADHD brain: A neuropsychotherapeutic perspective. *Frontiers in Psychiatry, 7,* 117.

Baer, R. (2016). Assessment of mindfulness and closely related constructs: Introduction to the special issue. *Psychological Assessment, 28*(7), 787–790.

Baer, R. A., Smith, G. T., Lykins, E., Button, D., Krietemeyer, J., Sauer, S., Walsh, E., . . . Williams, J. M. (2008). Construct validity of the Five Facet Mindfulness Questionnaire in meditating and nonmeditating samples. *Assessment, 15*(3), 329–342.

Baijal, S., & Gupta, R. (2008). Meditation-based training: A possible intervention for attention deficit hyperactivity disorder. *Psychiatry (Edgmont), 5*(4), 48–55.

Barkley, R. A. (1997). Behavioral inhibition, sustained attention, and executive functions: Constructing a unifying theory of ADHD. *Psychological Bulletin, 121*(1), 65–94.

Barkley, R. A. (2010). Deficient emotional self-regulation is a core component of attention-deficit/hyperactivity disorder. *Journal of ADHD and Related Disorders, 1*(2), 5–37.

Barkley, R. A., Murphy, K. R., & Fischer, M. (2008). *ADHD in adults: What the science says.* New York: Guilford Press.

Becker, K. D., Chorpita, B. F., & Daleiden, E. L. (2011). Improvement in symptoms versus functioning: How do our best treatments measure up? *Administration and Policy in Mental Health and Mental Health Services Research, 38*(6), 440–458.

Bishop, S. R., Lau, M., Shapiro, S., Carlson, L., Anderson, N. D., Carmody, J., . . .

Devins, G. (2004). Mindfulness: A proposed operational definition. *Clinical Psychology: Science and Practice, 11*(3), 230–241.

Black, D. S. (2014). Mindfulness-based interventions: An antidote to suffering in the context of substance use, misuse, and addiction. *Substance Use and Misuse, 49*(5), 487–491.

Black, D. S., Milam, J., & Sussman, S. (2009). Sitting-meditation interventions among youth: A review of treatment efficacy. *Pediatrics, 124*(3), e532–e541.

Bögels, S., Hoogstad, B., van Dun, L., de Schutter, S., & Restifo, K. (2008). Mindfulness training for adolescents with externalizing disorders and their parents. *Behavioral and Cognitive Psychotherapy, 36*(2), 193–209.

Bögels, S. M., Lehtonen, A., & Restifo, K. (2010). Mindful parenting in mental health care. *Mindfulness (NY), 1*(2), 107–120.

Bohlmeijer, E., Prenger, R., Taal, E., & Cuijpers, P. (2010). The effects of mindfulness-based stress reduction therapy on mental health of adults with a chronic medical disease: A meta-analysis. *Journal of Psychosomatic Research, 68*(6), 539–544.

Boonstra, A. M., Oosterlaan, J., Sergeant, J. A., & Buitelaar, J. K. (2005). Executive functioning in adult ADHD: A meta-analytic review. *Psychological Medicine, 35*(8), 1097–1108.

Bowen, S., Witkiewitz, K., Clifasefi, S. L., Grow, J., Chawla, N., Hsu, S. H., . . . Larimer, M. E. (2014). Relative efficacy of mindfulness-based relapse prevention, standard relapse prevention, and treatment as usual for substance use disorders: A randomized clinical trial. *JAMA Psychiatry, 71*, 547–556.

Brewer, J. A., Worhunsky, P. D., Gray, J. R., Tang, Y. Y., Weber, J., & Kober, H. (2011). Meditation experience is associated with differences in default mode network activity and connectivity. *Proceedings of the National Academy of Sciences of the USA, 108*(50), 20254–20259.

Buitelaar, J. K. (2017). Optimising treatment strategies for ADHD in adolescence to minimise "lost in transition" to adulthood. *Epidemiology and Psychiatric Sciences, 17*, 1–5.

Burke, C. A. (2010). Mindfulness-based approaches with children and adolescents: A preliminary review of current research in an emergent field. *Journal of Child and Family Studies, 19*(2), 133–144.

Cairncross, M., & Miller, C. J. (2016, February 2). The effectiveness of mindfulness-based therapies for ADHD: A meta-analytic review. *Journal of Attention Disorders*. [Epub ahead of print]

Carboni, J. A., Roach, A. T., & Fredrick, L. D. (2013). Impact of mindfulness training on the behavior of elementary students with attention-deficit/hyperactive disorder. *Research in Human Development, 10*(3), 234–251.

Cassone, A. R. (2015). Mindfulness training as an adjunct to evidence-based treatment for ADHD within families. *Journal of Attention Disorders, 19*(2), 147–157.

Chambers, R., Gullone, E., & Allen, N. B. (2009). Mindful emotion regulation: An integrative review. *Clinical Psychology Review, 29*(6), 560–572.

Chiesa, A., Calati, R., & Serretti, A. (2011). Does mindfulness training improve cognitive abilities?: A systematic review of neuropsychological findings. *Clinical Psychology Review, 31*(3), 449–464.

Chiesa, A., & Serretti, A. (2011). Mindfulness based cognitive therapy for psychiatric disorders: A systematic review and meta-analysis. *Psychiatry Research, 187*(3), 441–453.

Chiesa, A., & Serretti, A. (2014). Are mindfulness-based interventions effective for substance use disorders?: A systematic review of the evidence. *Substance Use and Misuse, 49*(5), 492–512.

Davidson, R. J., & Kaszniak, A. W. (2015). Conceptual and methodological issues in research on mindfulness and meditation. *American Psychologist, 70*(7), 581–592.

de Bruin, E. I., Blom, R., Smit, F. M., van Steensel, F. J., & Bögels, S. M. (2015). MYmind: Mindfulness training for youngsters with autism spectrum disorders and their parents. *Autism, 19*(8), 906–914.

Deplus, S., Billieux, J., Scharff, C., & Philippot, P. (2016). A mindfulness-based group intervention for enhancing self-regulation of emotion in late childhood and adolescence: A pilot study. *International Journal of Mental Health and Addiction, 14*(5), 775–790.

DeSole, L. (2011). Eating disorders and mindfulness [Special issue]. *Eating Disorders, 19*(1), 1–5.

Emilsson, M., Gustafsson, P. A., Öhnström, G., & Marteinsdottir, I. (2017). Beliefs regarding medication and side effects influence treatment adherence in adolescents with attention deficit hyperactivity disorder. *European Child and Adolescent Psychiatry, 26*(5), 559–571.

Evans, S., Ling, M., Hill, B., Rinehart, N., Austin, D., & Sciberras, E. (2018). Systematic review of meditation-based interventions for children with ADHD. *European Child and Adolescent Psychiatry, 27*(1), 9–27.

Farb, N. (2014). From retreat center to clinic to boardroom?: Perils and promises of the modern mindfulness movement. *Religions, 54*(4), 1062–1086.

Felver, J. C., Celis-de Hoyos, C. E., Tezanos, K., & Singh, N. N. (2016). A systematic review of mindfulness-based interventions for youth in school settings. *Mindfulness, 7*(1), 34–45.

Fjorback, L. O., Arendt, M., Ornbol, E., Fink, P., & Walach, H. (2011). Mindfulness-based stress reduction and mindfulness-based cognitive therapy: A systematic review of randomized controlled trials. *Acta Psychiatrica Scandinavica, 124*(2), 102–119.

Galla, B. M. (2016). Within-person changes in mindfulness and self-compassion predict enhanced emotional well-being in healthy, but stressed adolescents. *Journal of Adolescence, 49,* 204–217.

Goldin, P. R., & Gross, J. J. (2010). Effects of mindfulness-based stress reduction (MBSR) on emotion regulation in social anxiety disorder. *Emotion, 10*(1), 83–91.

Goodman, M. S., Madni, L. A., & Semple, R. J. (2017). Measuring mindfulness in youth: Review of current assessments, challenges, and future directions. *Mindfulness, 8,* 1409–1420.

Gratz, K. L., & Tull, M. T. (2010). Emotion regulation as a mechanism of change in acceptance- and mindfulness-based treatments. In R. A. Baer (Ed.), *Assessing mindfulness and acceptance processes in clients: Illuminating the theory and practice of change* (pp. 107–133). Oakland, CA: Context Press/New Harbinger.

Graziano, P. A., Reid, A., Slavec, J., Paneto, A., McNamara, J. P., & Geffken, G. R. (2015). ADHD symptomatology and risky health, driving, and financial behaviors in college: The mediating role of sensation seeking and effortful control. *Journal of Attention Disorders, 19*(3), 179–190.

Greenberg, M. T., & Harris, A. R. (2012). Nurturing mindfulness in children and youth: Current state of research. *Child Development Perspectives, 6*(2), 161–166.

Greeson, J., Garland, E. L., & Black, D. (2014). Mindfulness: A transtherapeutic approach for transdiagnostic mental processes. In A. Ie, C. T. Ngoumen, & E. J. Langer (Eds.), *The Wiley-Blackwell handbook of mindfulness* (pp. 533–562). Chichester, UK: Wiley.

Grossman, P. (2008). On measuring mindfulness in psychosomatic and psychological research. *Journal of Psychosomatic Research, 64*(4), 405–408.

Grossman, P. (2011). Defining mindfulness by how poorly I think I pay attention during everyday awareness and other intractable problems for psychology's (re)invention of mindfulness: Comment on Brown et al. (2011). *Psychological Assessment 23*(4), 1034–1040; discussion 1041–1036.

Guendelman, S., Medeiros, S., & Rampes, H. (2017). Mindfulness and emotion regulation: Insights from neurobiological, psychological, and clinical studies. *Frontiers in Psychology, 8,* 220.

Haydicky, J., Shecter, C., Wiener, J., & Ducharme, J. M. (2015). Evaluation of MBCT for adolescents with ADHD and their parents: Impact on individual and family functioning. *Journal of Child and Family Studies, 24*(1), 76–94.

Haydicky, J., Wiener, J., Badali, P., Milligan, K., & Ducharme, J. M. (2012). Evaluation of a mindfulness-based intervention for adolescents with learning disabilities and co-occurring ADHD and anxiety. *Mindfulness, 3*(2), 151–164.

Hayes, S. C., Follette, V. M., & Linehan, M. M. (Eds.). (2004). *Mindfulness and acceptance: Expanding the cognitive-behavioral tradition.* New York: Guilford Press.

Hayes, S. C., Luoma, J. B., Bond, F. W., Masuda, A., & Lillis, J. (2006). Acceptance and commitment therapy: Model, processes and outcomes. *Behaviour Reseach and Therapy, 44*(1), 1–25.

Hechtman, L., Swanson, J. M., Sibley, M. H., Stehli, A., Owens, E. B., Arnold, L. E., . . . MTA Cooperative Group. (2016). Functional adult outcomes 16 years after childhood diagnosis of attention-deficit/hyperactivity disorder: MTA results. *Journal of the American Academy of Child and Adolescent Psychiatry, 55*(11), 945–952.

Hervey, A. S., Epstein, J. N., & Curry, J. F. (2004). Neuropsychology of adults with attention-deficit/hyperactivity disorder: A meta-analytic review. *Neuropsychology, 18*(3), 485–503.

Hodgkins, P., Sasane, R., Christensen, L., Harley, C., & Liu, F. (2011). Treatment outcomes with methylphenidate formulations among patients with ADHD: Retrospective claims analysis of a managed care population. *Current Medical Research and Opinion, 27*(Suppl. 2), 53–62.

Hölzel, B. K., Lazar, S. W., Gard, T., Schuman-Olivier, Z., Vago, D. R., & Ott, U. (2011). How does mindfulness meditation work?: Proposing mechanisms of action from a conceptual and neural perspective. *Perspectives on Psychological Science, 6*(6), 537–559.

Howard, A. L., Strickland, N. J., Murray, D. W., Tamm, L., Swanson, J. M., Hinshaw, S. P., . . . Molina, B. S. (2016). Progression of impairment in adolescents with attention-deficit/hyperactivity disorder through the transition out of high school: Contributions of parent involvement and college attendance. *Journal of Abnormal Psychology, 125*(2), 233–247.

Kabat-Zinn, J. (1982). An outpatient program in behavioral medicine for chronic pain patients based on the practice of mindfulness meditation: Theoretical considerations and preliminary results. *General Hospital Psychiatry, 4*(1), 33–47.

Kabat-Zinn, J. (1990). *Full catastrophe living: Using the wisdom of your body and mind to face stress, pain, and illness.* New York: Deltacorte Press.

Kabat-Zinn, J., Lipworth, L., & Burney, R. (1985). The clinical use of mindfulness meditation for the self-regulation of chronic pain. *Journal of Behavioral Medicine, 8*(2), 163–190.

Kallapiran, K., Koo, S., Kirubakaran, R., & Hancock, K. (2016). Review: Effectiveness of mindfulness in improving mental health symptoms of children and adolescents: A meta-analysis. *Child and Adolescent Mental Health, 20*(4), 182–194.

Kang, C., & Whittingham, K. (2010). Mindfulness: A dialogue between Buddism and clinical psychology. *Mindfulness, 1*(3), 161–173.

Keng, S. L., Smoski, M. J., & Robins, C. J. (2011). Effects of mindfulness on psychological health: A review of empirical studies. *Clinical Psychology Review, 31*(6), 1041–1056.

Kiani, B., Hadianfard, H., & Mitchell, J. T. (2017). The impact of mindfulness meditation training on executive functions and emotion dysregulation in an Iranian sample of female adolescents with elevated attention-deficit/hyperactivity disorder symptoms. *Australian Journal of Psychology, 69*(4), 273–282.

Krisanaprakornkit, T., Ngamjarus, C., Witoonchart, C., & Piyavhatkul, N. (2010). Meditation therapies for attention-deficit/hyperactivity disorder (ADHD). *Cochrane Database of Systematic Reviews, 6*, CD006507.

Kuyken, W., Warren, F. C., Taylor, R. S., Whalley, B., Crane, C., Bondolfi, G., . . . Dalgleish, T. (2016). Efficacy of mindfulness-based cognitive therapy in prevention of depressive relapse: An individual patient data meta-analysis from randomized trials. *JAMA Psychiatry, 73*(6), 565–574.

Leonard, N. R., Jha, A. P., Casarjian, B., Goolsarran, M., Garcia, C., Cleland, C. M., . . . Massey, Z. (2013). Mindfulness training improves attentional task performance in incarcerated youth: A group randomized controlled intervention trial. *Frontiers in Psychology, 4*, 792.

Mak, C., Whittingham, K., Cunningham, R., & Boyd, R. N. (2018). Efficacy of mindfulness-based interventions for attention and executive function in children and adolescents—A systematic review. *Mindfulness, 9*(1), 59–78.

Marcus, S. C., & Durkin, M. (2011). Stimulant adherence and academic performance in urban youth with attention-deficit/hyperactivity disorder. *Journal of the American Academy of Child and Adolescen Psychiatry, 50*, 480–489.

Mehta, S., Mehta, V., Mehta, S., Shah, D., Motiwala, A., Vardhan, J., . . . Mehta, D. (2011). Multimodal behavior program for ADHD incorporating yoga and implemented by high school volunteers: A pilot study. *ISRN Pediatrics, 2011*, Article 780745.

Mehta, S., Shah, D., Shah, K., Mehta, S., Mehta, N., Mehta, V., . . . Mehta, D. (2012). Peer-mediated multimodal intervention program for the treatment of children with ADHD in India: One-year followup. *ISRN Pediatrics, 2012*, Article 419168.

Meppelink, R., de Bruin, E. I., & Bogels, S. M. (2016). Meditation or medication?: Mindfulness training versus medication in the treatment of childhood ADHD: A randomized controlled trial. *BMC Psychiatry, 16*, 267.

Metz, S. M., Frank, J. L., Reibel, D., Cantrell, T., Sanders, R., & Broderick, P. C. (2013). The effectiveness of the Learning to BREATHE program on adolescent emotion regulation. *Research in Human Development, 10*(3), 252–272.

Miller, C. J., & Brooker, B. (2017). Mindfulness programming for parents and teachers of children with ADHD. *Complementary Therapies in Clinical Practice, 28*, 108–115.

Mitchell, J. T., McIntyre, E. M., English, J. S., Dennis, M. F., Beckham, J. C., & Kollins, S. H. (2017). A pilot trial of mindfulness meditation training for ADHD in adulthood: Impact on core symptoms, executive functioning, and emotion dysregulation. *Journal of Attention Disorders, 21*(13), 1105–1120.

Mitchell, J. T., Zylowska, L., & Kollins, S. H. (2015). Mindfulness meditation training for attention-deficit/hyperactivity disorder in adulthood: Current empirical support, treatment overview, and future directions. *Cognitive and Behavioral Practice, 22*(2), 172–191.

Modesto-Lowe, V., Farahmand, P., Chaplin, M., & Sarro, L. (2015). Does mindfulness meditation improve attention in attention deficit hyperactivity disorder? *World Journal of Psychiatry, 5*, 397–403.

Mukerji Househam, A., & Solanto, M. V. (2016). Mindfulness as an intervention for ADHD. *ADHD Report, 24*(2), 1–13.

Murrell, A. R., Steinberg, D. S., Connally, M. L., Hulsey, T., & Hogan, E. (2015). Acting out to ACTing on: A preliminary investigation in youth with ADHD and comorbid disorders. *Journal of Child and Family Studies, 24*(7), 2174–2181.

Nolan, E. E., & Gadow, K. D. (1997). Children with ADHD and tic disorder and their classmates: Behavioral normalization with methylphenidate. *Journal of the American Academy of Child and Adolescent Psychiatry, 36*(5), 597–604.

Pallozzi, R., Wertheim, E., Paxton, S., & Ong, B. (2017). Trait mindfulness measures for use with adolescents: A systematic review. *Mindfulness, 8*(1), 110–125.

Pellow, J., Solomon, E. M., & Barnard, C. N. (2011). Complementary and alternative medical therapies for children with attention-deficit/hyperactivity disorder (ADHD). *Alternative Medicine Review, 16*(4), 323–337.

Perry-Parrish, C., Copeland-Linder, N., Webb, L., Shields, A. H., & Sibinga, E. M. (2016). Improving self-regulation in adolescents: Current evidence for the role of mindfulness-based cognitive therapy. *Adolescent Health, Medicine and Therapeutics, 7,* 101–108.

Poletti, M. (2009). Adolescent brain development and executive functions: A prefrontal framework for developmental psychopathologies. *Clinical Neuropsychiatry: Journal of Treatment Evaluation, 6*(4), 155–165.

Quach, D., Mano, K. J., & Alexander, K. (2016). A randomized controlled trial examining the effect of mindfulness meditation on working memory capacity in adolescents. *Journal of Adolescent Health, 85*(5), 489–496.

Renshaw, T. L., & Cook, C. R. (2016). Introduction to the Special Issue: Mindfulness in the schools—Historical roots, current status, and future directions. *Psychology in the Schools, 54*(1), 5–12.

Searight, H. R., Robertson, K., Smith, T., Perkins, S., & Searight, B. K. (2012). Complementary and alternative therapies for pediatric attention deficit hyperactivity disorder: A descriptive review. *ISRN Psychiatry, 2012,* Article 804127.

Segal, Z. V., Williams, J. M. G., & Teasdale, J. D. (2002). *Mindfulness-based cognitive therapy for depression: A new approach to preventing relapse.* New York: Guilford Press.

Shaw, P., Stringaris, A., Nigg, J., & Leibenluft, E. (2014). Emotion dysregulation in attention deficit hyperactivity disorder. *American Journal of Psychiatry, 171*(3), 276–293.

Sibley, M. H., Graziano, P. A., Kuriyan, A. B., Coxe, S., Pelham, W. E., Rodriguez, L., . . . Ward, A. (2016). Parent–teen behavior therapy + motivational interviewing for adolescents with ADHD. *Journal of Consulting and Clinical Psychology, 84*(8), 699–712.

Sibley, M. H., Kuriyan, A. B., Evans, S. W., Waxmonsky, J. G., & Smith, B. H. (2014). Pharmacological and psychosocial treatments for adolescents with ADHD: An updated systematic review of the literature. *Clinical Psychology Review, 34*(3), 218–232.

Sibley, M. H., Pelham, W. E., Jr., Molina, B. S., Gnagy, E. M., Waschbusch, D. A., Garefino, A. C., . . . Karch, K. M. (2012). Diagnosing ADHD in adolescence. *Journal of Consulting and Clinical Psychology, 80*(1), 139–150.

Singh, N. N., Lancioni, G. E., Karazsia, B. T., Felver, J. C., Myers, R. E., & Nugent, K. (2016). Effects of Samatha meditation on active academic engagement and math performance of students with attention deficit/hyperactivity disorder. *Mindfulness, 7*(1), 68–75.

Tan, L. B. (2016). A critical review of adolescent mindfulness-based programmes. *Clinical Child Psychology and Psychiatry, 21*(2), 193–207.

Tan, L. B., & Martin, G. (2016). Mind full or mindful: A report on mindfulness and psychological health in healthy adolescents. *International Journal of Adolescence and Youth, 21*(1), 64–74.

Tang, Y. Y., Holzel, B. K., & Posner, M. I. (2015). The neuroscience of mindfulness meditation. *Nature Reviews Neuroscience, 16*(4), 213–225.

Tang, Y. Y., & Posner, M. I. (2013). Special issue on mindfulness neuroscience. *Social Cognitive and Affective Neuroscience, 8*(1), 1–3.

Teper, R., Segal, Z. V., & Inzlicht, M. (2013). Inside the mindful mind: How mindfulness enhances emotion regulation through improvements in executive control. *Current Directions in Psychological Science, 22*(6), 449–454.

Van Dam, N. T., van Vugt, M. K., Vago, D. R., Schmalzl, L., Saron, C. D., Olendzki, A., . . . Meyer, D. E. (2018). Mind the hype: A critical evaluation and prescriptive agenda for research on mindfulness and meditation. *Perspectives on Psychological Science, 13*(1), 36–61.

van de Weijer-Bergsma, E., Formsma, A. R., de Bruin, E. I., & Bögels, S. M. (2012). The effectiveness of mindfulness training on behavioral problems and attentional functioning in adolescents with ADHD. *Journal of Child and Family Studies, 21*(5), 775–787.

van der Oord, S., Bögels, S. M., & Peijnenburg, D. (2012). The effectiveness of mindfulness training for children with ADHD and mindful parenting for their parents. *Journal of Child and Family Studies, 21*(1), 139–147.

van Stralen, J. (2016). Emotional dysregulation in children with attention-deficit/hyperactivity disorder. *Attention Deficit and Hyperactivity Disorders, 8*(4), 175–187.

VanderDrift, L. E., Antshel, K. M., & Olszewski, A. K. (2017, May 1). Inattention and hyperactivity–impulsivity: Their detrimental effect on romantic relationship maintenance. *Journal of Attention Disorders.* [Epub ahead of print]

Zenner, C., Herrnleben-Kurz, S., & Walach, H. (2014). Mindfulnesss-based interventions in schools—A systematic review and meta-analysis. *Frontiers in Psychology, 5,* 603.

Zhang, D., Chan, S. K. C., Lo, H. H. M., Chan, C. Y. H., Chan, J. C. Y., Ting, K. T., . . . Wong, S. Y. S. (2017). Mindfulness-based intervention for Chinese children with ADHD and their parents: A pilot mixed-method study. *Mindfulness, 8*(4), 859–872.

Zoogman, S., Goldberg, S. B., Hoyt, W. T., & Miller, L. (2015). Mindfulness interventions with youth: A meta-analysis. *Mindfulness, 6*(2), 290–302.

Zylowska, L., Ackerman, D. L., Yang, M. H., Futrell, J. L., Horton, N. L., Hale, T. S., . . . Smalley, S. L. (2008). Mindfulness meditation training in adults and adolescents with ADHD: A feasibility study. *Journal of Attention Disorders, 11*(6), 737–746.

CHAPTER 18

Medication for Adolescents with ADHD

From Efficacy and Effectiveness to Autonomy and Adherence

William B. Brinkman
Tanya E. Froehlich
Jeffery N. Epstein

The American Academy of Pediatrics Clinical Practice Guideline for attention-deficit/hyperactivity disorder (ADHD) states that for adolescents, the clinician "should prescribe FDA-approved medications for ADHD with the assent of the adolescent and may prescribe behavior therapy as treatment for ADHD, preferably both" (Wolraich et al., 2011). Given the centrality of medication as an ADHD treatment modality, we review in this chapter the evidence underlying ADHD medication prescription in the adolescent age group, including effects on core ADHD symptoms and impairments, as well as side effects and possible adverse consequences, such as misuse and diversion. In addition, ADHD medication adherence in adolescence and its relationship to the developmental tasks of this age group are discussed. Furthermore, we provide recommendations to the clinician when prescribing ADHD medications to adolescents, including strategies to improve medication adherence and reduce possible negative sequelae.

Medication Efficacy and Effectiveness

It is noteworthy that several randomized controlled trials have been conducted with adolescents to specifically examine whether the effects of ADHD medication documented at younger ages (MTA Cooperative Group, 1999) are similar in this population. Clinically significant reductions in ADHD symptoms have been demonstrated for extended release methylphenidate in osmotic (Wilens, McBurnett, et al., 2006) and transdermal release formulations (Findling et al., 2010), extended release amphetamine formulations containing mixed amphetamine salts (Spencer et al., 2006) and lisdexamfetamine (Findling et al., 2011), and atomoxetine (Wilens, Kratochvil, Newcorn, & Gao, 2006). Across all of these studies, the beneficial effects of medication on ADHD symptoms in adolescents with ADHD are consistent in magnitude with studies of children at other ages (Chan, Fogler, & Hammerness, 2016). Compared to stimulants and atomoxetine, smaller reductions in ADHD symptoms have been noted in adolescents with ADHD who are treated with extended release guanfacine (Wilens et al., 2015).

In addition to ADHD symptom reduction, there is evidence that medication reduces functional impairments among adolescents. Some of these medication studies were conducted in the context of ADHD summer treatment programs in which investigators had the opportunity to directly observe the behavior of adolescents in authentic settings (e.g., classroom, team sporting events) while teens participated in a double-blind placebo-controlled trial of ADHD medication. For example, counselor-observed social behavior of adolescents with ADHD improved when taking medication compared to placebo (Smith, Pelham, Evans, et al., 1998). Moderate to large medication effect sizes were also noted for adolescent academic performance, such as note taking quality, quiz and worksheet scores, written language usage and productivity, on-task behavior, and percentage of work completed (Evans et al., 2001; Smith, Pelham, Gnagy, & Yudell, 1998). A large retrospective cohort study of individuals in Sweden who had taken multiple entrance tests and used ADHD medications intermittently showed that test scores were higher during medicated periods versus nonmedicated periods, after researchers adjusted for age and practice effects (Lu et al., 2017). In a naturalistic follow-up of the Multimodal Treatment of ADHD (MTA) study, continued medication use predicted better math achievement but no other academic outcomes (e.g., grade point average, reading achievement) when participants were ages 13–18 years (Molina et al., 2009).

Driving is another behavior of importance during adolescence and diagnosis with ADHD is associated with high risk driving behaviors (Jillani & Kaminer, 2016; see Garner, Chapter 12, this volume). There is evidence to suggest that ADHD medication may improve driving outcomes among adolescents with ADHD. A driver simulation study demonstrated that taking methylphenidate, compared to placebo, resulted in less time driving off the road, fewer instances of speeding, less erratic speed control, more time executing left turns, and less inappropriate use of brakes (Cox et al., 2006). Other reports suggest that on a population-level twenty to fifty percent of driving accidents in adolescent and adult males with ADHD could have been avoidable if they had been receiving medication (Chang, Lichtenstein, D'Onofrio, Sjolander, & Larsson, 2014; Chang et al., 2017).

While the MTA study failed to find a relationship between adolescent medication use and delinquency outcomes (Molina et al., 2009), some studies have suggested that medication use in individuals with ADHD may reduce the risk of criminality. Large, retrospective, population-based cohort studies in Sweden have documented lower rates of criminality in patients with ADHD during medication periods compared to nonmedication periods (Lichtenstein et al., 2012), as well as an association between psychostimulant receipt and lower likelihood of violent reoffending in individuals released from prison (Chang, Lichtenstein, Langstrom, Larsson, & Fazel, 2016). Of note, more than half of the individuals in these cohorts were adults at baseline, so the magnitude of benefit among adolescents specifically is unclear.

Many studies have examined whether a protective or predisposing association exists between ADHD medication use and development of substance use and related problems (see Kennedy, McKone, & Molina, Chapter 11, this volume). This remains a highly controversial topic, because the body of evidence is inconclusive. In 2013, Humphreys, Eng, and Lee published a meta-analysis of 15 studies. Across all substance types, results suggested comparable outcomes between children with and without medication treatment history for any substance use and abuse or dependence outcome. These studies include a wide range of ages, with subjects often enrolled during childhood or adolescence and followed into adulthood. Since this meta-analysis was conducted, there have been additional noteworthy publications. In naturalistic follow-up of the MTA study, ADHD medication use (i.e., randomized treatment assignment in childhood, medication use at follow-up, or cumulative stimulant use over 8 years of follow-up from childhood) was not related to substance use or substance use disorders by adolescence (Molina et al., 2013). However, large retrospective population-based cohort studies in Sweden (in which 45% of participants were ages 8–15 years at the start of study follow-up) have documented that patients with ADHD had lower rates of substance-related problems requiring care at an emergency department during periods when they were receiving medication compared to periods when not receiving medication (Chang, Lichtenstein, Halldner, et al., 2014). A study in the United States (in which 31% of participants were ages 13–17 years at the study's start) demonstrated similar findings (Quinn et al., 2017). Methodological differences across these studies examining the relationship between ADHD medication and developing substance use and related problems makes it challenging to synthesize the findings. Protective effects are hypothesized to act through a reduction in ADHD symptoms (e.g., impulsive decision making), oppositional defiant disorder (ODD) and conduct disorder (CD) symptoms, and/or a decreased need for self-medication (Khantzian, 1997; Wilens, Faraone, Biederman, & Gunawardene, 2003). Predisposing effects are hypothesized to act through child reliance on drug use as a coping strategy (Henker, Whalen, Blunt-Bugental, & Barker, 1981). Additional research elucidating the factors that make children with ADHD vulnerable to substance use and related problems may shed additional light on how ADHD medication use may influence these outcomes.

There is a similar controversy over the association between ADHD medication treatment and subsequent development of comorbid mental health conditions (see Becker & Fogleman, Chapter 9, this volume). Two studies reported a reduction in the long-term risk of depression (Biederman, Monuteaux, Spencer, Wilens, & Faraone, 2009; Daviss, Birmaher, Diler, & Mintz, 2008), while two other studies found no relationship (Jensen et al., 2007; Staikova, Marks, Miller, Newcorn, & Halperin, 2010). Large, retrospective population-based cohort studies in Sweden have documented reduced risks of depression (Chang, D'Onofrio, Quinn, Lichtenstein, & Larsson, 2016) and suicidal behavior (Chen et al., 2014) in individuals receiving ADHD medications. Despite these suggested benefits, clinicians should be alert to the possibility that their adolescents with ADHD may have unrecognized comorbid bipolar disorder, which can be unmasked by psychostimulant treatment. In a recent study, patients on methylphenidate monotherapy displayed an increased rate of manic episodes within 3 months of medication initiation (Viktorin et al., 2017).

MEDICATION SIDE EFFECTS

Treatment-emergent adverse effects reported in studies of ADHD medication in adolescents have mirrored those reported in other age groups. Methylphenidate- or amphetamine-containing stimulant medications compared to placebo increased the risk of reduced appetite, headache, irritability, abdominal pain, nausea, insomnia, and weight loss (Findling et al., 2010, 2011; Spencer et al., 2006; Wilens, McBurnett, et al., 2006). In addition to these risks, transdermal-release methylphenidate also had the risk of localized skin irritation (Findling et al., 2010). Nonstimulant medications containing atomoxetine or guanfacine compared to placebo increased the risk of nausea, decreased appetite, dizziness, abdominal pain, fatigue, headache, vomiting, and somnolence (Wilens, Kratochvil, et al., 2006; Wilens et al., 2015). Cardiovascular effects varied across ADHD medications. Stimulants were associated with a small mean increase in systolic and diastolic blood pressure and heart rate, whereas atomoxetine was not associated with vital sign changes, and guanfacine was associated with minor reductions in blood pressure and heart rate (Chan et al., 2016). The U.S. Food and Drug Administration (FDA; 2013) has issued warnings that methylphenidate products may rarely cause prolonged and sometimes painful erections known as priapism. In addition, stimulant medications can cause erectile dysfunction. Extended use of stimulant medication has also been associated with suppression of adult height (Swanson et al., 2017).

Medication Usage Patterns in Adolescents

Medication effectiveness in real-world settings is negatively impacted by poor adherence. Medication use declines dramatically after age 11 (Visser et al., 2014) even though most adolescents continue to demonstrate symptoms and functional impairment (Howard et al., 2016). Teens who continue to take medicine often take their medications inconsistently (i.e., only 50% of days covered with medicine) (Molina et al., 2009). Qualitative research suggests that some adolescents with ADHD start to use medication selectively based on their perceptions of whether it will be beneficial for specific tasks (Brinkman et al., 2012; Meaux, Hester, Smith, & Shoptaw, 2006). Unfortunately, at the same time that medication continuity declines, the outcomes of ADHD become increasingly consequential. For example, adolescents with ADHD, compared to their peers without ADHD, are more likely to drop out of school, use tobacco and illicit drugs, interact with the juvenile justice system, be treated for sexually transmitted infections, have motor vehicle accidents, and experience teenage pregnancies (Barkley, Fischer, Smallish, & Fletcher, 2006; Bussing, Mason, Bell, Porter, & Garvan, 2010; Curry et al., 2017; Molina et al., 2009). Given that medication has beneficial effects on adolescent performance across a variety of domains (e.g., social skills, academic tasks, driving performance, mental health; Chan et al., 2016; Cox et al., 2006; Evans et al., 2001; Smith, Pelham, Evans, et al., 1998), poor medication continuity may represent a significant public health problem.

Developmental Influences on Medication Adherence

Developmental changes during adolescence likely contribute to this decline in ADHD medication continuity. Normal adolescent development involves the maturation of cognitive capacities and behavioral–emotional self-regulation and the need to develop independence in the face of increasingly complex demands. These processes compound the challenges experienced by individuals with ADHD due to their deficits in executive functioning, as well as heightened impulsivity. In order to understand the relationship between the developmental maturation process in adolescence and ADHD medication adherence, it is useful to examine the unified theory of behavior change (UTBC; Fishbein, Triandis, Kanfer, Becker, & Middlestadt, 2001), which is a conceptual model that can help explain the mechanism underlying medication adherence and guide the development of interventions to improve the continuity of treatment (Chacko, Newcorn, Feirsen, & Uderman, 2010).

The UTBC identifies two broad processes in behavioral change (see Figure 18.1): preintention factors and implementation factors. The preintention factors domain focuses on five determinants of an individual's willingness, intention, or decision to perform a critical behavior (see left portion of Figure 18.1).

1. *Expectations* refer to an individual's perceived advantages and disadvantages of performing the behavior. For example, in the case of taking a medication, an adolescent might believe with varying degrees of certainty that a medication will help him or her pay attention at school, but he or she may also believe that these benefits may be outweighed by other negative

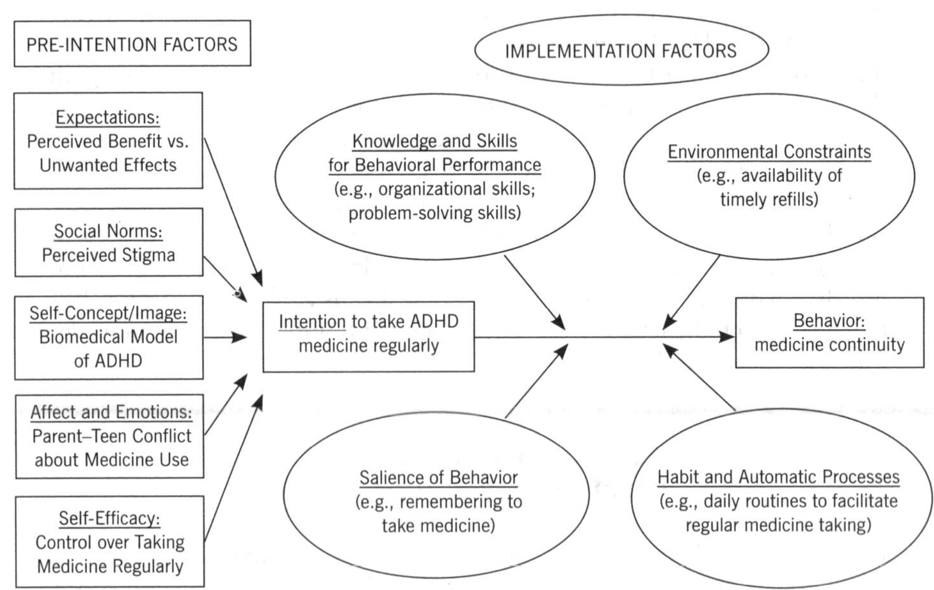

FIGURE 18.1. UTBC model adapted for medication continuity among adolescents with ADHD.

consequences (e.g., side effects). Unfortunately, typical adolescents' perceptions of their invincibility, combined with the positive illusory bias seen in some individuals with ADHD, may lead teens with ADHD to overestimate their capabilities and underestimate their need for continued medication treatment (Owens, Goldfine, Evangelista, Hoza, & Kaiser, 2007). On the other hand, heightened body awareness during adolescence may magnify teens' perceptions of side effects (Brinkman et al., 2012; Meaux et al., 2006).

2. *Social norms* include two components: (a) the adolescent's perceptions about what his or her parents think he or she should do with respect to the behavior (i.e., taking medicine), and (b) the adolescent's perceptions about whether his or her peers would also approve of and/or perform the behavior. Given the primacy placed on fitting in with one's peer group during adolescence, it is not surprising that many adolescents eschew taking ADHD medications due to perceived stigma (Pescosolido, Perry, Martin, McLeod, & Jensen, 2007).

3. *Self-concept and image* considerations refer to an individual's concept of him- or herself and whether performing the behavior is consistent with or contradicts his or her self-image, rendering the behavior more or less attractive. An individual who strongly feels that ADHD is a biomedical condition that requires biomedical treatment and that he or she is the type of person who always takes action to improve his or her health will be more likely to take medicine for ADHD than one who does not (Leslie, Plemmons, Monn, & Palinkas, 2007). However, as we noted earlier, an adolescent influenced by positive illusory bias may not recognize and therefore accept that he or she has ADHD and therefore requires treatment.

4. *Affect and emotions* refers to an individual's affective and emotional reactions to behavioral performance. Given the drive for autonomy and individuation from one's parents during adolescence, teens with ADHD may have a strongly negative emotional reaction to taking medicine, because they equate it to a battle with their parents for control (Miller & Jawad, 2014). Indeed, adolescents with ADHD may be more likely to resist help from others when support is still needed (Chan et al., 2016). In addition, adolescent–parent conflict often flows from differences of opinion about the benefit of medicine, with parents worrying that adolescents are shortsighted in their goals and overestimate their competence compared to objective criteria (Brinkman et al., 2009; Owens et al., 2007). Conversely, adolescent involvement in decision making (e.g., an adolescent expressing an opinion, a parent listening to adolescent, adolescent and parent negotiating) has been related to higher levels of treatment regimen adherence in chronic conditions such as diabetes (Miller & Jawad, 2014).

5. *Self-efficacy* refers to one's beliefs that one can perform the behavior, and how easy/difficult it is to perform the behavior. Thus, an adolescent who believes that he or she can easily take medicine regularly within their daily routines will be more willing to do so (i.e., higher self-efficacy beliefs result in stronger behavioral intentions).

Each of these five factors predicts variation in behavioral intentions or the decisions whether to perform specific behaviors such as taking one's medications.

The second set of UTBC processes—implementation factors—affects whether strong behavioral intentions are actually carried out (see right side of Figure 18.1).

1. This variable pertains to the requisite *knowledge and skills for behavioral performance*: An individual who may intend to take ADHD medicine regularly may subsequently find that he or she does not have the skills needed to take medicine every day. For example, some adolescents struggle to swallow pills. Adolescents with ADHD may also lack the organizational and/or problem-solving skills needed to take medicine reliably due to delays in their executive functioning skills that often go unrecognized by parents who expect age-appropriate self-care skills.

2. This variable is the *environmental constraints* that may render behavioral performance difficult or impossible. For example, adolescents taking ADHD medicine are often dependent on their parent(s) to obtain medicine refills. This is often relevant, because parents of adolescents with ADHD are more likely to have ADHD and/or depression (Chronis et al., 2003) which may interfere with their ability to support medication continuity by obtaining timely refills.

3. It is important that the person does not forget to enact the third variable, *salience of the behavior*. Even when salience is present, forgetting can be a challenge for adolescents with ADHD, who often experience working memory challenges. Forgetting to take medicine appears to cause more problems in adolescence than in childhood (Brinkman, Simon, & Epstein, 2018) likely due to parents playing a less of a role providing reminders and directly observing medication taking during adolescence.

4. Finally, the variable *habit and automatic processes* may influence behavior. For example, by force of habit, a person who has developed a routine to help him or her remember to obtain and take their medicine regularly will be more likely to sustain this behavior when competing intentions are activated and distractions are present. Unfortunately, following routines is a prevalent challenge for individuals with ADHD.

Evidence for Preintention Factors Influencing ADHD Medication Continuity

One study analyzed data from the MTA study to determine the prevalence of factors that impact adolescents' intentions to take medicine regularly (Brinkman et al., 2018). Twelve years after enrolling in the MTA, participants completed a survey reporting their age when they last stopped taking medicine for a month or more and their reasons for stopping. Seventy-seven percent of participants with a history of taking ADHD medicine (286/372) reported last stopping medicine for a month or longer during childhood (ages 5–12; $n = 115$) or adolescence (ages 13–18; $n = 171$). The average age when participants last stopped taking medication was 13.3 years (standard deviation of 3.0 years). The most commonly endorsed reasons for stopping medicine related to questioning whether medicine was still needed (69%) or whether it helped (56–82%). Reasons related to concerns about side effects were endorsed by 35–50% of adolescents. Some teens describe feeling "zoned out," less social, less creative, and/or more irritable, or they may experience other somatic side effects (e.g., headache) (Brinkman et al., 2012; Knipp, 2006; Meaux et al., 2006; Singh et al., 2010). Logistical barriers to getting or taking medicine (e.g., cost, getting prescriptions) were less common (all < 7%). Participants also endorsed social concerns (20%) or stigma (13%) as reasons for stopping medicine. The most commonly endorsed reasons that adolescents restarted medicine related to recognition that medicine was helping at school or work (86%), with 45% of adolescents coming to realize that they still needed medicine after they had stopped taking it (Brinkman et al., 2017). The validity of these reasons for stopping and/or re-starting medicine are supported by past qualitative research (Brinkman et al., 2009; Brinkman et al., 2012; Charach, Yeung, Volpe, Goodale, & Dosreis, 2014; Hansen & Hansen, 2006; Knipp, 2006; Leslie et al., 2007; Meaux et al., 2006), but the MTA analysis is the first to provide an estimate of the prevalence of these issues (Brinkman et al., 2018). For both stopping and restarting medication, the proportion endorsing some reasons differed by age range, with the overall pattern suggesting that parental involvement in stopping and restarting medications decreased with age. Regarding age-related differences in reasons for stopping, five items suggest that parental support for medication decreased (i.e., "My parents wanted to find out if I could manage without it," "My parents decided to stop it") and autonomy increased (i.e., "I wanted to find out if I could manage without it," "I kept forgetting to take it," "I was tired of taking it") as participant age increased. Based on parent and/or participant responses on the Columbia Impairment Rating Scale and the Impairment Rating Scale, 98% of participants continued to have functional impairment after stopping the medicine. Problems with schoolwork were the most commonly reported impairment. In summary, adolescent–parent expectations about medicine appear to play a critical role in shaping intention to take ADHD medicine regularly.

Evidence for Implementation Factors Influencing ADHD Medication Continuity

Qualitative research studies involving focus groups with adolescents with ADHD (n = 44) (Brinkman et al., 2012) and parents (n = 52) (Brinkman et al., 2009) have shed light on the implementation factors that influence ADHD medication continuity. One study finding was that some adolescents struggle with swallowing pills. Parental involvement in medication taking ranged from providing direct supervision to providing reminders, to providing no supervision. Adolescent responsibility for taking medication increased with age. However, many adolescents acknowledged that forgetting to take their medication was still an issue. Indeed, the organizational difficulties experienced by many adolescents with ADHD and their parents, who are at higher risk for ADHD themselves (Chronis et al., 2003), are a significant barrier to reliably obtaining refills before medicine runs out and taking medicine regularly. Moreover, parents often benefit from training on how to set goals, and use behavioral contracts and rewards/consequences to encourage desired behaviors from their children with ADHD (Chronis, Jones, & Raggi, 2006), though these approaches have not been applied to ADHD medication continuity. Furthermore, many teens with ADHD are given the day-to-day responsibility for taking medication and are increasingly without the safety net of parental supervision (Brinkman et al., 2012, 2018) despite their well-documented challenges with organization and planning.

Strategies to Improve Medication Continuity

The heterogeneous nature of teens' reasons for stopping medicine makes efforts to support medication continuity challenging. Different reasons are relevant at different times for different teens, and tailored interventions are needed to meet the needs of each individual. Nonetheless, some generally recommended practices can be espoused, such as employing collaborative decision making between parents and children (White, 1996; Wills, Blechman, & McNamara, 1996). Teen involvement in medical decisions may positively impact self-efficacy, satisfaction with medical care, adherence, and, ultimately, the transition to adult health care (McCabe, 1996; Miller & Jawad, 2014; Schmidt, Petersen, & Bullinger, 2003; Walker & Doyon, 2001; White, 1996; Wills et al., 1996). Of note, all major ADHD clinical practice guidelines recommend physician-supervised trials of stopping adolescents' medicine to assess continued need for and benefit from medicine (American Academy of Pediatrics, 2011; Pliszka, 2007). While underutilized in clinical practice, this strategy is ideal when an adolescent or parent questions whether medicine helps or is still needed, as it targets the UTBC preintention factors of adolescent and parent expectations and affect/emotions. Guidelines provide practical advice on the conduct of such trials that differentiate these from the common clinical practice of stopping medication during summer or holiday breaks from school: (1) Consider this when the patient is stable and doing well; (2) conduct this when the patient is not undergoing a transition (e.g., when the adolescent has fully acclimatized to class schedule and responsibilities); (3) avoid at the beginning of any school year, especially the start of junior or senior high school; (4) discontinue medication for 2–4 weeks; and (5) identify and monitor target outcomes closely.

Indeed, approaches to enable teens with ADHD to more objectively assess benefit/need is appealing for many reasons. First, objective measures of outcome may help address the unrealistically high self-views of performance (i.e., positive illusory bias) that have been observed in a sizable subset of teens with ADHD (Owens et al., 2007). Second, measuring proximal outcomes that matter to teens and parents might detect an early signal of the continued need for and benefit from medicine, potentially averting sentinel events (e.g., class failure, auto accident). Third, structured trials on or off medicine could provide a concrete way for teens and parents to work together, which might defuse parent–teen conflict about medicine taking. Research is needed to determine how best to engage teens and parents in this activity, which requires collaboration on the selection of goals and target outcomes from multiple perspectives (e.g., teen, parent, and physician) and the capacity to systematically measure and track outcomes over time. The trial on or off medicine is designed to reduce ambivalence about medicine (i.e., document improvement with medication among teens that still benefit from it), which may motivate self-directed changes to support medication continuity. Research on structured trials on or off medicine needs to examine whether this strategy increases collaborative decision making about continuing medicine and averts sentinel events (e.g., grade failure, delinquency, driving accidents).

Enabling teens (and possibly parents) to interact with their peers is a potentially important source of support. Existing mentoring programs for youth with ADHD, such as Eye to Eye (*http://eyetoeyenational.org*), which pairs preadolescents with college students with ADHD, may be an effective way of providing social support and anticipatory guidance for ADHD management. In addition, Internet-based media have potential as a powerful way to combat stigma and promote positive social norms. There are hundreds of videos available on YouTube related to ADHD (Kang, Ha,

& Velasco, 2017). Some videos share information about successful people with ADHD. Other videos feature celebrities talking about how medication helps them manage ADHD. Still other videos, such as *TED Talks,* feature adolescents and adults discussing how they have made sense of ADHD and have been successful managing ADHD symptoms. Efforts are needed to identify the videos that adolescents find most engaging and help normalize ADHD and medication taking, both for teens with ADHD themselves and their peers.

Other practical strategies are available to overcome common challenges posed by medication adherence implementation factors. Simplifying the medication regimen by prescribing once-a-day extended release medication has been associated with increased medication continuity (Marcus, Wan, Kemner, & Olfson, 2005). However, forgetting to take medicine remains a common challenge (Brinkman et al., 2018). Daily alarm reminders, text message reminders, and other interventions to embed pill taking in a teen's daily routine, with a level of parent supervision commensurate to the teen's developmental and organizational capacities, hold promise to improve medication continuity. We provide two case examples illustrating how clinicians can help support medication continuity for adolescents with ADHD in Table 18.1.

Diversion and Misuse of ADHD Medications

Strategies to improve ADHD medication adherence in teens are also critically needed due to the growing problem of psychostimulant diversion and misuse. Specifically, adolescents who are in conflict with their parents and no longer desire to take ADHD medications often rebel by conducting covert trials off medicine (Brinkman et al., 2012). In these cases, parents continue to refill ADHD medication that is not being taken by their adolescents, and is therefore available for diversion or misuse. As many as 20% of young teens with ADHD report that they diverted (e.g., gave away, traded, or sold) their ADHD medication to someone for whom it was not prescribed (McCabe, West, Teter, et al., 2011). In addition, 20% of teens with ADHD reported that they misused their ADHD medicine (e.g., took too much, intentionally got high, or used it to increase alcohol or other drug effects) (McCabe, West, Cranford, et al., 2011). The impact of stimulant misuse is significant. Calls to Poison Control Centers related to teens' stimulant misuse increased by 76% from 1998 to 2005 (Setlik, Bond, & Ho, 2009) and emergency department (ED) visits related to stimulant misuse tripled between 2005 and 2010 (Substance Abuse and Mental Health Services Administration, 2013). The combined prevalence of diversion or misuse likely approaches 30% in young teens prescribed ADHD medicines

TABLE 18.1. Two Hypothetical Examples to Illustrate How Clinicians Can Help Support Medication Continuity

Case Study 1: Pediatrician addresses preintention factors.

- John is 12 years old. He expresses uncertainty about whether medicine is still needed or helpful, but his mother is convinced medicine still helps and is worried that his school performance will suffer if he stops taking medicine.
- Their pediatrician, Dr. Smith, recommends conducting a supervised trial on or off medicine to help resolve this uncertainty.
- John, his mother, and Dr. Smith discuss outcome measures that each would like to track during the trial on or off medicine. John wants to track the number of positive interactions he has with his friends at school. His mother wants to track the accuracy in homework assignments. Dr. Smith wants to track symptoms of inattention reported by John, his mother, and his math teacher.
- Dr. Smith reviews the ground rules for trial on or off medicine. The trial will start after the first set of tests have been completed. For the first 2 weeks, outcomes will be assessed while John is taking his medicine. His mother will directly observe his medicine taking these 2 weeks to make sure that he doesn't forget. The next 2 weeks, he won't take his medicine. John and his mother will return with the outcome measures they collect during all 4 weeks. John and his mother sign a behavioral contract agreeing to these rules.
- After the trial is complete, the data suggest that inattention increased and homework accuracy decreased after stopping medicine. However, John reported more positive social interactions when off medicine, and he and his mother noticed he had fewer problems with feeling irritable.
- Based on these data, Dr. Smith suggested that John resume medication but at a slightly lower dosage to see whether he receives adequate benefit while minimizing the adverse effects of medication on social interactions that John reported.

Case Study 2: Psychologist addresses implementation factors.

- Mary is 15. She indicates that she forgets to take medicine a couple of times per week when she is rushing to get to the bus stop in the morning. Her father admits that she often runs out of medicine before he remembers to request a refill.
- Their psychologist, Dr. Jones, suggests they try using an app to help keep them organized.
- Mary selects an app that provides alerts to remind her to take her long-acting medicine at 6:30 A.M. and her short-acting medicine at 4:30 P.M. The app also allows her to track whether she successfully took her medications.
- Her father selects an app that will send him monthly reminders to request a refill from the doctor's office. He can also track his progress using the app.
- When they return to Dr. Jones 2 months later, it is clear that the apps have been helpful. Mary's father was able to get refills before she ran out of medicine, and Mary didn't miss her morning dose on any school days. However, she's been less consistent taking her medicine at 4:30 P.M., because she goes straight from school to her piano lesson on Wednesdays.
- Dr. Jones helps Mary and her father develop a contingency plan to ensure that he brings the medicine with him when he picks her up at school on Wednesday afternoons.

(McCabe, West, Teter, et al., 2011; McCabe, West, Cranford, et al., 2011) and dramatically increases to over 50% among college students (Sepulveda et al., 2011).

STRATEGIES TO DECREASE DIVERSION AND MISUSE

To date, no interventions have been described or shown to curb diversion or misuse of ADHD medications. However, practical recommendations have been proposed. Because stimulant medications can be misused to get high or accentuate the effects of alcohol or other drugs, the American Academy of Pediatrics ADHD Clinical Practice Guideline suggests that clinicians consider prescribing nonstimulant medications (e.g., atomoxetine) that have no abuse potential, or stimulant medications with less abuse potential, such as lisdexamfetamine, transdermal methylphenidate, or osmotic-release methylphenidate (Wolraich et al., 2011). Indeed, it is much harder to extract the stimulants from these preparations in order to get high, which may decrease the likelihood that they are misused in this way by adolescents with ADHD or diverted for this purpose. However, it should be noted that this approach to prescribing may alienate adolescents who use medication selectively depending on perceived need to complete daily tasks (e.g., tests, team sports) (Brinkman et al., 2012). Such adolescents may prefer the flexibility offered by immediate release stimulant preparations that are relatively short acting (i.e., 4- to 6-hour duration). Whether selective use of stimulant medication constitutes effective self-management or misuse of a prescription medication is debatable, but awareness of selective use is important for physicians and parents, so that medication can be a continued topic of discussion given the chronic nature of ADHD.

Pleasure seeking is not the only driver of stimulant medication diversion. In fact, most individuals who take these medicines without a prescription are motivated by improved academic performance and would still value extended release stimulants (Rabiner et al., 2009; Teter, McCabe, LaGrange, Cranford, & Boyd, 2006). Adolescents with ADHD who divert their medication may do so for a variety of reasons. Some may be interested in profiting from the sale of their medicine. Others may simply be trying to help a friend or family member who appears to need or desires the medicine. It is also possible that adolescents with ADHD feel pressured to divert their prescription stimulants. The relationship between diversion and peer victimization warrants further investigation (Epstein-Ngo et al., 2016). Similar to the challenge of improving medication continuity, decreasing diversion and misuse of stimulant medication will likely require interventions tailored to fit the individual's needs and circumstances.

Conclusion

The vast majority of children with ADHD continue to experience symptoms and impairment through adolescence. Although adolescents obtain similar benefits from ADHD medications as younger children, adherence to medication among adolescents is poor. Decisions about continued medication use should be guided by physician-supervised structured trials on or off medication in which adolescents, parents, and physicians collaborate to identify salient outcomes to monitor. Research is needed to determine how best to engage in this activity and other strategies to support medication treatment among those who still benefit. Research is also needed to decrease diversion and misuse of ADHD medications among adolescents. Ultimately, addressing the interrelated areas of medication continuity, diversion, and misuse is essential to improve outcomes for adolescents with ADHD.

References

American Academy of Pediatrics. (2011). Implementing the key action statements: An algorithm and explanation for process of care for the evaluation, diagnosis, treatment, and monitoring of ADHD in children and adolescents. Retrieved October 13, 2013, from *http://pediatrics.aappublications.org/content/suppl/2011/10/11/peds.2011-2654.DC1/zpe611117822p.pdf.*

Barkley, R. A., Fischer, M., Smallish, L., & Fletcher, K. (2006). Young adult outcome of hyperactive children: Adaptive functioning in major life activities. *Journal of the American Academy of Child and Adolescnt Psychiatry, 45*(2), 192–202.

Biederman, J., Monuteaux, M. C., Spencer, T., Wilens, T. E., & Faraone, S. V. (2009). Do stimulants protect against psychiatric disorders in youth with ADHD?: A 10-year follow-up study. *Pediatrics, 124*(1), 71–78.

Brinkman, W. B., Sherman, S. N., Zmitrovich, A. R., Visscher, M. O., Crosby, L. E., Phelan, K. J., & Donovan, D. F. (2009). Parental angst making and revisiting decisions about treatment of ADHD. *Pediatrics, 124,* 580–589.

Brinkman, W. B., Sherman, S. N., Zmitrovich, A. R., Visscher, M. O., Crosby, L. E., Phelan, K. J., & Donovan, E. F. (2012). In their own words: Adolescent views on ADHD and their evolving role managing medication. *Academic Pediatrics, 12*(1), 53–61.

Brinkman, W. B., Simon, J. O., & Epstein, J. N. (2018). Reasons why children and adolescents with attention-deficit/hyperactivity disorder stop and restart taking medicine. *Academic Pediatrics, 18*(3), 273–280.

Bussing, R., Mason, D. M., Bell, L., Porter, P., & Garvan, C. (2010). Adolescent outcomes of childhood attention-deficit/hyperactivity disorder in a diverse community sample. *Journal of the American Academy of Child and Adolescent Psychiatry, 49*(6), 595–605.

Chacko, A., Newcorn, N., Feirsen, N., & Uderman, J. Z. (2010). Improving medication adherence in chronic pediatric health conditions: A focus on ADHD in youth. *Current Pharmaceutical Design, 16*(22), 2416–2423.

Chan, E., Fogler, J. M., & Hammerness, P. G. (2016). Treatment of attention-deficit/hyperactivity disorder in adolescents: A systematic review. *Journal of the American Medical Association, 315*(18), 1997–2008.

Chang, Z., D'Onofrio, B. M., Quinn, P. D., Lichtenstein, P., & Larsson, H. (2016). Medication for attention-deficit/hyperactivity disorder and risk for depression: A nationwide longitudinal cohort study. *Biological Psychiatry, 80*(12), 916–922.

Chang, Z., Lichtenstein, P., D'Onofrio, B. M., Sjolander, A., & Larsson, H. (2014). Serious transport accidents in adults with attention-deficit/hyperactivity disorder and the effect of medication: A population-based study. *JAMA Psychiatry, 71*(3), 319–325.

Chang, Z., Lichtenstein, P., Halldner, L., D'Onofrio, B., Serlachius, E., Fazel, S., . . . Larsson, H. (2014). Stimulant ADHD medication and risk for substance abuse. *Journal of Child Psychology and Psychiatry, 55*(8), 878–885.

Chang, Z., Lichtenstein, P., Langstrom, N., Larsson, H., & Fazel, S. (2016). Association between prescription of major psychotropic medications and violent reoffending after prison release. *Journal of the American Medical Association, 316*(17), 1798–1807.

Chang, Z., Quinn, P. D., Hur, K., Gibbons, R. D., Sjolander, A., Larsson, H., & D'Onofrio, B. M. (2017). Association between medication use for attention-deficit/hyperactivity disorder and risk of motor vehicle crashes. *JAMA Psychiatry, 74*(6), 597–603.

Charach, A., Yeung, E., Volpe, T., Goodale, T., & Dosreis, S. (2014). Exploring stimulant treatment in ADHD: Narratives of young adolescents and their parents. *BMC Psychiatry, 14,* 110.

Chen, Q., Sjolander, A., Runeson, B., D'Onofrio, B. M., Lichtenstein, P., & Larsson, H. (2014). Drug treatment for attention-deficit/hyperactivity disorder and suicidal behaviour: Register based study. *British Medical Journal, 348,* g3769.

Chronis, A. M., Jones, H. A., & Raggi, V. L. (2006). Evidence-based psychosocial treatments for children and adolescents with attention-deficit/hyperactivity disorder. *Clinical Psychology Review, 26*(4), 486–502.

Chronis, A. M., Lahey, B. B., Pelham, W. E., Jr., Kipp, H. L., Baumann, B. L., & Lee, S. S. (2003). Psychopathology and substance abuse in parents of young children with attention-deficit/hyperactivity disorder. *Journal of the American Academy of Child and Adolescent Psychiatry, 42*(12), 1424–1432.

Cox, D. J., Merkel, R. L., Moore, M., Thorndike, F., Muller, C., & Kovatchev, B. (2006). Relative benefits of stimulant therapy with OROS methylphenidate versus mixed amphetamine salts extended release in improving the driving performance of adolescent drivers with attention-deficit/hyperactivity disorder. *Pediatrics, 118*(3), e704–e710.

Curry, A. E., Metzger, K. B., Pfeiffer, M. R., Elliott, M. R., Winston, F. K., & Power, T. J. (2017). Motor vehicle crash risk among adolescents and young adults with attention-deficit/hyperactivity disorder. *JAMA Pediatrics, 171*(8), 756–763.

Daviss, W. B., Birmaher, B., Diler, R. S., & Mintz, J. (2008). Does pharmacotherapy for attention-deficit/hyperactivity disorder predict risk of later major depression? *Journal of Child and Adolescent Psychopharmacology, 18*(3), 257–264.

Epstein-Ngo, Q. M., McCabe, S. E., Veliz, P. T., Stoddard, S. A., Austic, E. A., & Boyd, C. J. (2016). Diversion of ADHD stimulants and victimization among adolescents. *Journal of Pediatric Psychology, 41*(7), 786–798.

Evans, S. W., Pelham, W. E., Smith, B. H., Bukstein, O., Gnagy, E. M., Greiner, A. R., . . . Baron-Myak, C. (2001). Dose–response effects of methylphenidate on ecologically valid measures of academic performance and classroom behavior in adolescents with ADHD. *Experimental and Clinical Psychopharmacology, 9*(2), 163–175.

Findling, R. L., Childress, A. C., Cutler, A. J., Gasior, M., Hamdani, M., Ferreira-Cornwell, M. C., & Squires, L. (2011). Efficacy and safety of lisdexamfetamine dimesylate in adolescents with attention-deficit/hyperactivity disorder. *Journal of the American Academy of Child and Adolescent Psychiatry, 50*(4), 395–405.

Findling, R. L., Turnbow, J., Burnside, J., Melmed, R., Civil, R., & Li, Y. (2010). A randomized, double-blind, multicenter, parallel-group, placebo-controlled, dose-optimization study of the methylphenidate transdermal system for the treatment of ADHD in adolescents. *CNS Spectrums, 15*(7), 419–430.

Fishbein, M. H. C., Triandis, H. C., Kanfer, F. H., Becker, M., & Middlestadt, S. E. (2001). Factors influencing behavior and behavior change. In A. Baum, T. A. Revenson, & J. E. Singer (Eds.), *Handbook of health psychology* (pp. 1–17). Mahwah, NJ: Erlbaum.

Hansen, D. L., & Hansen, E. H. (2006). Caught in a balancing act: Parents' dilemmas regarding their ADHD child's treatment with stimulant medication. *Qualitative Health Research, 16*(9), 1267–1285.

Henker, B., Whalen, C. K., Blunt-Bugental, D., & Barker, C. (1981). Licit and illicit drug use patterns in stimulant-treated children and their peers. In K. D. Gadow & J. Loney (Eds.), *Psychosocial aspects of drug treatment for hyperactivity* (pp. 443–462). Boulder, CO: Westview.

Howard, A. L., Strickland, N. J., Murray, D. W., Tamm, L., Swanson, J. M., Hinshaw, S. P., . . . Molina, B. S. (2016). Progression of impairment in adolescents with attention-deficit/hyperactivity disorder through the transition out of high school: Contributions of parent involvement and college attendance. *Journal of Abnormal Psychology, 125*(2), 233–247.

Humphreys, K. L., Eng, T., & Lee, S. S. (2013). Stimulant medication and substance use outcomes: A meta-analysis. *JAMA Psychiatry, 70*(7), 740–749.

Jensen, P. S., Arnold, L. E., Swanson, J. M., Vitiello, B., Abikoff, H. B., Greenhill, L. L., . . . Hur, K. (2007). 3-year follow-up of the NIMH MTA study. *Journal of the American Academy of Child and Adolescent Psychiatry, 46*(8), 989–1002.

Jillani, S. A., & Kaminer, Y. (2016). High risk driving in treated and untreated youth with attention deficit hyperactivity disorder: Public health implications. *Adolescent Psychiatry, 6*(2), 89–99.

Kang, S., Ha, J. S., & Velasco, T. (2017). Attention deficit hyperactivity disorder on YouTube: Framing, anchoring, and objectification in social media. *Community Mental Health Journal, 53*(4), 445–451.

Khantzian, E. J. (1997). The self-medication hypothesis of substance use disorders: A reconsideration and recent applications. *Harvard Review of Psychiatry, 4*(5), 231–244.

Knipp, D. K. (2006). Teens' perceptions about attention deficit/hyperactivity disorder and medications. *Journal of School Nursing, 22*(2), 120–125.

Leslie, L. K., Plemmons, D., Monn, A. R., & Palinkas, L. A. (2007). Investigating ADHD treatment trajectories: Listening to families' stories about medication use. *Journal of Devopmental and Behavioral Pediatrics, 28*(3), 179–188.

Lichtenstein, P., Halldner, L., Zetterqvist, J., Sjolander, A., Serlachius, E., Fazel, S., . . . Larsson, H. (2012). Medication for attention deficit-hyperactivity disorder and criminality. *New England Journal of Medicine, 367*(21), 2006–2014.

Lu, Y., Sjolander, A., Cederlof, M., D'Onofrio, B. M., Almqvist, C., Larsson, H., & Lichtenstein, P. (2017). Association between medication use and performance on higher education entrance tests in individuals with attention-deficit/hyperactivity disorder. *JAMA Psychiatry, 74*(8), 815–822.

Marcus, S. C., Wan, G. J., Kemner, J. E., & Olfson, M. (2005). Continuity of methylphenidate treatment for attention-deficit/hyperactivity disorder. *Archives of Pediatric and Adolescent Medicine, 159*(6), 572–578.

McCabe, M. A. (1996). Involving children and adolescents in medical decision making:

Developmental and clinical considerations. *Journal of Pediatric Psychology, 21*(4), 505–516.

McCabe, S. E., West, B. T., Cranford, J. A., Ross-Durow, P., Young, A., Teter, C. J., & Boyd, C. J. (2011). Medical misuse of controlled medications among adolescents. *Archives of Pediatric and Adolescent Medicine, 165*(8), 729–735.

McCabe, S. E., West, B. T., Teter, C. J., Ross-Durow, P., Young, A., & Boyd, C. J. (2011). Characteristics associated with the diversion of controlled medications among adolescents. *Drug and Alcohol Dependence, 118*(2–3), 452–458.

Meaux, J. B., Hester, C., Smith, B., & Shoptaw, A. (2006). Stimulant medications: A trade-off?: The lived experience of adolescents with ADHD. *Journal for Specialists in Pediatric Nursing, 11*(4), 214–226.

Miller, V. A., & Jawad, A. F. (2014). Relationship of youth involvement in diabetes-related decisions to treatment adherence. *Journal of Clinical Psychology in Medical Settings, 21*(2), 183–189.

Molina, B. S. G., Hinshaw, S., Arnold, L. E., Swanson, J., Pelham, W., Hechtman, L., . . . MTA Cooperative Group. (2013). Adolescent substance use in the Multimodal Treatment Study of Attention-Deficit/Hyperactivity Disorder (ADHD) (MTA) as a function of childhood ADHD, random assignment to childhood treatments, and subsequent medication. *Journal of the American Academy of Child and Adolescent Psychiatry, 52*(3), 250–263.

Molina, B. S. G., Hinshaw, S. P., Swanson, J. M., Arnold, L. E., Vitiello, B., Jensen, P. S., . . . Houck, P. R. (2009). The MTA at 8 years: Prospective follow-up of children treated for combined-type ADHD in a multisite study. *Journal of the American Academy of Child and Adolescent Psychiatry, 48*(5), 484–500.

MTA Cooperative Group. (1999). A 14-month randomized clinical trial of treatment strategies for attention-deficit/hyperactivity disorder: Multimodal Treatment Study of Children with ADHD. *Archives of General Psychiatry, 56*(12), 1073–1086.

Owens, J. S., Goldfine, M. E., Evangelista, N. M., Hoza, B., & Kaiser, N. M. (2007). A critical review of self-perceptions and the positive illusory bias in children with ADHD. *Clinical Child and Family Psychology Review, 10*(4), 335–351.

Pescosolido, B. A., Perry, B. L., Martin, J. K., McLeod, J. D., & Jensen, P. S. (2007). Stigmatizing attitudes and beliefs about treatment and psychiatric medications for children with mental illness. *Psychiatric Services, 58*(5), 613–618.

Pliszka, S. (2007). Practice parameter for the assessment and treatment of children and adolescents with attention-deficit/hyperactivity disorder. *Journal of the American Academy of Child and Adolescent Psychiatry, 46*(7), 894–921.

Quinn, P. D., Chang, Z., Hur, K., Gibbons, R. D., Lahey, B. B., Rickert, M. E., . . . D'Onofrio, B. M. (2017). ADHD medication and substance-related problems. *American Journal of Psychiatry, 174*(9), 877–885.

Rabiner, D. L., Anastopoulos, A. D., Costello, E. J., Hoyle, R. H., McCabe, S. E., & Swartzwelder, H. S. (2009). Motives and perceived consequences of nonmedical ADHD medication use by college students: Are students treating themselves for attention problems? *Journal of Attention Disorders, 13*(3), 259–270.

Schmidt, S., Petersen, C., & Bullinger, M. (2003). Coping with chronic disease from the perspective of children and adolescents—a conceptual framework and its implications for participation. *Child: Care, Health and Development, 29*(1), 63–75.

Sepulveda, D. R., Thomas, L. M., McCabe, S. E., Cranford, J. A., Boyd, C. J., & Teter, C. J. (2011). Misuse of prescribed stimulant medication for ADHD and associated patterns of substance use: Preliminary analysis among college students. *Journal of Pharmacy Practice, 24*(6), 551–560.

Setlik, J., Bond, G. R., & Ho, M. (2009). Adolescent prescription ADHD medication abuse is rising along with prescriptions for these medications. *Pediatrics, 124*(3), 875–880.

Singh, I., Kendall, T., Taylor, C., Mears, A., Hollis, C., Batty, M., & Keenan, S. (2010). Young people's experience of ADHD and stimulant medication: A qualitative study for the NICE guideline. *Child and Adolescent Mental Health, 15*(4), 186–192.

Smith, B. H., Pelham, W. E., Evans, S., Gnagy, E., Molina, B., Bukstein, O., . . . Willoughby, M. (1998). Dosage effects of methylphenidate on the social behavior of adolescents diagnosed with attention-deficit hyperactivity disorder. *Experimental and Clinical Psychopharmacology, 6*(2), 187–204.

Smith, B. H., Pelham, W. E., Gnagy, E., & Yudell, R. S. (1998). Equivalent effects of stimulant treatment for attention-deficit hyperactivity disorder during childhood and adolescence. *Journal of the American Academy of Child and Adolescent Psychiatry, 37*(3), 314–321.

Spencer, T. J., Wilens, T. E., Biederman, J., Weisler, R. H., Read, S. C., & Pratt, R. (2006). Efficacy and safety of mixed amphetamine salts extended release (Adderall XR) in the management of attention-deficit/hyperactivity disorder in adolescent patients: A 4-week, randomized, double-blind, placebo-controlled, parallel-group study. *Clinical Therapeutics, 28*(2), 266–279.

Staikova, E., Marks, D. J., Miller, C. J., Newcorn, J. H., & Halperin, J. M. (2010). Childhood stimulant treatment and teen depression: Is there a relationship? *Journal of Child and Adolescent Psychopharmacology, 20*(5), 387–393.

Substance Abuse and Mental Health Services Administration. (2013). Emergency department visits involving attention deficit/hyperactivity disorder stimulant medications. Retrieved from *www.samhsa.gov/data/2k13/dawn073/sr073-add-adhd-medications.htm.*

Swanson, J. M., Arnold, L. E., Molina, B. S., Sibley, M. H., Hechtman, L. T., Hinshaw, S. P., . . . MTA Group. (2017). Young adult outcomes in the follow-up of the multimodal treatment study of attention-deficit/hyperactivity disorder: Symptom persistence, source discrepancy, and height suppression. *Journal of Child Psychology and Psychiatry, 58*(6), 663–678.

Teter, C. J., McCabe, S. E., LaGrange, K., Cranford, J. A., & Boyd, C. J. (2006). Illicit use of specific prescription stimulants among college students: Prevalence, motives, and routes of administration. *Pharmacotherapy, 26*(10), 1501–1510.

U.S. Food and Drug Administration. (2013). FDA Drug Safety Communication: FDA warns of rare risk of long-lasting erections in males taking methylphenidate ADHD medications and has approved label changes. Retrieved August 31, 2017, from *www.fda.gov/Drugs/DrugSafety/ucm375796.htm.*

Viktorin, A., Ryden, E., Thase, M. E., Chang, Z., Lundholm, C., D'Onofrio, B. M., . . . Landen, M. (2017). The risk of treatment-emergent mania with methylphenidate in bipolar disorder. *American Journal of Psychiatry, 174*(4), 341–348.

Visser, S. N., Danielson, M. L., Bitsko, R. H., Holbrook, J. R., Kogan, M. D., Ghandour, R. M., . . . Blumberg, S. J. (2014). Trends in the parent-report of health care provider-diagnosed and medicated attention-deficit/hyperactivity disorder: United States, 2003–2011. *Journal of the American Academy of Child and Adolescent Psychiatry, 53*(1), 34–46.

Walker, N. E., & Doyon, T. (2001). "Fairness and reasonableness of the child's decision": A proposed legal standard for children's participation in medical decision making. *Behavioral Sciences and the Law, 19*(5–6), 611–636.

White, F. A. (1996). Parent–adolescent communication and adolescent decision-making. *Journal of Family Studies, 2,* 41–56.

Wilens, T. E., Faraone, S. V., Biederman, J., & Gunawardene, S. (2003). Does stimulant therapy of attention-deficit/hyperactivity disorder beget later substance abuse?: A meta-analytic review of the literature. *Pediatrics, 111*(1), 179–185.

Wilens, T. E., Kratochvil, C., Newcorn, J. H., & Gao, H. (2006). Do children and adolescents with ADHD respond differently to atomoxetine? *Journal of the American Academy of Child and Adolescent Psychiatry, 45*(2), 149–157.

Wilens, T. E., McBurnett, K., Bukstein, O., McGough, J., Greenhill, L., Lerner, M., . . . Lynch, J. M. (2006). Multisite controlled study of OROS methylphenidate in the treatment of adolescents with attention-deficit/hyperactivity disorder. *Archives of Pediatrics and Adolescent Medicine, 160*(1), 82–90.

Wilens, T. E., Robertson, B., Sikirica, V., Harper, L., Young, J. L., Bloomfield, R., . . . Cutler, A. J. (2015). A randomized, placebo-controlled trial of guanfacine extended release in adolescents with attention-deficit/hyperactivity disorder. *Journal of the American Academy of Child and Adolescent Psychiatry, 54*(11), 916–925.

Wills, T., Blechman, E., & McNamara, G. (1996). Family support, coping, and competence. In E. M. Hetherington & E. A. Blechman (Eds.), *Stress, coping, and resiliency in children and families* (pp. 107–133). Mahwah, NJ: Erlbaum.

Wolraich, M., Brown, L., Brown, R. T., DuPaul, G., Earls, M., Feldman, H. M., . . . Visser, S. (2011). ADHD: Clinical practice guideline for the diagnosis, evaluation, and treatment of attention-deficit/hyperactivity disorder in children and adolescents. *Pediatrics, 128*(5), 1007–1022.

Index

Note. f or *t* following a page number indicates a figure or table.

B

D

J

K

L

M

N

O

P

R

S

T